FIRST AID FOR THE® WARDS

Fifth Edition

TAO LE, MD, MHS
Associate Clinical Professor of Medicine and Pediatrics
Chief, Section of Allergy and Immunology
Department of Medicine
University of Louisville

VIKAS BHUSHAN, MD
Diagnostic Radiologist
Los Angeles

JAMES S. YEH, MD
Resident Physician
Clinical Fellow in Medicine
Cambridge Health Alliance
Harvard Medical School

McGraw Hill Medical

New York Chicago San Francisco Lisbon London Madrid Mexico City
Milan New Delhi San Juan Seoul Singapore Sydney Toronto

The McGraw-Hill Companies

First Aid for the® Wards, Fifth Edition

2 3 4 5 6 7 8 9 0 CTP/CTP 17 16 15 14

ISBN 978-0-07-176851-1
MHID 0-07-176851-3
ISSN 1557-4083

NOTICE

Medicine is an ever-changing science. As new research and clinical experience broaden our knowledge, changes in treatment and drug therapy are required. The authors and the publisher of this work have checked with sources believed to be reliable in their efforts to provide information that is complete and generally in accord with the standards accepted at the time of publication. However, in view of the possibility of human error or changes in medical sciences, neither the authors nor the publisher nor any other party who has been involved in the preparation or publication of this work warrants that the information contained herein is in every respect accurate or complete, and they disclaim all responsibility for any errors or omissions or for the results obtained from use of the information contained in this work. Readers are encouraged to confirm the information contained herein with other sources. For example and in particular, readers are advised to check the product information sheet included in the package of each drug they plan to administer to be certain that the information contained in this work is accurate and that changes have not been made in the recommended dose or in the contraindications for administration. This recommendation is of particular importance in connection with new or infrequently used drugs.

This book was set in Electra LH by Rainbow Graphics.
The editors were Catherine A. Johnson and Christina M. Thomas.
The production supervisor was Jeffrey Herzich.
Project management was provided by Rainbow Graphics.
China Translation & Printing Services, Ltd., was printer and binder.

This book is printed on acid-free paper.

DEDICATION

To all our contributors, who took time to share their experience,
advice, and humor for the benefit of students

and

To our families, friends, and loved ones, who endured and assisted
in the task of assembling this guide.

Contents

CONTRIBUTING AUTHORS

EIKE BLOHM, MD
Resident, Department of Emergency Medicine
University of Massachusetts at Worcester

VIVEK BUCH
Warren Alpert Medical School of Brown University
Class of 2013

JOHN HEGDE
Harvard Medical School
Class of 2013

KIMBERLY KALLIANOS, MD
Resident, Department of Radiology and Biomedical Imaging
University of California, San Francisco

AMANDA KUMAR, MD
Resident, Department of Anesthesia
Stanford University Medical Center

KARAN KUMAR, MD
Resident, Department of Pediatrics
Lucile Packard Children's Hospital
Stanford University Medical Center

TAUHEED ZAMAN, MD
Resident Physician, Department of Psychiatry
Cambridge Health Alliance
Clinical Fellow in Psychiatry
Harvard Medical School

IMAGE EDITOR

S. JARRETT WRENN, MD, PhD
Chief Resident, Department of Radiology and Biomedical Imaging
University of California, San Francisco

FACULTY REVIEWERS

ERIC BALIGHIAN, MD
Instructor, Department of Pediatrics
Johns Hopkins Hospital
St. Agnes Hospital
Johns Hopkins School of Medicine

SHARON BORD, MD
Instructor, Department of Emergency Medicine
Assistant Clerkship Director
Johns Hopkins Bayview Medical Center
Johns Hopkins School of Medicine

RONIT DEDESMA, MD
Instructor, Department of Psychiatry
Cambridge Health Alliance
Harvard Medical School

PRIYANK JAIN, MD
Instructor, Department of Medicine
Assistant Program Director, Medicine Residency Program
Associate Chief Hospitalist
Cambridge Health Alliance
Harvard Medical School

PETER JEPPSON, MD
Fellow in Urogynecology, Department of Obstetrics and Gynecology
Women and Infants Hospital
Warren Alpert Medical School of Brown University

JILL E. KASPER, MD
Instructor, Department of Pediatrics
Pediatric Liaison, HMS Cambridge Integrated Clerkship
Assistant Director, HMS MGH Pediatric Clerkship
Cambridge Health Alliance
Massachusetts General Hospital
Harvard Medical School

OLIVER KENDALL, MD
Instructor, Department of Neurology
Cambridge Health Alliance
Harvard Medical School

DAVENDER SINGH KHERA, MD
Instructor, Department of Neurology
Cambridge Health Alliance
Harvard Medical School

BENJAMIN MILLIGAN, MD
Instructor, Division of Emergency Medicine
Cambridge Health Alliance
Harvard Medical School

ALBERTO PUIG, MD, PhD, FACP
Assistant Professor, Department of Medicine
Hospitalist, Clinician Educator Service
Massachusetts General Hospital
Harvard Medical School

KETAN SHETH, MD, FACS
Instructor, Department of Surgery
Chief, Division of General Surgery
Cambridge Health Alliance
Harvard Medical School

RACHEL STARK, MD, MPH
Instructor, Department of Medicine
Associate Program Director, Medicine Residency Program
Cambridge Health Alliance
Harvard Medical School

STEPHEN C. YANG, MD
The Arthur B. and Patricia B. Modell Professor of Thoracic Surgery
Professor and Chief of Thoracic Surgery
Surgical Clerkship and Curriculum Director
The Johns Hopkins Medical Institutions
Johns Hopkins School of Medicine

Preface

The change from the passive and controlled environment of the classroom to the fast-paced and active world of the wards can be stressful, confusing, and downright frightening at times. The purpose of *First Aid for the Wards* is to help ease the transition wards students must make as they begin their clerkship rotations. This book is a student-to-student guide that draws on the advice and experiences of medical students who were successful on the wards. It is our hope to familiarize you with life on the wards and to pass on some of the "secrets of success" that we picked up along the way in our training. The facts and wisdom contained within this book are an amalgam of information we, the authors, wish we had known at the beginning of our third year of medical school. *First Aid for the Wards* has a number of unique features that make it an indispensable guide for MD, DO, and DPM students:

- An all-new color design for better learning.
- New, innovative flash cards embedded in the margins to reinforce key concepts.
- Hundreds of new color images and illustrations throughout the text.
- Insider advice from students on how to succeed on your clinical rotations.
- Sample H&P notes, daily progress notes, procedure notes, post-op notes, labor and delivery notes, and admission orders.
- Specific advice on how to give both concise and detailed oral patient presentations.
- Descriptions of typical daily responsibilities and interactions on each core rotation, including emergency medicine, internal medicine, pediatrics, obstetrics and gynecology, neurology, psychiatry, and surgery.
- A checklist of high-yield clinical topics in each chapter.

First Aid for the Wards is meant to be a survival guide rather than a comprehensive source of information. It should supplement information and advice provided by other students, house staff, and faculty. It is designed not to replace reference texts as a source of information but rather to provide some essential background information for each core ward rotation. Although the material has been reviewed by medical faculty and students, errors and omissions are inevitable. We urge readers to suggest improvements and identify inaccuracies. We invite students and faculty to continue sharing their thoughts and ideas to help us improve *First Aid for the Wards* (see How to Contribute, page xiii).

Louisville	Tao Le
Los Angeles	Vikas Bhushan
Cambridge	James S. Yeh

Acknowledgments

This collaborative project would not have been possible without the thoughtful comments, insights, and advice of the many medical students and faculty whom we gratefully acknowledge for their support in the development of *First Aid for the Wards*.

Special thanks to Andrea Fellows, our tireless editor; Selina Franklin; Louise Petersen; and the section editors, contributors, and faculty reviewers for bringing the book together under constant pressure. For continuing enthusiasm, support, and commitment to this project, thanks to our executive editor, Catherine Johnson. For remarkable editorial and production support, we thank David Hommel, Tina Castle, Susan Cooper, and the staff at Rainbow Graphics.

How to Contribute

First Aid for the Wards is a work in progress—a collaborative project that was refined through the many contributions and changes received from students and faculty. The authors and McGraw-Hill intend to update *First Aid for the Wards* so that the book grows both in quality and in scope while continuing to serve as a timely guidebook to survival and success on the wards. We invite you to participate in this process by passing on your own insights. Please send us:

- Tips for survival and success on the wards.
- New topics, diagrams, and tables that you feel should be included in the next edition.
- Mnemonics or algorithms you have used on the wards.
- Personal ratings and comments on books that you have used while on the hospital wards, including books that were not reviewed in this edition.
- Your medical school's handbook to the clerkships.
- Corrections and clarifications.

For each entry incorporated into the next edition, you will receive a **$10 Amazon.com gift certificate,** as well as a personal acknowledgment in the next edition. Significant contributions will be compensated at the discretion of the publisher.

The preferred way to submit suggestions and contributions is via the First Aid Team's blog at:

www.firstaidteam.com

Please also check **firstaidteam.com** for the latest updates and corrections.

You can also e-mail us directly at:

firstaidteam@yahoo.com

NOTE TO CONTRIBUTORS

All entries become properties of the authors and are subject to review and edits. Please verify all data and spelling carefully. In the event that similar or duplicate entries are received, only the first entry received will be used. Include a reference to a standard textbook to facilitate verification of the fact. Please follow the style, punctuation, and format of this edition if possible.

INTERNSHIP OPPORTUNITIES

The author team is pleased to offer part-time and full-time paid internships in medical education and publishing to motivated physicians. Internships may range from three months (eg, a summer) up to a full year. Participants will have an opportunity to author, edit, and earn academic credit on a wide variety of projects, including the popular First Aid series. Writing/editing experience, familiarity with Microsoft Word, and Internet access are required. For more information, e-mail a résumé or a short description of your experience along with a cover letter to the authors at **firstaidteam@yahoo.com.**

SECTION 1

INTRODUCTION TO THE WARDS

CHAPTER 1

GUIDE FOR WARDS SUCCESS

Introduction

For the past 2 years, you have learned medicine in classrooms, labs, and libraries. Yet while you may have shadowed a preceptor or practiced taking histories on the wards, in all probability you have not yet had any significant clinical experiences. That is all about to change. As a third-year medical student, you will be an integral part of a clinical team. You will now be given real responsibilities—and, yes, your own patients. The team you will be a part of will make medical decisions based on the clinical data you gather. So be thorough, diligent, and honest about what you have observed (or what you forgot to observe or ask; it's OK, you're here to learn).

In general, there are 4 levels at which a medical student functions on a team. During your first rotation, you may merely **report** data ("Mr. Smith's blood pressure is 150/80 mm Hg"). Once you have a bit of experience under your belt, you will then start to **interpret** ("That's a bit high") and later **manage** ("We should start Mr. Smith on an antihypertensive"). Finally, you should try to reach a level at which you can **educate** your peers ("Guidelines suggest that men who have both hypertension and BPH should receive an α-blocker such as prazosin as their first-line treatment rather than the traditional thiazide diuretic, as α-blockers treat both conditions at the same time").

KEY FACT

Strive to be an educator of both your peers and your patients.

The transition from classroom to wards will be one of the most exhilarating periods in your training, and the purpose of this book is to make that transition as smooth and stress free as possible.

In this section, we will offer advice to help you avert **common pitfalls** that many students encounter when starting clinical rotations. Some of these pitfalls include:

- Not understanding the responsibilities and expectations associated with the rotation
- Not seeking timely feedback
- Not using appropriate pocket references and clinical texts
- Not knowing what to study
- Failing to be a team player
- Not efficiently organizing and executing daily work
- Not sufficiently preparing for oral presentations
- Scheduling key rotations too early or too late

To prevent these mistakes, you must first understand the wards experience itself.

Who?

To succeed on the wards, you should understand how your team works and how you fit in. Toward this end, you should have 3 major goals:

- To function as a productive team member
- To care for your patients
- To learn

A medical team typically consists of the following members:

ATTENDING

As the head of the team, the attending is usually involved in the most critical treatment decisions affecting your patients, with the logistics of patient care typically left to the residents and interns. On certain surgical services, the chief resident acts as the head of the team and reports to several "attending" surgeons.

The attending is legally and morally responsible for the actions of each member of the team. He or she is therefore responsible for **educating and evaluating** the residents, interns, and medical students.

Your attending will interact with you primarily during morning rounds. In order to make a good impression, it is important to:

- Deliver buffed oral presentations.
- Submit a clear, **well-organized** admission note.
- Have a basic understanding of your patients' problems and the rationale behind the treatment plan of each.

RESIDENT

The residents (PGY-2 and up) are house officers who have completed internship. They work closely with the attending to formulate and manage treatment plans for your patients, and they oversee your daily activities. Residents are also responsible for teaching medical students and interns through didactics or informal "pimping." Subinterns often report directly to the residents. You can make a strong impression on your residents through your:

- **Concise** presentations on rounds
- Solid knowledge base concerning the illnesses commonly seen on the service
- Awareness of all changes in the status of your patient (eg, new CXR results)
- Hustle and effort in scut work

INTERN

The interns (PGY-1) carry out the practical aspects of patient care under the direct supervision of the residents. Because interns are usually overworked, they do little didactic teaching. Generally, however, interns are excellent sources of information on how to get tasks done **quickly and efficiently.** Junior medical students usually report directly to the interns.

Although interns are not always involved in grading, they will let the resident know how you're doing. You can score points with them by:

- Keeping your intern up to date on your patients
- Lightening the scut burden

KEY FACT

Intern rules: Eat when you can, sleep when you can, leave when you can.

KEY FACT

Interns can be your best friends, so keep them informed.

SUBINTERN

Subinterns are fourth-year medical students who carry the same responsibilities as interns. Subinterns do not evaluate or teach you, but they can often serve as a valuable source of clinical pearls and practical information.

NURSE

Ward nurses carry out physician orders and attend to the daily needs of the patient. They are often very knowledgeable about patient care and can give you the scoop on your patient when you preround in the morning. If nurses like you, they may also take the time to teach you important scut skills, such as placing Foley catheters or IV lines. For these reasons, a **good rapport with the nursing staff is critical** to a successful and enjoyable rotation. So make sure that you:

- Learn the names of the nurses caring for your patients.
- Always be respectful in discussing patient care with nurses.
- Always double-check with your resident if you are unsure about how a treatment plan should be carried out.
- Never leave a mess for the nurse to clean up.
- Always let nurses know if there is an important change in treatment or discharge plans.

KEY FACT

Nurses can make or break your rotation.

WARD CLERK

The ward clerk is usually in charge of administrative issues such as taking written orders off the charts, scheduling procedures, and completing discharge work on your patient. If a patient has been taken somewhere for a diagnostic study, the ward clerk often knows where that patient is and when he or she will return.

PHARMACIST

Staff pharmacists or pharmacy residents may also round with the team. Do not hesitate to hit them up for valuable information regarding toxicity, drug interactions, dosing in different disease states, and efficacy.

OTHER HOSPITAL STAFF

Other members of the hospital staff include physician assistants, nurse practitioners, nutritionists, physical therapists, social workers, respiratory therapists, phlebotomists, radiology technicians, and laboratory technicians.

- Tagging along with the phlebotomy team can quickly improve your blood draw and IV placement skills.
- Social workers provide patient counseling, psychosocial assessment, and housing or transportation arrangements.
- Some hospitals conduct multidisciplinary rounds to make sure that all team members are aware of the treatment and discharge plans for each patient.

When?

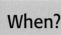

THE SCHEDULE—MEDICINE WARDS

The following is a general outline of the daily schedule for **medicine, pediatrics, neurology, and psychiatry.** Please refer to the chapters that follow for specific advice and information on each rotation.

MNEMONIC

SOAP format:

Subjective status
Objective status
Assessment
Plan

Prerounds: 7:00–8:00 A.M. During prerounds, note and evaluate all events that have affected your patient since you left the hospital the previous day (see Table 1-1). Allow 15–20 minutes per patient at first, and write all information down to make sure you don't forget any details. Thorough prerounding in **SOAP** format (see mnemonic) will help you complete the progress note quickly and efficiently.

Rounding: 8:00–11:00 A.M. During rounds, you will see and discuss patients with the team and give a very brief presentation (the "one-liner" and significant overnight events, lab results, etc.) on your old patients. After you present your plan, the team will create a "to-do" list for the day. Toward this goal:

- Have the patient charts available to write orders as you discuss the patient.
- Get your orders cosigned by the resident.
- Write down to-do tasks immediately to prevent subsequent confusion.

Whereas old patients are only briefly discussed during rounds, the admitting provider (you) will present new admissions to the team in considerable detail. So at the beginning of each rotation, you should inquire about your attending's preferences with regard to the length and level of detail of these presentations. Other tips are as follows:

- Make your presentation smooth, concise, and well organized!
- Read up on the illness you are presenting, particularly with regard to its clinical presentation, differential diagnosis, and treatment.
- Volunteer to present a relevant topic to your team. Preparing a brief handout on your patient's disease will demonstrate your interest in the subject. Alternatively, make sure you include a brief "teaching point" at the end of your presentation.

Work time (during/after rounds): This is when you and the intern crank out the scut. Speed and efficiency during this period determine when you and the intern will get to go home. With this in mind, be sure to **call in consults**

TABLE 1-1. Preround Checklist

- Ask the overnight nurse and cross-covering house officer for overnight events.
- Review the patient chart for any overnight events or consult notes.
- **Subjective:** Ask the patient how he or she feels.
- **Objective:** Check vital signs, perform a brief physical examination, and review new labs, culture results, study results, and radiographs.
- **Assessment:** Summarize the patient in 1 sentence (eg, Mr. Smith is a 79-year-old man with a history of ischemic cardiomyopathy who presented on 9/12 for a CHF exacerbation and is now clinically improved after 4 L diuresis).
- **Plan:** Formulate a plan for the patient for today, breaking it down by problem.

and order studies as early in the day as possible, as those requested later are often not done until the following day. Tasks often include the following:

- Scheduling studies (eg, CT scans)
- Requesting consults
- Performing procedures (eg, paracentesis)
- Completing discharge paperwork
- Writing progress notes

Noon conference: Noon–1:00 P.M. If your service offers a noon conference, you should attend it. Not only is there often free food, but the topics are generally bread-and-butter subjects geared toward house staff and medical students.

Afternoon work: 1:00 P.M.–? In the afternoon, you will finish your to-do list and your progress notes. On some days, there will be additional conferences or lectures geared toward medical students. At this time:

- Follow up on the results of any consults, studies, or labs that were ordered in the morning. Work with the intern to adjust your treatment plan accordingly.
- Be inquisitive. If you have some downtime and your resident has a few free moments, ask about a particular disease or diagnostic study you don't quite understand.
- Keep your patients informed. If you are following a particular patient, make sure he or she knows what the team is planning.

Signing out: Sign out at the end of the day to your intern or to the cross-covering intern on call.

- Make sure you communicate current problems, medications, and allergies.
- Highlight any details that need follow-up overnight (eg, "Please check the wound site at 10:00 P.M.").
- Document the patient's code status and relevant management issues. Does an IV need to be restarted overnight if it falls out? Do you need blood cultures to be sent if a patient spikes a fever overnight?

KEY FACT

A good sign-out is the mark of a good student.

THE SCHEDULE—SURGERY WARDS

The surgery day starts earlier and ends later than a typical medicine day. One or more days per week may also include clinic with an attending surgeon.

Prerounds: 5:00–6:00 A.M. This is just like medicine prerounds, except that your physical examination must include checking on wounds and drains for post-op patients. You may be expected to write progress notes before work rounds begin.

Work rounds: 6:00–7:30 A.M. Progress notes will be completed during work rounds. You may write a second round of progress notes during afternoon rounds. Surgical progress notes are typically much shorter than medicine progress notes.

Pre-op preparation: 7:30–8:00 A.M. You and a house officer will work with the anesthesiologist to prepare patients for surgery. Typical medical student duties include positioning the patient, placing urinary catheters, and prepping (eg, clipping hair, cleaning) the operative area.

Surgery: 8:00 A.M.–5:00 P.M. During surgery, your role may range from observation to retraction, suctioning, and tying and cutting sutures. This will be your primary exposure to attending surgeons.

- Read up on the patient history, the surgical indications, and the basics of the procedure the night before the surgery.
- Know your anatomy, as the OR is home to frequent pimping sessions.

KEY FACT

Pimp questions often fly fast and furious in the OR.

Floor work: 8:00 A.M.–5:00 P.M. When you are not in the OR, you will be doing daily scut work on your patients with the resident. This usually includes wound checks, removing staples, pulling chest tubes, and calling consults.

- Decide on a fair distribution of cases with your fellow medical students so that everyone gets some OR time and some floor time.
- Know your patients, and read up on their conditions. Understanding a disease and its treatment will help you anticipate the next steps in management.

"Afternoon" rounds: 5:00–7:30 P.M. These rounds generally start just after the last surgery of the day has ended. Afternoon rounds are usually more casual and abbreviated than morning rounds, and they allow the team to review the day's events and plan the next day.

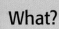

What?

PROCEDURES

You will typically learn procedures either by directly observing them as they are performed or by doing them under supervision (see Table 1-2). Reading about a procedure in a manual beforehand will maximize your learning experience, but remember that a procedure is more than just technique. You should be familiar with the indications, contraindications, and potential complications of each. Other tips include the following:

- Before performing any procedure, you must obtain a signed informed consent from the patient or the patient's representative. Informed consent includes explanations of the procedure, indications, risks, benefits, and alternative options. Check with your resident to determine whether you are allowed to consent a patient.

TABLE 1-2. Common Procedures for a Junior Student

Basic	Advanced
ABGs	Arthrocentesis
Blood culture	Central line placement
ECG	Chest tube insertion
IV placement	LP
NG tube placement	Obstetrical delivery
Surgical knots	Paracentesis
Suturing	Thoracentesis
Urine (Foley) catheterization	
Venipuncture	
Wound dressing changes	

- Have **everything you will need** at the bedside, and gather enough materials for multiple tries.
- Position the patient and yourself for comfort (eg, bed height, lighting).
- Remember universal precautions.
- Use drop cloths, and **clean up after yourself.** Discard all sharps appropriately.
- Write a procedure note for all procedures and place it in the chart.

CONSULTS

Your team will often call consults from specialty services. Obtaining a consult requires filling out a request form and calling the consultant to tell him or her about the patient. Additional tips are as follows:

- **Have a clear question to ask the consultant.** If you don't understand the reason for a consultation, clarify it with your resident **before calling.**
- Request consultations **early in the day.**
- Give the consultant a concise, 1-minute overview of the patient. Include patient identification, pertinent past medical history, pertinent medications, allergies, physical examination findings, and key lab and study results.

CHECKING LABS AND STUDIES

Check labs and study results during prerounds, in the afternoon, and whenever STAT labs or important studies are expected back. If a patient is unstable, labs should be checked more frequently. Any pertinent findings should be reported to the resident.

COMMUNICATING WITH PATIENTS AND FAMILIES

You will serve as the main communication link between the team and the patient. The following tips may help you learn to communicate effectively:

- **Respect your patients' privacy,** and do not discuss patients in public spaces.
- **Be compassionate** yet honest and direct. If you don't know the answer to a question, tell the family that you will check with the team and get back to them promptly.
- Immediately inform the patient of any upcoming studies or events.
- Have a resident or an attending help you break bad news to a patient or to his or her family.
- Choose a quiet time and a private location to talk to a patient.
- **Minimize technical jargon** and explain any medical terms you use.
- Always finish by asking, "Do you have any questions?"

INDEPENDENT READING

Aside from didactic teaching sessions, you will be expected to learn through independent reading. Given that you will need to understand the rationale behind your patients' treatment plans, your first priority should be to read about the pathophysiology of their conditions. Next, you should read about other patients on your team who might have interesting and active issues. This will help keep you involved in patient discussions during rounds. Relevant sources of information include the following:

- **Handbooks.** When you have 5 minutes before rounds, use the time to quickly review a disease using a handbook. Classic examples are *The Washington Manual of Medical Therapeutics* and *Pocket Medicine: The Massachusetts General Hospital Handbook of Internal Medicine.*
- **Review books.** These reference books cover diseases in moderate detail and are meant to be read cover to cover during the course of a rotation. Examples include the First Aid Clerkship series and the Blueprints series.
- **Textbooks.** These tomes are comprehensive, highly detailed references. An example is *Harrison's Principles of Internal Medicine.*
- **Electronic references.** These useful resources are designed to give you a quick answer to your question. Examples include UpToDate (www.uptodate.com), AccessMedicine (www.accessmedicine.com), Micromedex (www.micromedex.com), and DynaMed (www.ebscohost.com/dynamed). Ask your medical institution which resources are available to you.
- **Journal articles.** Journal articles contain information 2–4 years more current than that found in a reference book. For constantly evolving diseases or recent therapeutic developments, literature searches are highly useful. If you find a relevant paper, it is highly appropriate to photocopy the document for your team.

HUMAN SUPPLY CABINET

Particularly for surgical rotations, students are often relied on to have common items on hand for the attending or house staff. Stocking your pockets with tape, tongue blades, extra gloves, and scissors will save time on rounds and earn you points with your team.

How?

ADMISSION H&P

Third-year medical students are generally expected to admit anywhere from 1 to 3 patients on a call night. Patients can be admitted through the ED or directly through a clinic, or they may be transferred from another service or an outside hospital. The resident will receive a call with a 1-line description of the patient such as "33-year-old African American female with abdominal pain." On the basis of this description, you should start formulating a differential diagnosis by the following means:

Review objective data. This includes any paperwork from paramedics or the ED. You should also do a brief chart biopsy focusing on discharge summaries from recent admissions and studies such as ECGs, recent echocardiograms, and past blood work.

Interview the patient. The history and physical (H&P) may be conducted as a team, or you may interview the patient alone. Remember to keep the interview focused and ask about pertinent positive and negatives in the history. Start with open-ended questions (eg, "What brought you to the hospital?") and then move toward more structured questions (eg, "Was the pain sharp or dull?"). Always do a complete review of systems (ROS) with every patient you see, asking about symptoms relating to all of the major organ systems.

KEY FACT

Two reasons not to do a rectal examination: (1) you don't have a finger, or (2) the patient doesn't have a rectum.

MNEMONIC

Admit orders–

ADC VANDALISM

Admit to
Diagnosis
Condition
Vitals
Allergies
Nursing orders
Diet
Activity
Labs
IV fluids
Special studies
Medications

Key:

ADA = American Diabetes Association

BNP = B-type natriuretic peptide

CBC = complete blood count

CHF = congestive heart failure

CMP = complete metabolic panel

CT = computed tomography

CXR = chest x-ray

D5 = 5% dextrose

ECG = electrocardiogram

I/O = intake/output

KVO = keep vein open

MI = myocardial infarction

NG = nasogastric

NKDA = no known drug allergies

NPO = nothing by mouth

NS = normal saline

PRN = as required

RR = respiratory rate

SBP = systolic blood pressure

T = temperature

TED = thromboembolic deterrent (stockings)

Conduct a thorough physical examination. Practice your physical examination skills, and try to use the same sequence at all times. Ask for supervision and feedback from your residents.

Present your patient. Give a short, 3- to 5-minute presentation to your resident, including your leading diagnoses. Your resident may be able to help you polish your presentation and flesh out your assessment and plan (A&P) for your admit note.

ADMIT ORDERS

Admit orders should be entered **before** your admit note is completed. Once you have a working diagnosis and a skeletal management plan, begin entering orders. Many hospitals with electronic order entry have automated admission order sets, but it is important to be able to write out admit orders as well. Use the mnemonic **ADC VANDALISM** as a guide to help you formulate your orders. Shown below is an example of an admit order for a patient admitted with pneumonia.

SAMPLE ADMIT ORDER

6/10/11 12:02 P.M.

ADMIT TO: Ward, service, your name/intern's name, beeper number.

DIAGNOSIS: If there is no clear diagnosis, give the 2 or 3 most likely suspects (eg, pulmonary embolism vs. CHF exacerbation), the presenting complaint (eg, chest pain), or the diagnoses you are trying to exclude (eg, rule out MI).

CONDITION: Options include satisfactory, stable, fair, guarded, and critical.

VITALS: Options include per routine, q 4 h, q 1 h, q shift.

ALLERGIES: Mention the specific reaction to the drug (eg, rash); note NKDA if no allergies.

NURSING ORDERS: Consider strict I/Os, oxygen, daily weights, telemetry, glucose checks, Foley catheter, NG tube, and TED stockings.

DIET: Options include regular, 1800-cal ADA, low sodium, soft mechanical, and NPO.

ACTIVITY: Options include ad lib, out of bed to bathroom (with assistance), out of bed to chair, strict bed rest, and ambulation with crutches.

LABS: Consider specific labs relevant to the patient's presenting complaint (eg, pro-BNP, D-dimer). Most patients get routine A.M. labs (CBC, CMP, etc.).

IV FLUIDS: Specify heparin lock, KVO, or type of solution (eg, D5, NS, D5 1/2 NS) and rate of infusion (eg, D5 1/2 NS + 20 mEq/L KCl at 125 cc/hr).

SPECIAL STUDIES: ECG, CXR, CT, etc.

MEDICATIONS: Don't forget antibiotics and PRN medications.

NOTIFY HOUSE OFFICER: T > 38.4, pulse > 120 or < 50, SBP < 90 or > 180, RR < 8 or > 30, O_2 sat < 90%.

COMMON PRN MEDICATION ORDERS

Acetaminophen (Tylenol) 650 mg PO q 4 h PRN temp > 39°C

Bisacodyl (Dulcolax) 10 mg PO/PR QD PRN constipation

Diphenhydramine (Benadryl) 25 mg PO QHS PRN insomnia

Maalox 10–20 cc PO q 1–2 h PRN dyspepsia

Lorazepam (Ativan) 1–2 mg IM/IV q 6 h PRN anxiety/agitation

Promethazine (Phenergan) 25 mg PO/IM/IV q 4 h PRN nausea

Key:

IM = intramuscular

IV = intravenous

QD = every day

QHS = at bedtime

PO = by mouth

PR = by rectum

ADMIT NOTES

The amount of time you have to complete your admit note will depend on the policies of your service. Regardless of time and circumstance, however, you should have the admit note in the chart **before work rounds** the next morning. Use the time you have to learn more about the patient's condition and to develop a thorough management plan. The history of present illness (HPI) and the A&P are the most challenging portions of the admit note.

A well-written admit note is a testament to your thought processes and fund of knowledge. Some helpful ground rules are as follows:

- As you write the admit note, try to identify any missing information before you go back to the patient to ask more questions.
- Feel free to use common abbreviations, but avoid abbreviations that might be unrecognizable or easily mistaken for something else.
- Remember that all of your notes will become part of a legal record, so avoid making unprofessional or opinionated comments that are not relevant to the patient's care.
- Each page of your note should include the date and time as well as your name and signature.
- Neat handwriting wins points. Messy handwriting can always be improved by slowing down. There is little point to writing an illegible note.

HPI. Deciding which pieces of information belong in the HPI can be a difficult task. Some tips for helping you formulate your HPI include the following:

- Begin with the patient's name, age, sex, and race (if contributory). In your first sentence, also include **pertinent** past medical and surgical history as well as the chief complaint. For example: "Mr. Jones is a 49-year-old African American male with a past medical history of sarcoidosis who presents with a productive cough and chest pain of 3 days' duration."
- Do not forget to characterize the chief complaint. Use the **OLD CARS** mnemonic.
- Include **pertinent** positives and negatives that support your diagnosis, and rule out the other main suspects.
- **Tell a story.** Information should be presented in chronological order and should lead the reader toward the most likely diagnosis.
- If information in the patient's past medical history (PMH), family history (FH), or social history (SH) is pertinent to the reason for admission, it should be included in the HPI.

MNEMONIC

Characterizing the chief complaint–

OLD CARS

Onset
Location
Duration
Character
Alleviating/**A**mplifying factors
Radiation
Severity

A&P. In your A&P, start off with a brief summary of the case, including the presenting complaint, relevant symptoms, pertinent lab or imaging results, and your presumed diagnosis. Some attendings appreciate it if you outline your thought process by briefly discussing which parts of the H&P either support your presumptive diagnosis or make alternative diagnoses less likely. Take the time to read up on your patient's diagnosis and management as well as his or her other important medical problems. Ask your team if they would prefer that your A&P be presented by problem or by system. In general, problem-based approaches are used on general medical floors, whereas systems-based approaches are used in critical care settings.

For **each** problem or system, you should include a brief A&P. For the **primary** problem, explain (1) why you think this is the diagnosis, and (2) why the other possible diagnoses are less likely to be correct. Other incidental problems get a 1-line assessment. In the plan for each problem, outline your initial treatment plans (eg, medications, procedures) and any additional workup that needs to be done to further clinch the diagnosis.

Key:

A&O × 4 = alert and oriented to person, place, time, and situation

Ab = antibody

abx = antibiotics

ALT = alanine transaminase

AST = aspartate transaminase

BID = twice a day

BP = blood pressure

BRBPR = bright red blood per rectum

c̄ = with

CC = chief complaint

C/C/E = clubbing/cyanosis/edema

CN = cranial nerve

CTAB = clear to auscultation bilaterally

CV = cardiovascular

D/C = diarrhea/constipation

DOE = dyspnea on exertion

DTRs = deep tendon reflexes

EOMI = extraocular movements intact

EtOH = ethanol

F/C/S = fever/chills/sweating

GI = gastrointestinal

GU = genitourinary

HA = headache

SAMPLE ADMIT NOTE

MS-3 Admission H&P

Date and Time: 6/10/11, 1:30 P.M.

ID/CC: 42-year-old Caucasian woman, former IV drug user, HIV ⊕ c̄ CD4 count of 250, complains of 3 days of painful neck rash and diffuse itching.

HPI: Patient has been HIV ⊕ × 3 years, no opportunistic infections. She complains of a sudden-onset painful neck rash 2 days prior to admission. Noted vesicle formation on L neck and deltoid c̄ pruritus, as well as severe burning/stinging pain. Used warm compresses for symptomatic relief. She felt "drained" and stayed in bed × 2 days, denies any F/C/S, no N/V, no abdominal pain, no diarrhea. No arthralgias/myalgias, no cough, no SOB, no HA. She denies any vesicles on face. No ear pain; no eye pain or visual changes. She is unaware of any childhood history of chickenpox and denies any chemical or plant contacts or contact with others with similar symptoms. Denies any recent changes in medication.

PMH:

1. HIV ⊕ × 3 years. Last CD4: 250, 3 months ago. Denies any opportunistic infections.
2. Pneumonia 3–4 × in past 3 years. Hospitalized but cannot relate dates, durations, or diagnoses. Recalls having a chest CT in past and has never had to take prophylactic abx. Chart currently unavailable for review.
3. Cellulitis of extremities several times in the past. Patient is unable to recall details or dates.
4. HCV Ab ⊕

Meds: Indinavir 800 mg PO QID.

Zidovudine 300 mg PO BID.

ddC 0.75 mg PO TID.

All: NKDA.

FH: Noncontributory.

SH: Patient is homeless. Moved from Chicago to San Francisco 4 years ago. She is unmarried and has 4 children, no family on the West Coast. She is intermittently followed by the HIV clinic at San Francisco General Hospital; ⊕ tobacco 1 ppd × 20 years; ⊕ EtOH 1 pint vodka per day; no h/o withdrawal; ⊕ h/o IV drug use, none × 6 years.

ROS:

Constitutional: No fatigue/weakness, no N/V, no F/C, no night sweats, no recent weight change.

HEENT: Denies headaches, visual changes, blurry vision, hearing changes, tinnitus, vertigo, rhinorrhea, nasal congestion, epistaxis, or sore throat.

Neck: As noted above. No stiffness or masses.

CV: No chest pains, no palpitations, no DOE, no orthopnea.

Resp: No SOB, no cough, no wheezing.

GI: No recent change in appetite, no dysphagia, no jaundice, no abdominal pain, no D/C, no melena, no BRBPR.

GU: No sexual dysfunction, no dysuria, no hematuria, no polyuria, no stones, no nocturia, no frequency, no hesitancy; no genital sores, rashes, or discomfort.

Neuro: No seizures, no paresthesias, no numbness, no motor weakness, no difficulties with gait.

Extremities/MS: No edema, no joint stiffness, no change in ROM.

Endocrine: No heat/cold intolerance, no excessive sweating, no polyuria, no polydipsia.

Psychiatric: No depression, no change in sleep pattern, no change in motivation.

PE:

Gen: Somnolent, but arousable to alert state, in mild distress due to pain and pruritus.

VS: T 37.1 BP 111/80 HR 112 RR 18, 99% O_2 sat on 2 L NC.

Skin/hair/nails: Vesicular rash c̄ erythematous base, clustered, on L lateral and posterior neck and L deltoid, anterior to clavicle, stops at midline anterior and posterior.

HEENT: NC/AT, PERRL 4 → 3, EOMI, mild conjunctival injection bilat, TMs clear without vesicles, O/P is dry with poor dentition, no vesicles or open lesions, no thrush.

Neck: 1 posterior SCM node 1 × 1 cm on left, supple neck.

Breast: Deferred at this time per patient request.

Lungs: CTAB, no rales, no wheezes.

CV: Tachycardic, reg rhythm, normal S1/S2, no M/R/G. Palpable distal pulses.

Abd: Soft, NT, NABS, ND, no HSM.

GU: Deferred at this time per patient request.

HCV = hepatitis C

HEENT = head, eyes, ears, nose, and throat

HIV = human immunodeficiency virus

h/o = history of

HR = heart rate

HSM = hepatosplenomegaly

INR = International Normalized Ratio

MAE = moves all extremities

M/R/G = murmurs/rubs/gallops

MS = musculoskeletal

MVI = multivitamin infusion

NABS = normoactive bowel sounds

NC = nasal cannula

NC/AT = normocephalic/atraumatic

ND = nondistended

NT = nontender

N/V = nausea/vomiting

O/P = oropharynx

o/w = otherwise

PE = physical examination

PERRL 4 → 3 = pupils equal, round, and reactive to light from 4 mm to 3 mm

ppd = pack per day

PT = prothrombin time

PTT = partial thromboplastin time

QID = 4 times a day

ROM = range of motion

SCM = sternocleidomastoid

SOB = shortness of breath

T. bili = total bilirubin

TID = 3 times a day

TM = tympanic membrane

VS = vital signs

Ext: No C/C/E. Cool and dry. Numerous old needle-track scars.

Neuro: A&O × 4. CN II–XII intact. MAE, DTRs 2+ and symmetric, sensation intact. Normal and symmetric strength, tone, and bulk throughout.

Labs:

CBC: WBC 8.2; Hgb 13.3; Hct 40.0; Plt 297

Chem 7: Na 142; Cl 105; BUN 8; K 4.0; HCO_3 29; Cr 0.8; Glucose 92

T. bili 0.7; AST 38; ALT 20; alk phos 77

PT/INR/PTT: 12.4/1.2/32.2

Ca 8.3; Mg 2.3; phos 3.9; albumin 3.6; amylase 82

CXR: Increased interstitial markings, o/w ⊖.

A&P: 42-year-old woman c̄ HIV, presenting with likely herpes zoster in L C3/C4 dermatomal distribution.

1. **Herpes zoster:** The differential in this case is rather narrow given the history and presentation. A contact dermatitis is unlikely although a possibility. Given the specific dermatomal distribution, which stops at the midline, reactivation is far more likely than a 1° varicella infection. The patient's HIV status places her at risk for zoster dissemination. Admit for involvement of 2 contiguous dermatomes and monitor for signs of dissemination.

   Acyclovir 500 mg IV q 8 h.

   Benadryl 25–50 mg PO q 6 h PRN pruritus.

   TyCo#3 1–2 tabs PO q 4 h PRN pain.

   Isolation protocol to protect other immunocompromised patients on floor.
2. **HIV:** CD4 > 200, no h/o opportunistic infections.

   Continue current medications as noted above.

   Will arrange follow-up appointment with HIV clinic.
3. **EtOH:** Monitor for signs of EtOH withdrawal.

   Thiamine 100 mg IV.

   Folate 1 mg IV.

   MVI 1 amp IV.

   Ativan 1–2 mg IV q 1–2 h PRN agitation.
4. **Code status:** Patient is Full Code.
5. **Disposition:** Patient is homeless. Will consult social worker for discharge planning.

PROGRESS NOTES

A progress note is a daily written record of all events pertaining to a patient. An example is provided below. On medical-type services (including pediatrics, psychiatry, and neurology), progress notes are typically written in the afternoon. On surgical-type services (including OB/GYN), progress notes are written before work rounds in the morning. Make sure your intern or resident reviews and cosigns your notes. Most students write progress notes in SOAP format:

- **Subjective:** The patient's account of symptom changes, significant events over the last day, and physical complaints.
- **Objective:** Vital signs; a focused, brief physical examination; and any laboratory and study results.
- **A&P:** Your impression of the objective and subjective information and what the appropriate diagnostic and treatment regimen will be. Your plan should be concise and laid out so that someone else reading your note can easily understand the team's plan for your patient.

SAMPLE PROGRESS NOTE

Date and Time: 6/11/11, 10:00 A.M.

Hospital Day #2: Medicine Service

S: No events overnight. Patient "feels OK"; reports continued pruritus, although significantly improved since yesterday. Good sleep last night; good pain control. No other complaints. Has not noticed any progression of rash.

O: VS: T 36.6 BP 110/65 HR 90 RR 18, 97% O_2 sat on RA.

I/O: 950 cc/BR.

Skin: No change in distribution or size of vesicles on L neck/shoulder, although some have crusted over. No new vesicles on body.

HEENT: PERRL, EOMI, no conjunctival injection, TMs clear, no vesicles, O/P moist and clear.

Lungs: CTAB, no crackles, no wheezes.

CV: RRR, nl S1/S2, no M/R/G.

Abd: Soft, NT, ⊕ BS.

Labs:

WBC 7.9; Hb 12.8 / Hct 37.2; Plt 260

Na 134 | Cl 103 | BUN 8 / Glu 90
K 3.6 | HCO_3 25 | Cr 0.8

A&P: 42-year-old woman with herpes zoster, afebrile and comfortable, doing well.

1. **Herpes zoster:** No evidence of dissemination or spread to other dermatomes. Good pain control; tolerating IV acyclovir well.

   Atarax PRN pruritus.

   Continue IV acyclovir, TyCo#3.
2. **HIV:**

   Continue AZT, indinavir, and ddC.

   Plan to speak with HIV clinic today to arrange follow-up care.
3. **EtOH:** No sign of alcohol withdrawal at this time. Continue to monitor.
4. **Dispo:** Social worker to speak with patient this afternoon re housing and $.

Key:

BR = bathroom

BS = bowel sounds

nl = normal

RA = room air

RRR = regular rate and rhythm

PROCEDURE NOTES

A procedure note must be written and placed in the chart for any invasive procedure that is performed, including an LP, thoracentesis, paracentesis, and central line placement. The note should be concise and should document the date and time, indications, consent, preparation of the patient, anesthesia used (if any), details of the procedure, yield, any studies sent, and any complications.

> ***SAMPLE PROCEDURE NOTE***
>
> **Procedure:** Diagnostic LP.
>
> **Indication:** Suspected meningitis.
>
> **Consent:** Patient gave informed consent.
>
> **Complications:** None.
>
> Patient was placed in left lateral decubitus position with spine flexed, and the L4–L5 interspace was identified. Under sterile conditions, the area was prepared with Betadine and anesthetized with 1% lidocaine 5 cc. Spinal needle introduced into L4–L5 interspace without difficulty. Opening pressure 130 mm; 8 cc clear, nonturbid spinal fluid collected and sent for protein, glucose, Gram stain, cell count, culture. Patient tolerated the procedure well.

DAILY ORDERS

Make it clear to your team that you would like to write orders for your patients when possible (bearing in mind that these orders will be cosigned). This will give you valuable practice in prescription writing and drug dosing and will also help you stay current with your patient's treatment regimens. Tips include the following:

- Become familiar with your hospital's order entry system so that you can enter or write orders quickly without slowing the team down.
- Before writing orders, always double-check to make sure you have the right chart.
- When writing drug orders, always remember to consider patient weight and any medical conditions that may alter drug dosing (eg, hepatic or renal insufficiency).
- If the order is important, pass it on verbally to the nurse or the ward clerk. Check nursing records frequently to be sure orders were properly carried out.

KEY FACT

An intern will usually cosign everything you do—including orders and notes.

PRESCRIPTIONS

Prescriptions are most frequently needed in outpatient settings and before discharge in a hospital. Although you cannot sign prescriptions, you should ask to fill them in before they are signed. If you are not sure why a patient is being discharged on a particular medication, don't be afraid to ask. This will show that you are interested and are trying to understand the rationale behind the patient's care. When writing prescriptions:

- Make sure to include time and date, generic drug name, dose, route of delivery (PO, IV, IM, SQ), frequency, and signature. Remember that for a PRN prescription, you must also list the indication (eg, PRN pain). Include your printed name, title, and beeper number.
- Write legibly and be careful with the use of abbreviations.
- Have the prescription cosigned by a house officer immediately. Your signature alone is not sufficient.

SAMPLE PRESCRIPTION

Name: John Smith

Date of birth: 9/22/1953

Rx: Cephalexin 500 mg

Sig: Take 1 tab PO TID × 7 days (if a PRN medication, list indication)

Disp: Forty (write out "forty," especially for narcotics; otherwise adding a zero will get you 400 pills)

Refills: None (write it out)

Generic OK

THE FORMAL ORAL PRESENTATION

During your clerkships, no skill is more important to master than the delivery of a focused, fluent, and concise oral presentation. You will be called on to present patients under varied circumstances and time constraints for the rest of your professional life, so getting a good handle on this skill early is critical to success on the wards.

KEY FACT

Practice, practice, practice your presentation.

Confidence and brevity should be your goals for formal oral presentations. Most presentations can be given in **less than 7 minutes** and should focus on delivering only essential details. The presentation should follow the same format as your admit note but should omit superfluous information.

In general, more emphasis can be placed on the patient's *current* state (CC, HPI, PE, labs, A&P) than on past events (PMH, FH, SH). Each detail should give the audience insight into your decision-making process such that listeners can anticipate your A&P. Yet while the substance of your presentation is important, **do not forget about style.** Deliver your presentation with confidence, and pay attention to body language, eye contact, and posture. Don't just recite your H&P; instead, tell your team the patient's story.

KEY FACT

A well-done presentation is like a riveting story.

Each attending will have specific preferences with regard to the format and length of an oral presentation. Listen closely to the style and format of presentations given by the residents and interns over the first few days of your rotation. Some teams prefer patient-centered rounds, in which case you will present in front of your patient. Remember, too, that it is not your job to look smart in front of your patients but rather to involve them in their own care—so use layman's terms when feasible. The categories that follow should be addressed in any oral presentation.

Chief complaint (CC). This is the presenting symptom **according to the patient** as well as that symptom's **duration.** If, for example, a patient presents with shortness of breath and you make the diagnosis of congestive heart failure, the chief complaint is "shortness of breath for 3 days," not "congestive heart failure."

History of present illness (HPI). Begin with a **one-line** introduction that includes identifying information and the chief complaint (eg, "Mr. X is a 71-year-old diabetic male with long-standing hypertension who presents with a 2-day history of dyspnea, bilateral pedal edema, and chest pain"). Your oral HPI should be similar to your written HPI and should take the listener through the story of how the patient arrived at the hospital. Include only pertinent positives and negatives.

Review of systems (ROS). This should be very brief, as most pertinent information should already have been covered in the HPI.

Past medical history (PMH). Include all ongoing medical conditions and any pertinent past history (you do not need to mention a history of childhood chickenpox in an elderly man with an acute MI). Any past history that is relevant to the current admission should be included in the HPI.

Allergies/medications. You do not need to present the dosage for each medication, but have dosages written down in case you are asked for them.

Social history (SH). Include a brief social history, including a history of tobacco, alcohol, and drug use. Sexual histories are generally included only if they are relevant to the present admission.

Family history (FH). This section includes both positive and negative findings and should be very short, as any relevant information should already have been mentioned in the HPI.

Physical examination (PE). Always present a **focused physical examination,** elaborating only on relevant sections (eg, if you are rotating through neurology, your attending is unlikely to be interested in poor dentition). Avoid general, uninformative statements such as "The cardiac exam was unremarkable." Instead, briefly cover your specific physical findings: "No murmurs, rubs, or gallops were present on cardiac examination."

Labs/imaging. Some attendings prefer thorough reports of lab and imaging results, while others favor just hearing the highlights. If you are unsure, ask your attending in advance of the presentation. Make sure you have personally reviewed all imaging and ECGs so that you feel comfortable pointing out your findings to the team (have a copy of the ECG with you on rounds).

Assessment and plan (A&P). Begin with a short summary of the patient, tying together the most relevant points of your presentation and concluding with your most likely diagnosis. For example, "Mr. Smith is a 58-year-old man with known CAD and hypertension who presents with 1 hour of substernal chest pain radiating to the left jaw and troponin elevations to 7.3 without ischemic changes on ECG, consistent with an NSTEMI." If the diagnosis is unclear, present the 2 or 3 most likely diagnoses on your differential.

Again, you can present the A&P in the form of a problem or according to organ system. In either format, you should generate a list of the issues facing your patient and should then develop plans for both the acute and the long-term management of each issue. Finally, if you want to be a star, it is always impressive to present a brief discussion of a recent journal article on a management or diagnostic technique related to the admission.

THE BULLET PRESENTATION

The 1-minute bullet presentation is an extremely concise synopsis of the case presentation. You may give bullet presentations to your team during work rounds as well as to consultants or other health care providers who are unfamiliar with your patient. Practicing this skill with each patient you write up will help you filter information more easily.

- Summarize the history, physical examination, laboratory findings, and A&P sections into 1 sentence each.
- Include only the most pertinent positive and negative findings, usually encompassing anywhere from 15 to 20 facts about the case.

Tips for Wards Survival

So now you know what to do, when and how to do it, and whom to talk to when you have questions. Those are the basics, but to make the best use of your time on the wards, here are a few additional tips that might prove helpful.

EFFICIENT TIME MANAGEMENT

Although complicated patients will certainly make your days longer, ending your day at a reasonable hour ultimately depends on your ability to work closely with your team and efficiently execute your duties. Some people will swear that they have a "black cloud" hanging over them, meaning that for some reason they seem to be burdened with more work and more admissions than others. Not surprisingly, studies conducted to determine whether so-called black clouds really exist have found that people who claim to be affected by them are merely less efficient. Use the following tips to improve your time management skills:

Make a to-do list. Write down all tasks—even those that seem to be less important than others. Remember that you will be bombarded with multiple responsibilities while on the wards, so it is inevitable that you will forget something. Keeping a running list of all tasks, and checking them off as they are accomplished, will help ensure that everything gets done.

Prioritize your tasks. Think about what you need to do first to ensure that your patients do not stay in the hospital any longer than necessary. For example, consults and studies must be requested in the morning or they will not get done that day (see Table 1-3). If you plan to discharge a patient, take care of the paperwork and placement issues early. Also remember to eat and sleep whenever you get the chance. Lunch at 10:30 A.M. is far better than "lunch" at 7:00 in the evening!

Try to organize tasks by location. Always think about how to combine tasks on a single trip. For example, if you happen to be in radiology following up on a CXR for Patient A, you should also check off any other radiology chores

TABLE 1-3. Examples of Prioritized Tasks

Do Now	Do Next
Request consults	Write progress notes
Schedule studies	Check routine labs
Do discharge paperwork	Follow up on consults
Check STAT or crucial labs	Follow up on studies

you might have, such as looking at a head CT for Patient B or abdominal films for Patient C.

Learn to maximize the hospital information system. Remember that a good hospital information system can be your friend. Some systems can handle custom patient lists, print labs and problem lists, and even perform literature searches.

Keep scut essentials on board. Supply carts are always in the third place you look. So if you do find a mother lode of supplies, be sure to stock up on suture removal kits, blood-draw supplies, and other essentials you need to get through your scut so that you don't have to hunt for a supply cart every time you go to a different floor. Also be sure to carry a beeper. The easier you are to reach, the more you will stay involved with patient care. There is nothing worse than hanging around waiting for an admission without a pager when you could be in the library or call room instead.

ORGANIZATIONAL AIDS ("PERIPHERAL BRAINS")

KEY FACT

If you can't fit your organizational aid in your pocket, you risk misplacing it.

Another key to being an efficient medical student lies in having and using the right organizational aids. The pros and cons of the most popular organizational aids are discussed below.

Clipboards. Many students start out with a clipboard as their preferred mode of organization. Clipboards offer ample surface area on which to organize patient information and tasks, and they also have the ability to hold additional items such as progress notes, journal articles, and lab requests. However, clipboards are easy to lose and are easy to overstuff with miscellaneous papers.

Binders. Three-ring binders can be extremely helpful, particularly on medicine services, where a wealth of patient information is accumulated. Binder tabs can help you locate patient information quickly without necessitating that you shuffle through papers or cards. Remember, however, that binders can be bulky and can also be easily misplaced.

Data sheets. Many students prefer 8½ × 11-inch sheets that can be folded in half and put in the pocket. You can carry separate sheets for the patient's H&P and lab data. You can shop around for a format you like (ask your residents or fellow medical students) or make your own.

Note cards. Most house staff and senior students use note cards to organize their patients, scut lists, and clinical cheat sheets. Note cards are compact and slide easily into your pocket. Because of space considerations, note cards also force you to organize your thoughts and record only important information. In addition, they are much less obtrusive than other organizational aids when you are presenting. However, note cards may force you to use abbreviations and tiny print to the point at which your notes are barely legible. Here are some pointers regarding note cards:

- Blank note cards can often be found at the nurses' station.
- A ring binder or clip allows you to keep your cards together. You will need to punch holes in the cards. An alternative is to maintain a pocket-size spiral-bound notebook.
- Use a high-quality fine-point pen (eg, a Pilot fine ballpoint) to minimize "microglyphics." Do not use felt-tip pens, as they may run if your cards get wet.
- Consider using a card of a different color for the patient's admission H&P.

- Create an "if found" card with your name and pager number written on it. Losing your cards is like having an unscheduled lobectomy. You have not known true fear until you have misplaced your patient cards.
- Create a card with key phone numbers on it (eg, team pagers, lab, x-ray, nursing stations of each ward). This is critical, as it will save you time and will often help members of your team.

Your digital cerebrum. It is strongly advised that you carry either a smartphone or a tablet computer with you on the wards. This will allow you to quickly reference the Internet, calculate standardized risk scores for patients, determine correct medication dosages, access landmark studies, and the like. However, if you happen to look something up while on rounds, make sure your team knows that you are **not** just checking your Facebook page but are actively engaged in patient care. Please consult the Top-Rated Resources section for a list of recommended apps and Web pages.

SURVIVING CALL NIGHTS

The following tips will make call nights more pleasant and less stressful events:

- Bring a travel alarm, or use the alarm on your pager.
- Make an "on-call" bag with a toothbrush, a hairbrush, a razor, and a change of clothes if you are working in a clinic the next day.
- Bring snacks! Dried fruit or nuts are good options for late-night hunger.
- Bring a review/mini–reference book to learn about your patients' problems when you find you have downtime.
- Sleep when life lets you.

Evaluations

Your third-year evaluations are critical, as they make up the majority of your dean's letter. Residency directors who are seeking to recruit the best medical students begin by examining third- and fourth-year evaluations. So to do well on the wards, you will need to develop new skills: working with a team, communicating effectively, and understanding the nuances of clinical presentations. During the first 2 years, your fund of knowledge is everything—but during the clinical years, it is only one of many criteria by which you will be judged.

KEY FACT

Third-year evaluations are crucial to a successful residency application.

Written evaluations. Written evaluations are usually subjective assessments compiled by the attending or the senior resident. These assessments are intended to convey comments and observations of your performance on a given service. However, not all residents and attendings will be asked to evaluate you in writing, so it may be useful to try to determine who will be evaluating you before your rotation starts. Written evaluations are easily influenced by personal factors and can be dangerous, as they are often quoted verbatim in the dean's letter. A single interaction (be it positive or negative) can easily be seen by an attending as representative of your performance during the entire rotation.

Maximizing your evaluations. It is critical to stay on top of your evaluations by getting feedback from your attendings and residents at an early stage, before potentially negative information ends up in your written evaluations.

KEY FACT

Find out what your team expects of you on the first day of your rotation.

One study has shown that asking for verbal feedback before the resident or attending completes your written evaluation results in higher written evaluation marks. At the beginning of the rotation, you should thus ask both your attending and your resident to define their expectations. Then, 2 weeks into the rotation, reconvene with your attending as well as with your resident to determine if you are fulfilling their expectations and if there are any areas in which you might improve (eg, notes, rounds, procedures, communication). Sit down with your attending and resident at the end to review your performance. Your persistence will not only provide invaluable feedback but also demonstrate initiative that will not go unnoticed.

Within weeks, the clerkship office should have written evaluations on file. Visit the office to review them; with any luck at all, the results will be pleasant. However, if you believe your evaluation is an inaccurate representation of your performance, now is the time to bring it to the attention of the clerkship director or the dean. By the time dean's letters are written during the summer of your fourth year, it may be too late to change an evaluation.

Do not allow evaluations to affect your self-perception, as they can vary widely. However, do not ignore trends or patterns that emerge, as they more or less reflect the consensus perception of your performance.

HONORS/GRADES

Most schools have a grading system of one sort or another—such as "honors/pass/fail" or the traditional letter grading system—with which to gauge your clinical performance. Make sure you have a clear understanding of the criteria for achieving honors and top grades. Looking at an evaluation form can tell you what specific skills and performance criteria will be used to judge you. In addition, keep in mind that getting honors is not necessarily everything. Although honors are certainly helpful for residency, it is far more important that you perform consistently well on rotations, as such performance will be reflected in your dean's letter.

Your final grade in a rotation usually reflects both your performance on the wards and your grade on a final examination. Basic clerkships usually use the National Board of Medical Examiners (NBME) subject test, also known as the shelf exam—a 100-question standardized test administered to students at medical schools throughout the country. Because you will not be judged on your clinical skills alone, it is important to make time to study for this examination independently.

LETTERS OF RECOMMENDATION

If your attending wrote you a glowing evaluation or has given you consistently positive feedback, you might consider asking for a letter of recommendation while details of your valor are still fresh in his or her mind. Letters of recommendation are used when you apply for residency positions. If you ask for a letter early in the third year, ask the attending to update the letter when your career path is better defined. In general, it may be advisable to ask upperclassmen (or women) which attendings are known to write good letters. Have a CV and a draft of your personal statement ready when asking for a letter, as the attending will most likely request such documents so that they will have some material to work with other than their interaction with you in the hospital.

Difficult Situations

The junior student is faced with a host of new situations that may require social and political savvy. Unfortunately, medical students are typically at the bottom of the totem pole and have little political leverage. At the same time, however, failure to handle difficult situations can lead to anything from simple embarrassment to patient endangerment.

Do not hesitate to seek help if circumstances on the wards become overwhelming. The wards can be a very stressful environment, so bear in mind that getting help is not a sign of weakness but rather a testament to your ability to understand your limitations. The 3 main sources of stress for medical students are academic pressures, social issues, and financial problems. Try to recognize your own stressors. If necessary, seek help from your medical school, as doing so will not reflect negatively on your evaluations or dean's letter; schools are more concerned with your well-being than anything else. Most institutions will also have discreet counseling services available to you at little or no cost. Remember, too, that your fellow classmates are in the same situation and may well be facing similar issues. So this is a time to reach out to others and talk about your feelings, concerns, and fears.

KEY FACT

Confidential counseling is available.

NEEDLESTICKS

Being stuck by a needle or a similar sharp is cause for significant concern in the health care field. Because you are inexperienced with handling sharps, you are at a higher risk of incurring needlesticks. Following these tips will reduce your chances of being stuck:

- Always practice universal precautions, treating all body fluids as if they are potentially infectious. Wear gloves when handling blood products, protect your eyes against splashes, and wear a gown to protect yourself from contamination. Substances that require universal precautions include blood; maternal milk, semen, and vaginal secretions; and cerebrospinal, synovial, peritoneal, pleural, pericardial, and amniotic fluids.
- Don't rush. Slow down and think about what you are doing. Be especially careful in the ER and in surgery, where needles and other sharps are being passed around you.
- Dispose of contaminated sharps immediately using the nearest sharps container. Remember that you are responsible for your own sharps. Never simply leave a needle on a table or a bed, as you may forget that it is there or someone else may be stuck by it. If you absolutely must put a contaminated sharp down, announce that you are doing so ("Sharp on the table") so that others can be made aware of it. If others are in the room when you are carrying a sharp to the disposal container, let them know you are carrying a sharp.
- Never recap, bend, or break any needles/sharps.
- Don't force a needle into a sharps container that is full.
- Get vaccinated against HBV!

KEY FACT

Treat all body fluids as if they are potentially infectious. Never recap, bend, or break a sharp.

Despite your best efforts, the unthinkable may still occur. So if you are ever stuck by a contaminated sharp, try to remember the following:

- Don't panic. Take a deep breath.
- Make sure the patient is safe, and discard the sharp properly.
- Wash the involved area with soap and water or Betadine.

KEY FACT

Always report a needlestick.

- Call the Needlestick Hotline or present to employee health or the ED as soon as possible, and inform one of your team members. Report exactly what happened and follow the appropriate protocol. This will facilitate blood testing, counseling, and possible HIV prophylactic treatment.

Do not hesitate to speak with team members, fellow students, friends and family, or counselors about what happened. A needlestick can be extremely traumatizing (in many ways, it can be like a brush with death). If you feel you need to leave early to go home, tell your resident.

ABUSIVE OR INAPPROPRIATE HOUSE OFFICERS

House staff typically work long hours and lead hectic lifestyles. However, that does not give them the right to vent their frustrations on you. Issues of abuse can, of course, be problematic given that you are likely being evaluated by the offending team member—but if an abusive situation does not resolve, you should bring it to the attention of your clerkship director or student dean. Avoid reporting the issue to the attending, as doing so may further disrupt the dynamics of the team.

On the other hand, you may receive unwanted attention from a coworker, such as being asked out for a drink by the resident. You may avert an awkward situation by suggesting that the entire team go out for drinks. If the resident is insistent, you may have to be more direct. If this leads to a negative working relationship, you may need to bring the issue to the attention of the clerkship director or the student dean in order to protect yourself from any unfair evaluations that may result.

INAPPROPRIATE PROCEDURES

Be aggressive in volunteering for any procedures that may be appropriate to your skill level (residents love highly motivated students). However, do not allow yourself to be pushed into performing a procedure with which you are uncomfortable, as this can pose a danger both to you and to your patient and will not make for an optimal learning situation. If you do not feel comfortable performing a procedure, it is acceptable to say, "I'm not comfortable with this procedure. Can you walk me through it, or can I watch this procedure and perform the next one?"

OVERLY COMPETITIVE CLASSMATES (AKA "GUNNERS")

The desire to achieve recognition and to get good grades can cloud your classmates' better judgment—and sometimes your own. When there is more than 1 student to a team, a sense of do-or-die competition may arise, leading to excessive "brown-nosing" or backstabbing behavior. This way of thinking must be curbed at the very start of a rotation. Your classmates are some of the most valuable resources you have, and their cooperation and support are integral to learning and excelling on the wards. Also remember that residents and attendings have themselves been junior students and can easily recognize overly competitive behavior. So take the initiative—keep your classmates informed of scheduled events, share procedures and information, and teach one another. Address backstabbing behavior immediately and firmly. If the pattern persists, bring it to the attention of your intern or resident. Always maintain the moral high ground; you'll sleep better at night.

KEY FACT

Learn to trust and depend on your classmates.

PATIENT DEATH

Despite your best efforts to the contrary, some of your patients will inevitably die while under your care. The first patient death you experience can be particularly daunting, especially if you have developed personal attachments to the patient. If this is the case, you should consider discussing the patient's death with your team or with other students who are receptive. Good social and family support can also be of benefit. Seek confidential counseling if necessary. As you continue your clinical training, you will learn to deal more effectively with patient death. However, do not distance yourself from the patient so much that you lose the human perspective.

KEY FACT

The first few patient deaths you encounter can often be very difficult to deal with.

SEXUAL HARASSMENT

The power structure of a medical team can lead to abuses of attending and house staff privileges. Female students are especially vulnerable to snide remarks and outright inappropriate behavior. However, confronting the offender immediately is an option that should be exercised only if you feel you can handle it. In any case, you should document the event(s) clearly and unambiguously, record the exact circumstances and nature of the incident(s), and identify any witnesses. Then make an appointment to see your student dean as soon as possible, and review the school's written policies on the subject. Your dean should be able to confidentially evaluate the information and determine the best course of action. Your school may also have a sexual harassment prevention office or a dean or ombudsperson in charge of a sexual harassment protocol.

Sexual harassment is a highly charged issue, so you should seek as many backers as possible before you confront an offender. If you decide that the degree of harassment you are experiencing is mild, you may elect to tolerate it or wait until the rotation is over for the sake of preserving your evaluation and your team dynamics. However, it is advisable that you continue to document all offending incidents in the event that you do change your mind and decide to act. At the end of the rotation, consider using evaluation forms to state your case so that you can help prevent similar behavior in the future.

KEY FACT

Document harassment. Then see your student dean.

DIFFICULT OR VIOLENT PATIENTS

Not all patients are pleasant and enjoyable to work with. To the contrary, patients can sometimes be manipulative, hostile, verbally abusive, and even violent. Often, however, such negative behavior is a physical manifestation of the patient's anger and frustration. So do not take anything personally. You don't have to like every patient you care for, but each deserves your best efforts and respect. You should also use common sense when dealing with difficult patients. Never hesitate to call on more experienced house staff to intervene when situations escalate. And never, ever retaliate against a patient. When dealing with agitated or potentially violent patients, bear the following in mind:

- Remember that your own safety must come first.
- Never let the patient get between you and the door.
- Keep the door open.
- Visit the patient only with a nurse or house officer.
- Assess restraint status.
- Rule out reversible causes of increased agitation and lability.
- Don't let your dislike for a patient compromise his or her care.

KEY FACT

Personal safety is a priority with potentially violent patients.

DIFFICULT FAMILY MEMBERS

Having a sick loved one in the hospital places considerable stress on family members and friends, and sometimes the anger, frustration, and sadness they feel are redirected toward you. So again, do not take anything personally. When dealing with family members, find out who the chief decision maker is, especially if the patient is incapacitated or is not competent to make his or her own decisions. Do not, however, let family members push you into speculating about a treatment course. If you are unsure about anything, check with your team before giving the family a definitive answer. Again, recognize when to seek help from your team or a social worker in order to defuse highly charged or emotional situations. And above all, do **not** disclose medical information to family members unless you have the patient's permission to do so.

"NARCOLEPSY"

During your preclinical years, no one ever noticed if you fell asleep after lunch in the middle of a lecture. On the wards, however, everyone will notice you if you doze off. Although falling asleep occasionally is understandable given your state of frequent exhaustion, constant snoozing is certain to leave a bad impression. The best remedy is to get more sleep. Some students become staunch believers in coffee as an antidote to fatigue; however, be aware that caffeine withdrawal is a real clinical syndrome! Another option is to remain standing during rounds and conferences. Although this may raise a few eyebrows, remember that it is your learning (and to some extent your evaluation) that is at stake. If you can sneak in a quick nap (20–30 minutes), do so if you are having trouble concentrating. Do not drive home if you are unable to stay awake, as automobile accidents are a major cause of morbidity and mortality among exhausted residents, and you are not immune.

KEY FACT

Do whatever it takes to stay awake.

PERSONAL ILLNESS

As students slip into the role of health care provider, they often come to believe that they themselves are not allowed to get sick. In reality, it is a wonder that students do not get sick more often given the long work hours and relentless stress they face. When you do get sick, however, your first priority must be your own health. You cannot provide good patient care while sick, and you may transmit your illness to your patients. With this in mind, do not dwell on your clinical responsibilities while you are ill; your team will likely get the job done just fine without your help. However, use your judgment when calling in sick, as some house staff will inevitably think less of your dedication to the team if you choose to do so. When sick, immediately page your resident or intern and let them know when you hope to return. If you are out for more than a day, try to keep track of events with your patients by speaking to your team once a day. This will help you slide back into the ward routine with minimal confusion. Use the downtime to catch up on reading.

KEY FACT

No one can blame you for getting sick.

TIME OFF FOR PERSONAL OBLIGATIONS

When you need time off to attend to personal obligations such as a wedding, make arrangements with your resident or clerkship administration as far in advance as possible, preferably at the beginning of the rotation. Some clerkships will have policies in place for these events. During your fourth-year rotations, you will also have to take time off for residency interviews. Whenever possible, try to arrange your call nights around the event. If this is not feasible, make up the call day elsewhere in the rotation. Try to limit major time off to once a rotation. Of course, there will also be situations in which you unexpectedly need time off, such as a family illness or a death. Here again, give your team as much advance notice as possible, even if it is just a day. Everyone will understand. As with personal illness, try to keep track of your patients' events if you can. Otherwise, come in the evening before or very early in the morning of your next workday to review patient notes.

STRATEGIES FOR MENTAL AND PHYSICAL HEALTH

Clinical clerkships are highly taxing, but you must make a conscious effort to balance work and rest, as ignoring your body's needs will eventually compromise your clinical performance. Remember that your own health must come first, as you are no help to the team if you are ill. Much of the following advice is considered so basic that it is actually ignored.

Streamline and/or delegate household chores when possible. Consider using an automatic bill-payment service. Chip in for a bimonthly cleaning service. Schedule household chores while you are on an easier rotation in exchange for having your roommate or spouse do them during the more time-consuming services. Make sure your roommate or spouse understands how difficult your schedule will be on the wards.

Stay grounded in friends and family. Your friends and family have been there for you during the preclinical years, but you'll need their support and companionship more than ever during the clerkships. Given the long hours you may be keeping, it may become difficult to stay in touch at times, especially since many of your friends may be classmates who are as overwhelmed as you are. Nonetheless, be sure to make a solid attempt to return phone messages and to remember birthdays, anniversaries, and the like.

Eat well. It is a well-known fact that hospital food and most lunches at noon conferences are considered risk factors for cardiovascular disease. Remember, however, that you can still be picky without sacrificing speed. In addition, you should eat when you can. Being well fed is key to maintaining a high energy level. Load up with complex carbohydrates instead of fat and sugar snacks.

Exercise. "No kidding," you might say—but getting exercise can be especially problematic when you're exhausted from a long day on the wards. It's even worse if you view exercise as yet another chore. To circumvent these problems, you should try to find an activity that you enjoy, be it walking or basketball. Exercising with a friend can help keep you committed and can make the activity more social. You might also consider joining a 24-hour gym so that you can work out during those rare hours in which you are free. Another option is to keep a treadmill or a bike at home so that you can work out while watching TV or reading.

Find healthy ways to deal with stress. Unfortunately, the incidence of alcohol and substance abuse is higher among medical students and medical graduates than in the general population. This abuse grows most rapidly between the second and fourth years of medical school. You should thus recognize that you are entering a significantly vulnerable group and be prepared to deal with stress in ways other than using alcohol and drugs. Find a nonmedical activity—such as reading, running, or painting—that can help you escape the stress of medical school every once in a while. Put it on your schedule and make sure to do it for your health!

KEY FACT

Practice what you preach—stay healthy.

Maximizing Your Potential

Although you may think that starting on the wards is akin to getting tossed to the wolves, remember that you are not going in empty-handed. You need to be aware of several advantages that you can maximize to work in your favor.

ENTHUSIASM

House staff may have a deeper fund of knowledge than you as well as more experience under their belts, but you can easily match or even surpass them when it comes to hustle, effort, getting there early, and staying late. Team members are often impressed by enthusiastic students, as are patients.

TIME

The house staff's time is very precious. You, on the other hand, have plenty of time on your hands. So while the house officers have to do brief H&Ps, you have the opportunity and privilege to really learn about your patients. This often allows you to ferret out bits of information on H&Ps that can contribute to—or sometimes even significantly alter—patient management. If your patients are frustrated at having to repeat their entire histories, be sure to remind them that you will be able to give them more time than anyone else on the team.

BASIC SCIENCE KNOWLEDGE

Not too long ago, you completed one of the most arduous tasks of medical school: passing the United States Medical Licensing Examination (USMLE) Step 1. Believe it or not, some of the minutiae that you memorized at that time are still buried somewhere in your unconscious and will resurface when you least expect it. By contrast, the interns and residents on your team are years away from their basic science classes. So don't be surprised if you can show them a thing or two on rounds (of course, don't make a habit of making your resident look dumb in front of the attending, or you may be less than pleased with your evaluation). Remember that discreetly feeding the tired intern or resident factoids for attending rounds will help them look good and will also build your reputation as a "team player."

"LOW" EXPECTATIONS

Remember that you are **not** expected to know the answer to every question, nor are you expected to know the set of orders written for a rule-out-MI protocol with your first patient. You will find to your surprise that residents are often impressed by your level of knowledge even when you consider a question to be a relatively simple one. You are, however, expected to care about your patients and to make a sincere effort to be a contributing member of the team. As long as you show your resident that you are trying to be productive, he or she will be satisfied.

Getting Off to a Good Start

To further maximize your wards experience, here are some preparatory measures you can take in the months and weeks before your first rotation starts.

SCHEDULING ROTATIONS

In the spring of your second year, you will go through the process of scheduling your third-year clerkships. Many schools have rotations prescheduled on tracks, in which case your only task is to choose a track, usually by lottery. Fortunately, there are only a few guidelines you need to know when scheduling your third-year clerkships.

Do not do your most likely specialty first. During the first few weeks of your clerkships, you won't even know where the bathroom is, let alone competently function as a health care provider. It is therefore important to give yourself a chance to get the general feel of the hospital wards, to understand the role you will play, and to become comfortable presenting patients and writing notes. With this in mind, your first rotation should be in a field that you are not likely to enter. For example, most students do not end up going into neurology; however, neurology (as opposed to psychiatry) has the look and feel of a medicine rotation. You should also make sure every member of your team knows that this is your first rotation; that way, they are likely to be more pleasant and forgiving.

Do not do your most likely specialty last. You will be scheduling your senior clerkships in the spring of your third year. If you're interested in pediatrics, you will want to have completed your junior pediatrics clerkship before that crucial scheduling period so that you can decide if and when you will be taking any senior pediatrics rotations.

Avoid back-to-back tough rotations. This is a soft rule, especially if you've decided that you have no career interests in one of the tougher specialties. However, you should be concerned about the possibility of burnout when "killer" rotations get scheduled together. So remember to strategically schedule vacation time after especially difficult rotations to give yourself a chance to unwind.

Schedule an easy rotation before your most likely specialty rotation. Also a soft rule, this gives you time to relax and do some preemptive reading before you start that big rotation. Some students even recommend taking a little vacation time before a key rotation to do some heavy-duty reading.

CHOOSING ROTATION SITES

Your rotations occur in a variety of hospital and clinical settings. Each type of setting has characteristics that will color your clinical experience. Consult senior students regarding the pros and cons of each site, including key attendings to seek out or avoid. The generalizations below don't always apply but should give you an idea of what to expect.

County. The county hospital is typically very busy yet understaffed and usually serves the urban poor. Chaos seems to be the baseline rule as interns and residents battle high patient loads and constant fatigue. In this "all hands on deck" state, you can expect to have more responsibility and hands-on procedures but less guidance and didactic teaching. You can excel in this environment by serving as the perfect "scut monkey," taking care of all those little (but necessary) patient-care tasks. This will help get your team's census down before the next on-call onslaught. The discharge of county hospital patients tends to be more difficult and time consuming owing to their social situations, so social workers will often become your best allies as you struggle to get your patients out of the hospital.

Department of Veterans Affairs (VA). The VA population is unique, consisting mostly of older men. Because the population is somewhat demographically restricted, you will also see the same diseases over and over again, including the following:

- CHF
- MI
- COPD
- Lung cancer
- Diabetes
- Arrhythmias
- GI bleeding
- Peripheral vascular disease

You should definitely read up on these diseases before you go to the VA. You should also be aware that VA patients often remain in house because of placement issues (where will the patient go after discharge?) rather than medical problems. So if you neglect discharge planning, you may end up with a large yet inactive census.

One great thing about the VA is that its electronic medical records link together all VA institutions. This centralization greatly simplifies the process of retrieving a patient's data from previous visits—meaning that you don't have to haggle with another hospital's medical record department. It is also a great instrument for research.

Academic/university center. Ivory-tower medicine has its own unique approach toward treating patients. Medical and surgical services are top-heavy with consultants and fellows. As a result, residents and interns are often deprived of procedures, leaving even less for you to do than would be the case in other settings. In addition, university hospitals are often tertiary and quaternary referral centers, which means that they often get those "zebra" cases that stump the community physicians. So be prepared to spend some quality time with PubMed.

The high staff-to-patient ratio at academic centers also means that much of your time will be spent rounding and discussing the latest treatment for your patient's disease. You can stay ahead of the game by pulling current review papers in the literature for yourself and for the team. The quality of didactics is typically best in the academic center but can sometimes stray into the realm of cutting-edge research and basic science.

Finally, you should bear in mind that a lot of the bigwigs at your school can be found in the academic center. Many students schedule key core and senior rotations there to rub elbows with the academic gods. Scoring an enthusiastic letter of recommendation from them can make your residency application more impressive.

Community hospital. Nonacademic centers often differ significantly from university hospitals. In the community setting, you will mostly see "bread-and-butter" cases, which can be very beneficial to medical students who are learning the basics of medicine. There are fewer esoteric diseases ("zebras") found here, as most patients with uncommon diseases seek help at tertiary referral centers. However, that doesn't mean you will never encounter any "zebras" at community hospitals, so maintain your index of suspicion. Treatment at community hospitals usually follows clinical guidelines, as there are few experimental treatments available.

Outpatient clinic. Reforms in medical education will lead to more time spent seeing patients in the outpatient clinic. In an outpatient setting, residents can see half a dozen patients in an afternoon; you'll be lucky if you manage to see 3 patients in the same amount of time given that you are still learning and not yet as efficient. Keys to becoming a well-regarded outpatient clerk include obtaining a focused H&P guided by past clinic notes and studies, as well as making a succinct presentation with pertinent positives and negatives that allow your resident or attending to clearly assess the problem. It is also crucial to learn the important things to ask and document as well as the nonessential information that is better left out, as time and efficiency are of the essence.

Outpatient medicine differs from inpatient care in that tests must be ordered in a way the accommodates the patient's schedule. So bear in mind that you cannot order all the tests you need at once and expect to get them back the same day. In this setting, you will also learn the frustration of patient noncompliance and missed appointments (think about that the next time you decide to blow off your dental appointment).

BEFORE YOU START ON THE WARDS

Months before starting on the wards. A few months prior to your rotation, you should consider the following:

- Order an extra white coat or two from the AMA catalog. These coats have huge pockets both inside and out.
- Gather your medical supplies. Find a stethoscope that is light, yet one you can actually hear with. Go to the bookstore and test some out on your own heart, lungs, and belly; you're sure to get some strange looks, but doing so will help you decide whether you really need that Littmann Cardiology III.
- Remember that equipment is less costly when ordered in bulk through medical schools. You may also want to buy a cheap stethoscope to use as an "extra" in case your good one walks off one day and you have no time to replace it. You should also buy a clip-on name tag for your stethoscope so that if it does happen to disappear, you may eventually be reunited.

One week before. You will feel less lost on the first day if you follow these general rotation-specific guidelines:

- If you're starting neuro, practice the neuro examination.
- If you're starting psych, practice or review the psych interview.
- If you're starting medicine, review normal values and the H&P.
- If you're starting surgery, review knots, sutures, and what goes in a pre-op, brief-op, post-op, and progress note.
- Read the appropriate chapter in *First Aid for the Wards*.

The night before. On the night before the start of your rotation, you should observe the following guidelines:

- Set out everything you will need to bring with you. Chances are that there is no safe place to leave anything in the hospital on your first day, so don't bring too much. Remember to bring your ID, your white coat, your name tag, some money, extra pens, your stethoscope, a pharmacopoeia (for all rotations, because it is tiny and will quickly translate all those brand names into generic names), and your beeper (memorize the number so that you can give it out).
- Set your alarm half an hour early, especially if you're not sure how to get either to the hospital or to your floor.
- Make sure you know where to go and when to get there. If in doubt, ask classmates who are on your team, or page a resident on the team.
- Recheck your alarm, especially the volume and the A.M./P.M. settings.

The first day. On the first day of your wards experience, be sure to do the following:

- Arrive early.
- Make sure every member of your team knows that this is your first rotation. That way, they are likely to be more tolerant toward you and to pay more attention to teaching you hospital basics, such as how to read a nursing chart, get labs or cultures off the computer, or page someone.
- Don't leave until the chief resident says to leave.
- If in doubt, ask when and where rounds will be the next day. Especially for surgery and medicine, bring an on-call bag with a toothbrush and toothpaste, underwear, socks, any medication you are on, and earplugs. Leave this gear in your car in case you are on call that first night.

CHAPTER 2

PRACTICAL INFORMATION FOR ALL CLERKSHIPS

This chapter reviews some key high-yield skills and information that you will need to acquire regardless of the rotation you are on. Topics include how to read a chest x-ray (CXR), how to make sense of an ECG, how to manage your patients' fluids and electrolytes, and how to interpret acid-base problems. The final section outlines key abbreviations with which you should be familiar as well as key formulas that you may need to use in order to solve common clinical problems.

The most important thing you can do when learning the high-yield skills and knowledge presented in this chapter is to create a systematic approach. Whether you are solving an acid-base problem or interpreting a CXR, you will be far less likely to miss something essential if you are systematic. There are many different ways to approach each of these skills, so find one that you are comfortable with and stick to it. Consistency is key to comprehensive and accurate readings. Your residents and attendings will be impressed!

KEY FACT

Be systematic in problem solving.

Reading Key Studies

THE CXR

Many of your patients in the hospital and ED will require a CXR. Although a formal reading will be completed by a radiologist, it is important that you learn the basics of CXR interpretation.

There are many different ways to approach a CXR. Again, the key here is to be systematic. When your attending asks for your impression of the study, you will earn points by walking through it step by step. One basic approach will be discussed below. First, however, you should become familiar with a few common ways of making a chest film. Most of the studies you see will be among the following:

- **Anteroposterior (AP):** X-rays pass through the patient from front to back (anterior to posterior). Since the heart is farthest from the film (the film is placed behind the patient as the x-ray is taken), AP films often falsely enlarge heart size. For this reason, AP films are less than ideal and are typically used when the patient cannot stand up (eg, when portable films are obtained in an ICU patient).
- **Posteroanterior (PA):** X-rays pass through the patient from back to front (posterior to anterior). These films yield a more accurate estimate of heart size.
- **Lateral:** Typically, the patient's left side is facing the film to prevent cardiac distortion. The lateral projection is named according to the side closest to the film (eg, left lateral). These films are used to pinpoint the location of abnormalities seen on AP/PA films; to assess AP diameter; and to check the posterior costophrenic angles for small (< 250-cc) effusions.
- **Decubitus:** Patients are lying on their sides (eg, in a left decubitus film, the left side faces down). These films are used to evaluate the presence of free air or fluid (eg, pleural effusion or pneumothorax).

When you set out to interpret a CXR, you should always begin by checking the patient's name and the date to ensure that you are looking at the correct film. No matter how stellar your interpretation may be, it won't count for much if you have the wrong patient! Next, begin to assess the film systematically using the **A-B-C-D** sequence (see Table 2-1).

TABLE 2-1. The A-B-C-D Sequence

Step	Process
Assessment	■ Assess the quality of the film using the mnemonic **PIER**: ■ **P**osition: Is this a supine AP film? PA? Lateral? ■ **I**nspiration: Count the posterior ribs. You should see 8–9 ribs with a good inspiratory effort. ■ **E**xposure: Well-exposed films have good lung detail and show a detailed outline of the spinal column. Overpenetration leads to a dark film with more spinal detail. Underpenetrated films are whiter with little spinal detail. ■ **R**otation: The space between the medial clavicle and the margin of the adjacent vertebrae should be roughly equal on each side. ■ Also look for indwelling lines or objects (eg, endotracheal tube, feeding tube, airway obstruction) that may reveal clues to the pathology in the film.
Bones and soft tissues	■ Scan the bones for symmetry, fractures, osteoporosis, or metastatic lesions. Evaluate the soft tissues for foreign bodies, edema, or subcutaneous air.
Cardiac	■ Evaluate heart size. The heart should be < 50% of the chest diameter on PA films and < 60% on AP films. ■ Check for heart shape, calcifications, and prosthetic valves.
Diaphragms	■ Check the diaphragms for position (the right is slightly higher than the left due to the liver) and shape (they may be flat in asthma or COPD). ■ Look below the diaphragms for free air (a sign of bowel perforation).
Effusions	■ Pleural effusions may be large and obvious or small and subtle. Always check the costophrenic angles for sharpness (blunted angles may indicate small effusions). ■ Check a lateral film for small posterior effusions.
Fields/Fissures	■ Check lung fields for infiltrates (interstitial vs. alveolar), masses, consolidation, air bronchograms, pneumothoraces, and vascular markings. Vessels should taper and should be almost invisible at the lung periphery. ■ Evaluate the major and minor fissures for thickening or fluid.
Great vessels	■ Check aortic size and shape and the outlines of pulmonary vessels. The aortic knob should be clearly seen.
Hilar/mediastinal area	■ Evaluate the hila for lymphadenopathy, calcifications, and masses. The left hilum is normally higher than the right. Check for widening of the mediastinum (which may indicate a mass effect or tension pneumothorax). In children, be careful not to mistake the thymus for a mass.
Impression	■ Always formulate a preliminary impression of the film. Even if it is incorrect, it will show that you have been thinking. However, the impression comes at the very end, and you should not editorialize your x-ray read.

THE ECG

Many books teach a detailed approach toward interpreting an ECG (see Top-Rated Review Resources). However, it is important to have a basic method for quickly scanning an ECG on the spot. There are many different methodologies with which to accomplish this goal, so again, pick one you like and stick with it. One basic approach is presented in Table 2-2.

> **KEY FACT**
>
> Each small box on an ECG is 0.04 second and each large box is 0.2 second.

Most studies you see will be 12-lead ECGs. Before you begin your reading, check the standardization mark. In a standard ECG set at 25 mm/sec, each

TABLE 2-2. ECG Interpretation

VARIABLE	METHOD OF ASSESSMENT
Rate	■ Estimate heart rate by counting the number of large boxes between consecutive R waves. The rate is roughly equal to 300 divided by this number. ■ Rates > 100 are tachycardia; those < 60 are bradycardia. ■ For tracings in which the rate appears irregular, you can count the number of RR intervals in 6 seconds and multiply that number by 10 to estimate the rate.
Rhythm	■ Identify the basic rhythm and look for abnormal waves, irregularities, or pauses. ■ Check for sinus rhythm. Is there a single P wave before each QRS complex? Is there a single QRS after each P wave? Do all the P waves look alike? Are the P waves upright in lead II and inverted in lead aVR? ■ Check for ectopic beats (premature atrial or ventricular contractions). ■ Check the RR intervals for regularity of rhythm. If the baseline appears jagged and consecutive RR intervals vary in duration (an irregularly irregular rhythm), the tracing suggests atrial fibrillation.
Axis	■ For a quick assessment of the axis, look at the QRS complexes in leads I and II. If both are predominantly upright, then the axis is normal—that is, between –30 degrees and +90 degrees. See Figure 2-1 for the diagnosis of axis deviation.

Intervals	■ Check the PR interval for AV block (> 0.2 sec). The classification of AV blocks is discussed in Table 2-3.
	■ Check the QRS for bundle branch block (> 0.12 sec).
	  ■ Right bundle branch block (RBBB): RSR′ ("rabbit ears" pattern) in V_1 and V_2; wide S in I and V_6.
	  ■ Left bundle branch block (LBBB): RR′ ("slurred" pattern) in I and V_6; wide S in V_1.
	■ Check the QT interval using the corrected interval: QTc = QT/RR. For a quick check, the QT interval should be less than half of the RR interval.

Hypertrophy (atrial)	■ Right atrial abnormality (RAA): Biphasic P in V_1, peaked first portion, > 2.5-mm height, or > 1 × 1 mm = "p pulmonale." Remember, **right** is **height.** ■ Left atrial abnormality (LAA): Biphasic P in V_1, wide/⊖ terminal portion, > 0.8-mm duration = "p mitrale." Remember, **left** is **length.**
Hypertrophy (ventricular)	■ Right ventricular hypertrophy (RVH): R > S in V_1; S persists in V_5 and V_6; right axis deviation; widened QRS interval. ■ Left ventricular hypertrophy (LVH): Amplitude of S in V_1 + R in V_5 > 35 mm; left axis deviation; wide QRS; inverted/asymmetric T wave. There are other diagnostic criteria, but this one is easiest to remember.

Infarction	■ Look for Q waves (old transmural infarct), inverted T waves, and ST-segment elevation or depression.
	■ Significant Q wave = 1 mm wide or more than one-third the amplitude of QRS.
	■ An inverted T wave may point to ischemia (may be difficult to rule out without an old ECG).
	■ ST-segment depression may mean ischemia or subendocardial infarct (non-ST-elevation MI).
	■ Localize the infarct:
	  ■ Inferior MI (dominant coronary, usually right): II, III, aVF.
	  ■ Lateral MI (left circumflex): I, aVL, V_5, V_6.
	  ■ Anterior MI (left anterior descending): V_1–V_4.
	  ■ Posterior MI (right coronary): Large R and ST depression in V_1, V_2.
	  ■ Septal MI: V_2, V_3.

Electrolyte abnormalities	■ Hyperkalemia: Peaked T waves → short PR interval → loss of P wave → wide QRS → sine wave. ■ Hypokalemia: Flat T wave → U wave → prominent U wave. ■ Hypercalcemia: Short QT interval. ■ Hypocalcemia and hypomagnesemia: Prolonged QT interval → torsades de pointes.

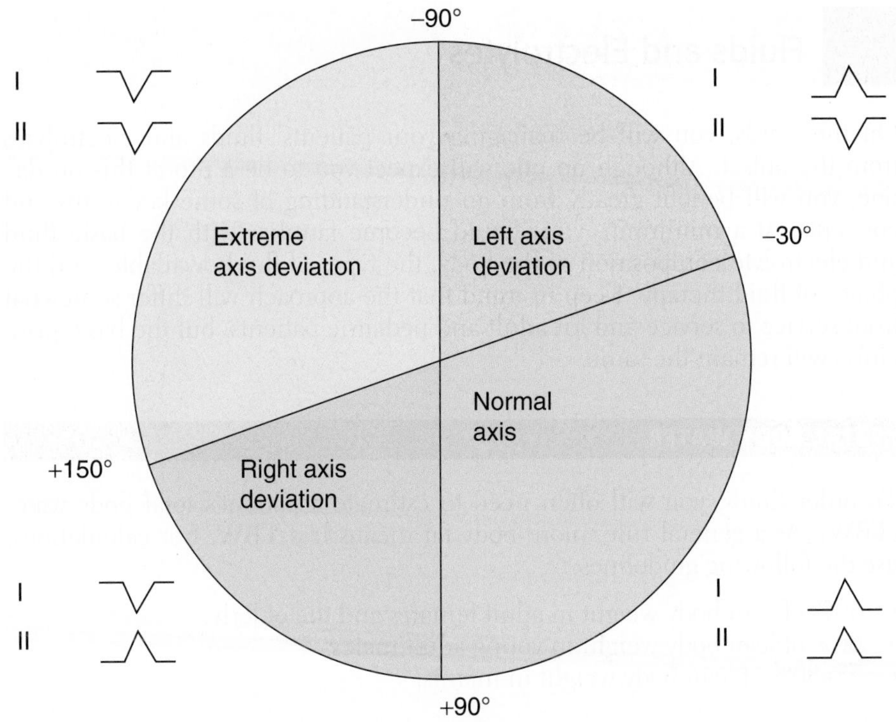

FIGURE 2-1. Quick method of axis determination.

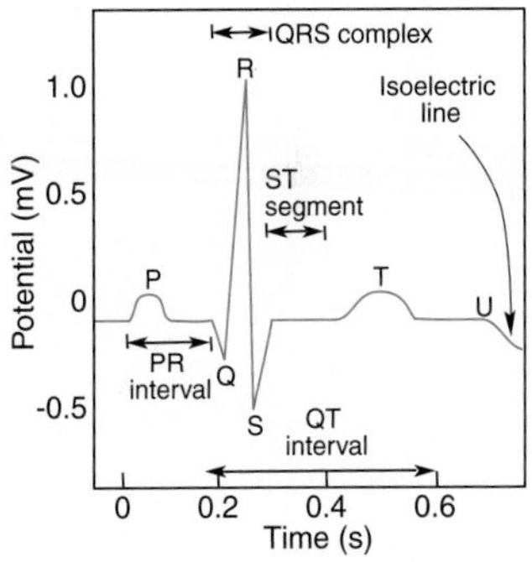

FIGURE 2-2. Sample ECG tracing.

small box represents 0.04 second, and each large box (composed of 5 small boxes) represents 0.2 second. See Figure 2-2 for the identification of the elements of an ECG tracing. Table 2-3 outlines the 3 degrees of atrioventricular (AV) block.

TABLE 2-3. Degrees of AV Block

DEGREE	CHARACTERISTICS
First degree	Prolonged PR interval (> 0.2 sec) with normal tracing.
Second degree	
Mobitz type I (Wenckebach)	Progressive lengthening of the PR interval until a QRS is dropped.
Mobitz type II	Consistent ratio of conducted to dropped QRS complexes. Requires a pacemaker.
Third degree	Complete dissociation between atrial and ventricular rates. Requires a pacemaker.

Fluids and Electrolytes

On the wards, you will be managing your patients' fluids and electrolytes from the outset. Although no one will expect you to be a pro at this on day one, you will benefit greatly from an understanding of some key terms and concepts. At a minimum, you should become familiar with the basic fluid and electrolyte composition of the body, the types of fluids available, and the phases of fluid therapy. Keep in mind that the approach will differ somewhat from service to service and for adult and pediatric patients, but the basic principles will remain the same.

TOTAL BODY WATER

To order fluids, you will often need to estimate a patient's total body water (TBW). As a general rule, more body fat means less TBW. For calculations, use the following guidelines:

- 50% of lean body weight in adult females and the elderly.
- 60% of lean body weight in young adult males.
- 75–80% of lean body weight in infants.

FLUID COMPARTMENTS

The TBW is distributed between the intracellular (two-thirds) and extracellular (one-third) compartments. Extracellular fluid is further distributed between the interstitial (three-fourths) and intravascular (one-fourth) spaces. Fluid distribution can also be calculated as a percentage of body weight (BW):

- Intracellular water accounts for 40% of BW.
- Extracellular water accounts for 20% of BW.
- Interstitial water accounts for 15% of BW.
- Blood volume in adults accounts for 7% of BW.
- Blood volume in children accounts for 8% of BW.

IV FLUIDS

You will have different types of fluids from which to choose in the hospital. Isotonic fluids include normal saline (NS) and lactated Ringer's (LR), which are frequently used for acute resuscitation; these are the best fluids to use for increasing intravascular volume. Note that resuscitation fluids do not contain dextrose, as dextrose can cause hyperglycemia and osmotic diuresis. Typically, LR is also a maintenance fluid of choice on surgical services. The lactate is converted by the liver into HCO_3. As a result, **this fluid should be avoided in patients with metabolic or respiratory alkalosis.**

KEY FACT

NS and LR are used for acute resuscitation.

In general, maintenance fluids contain added dextrose and potassium. Dextrose prevents the breakdown of muscle for energy needs, provides fuel for the Krebs cycle, and prevents ketoacidosis. "D5" means 5% dextrose solution, and "D5W" means dextrose in water. Potassium should be added only if the patient has adequate urine output. The components of common fluids are listed in Table 2-4, expressed in milliequivalents per liter (mEq/L). Normal plasma osmolarity ranges from 280 to 300.

KEY FACT

Don't add potassium until you know that the patient's kidneys work.

TABLE 2-4. Components of Common Fluids

FLUIDS	Na	Cl	K	HCO_3	Ca
Crystalloids					
NS	154	154			
D5NS	154	154			
½ NS	77	77			
D5 ½ NS	77	77			
D5 ¼ NS	39	39			
D5W					
LR	130	109	4	28	3
3% NaCl	513	513			
Colloids					
Hespan	154	154			
Plasmanate	145	100	0.25		
25% albumin	130–160	130–160	1		

FLUID AND ELECTROLYTE THERAPY

The important elements of complete fluid therapy are acute resuscitation, the provision of maintenance fluids, the replacement of ongoing losses, and the replacement of deficits. Some patients will present in an acutely dehydrated state and will require resuscitation and deficit replacement, while others may be admitted for an elective surgical procedure and will require only maintenance fluids. Keep in mind that fluids are ideally maintained by mouth; don't add fluids just because a patient is in the hospital.

Fluid resuscitation. If a patient is significantly volume depleted, the first goal will be to rapidly replenish intravascular volume. It is important to recognize that the extent of clinical symptoms will depend not only on the volume lost but also on the rate of loss. Patients who have a gradual volume contraction may be well compensated, while those with rapid volume loss may go into hypovolemic shock. Signs of dehydration are not obvious until a patient has lost a significant volume, so be sure to routinely assess volume status in all patients, especially those who are vulnerable populations or have altered mental status. Remember that patients with burns or infections are likely to be more severely dehydrated at baseline and will need much more fluid than the average patient.

In adults, the standard resuscitation fluid is LR or NS. In a severely dehydrated adult, a 1- to 2-L bolus may be given over 30–120 minutes. If the patient has a history of cardiac disease with a ↓ ejection fraction, a slower rate is recommended, and the patient should be monitored for signs of heart failure.

In children, you can ask parents about recent intake (bottle- or breastfeeding) and output (fewer than 4–5 wet diapers in 24 hours suggests dehydration). You should evaluate physical signs of dehydration, which are outlined in Table 2-5.

Mild to moderate dehydration in children may be treated with oral rehydration therapies such as Pedialyte or Ricelyte, which contain approximately

TABLE 2-5. Clinical Manifestations of Dehydration

SIGNS/SYMPTOMS	MILD DEHYDRATION	MODERATE DEHYDRATION	SEVERE DEHYDRATION
Weight loss	5%	10%	15%
Pulse	Normal or slightly ↑	↑	↑↑
Blood pressure	Normal	Normal to orthostatic	Orthostatic to shock
Tears	Present	↓	Absent; sunken eyes
Mucous membranes	Normal	Dry	Parched
Mental status	Normal	Altered	Depressed
Anterior fontanelle (in children)	Normal	Normal to sunken	Sunken
Skin	Capillary refill < 2 sec	Delayed capillary refill 2–4 sec; ↓ turgor	Very delayed capillary refill, > 4 sec, cool skin, acrocyanosis
Urine specific gravity	1.020	> 1.020, oliguria	Maximal, oliguria or anuria
Estimated fluid deficit	< 50 mL/kg	50–100 mL/kg	> 100 mL/kg

45–90 mEq/L of sodium, 20 mEq/L of potassium, 20 g/L of glucose, and 30 mEq/L of citrate or bicarbonate. IV fluid boluses with isotonic crystalloid (NS or LR) are used to rapidly expand intravascular volume within the following guidelines:

- **Mild dehydration:** 10 cc/kg bolus over 1 hour.
- **Moderate dehydration:** 20 cc/kg bolus over 1 hour.
- **Severe dehydration or shock:** 30–50 cc/kg over 1 hour.
- Reassess urine output and clinical status and rebolus as necessary.

KEY POINT

THREE-FOR-ONE RULE

To replace 1 L of intravascular volume, you should give 3 L of isotonic solution. After 1–2 hours, 1 L of isotonic solution redistributes such that only 300 mL remains in the intravascular space. Colloid solutions remain in the intravascular space for a longer period but are quite expensive and should be used only in appropriate clinical settings (eg, in edematous patients).

Maintenance fluids. People in the hospital often order IV fluids on the basis of average fluid requirements. For example, an average order for an adult is D5 ½ NS with 20 mEq/L of KCl at 125 cc/hr. You can also calculate the exact water and electrolyte needs of a given patient, which will be more accurate if your patient differs from the standard 70-kg male. Maintenance fluid requirements ↑ under certain conditions, such as burns, hyperventilation, sweating, fever, hyperthyroidism, renal disease, and GI losses. Water requirements are calculated using the following methods (see Table 2-6 for electrolyte requirements):

TABLE 2-6. Electrolyte Requirements

	ADULTS	CHILDREN
Na	80–120 mEq/day	3–5 mEq/kg/day or per 100 mL fluid
K	50–100 mEq/day	1–2 mEq/kg/day or per 100 mL fluid
Cl	80–120 mEq/day	3 mEq/kg/day or per 100 mL fluid
Glucose	100–200 g/day	100–200 mg/kg/hr

1. **Holliday-Segar method (100/50/20 rule):**
   - Administer 100 mL/kg/day for the first 10 kg of weight.
   - Add 50 mL/kg for the next 10 kg.
   - Add 20 mL/kg for each kilogram over 20.
   - **Sample calculation:** A 70-kg adult would need (100 × 10) + (50 × 10) + (20 × 50) = 2500 mL/day.
2. **Hourly fluids (4/2/1 rule):**
   - Administer 4 mL/kg/hr for the first 10 kg.
   - Add 2 mL/kg for the next 10 kg.
   - Add 1 mL/kg for each kilogram over 20.
   - **Sample calculation:** A 70-kg adult would need (4 × 10) + (2 × 10) + (1 × 50) = 110 mL/hr.

KEY FACT

A rough estimate of fluid requirements is weight + 40 = mL/hr.

KEY POINT

SAMPLE MAINTENANCE FLUID CALCULATION

- **Patient:** A 24-kg child is admitted for elective surgery.
- **Maintenance fluids:** (100 × 10) + (50 × 10) + (20 × 4) = 1580 mL/day = 65.8 mL/hr.
- **Maintenance electrolytes:**
  - Na = 3 mEq/100 m × 1580 mL/day = 47.4 mEq/day.
  - K = 2 mEq/100 mL × 1580 mL/day = 31.6 mEq/day.
- **Answer:** ¼ NS provides 34 mEq/L of NaCl. If a child requires approximately 1.5 L/day, that child will receive 51 mEq of NaCl, which satisfies his requirement. The addition of 20 mEq of KCl to each liter (after the first void) will provide 30 mEq/day.
- **Appropriate fluid order:** D5 ¼ NS + 20 mEq/L KCl to run at 65 mL/hr.

Replace ongoing losses. Evaluate the volume and composition of fluids lost through diarrhea, vomiting, chest tubes, or various other sources. Try to replace losses "cc for cc" with fluids of similar composition. The average composition of body fluids can be found in many pocket guides and textbooks.

Deficit therapy. The replacement of existing deficits will depend on the degree of dehydration (established by the history and examination) and on the type of dehydration (established by serum sodium, and generally classified as isonatremic, hyponatremic, or hypernatremic). Although a complete discussion of volume and electrolyte imbalances lies beyond the scope of this book, there are some basic facts that you should know.

Deficit replacement generally takes place at a rate proportional to the rate of loss. In a patient with 2 L of acute blood loss, IV fluids should be given rapidly in the resuscitation phase. By contrast, in a patient with well-compensated chronic hypernatremic dehydration, replacement should be undertaken slowly to avert rapid fluid shifts and potential complications. Further distinctions are as follows:

- **Isonatremic dehydration (Na 130–150 mEq/L):** This is the most common form of dehydration and involves a net loss of isotonic fluid. Begin treatment by estimating the fluid deficit based on the degree of dehydration (eg, mild = approximately 5% BW). Some clinicians replace the entire deficit with isotonic solution; standard therapy is D5 ¼ NS in small children and D5 ½ NS in older children and adults. After urination, 10–20 mEq of KCl can be added. Half of the deficit should be replaced over 8 hours and the remainder over 16 hours.
- **Hyponatremic dehydration (Na < 130 mEq/L):** There is a net loss of solute, so an additional sodium deficit must be replaced. The formula for calculating the sodium deficit is as follows:

  $$\text{Na deficit (mEq)} = (\text{desired Na} - \text{measured Na}) \times 0.6 \times \text{weight (kg)}$$

  This sodium should be added to the patient's other fluid and electrolyte needs. Again, half of the deficit can be replaced over 8 hours and the remainder over 16 hours. In chronic, severe hyponatremia, however, serum sodium should not be ↑ by > 2 mEq/L/hr or 10–12 mEq/L/day because of the risk of central pontine myelinolysis. In a symptomatic patient (eg, a patient who has CNS symptoms), 3% NaCl may be given in an ICU setting to ↑ Na to > 120 mEq/L. The remainder of fluid replacement should proceed slowly with NS. In general, free water should also be restricted.
- **Hypernatremic dehydration (Na > 150 mEq/L):** There is a net loss of water relative to solute. This is typically due to ↓ fluid intake in the presence of ↑ insensible losses (eg, fever, burns) but may also be due to excess salt intake. Treatment involves replacement of the free-water deficit, which is calculated using the following formula:

  $$\text{Water deficit (L)} = \text{TBW} \times (\text{actual Na} - \text{desired Na})/\text{desired Na}$$

  Correction must be undertaken cautiously, as cerebral edema, seizures, and CNS injury may result if sodium is corrected too rapidly (> 0.5–1.0 mEq/L/hr). Sodium may be lowered by 10–15 mEq/L/day, not to exceed 25 mEq/L/24 hr. General guidelines suggest using D5 ½ NS, D5 ¼ NS, or D5W to correct half of the free-water deficit over 24 hours. The remaining deficit may then be corrected over the following 48–72 hours. Begin replacing potassium after the patient urinates, and remember to replace ongoing losses and to provide maintenance fluids.

Acid-Base Calculations

On almost every rotation you embark on, you will be asked to evaluate the acid-base status of a patient. You will be sure to impress your residents and attendings if you can rapidly interpret your patient's acid-base status as well as

TABLE 2-7. Method for Defining 1° Acid-Base Disturbances

pH	P_{CO_2}	HCO_3^-	1° Disturbance
< 7.36	↑	↑ or ↔	Respiratory acidosis
	↓ or ↔	↓	Metabolic acidosis
	↑	↓	Combined respiratory and metabolic acidosis
> 7.44	↓	↓ or ↔	Respiratory alkalosis
	↑ or ↔	↑	Metabolic alkalosis
	↓	↑	Combined respiratory and metabolic alkalosis

provide a differential diagnosis for your patient's condition. Presented below is a systematic approach to acid-base problems.

Two essential laboratory results are necessary for interpreting acid-base problems: an arterial blood gas (ABG) and an electrolyte panel. Using these studies, you will ask yourself 4 major questions:

1. **Does the patient have an acidemia (pH < 7.36) or an alkalemia (pH > 7.44)?** Normal pH is 7.40.
2. **Is the 1° disturbance metabolic or respiratory?** First look at the P_{CO_2} (normal value 40). If the P_{CO_2} has shifted in the opposite direction of pH (eg, P_{CO_2} ↑ when pH ↓), then you know that the 1° disturbance is respiratory. If not, look at the HCO_3 (normal value 24). If the HCO_3 has shifted in the same direction as the pH, then the 1° disturbance is metabolic. See Table 2-7 for an algorithm with which to define the 1° disturbance.
3. **Is compensation for the 1° disturbance appropriate?** See Table 2-8.

TABLE 2-8. Methods of Compensation for 1° Disturbance

1° Disturbance	Compensatory Mechanism	Calculating Appropriate Compensation	Compensation Is Inappropriate
Metabolic acidosis	P_{CO_2}	▪ $P_{CO_2} = 1.5 \times HCO_3^- + 8 +/- 2$ (Winter's formula) ▪ P_{CO_2} = last 2 digits of pH ▪ P_{CO_2} ↑ by 10 for every ↓ in HCO_3^- by 10	If actual P_{CO_2} is: ▪ Higher, there is also a respiratory acidosis ▪ Lower, there is also a respiratory alkalosis
Metabolic alkalosis	P_{CO_2}	▪ $P_{CO_2} = 0.9 \times HCO_3^- + 9$ ▪ $\Delta P_{CO_2} = 0.6 \times HCO_3^-$ ▪ P_{CO_2} ↑ by 7 for every ↑ in HCO_3^- by 10	If actual P_{CO_2} is: ▪ Higher, there is also a respiratory acidosis ▪ Lower, there is also a respiratory alkalosis
Respiratory acidosis	HCO_3^-	▪ Acute: HCO_3^- ↑ by 1 for every ↑ in P_{CO_2} by 10 ▪ Chronic: HCO_3^- ↑ by 4 for every ↑ in P_{CO_2} by 10	If actual HCO_3^- is: ▪ Higher, there is also a metabolic alkalosis ▪ Lower, there is also a metabolic acidosis
Respiratory alkalosis	HCO_3^-	▪ Acute: HCO_3^- ↓ by 2 for every ↓ in P_{CO_2} by 10 ▪ Chronic: HCO_3^- ↓ by 5 for every ↓ in P_{CO_2} by 10	If actual HCO_3^- is: ▪ Higher, there is also a metabolic alkalosis ▪ Lower, there is also a metabolic acidosis

TABLE 2-9. Determination of Acidosis Type

ΔAG	ΔHCO_3^-	TYPE
0 +/– 2	> ΔAG	NAG acidosis
> 2	= ΔAG	AG acidosis
> 2	> ΔAG	Combined NAG and AG acidosis

KEY FACT

Compensating mechanisms never overcompensate or compensate completely.

4. **Is there an anion-gap (AG) acidosis?** Regardless of whether you initially identified a metabolic acidosis, always check for an AG acidosis. A normal anion gap is 12.
   a. Calculate the patient's AG.
   b. Calculate ΔAG: ΔAG = calculated AG – normal AG.
   c. Calculate ΔHCO_3^-: $\Delta HCO_3^- = [HCO_3^-]_{plasma} - [HCO_3^-]_{normal}$.
   d. Refer to Table 2-9 to determine if the patient has AG acidosis, non-anion-gap (NAG) acidosis, or combined metabolic acidosis.

Some examples are as follows:

1. **Lab values:** pH = 7.11, P_{CO_2} = 16, HCO_3^- = 5, Na^+ = 140, K^+ = 4.0, Cl^- = 115.
   Step 1: Does the patient have an acidemia or an alkalemia?
   pH = 7.11, so the patient is acidemic.
   Step 2: Is the 1° disturbance metabolic or respiratory?
   P_{CO_2} = 16, which is lower than normal. P_{CO_2} has moved in the same direction as pH (ie, down), so the 1° disturbance is not respiratory but metabolic. Consistent with a metabolic etiology, we see that HCO_3^- = 5, which indicates that the major base, bicarbonate, is ↓. We conclude that this patient's 1° disturbance is a metabolic acidosis.
   Step 3: Is the compensation for the 1° disturbance appropriate?
   For a metabolic acidosis, we expect that $P_{CO_2} = 1.5 \times HCO_3^- + 8$ +/– 2. So in this case, we would expect that $P_{CO_2} = 1.5 \times 5 + 8$ +/– 2 = 15.5 +/– 2. We therefore conclude that the compensation is appropriate.
   Step 4: Is there an AG acidosis?
   First we calculate the AG: 140 – 115 – 5 = 20. ΔAG therefore equals 8. ΔHCO_3^- = 19. Since ΔHCO_3^- is greater than ΔAG, we conclude that there is a combined AG and NAG metabolic acidosis.
   SOLUTION: Combined AG and NAG metabolic acidosis.
2. **Lab values:** pH = 7.67, P_{CO_2} = 30, HCO_3^- = 34, Na^+ = 140, K^+ = 3.0, Cl^- = 94.
   Step 1: Does the patient have an acidemia or an alkalemia?
   pH = 7.67, so the patient is alkalemic.
   Step 2: What is the 1° disturbance?
   P_{CO_2} = 30, which is lower than normal. P_{CO_2} has moved in the opposite direction from pH, so we can conclude that the 1° disturbance is respiratory. We also check HCO_3^- to determine if there is a combined 1° disturbance. HCO_3^- = 34, which indicates that the major base, bicarbonate, is ↑. We therefore conclude that there is also a 1° metabolic alkalosis.
   Step 3: Is the compensation appropriate?
   For a respiratory alkalosis, we expect HCO_3^- to ↓ 2–5 mEq/L for every 10-mm Hg ↓ in P_{CO_2}. We would therefore expect HCO_3^- to be be-

tween 19 and 22. HCO_3^- = 34, which is higher than expected, so we once again confirm that there is a metabolic alkalosis in addition to the respiratory alkalosis.

Step 4: Is there an AG acidosis?

First we calculate the AG: 140 – 94 – 34 = 12. ΔAG therefore equals zero, and we can conclude that there is no underlying AG metabolic acidosis.

SOLUTION: Combined 1° respiratory and metabolic alkalosis.

Antibiotic Therapy

Patients with bacterial infections can present anywhere from almost asymptomatic (eg, latent TB) to critically ill (eg, sepsis). In most cases, it will take days until bacterial culture results and antibiotic susceptibility patterns become available—and in all candor, some patients' life expectancy in the absence of antibiotic therapy may not exceed more than half an hour (eg, meningococcal meningitis). Therefore, it is common practice to start **empiric** antibiotic therapy based on the bacterium that is **most likely** to have caused the patient's illness. Only when culture results become available can the antibiotic therapy be narrowed.

KEY FACT

Antibiotic therapy is like fighting zombies: Use a shotgun in critical situations and a sniper rifle once you have identified your target.

The following are some general guidelines you can use when selecting empiric antibiotic therapy.

- **Therapy > diagnosis:** In a critically ill patient (eg, one with bacterial meningitis), give antibiotics without delay. To be sure, doing so may sterilize the CSF or blood, thereby preventing you from getting any culture data—but in general, it's better to tell a patient on discharge that you don't know what bug made him sick than to tell the patient's family exactly what pathogen he died from.
- **Route of administration:** Critically ill patients require IV antibiotics, as intravenously administered antibiotics have an almost immediate onset of action. In other cases, oral antibiotics may be considered (especially if the patient is safe to be discharged). In all instances, however, make sure the antibiotic you are prescribing can reach the target tissue (eg, oral vancomycin has 0% bioavailability in the blood but is great for some GI infections for that very reason).
- **Patient allergies:** A patient with penicillin allergy has a 10% chance of having an allergic reaction to cephalosporins (cross-reactivity). Of course, other β-lactam antibiotics may trigger allergic reactions as well.
- **Pregnancy status:** Trimethoprim, sulfonamides, clarithromycin, and quinolones are contraindicated in pregnancy owing to the harmful effects they may have on the fetus.
- **Patient age:** Some illnesses are more typical in certain age groups (eg, *Listeria monocytogenes* in the very young and very old). However, side effects may also differ with age; for example, kernicterus due to sulfa-containing antibiotics may occur in newborns but not in adults.
- **Patient comorbidities:** Patients with ↓ renal or hepatic function may require adjusted dosing. Telithromycin, aminoglycosides, colistin, and clindamycin may exacerbate myasthenia gravis to the point of respiratory failure.

Table 2-10 lists common bacterial infections, the most common pathogens associated with each, and initial antibiotic therapy for each. Bear in mind that

TABLE 2-10. Empiric Antibiotic Selection

Diagnosis	Common Pathogens	Empiric Antibiotics	Alternatives
Bacterial meningitis	*Pneumococcus* *Meningococcus* *Listeria monocytogenes*	Ceftriaxone IV + vancomycin IV + ampicillin IV (if *Listeria* is suspected)	Vancomycin IV + aztreonam IV + TMP/SMX IV
Community-acquired pneumonia	*Pneumococcus* *H influenzae* *Legionella* *Mycoplasma pneumoniae*	Ceftriaxone IV + azithromycin IV	Levofloxacin IV
Hospital-acquired pneumonia	*Pseudomonas aeruginosa* *S aureus* Gram-⊖ rods	Piperacillin/tazobactam IV + tobramycin IV	Levofloxacin IV + tobramycin IV or cefepime
Cellulitis	*S aureus* *Streptococcus*	Cefazolin IV	Clindamycin IV
Surgical site infection	*S aureus* *Streptococcus* Gram-⊖ organisms If GI tract: anaerobes, enterococci	Piperacillin/tazobactam IV + vancomycin IV	Levofloxacin IV + vancomycin IV + metronidazole IV
IV catheter–associated bacteremia	*S aureus* *Staphylococcus epidermidis* *P aeruginosa*	Vancomycin IV + piperacillin/ tazobactam IV	Vancomycin IV + aztreonam IV
UTI	*E coli* Enterococci	Ampicillin IV + gentamicin IV	Levofloxacin IV + gentamicin IV
UTI (Foley associated)	*E coli* *Klebsiella* *Pseudomonas*	Piperacillin/tazobactam IV + gentamicin IV	TMP/SMX IV + gentamicin IV

local resistance patterns vary, and the antibiotic guidelines of your hospital may differ.

Insulin Orders

You will see many patients on the wards who require insulin to maintain their blood glucose levels within the normal range. There are 2 general types of insulin with which you should be familiar: long acting and short acting.

- **Long-acting insulin** (eg, detemir, glargine) is given to a patient to maintain basal requirements throughout the day.
- **Short-acting insulin** (eg, aspart, regular insulin) is given in anticipation of a carbohydrate load.

You may need to write orders for insulin while on the wards. There are 3 different ways to determine the daily insulin requirement of your patient:

- If the patient is on insulin at home, ask what his or her daily dose is. Use this method only if you think your patient is able to provide accurate information.
- Alternatively, you can cover the patient on short-acting insulin for a period of 24 hours and then determine how much insulin he or she required during this time period and adjust accordingly.
- You can roughly estimate the total daily insulin need by dividing the patient's body weight (in kilograms) by 2.

Once you have determined the total daily insulin requirement, divide the total daily insulin need evenly into basal and prandial insulin. An example is given below.

Sensitivity to insulin varies among patients. A thin patient who has never received insulin before will need less (multiply body weight by 0.2), while a morbidly obese patient may have significant insulin resistance and may thus require more (multiply body weight by 0.6). The traditional thinking has been that a patient with high blood glucose in the morning needs less insulin at night, not more. It was hypothesized that hypoglycemia at night leads to catecholamine release, which raises glucose levels in the morning (the Somogyi effect). However, with the advent of continuous glucose monitoring, data have emerged that contradict this hypothesis. Prove your resident wrong if he or she tries to pimp you on this! (Hint: *Diabetologia*, Volume 48, Number 11, pp. 2437–2438.)

KEY POINT

DETERMINING INSULIN REQUIREMENTS

Mrs. Jones weighs 120 kg. Her daily insulin requirement is $0.5 \times 120 = 60$ units. She should receive half of that (30 units) as long-acting insulin. In addition, she will receive 10 units of short-acting insulin with each of her meals (10 units per meal × 3 meals = 30 units).

Patient Emergencies

One of a student's worst nightmares centers on the prospect of being alone with a patient when something bad happens. In such a situation, the primary rule is, "Don't panic!" Instead, immediately call for help (ie, yell, "Nurse, I've got a problem!"). We cover basic CPR here, but please refer to the Emergency Medicine chapter for information on other patient emergencies.

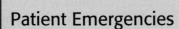

KEY FACT

In an emergency, immediately call for help.

CARDIOPULMONARY ARREST

In the event of cardiopulmonary arrest, check for patient responsiveness first. In a loud voice, ask the patient, "Are you okay?" while shaking him or her. If the patient is unresponsive and does not pass the "eyeball test" (ie, if he or she looks very sick), do not hesitate to call a Code Blue. Once you do this, you will get all the help you ever wanted. However, you will still have some very stressful moments when you are by yourself.

It should also be noted that the 2010 AHA adult CPR guidelines instruct providers to **assess circulation first** (ie, follow C-A-B, not the old A-B-C). So if the patient is without a pulse, start CPR and don't waste time assessing the airway.

KEY POINT

C-A-B / D-E-F SEQUENCE

Circulation	If the patient does not have a pulse, compress the chest at 100 compressions per minute.
Airway	Ensure airway patency (clear the bronchotracheal tract).
Breathing	If the patient is not breathing, begin intermittent positive-pressure ventilation.
Drugs/fluids	Place an IV line, push epinephrine and other drugs as indicated, and get a fingerstick glucose (blood sugar).
ECG	Monitor cardiac rhythms.
Fibrillation	Defibrillate. Note, however, that as soon as the defibrillator is attached to the patient, everything else stops regardless of what part of the cycle you are in. Certain arrhythmias need urgent defibrillation (VT, VF).

KEY FACT

Most adults stop breathing because their hearts stop. Most children's hearts stop because they are not breathing.

Circulation. Check the carotid pulses, one at a time, on both sides. Peripheral pulses are not reliable in these situations. If pulses are absent, initiate CPR. In adults and children, use the heel of your hand to compress the sternum 2 inches at the level of the nipples at a rate of 100 bpm. In infants, use the tips of the middle and ring fingers to compress the sternum 1 inch at a rate of at least 100 bpm. The ratio of compressions to breaths in adults is 30:2.

Once the patient is intubated, do **not** interrupt your compressions for breaths; just keep pumping. In the hospital, patients have a tendency to be placed on rather compressible mattresses. If this is the case, you **must** get a CPR board underneath them, or else you will risk giving CPR to the mattress. Lower the bed to the lowest position (most beds have a CPR lever) and have someone bring you a stepstool so that your compressions are truly vertical. Then, after 2 minutes, have someone take over compressions (studies have shown that fatigue compromises the efficacy of compressions). You should also attach defibrillator pads and check the rhythm on the monitor, as this may indicate which ACLS pathway is applicable and whether the patient needs immediate defibrillation.

Airway. Once it has been established that the patient has a pulse, determine if he or she has a patent airway. If the patient speaks or screams, don't worry about the airway; you can safely assume that it's patent. But do worry if the patient has a muffled or hoarse voice (indicating impeding airway compromise). If the patient's airway is not patent, adjust it with a backward head tilt (if a C-spine injury is not suspected) or a forward jaw thrust (if a C-spine injury is suspected) and reassess breathing.

Breathing. If the patient is still not breathing, provide bag-mask ventilation. If he or she is already intubated, be sure to listen with the stethoscope for bilateral breath sounds.

If asystole is detected by ECG in > 1 lead, continue CPR. The patient must be intubated. An IV is started immediately, and 1 mg of epinephrine is pushed every 3–5 minutes. If you arrive late to a code and the room is already crowded, be the timekeeper. Alert the person running the code every time 2 minutes are up.

If a ventricular fibrillation (VF) or ventricular tachycardia (VT) is detected with a ventricular rate of > 150 bpm, asynchronous cardioversion (defibrillation) is necessary. Although stable VT may be treated with medication, a patient with VF or unstable VT (ie, low BP or no pulse) should be treated immediately with electrocardioversion.

By the way—kudos for reading the entire introductory chapter! It takes a diligent and studious person to not just skip to the "relevant" chapter. You'll be a better physician for it.

Other Key Facts and Formulas

FORMULAS

- Mean arterial blood pressure (MAP) = DBP + [(SBP – DBP)/3], where DBP = diastolic blood pressure and SBP = systolic blood pressure.
- A-a (alveolar-arterial) oxygen gradient $= PAO_2 - PaO_2$
  $= [(pAtm - pH_2O) \times FiO_2 - (PaCO_2/RQ)] - PaO_2$
  $= [(713 \times FiO_2) - (PaCO_2/0.8)] - PaO_2$
  Normal $FiO_2 = 0.21$; normal A-a gradient = 5–15 mm or the upper limit of (age/4) + 4.
- Cerebral perfusion pressure (CPP) = MAP – ICP.

ELECTROLYTES

- Osmolality = 2 × serum Na + serum glucose / 18 + BUN/2.8.
- Normal plasma osmolality = 275–295 mOsm/kg.
- Corrected Ca $= Ca_{plasma} + 0.8 \times$ (normal albumin – patient's albumin) $= Ca_{plasma} + 0.8 \times (4 -$ serum albumin).
- Corrected $Na_{plasma} = Na_{plasma} + (\text{glucose} - 100) \times 0.0016$.
- Corrected $Na_{plasma} = Na_{plasma} + 0.2 \times$ triglycerides (g/L).
- Corrected $Na_{plasma} = Na_{plasma} + 0.025 \times$ protein (g/L).
- TBW = k × weight (kg), where k = 0.6 in men and 0.5 in women.
- Stool osmotic gap = stool osmolality $- 2(Na_{stool} + K_{stool})$, where < 50 osm is consistent with secretory diarrhea and > 125 osm is consistent with osmotic diarrhea.

ACID-BASE EQUATIONS

- $AG = Na_{plasma} - (Cl_{plasma} + HCO_3^-{}_{plasma})$.
- Urine $AG = Na_{urine} + K_{urine} - Cl_{urine}$.
- $pH = 6.1 + \log (HCO_3^- / 0.03 \times PCO_2)$.

RENAL FUNCTION

- Fractional excretion of sodium (Fe_{Na})
  $= (Na_{urine}/Na_{plasma}) / (Cr_{urine}/Cr_{plasma}) \times 100$ or
  $= (Na_{urine} \times Cr_{plasma}) / (Na_{plasma} \times Na_{urine}) \times 100$.
- Creatinine clearance (CrCl) = (Cr_{urine} × urine volume in mL) / (Cr_{plasma} × time in minutes).
- Expected CrCl = [(140 – age) × weight (kg) × 0.85 for females] / (72 × Cr_{plasma}), where Cr_{plasma} is in mg/dL.

STATISTICS

		Test	
		+	–
Disease	+	A	B
	–	C	D

- Sensitivity = A / (A + B).
- Specificity = D / (C + D).
- False positive rate = C / (A + C).
- False negative rate = B / (B + D).
- Positive predictive value = A / (A + C).
- Negative predictive value = D / (B + D).
- Positive likelihood ratio = sensitivity / (1 – specificity).
- Negative likelihood ratio = (1 – sensitivity)/specificity.
- Absolute risk reduction (ARR) = disease rate without intervention – disease rate with intervention = A / (A + B) – C / (C + D).
- Relative risk reduction (RRR) = ARR / disease rate without intervention = [A / (A + B)] / [C / (C + D)].
- Number needed to treat (NNT) = 1 / ARR.

COMMON ABBREVIATIONS

Numbers

Ṫ	one	
ṪṪ	two	
ṪṪṪ	three	
$\overline{ss}$	one-half	*semis*

Dosing Schedule

bid	twice a day	(*bis in die*)
hs	at bedtime	(*hora somni*)
tid	3 times a day	(*ter in die*)
÷	divided doses	
q	each, every	(*quaque*)
q6h	every 6 hours	(*quaque 6 hora*)
qac	before each meal	(*quaque ante cibum*)
qd	every day	(*quaque die*)
qh	every hour	(*quaque hora*)
qid	4 times a day	(*quater in die*)

qod	every other day	
pc	after meals	(*post cibos*)
prn	as needed	(*pro re nata*)

Routes of Administration

IM	intramuscular	
inj	injection	
IV	intravenous	
PO	by mouth	(*per os*)
PR	by rectum	(*per rectum*)
SL	sublingual	
SQ	subcutaneous	

Medication Preparations

amp	ampule	(*ampulla*)
caps	capsules	(*capsula*)
gtt	drops	(*guttae*)
liq	liquid	(*liquor*)
sol	solution	(*solutio*)
supp	suppository	(*suppositorium*)
susp	suspension	
tab	tablet	(*tabella*)
ung	ointment	(*unguentum*)

Prepositions

a	before	(*ante*)
p	after	(*post*)
s	without	(*sine*)
x	except	(*excipio*)

Miscellaneous

ad lib	at pleasure	(*ad libitum*)
disp	dispense	(*dispensia*)
NPO	nothing by mouth	(*nil per os*)
OD	right eye	(*oculus dexter*)
OS	left eye	(*oculus sinister*)
OU	both eyes	(*oculus uterque*)
qs	to a sufficient quantity	(*quantum sufficit*)
Rx	prescription, take	(*recipe*)
sig	label, or let it be printed	(*signa*)
stat	immediately	(*statim*)

SECTION 2

CORE CLERKSHIPS

CHAPTER 3

EMERGENCY MEDICINE

Ward Tips

Welcome to the emergency department (ED)! Emergency medicine (EM) is a popular clerkship as well as a "hot" field in medicine. This rotation allows students to see a broad spectrum of patients and diseases while also being given the opportunity to be the first to diagnose and treat those patients. In the course of this rotation, you will be given a chance to do procedures, practice primary and critical care, and participate in traumas and resuscitations. Regardless of the field you enter, aspects of it will be found in EM, and many of your patients will come from the ED. So take advantage of this learning opportunity and enjoy the rotation. You will see it all in the ED!

WHAT IS THE ROTATION LIKE?

EM is usually a required clerkship or elective of 3 or 4 weeks' duration, depending on the medical school involved. Your prior rotations and experiences will prove particularly useful in this rotation. You will be the first to see the patient and will decide which tests to order, and you will also be the one who renders a diagnosis and determines whether the patient is sick enough to be admitted into the hospital. For these reasons, your experience and confidence level will to a large extent dictate your ability to contribute to, and get the most out of, this rotation.

For many students, the EM rotation may present the most patient responsibility you will encounter during medical school. While on this rotation, you will see diseases affecting every system—be it neurologic, psychiatric, GI, endocrine, cardiac, respiratory, or urologic. You must therefore have a broad knowledge base to help you communicate effectively with the various services to which you may admit or with which you may request a consultation. Depending on the ED at your institution, you may also see adult and pediatric patients in the same or separate areas. This wide variation in disease severity and patient population may be why many students prefer to schedule this rotation after they have completed the majority of their other basic clerkships—especially if they are contemplating a career in EM.

> **KEY FACT**
>
> EM will challenge you to draw on your knowledge of a variety of specialties and patient populations.

Remember, anything can happen in the ED! As Dr. Frederick Levy of the Johns Hopkins Hospital stated, "I think the most important point that a student or resident can learn in EM is the adage, 'Absence of proof is not proof of absence.' It's not the MI in a 70-year-old diabetic, hypertensive male with the Levine sign that we miss; it's the 40-year-old with 1 or 2 risk factors and a normal ECG. Similarly, many patients with appendicitis may have unexplained RLQ tenderness but may be hungry and afebrile with a normal WBC." With this in mind, here are some tips on how to maximize your efficiency on this rotation.

- **Patient evaluations:**
  - **Be thorough yet efficient.** Remember that working up a patient in the ED is unlike doing a history and physical (H&P) during an inpatient service. The difference lies in the fact that in the ED, you have a limited amount of time at your disposal as well as many more patients waiting to be seen. So while some patients in the ED may well have a litany of problems, it is critical that you **isolate their chief complaint** and identify their most acute issue as soon as you can. You should not take more than 10 minutes for the history and 5 minutes for the physical examination. Within the first few minutes of your encounter with a

patient, you must determine whether the patient is "sick" or "not sick." Of course, most (but not all) patients presenting to the ED have some kind of illness, but try to get a "gestalt" of whether or not your patient is in serious trouble, as this determination will likely change the course of what you do.
  - **Develop a focused differential** of things that may kill the patient or that you cannot afford to miss. This is called the "differential of consequence" (DOC). For example, if your patient comes into the ED with left-sided chest pain, don't waste time and energy on ruling out shingles. Instead, focus on things like MI, pulmonary embolism (PE), pneumonia, and pericarditis. Once you have your DOC, think of which tests you can order in the ED to confirm these conditions or rule them out. Bear in mind, however, that tests ordered in the ED must have a quick (less than 2-hour) turnaround time. While you are in the ED, you won't be able to send a complete autoantibody panel (as you would on your medicine rotation) to find out if your patient's pericarditis is caused by lupus.
  - **Remember Occam's razor.** This principle, also known as the "law of parsimony," states that a single explanation for multiple symptoms is more likely to be true than multiple explanations. For example, a patient with fever and chest pain is more likely to have pneumonia than an MI and a URI at the same time.
  - **Learn to prioritize.** You should work on prioritizing your patients by disease severity. The ED is not a "first-come, first-served" environment. Prioritizing also means that at times, treatment comes before taking a history. Don't hold back an asthmatic's albuterol nebulizer just so that you can obtain a comprehensive social history. Prioritize your own needs as well; eat and sleep when you get the chance.
- **Presentations:** Regardless of whether you will present to a resident or the attending, be succinct. A presentation that takes more than 2 minutes is too long. Start with the patient's name, age, and pertinent past medical history, and then give a focused description of the problem. At the end of the history of present illness, briefly mention pertinent positives/negatives from the review of systems. Next, list pertinent positive and negative findings from your physical examination along with relevant lab values (if available). Finish with your preliminary diagnosis (put your money down!) and your differential. Suggest which studies are needed to rule various conditions in or out. Make sure you have pen and paper ready, as your resident/attending may tell you what else you should consider, which tests are and are not appropriate, and the like. Finally, once you have presented the patient, don't just forget about him or her. Follow up on the studies you've ordered and adjust your diagnosis accordingly.
- **Signing out:** Learning to sign out a patient is a valuable skill learned during the EM rotation. When your shift ends, you will be expected to give a quick and concise summary of your patients to the party taking over care for you. Be sure to efficiently describe the chief complaint, interventions thus far, pending work/lab results/consults, and disposition plans. It is generally poor form to sign out things that you would not really want to do yourself, such as rectal or pelvic examinations.
- **Trauma:** You will probably be involved in traumas as they come into the ED. Although these may occur at any time, you should be alerted by overhead announcements or pagers with the estimated time of arrival. If you are participating in trauma resuscitation, you should observe the following guidelines:
  - Be sure to gown up properly, making appropriate use of eye shields and gloves.
  - Be calm and ready to help in any capacity you can.

KEY FACT

There are 3 kinds of patients in the ED: those who will die regardless of what you do, those who will live regardless of what you do, and those who will live **because** of what you do.

- Although the environment surrounding a trauma may seem hectic, there should be a resident at the foot of the bed giving orders. This may be an ED resident or a trauma surgery resident, depending on your institution. The student's role during a trauma may be very limited, but each case represents an opportunity for you to learn—even if staying out of the way is your primary responsibility.
- Good things for a medical student to do during a trauma include cutting off clothes (just don't cut any ECG leads), doing compressions during CPR, and gathering more information from family members. Once you have seen a few traumas, ask your team if they would be comfortable letting you do the primary survey (**C**irculation, **A**irway, **B**reathing, or CAB).
- Anticipate the needs of your team. During rapid-sequence intubation, for example, ask if the physician needs cricoid pressure. In a patient with head trauma, have the otoscope ready so that hemotympanum can be ruled out. Check with the radiologist to determine whether the CT scanner is ready.
- Don't take things personally if people don't say "please" or "thank you" at this time. Treating a trauma can be a stressful event, and teaching comes secondary to saving a life during trauma resuscitation.

HOW IS THE DAY SET UP?

Most EM rotations consist of a certain number of 8-, 10-, or 12-hour shifts. When you initially arrive, patients already in the ED will be signed out to you by other medical students or residents. When assuming the care of a patient, be sure you know that patient's history and pertinent examination findings so that changes in his or her condition can be assessed adequately should a change in disposition be required. In addition, make sure you are aware of all procedures that need to be done and labs that are pending.

KEY FACT

Never sign out a pelvic or rectal examination to a colleague.

You should also take steps to familiarize yourself with your ED's etiquette regarding sign-out. In virtually every institution, it is poor form to sign out the less glamorous procedures. However, there is significant variability among institutions with regard to other procedures, with some facilities requiring that you perform all procedures before sign-out and others expecting you to leave outstanding procedures for the next shift. Of course, many students find it worthwhile to remain after their shift has ended to complete unfinished procedures, regardless of the prevailing norm. Depending on the ED, new patients may be triaged and assigned to a care area for which you are responsible or, alternatively, you may pick up new cases from a stack of unseen patients. Regardless of your institution's procedure for acquiring new patients, you should be sure to make the attending and residents aware of your presence, as they will often allow you to "cherry-pick" interesting patients, seek you out for procedures, and recommend the best area for you to work.

Be proactive about getting new patients. Find out which patients have not yet been seen and request permission to go see them. Be a go-getter.

HOW DO I EXCEL IN EMERGENCY MEDICINE?

For medical students, the key to excelling in EM is to be thorough yet efficient. Overcrowding is a major concern in EM, so moving patients through the ED is vital. For this reason, you will need to rapidly distinguish patients who require admission and immediate treatment from those who are safe to wait for test results or may just need reassurance and outpatient referral.

In your efforts to maximize your efficiency, much of your time will be spent "doing things" for your patients rather than "sitting and talking" about them. With this in mind, the paragraphs that follow offer guidelines on how to excel on this rotation.

- **Get along with the team.** Always maintain a positive attitude. During a long shift, remaining upbeat and helpful will make you shine. Also remember that in the ED, you may work one-on-one with the nurses more often than you do with your fellow students and residents. So be sure to get on their good side, as they will be able to teach you a great deal. Nurses not only can make or break your rotation but can also make you look great by updating you on your patients and helping you with ordering prior to presentations. In return, if the nurse is busy, don't be afraid to help a patient with a urinal, strip the sheets off a stretcher after patient discharge, etc.
- **Know your patients.** Be sure you are aware of your patients' conditions and vitals at all times. You want to be the first to know if your patients are decompensating or improving. Also remember to keep on top of the tests you ordered, as your approach toward management will often hinge on the results of those tests. In addition, residents will gain confidence in your abilities when you can keep them apprised of your patients' status.
- **Be assertive.** Assertiveness is key to furthering your education as well as to scoring points with the people who evaluate you. So ask good and well-thought-out questions; know other patients on the service (for your own learning and in case you are asked to fill in); take the initiative to ask for demonstrations of procedures; volunteer for drawing blood (you need to practice anyway); and, at the end of each shift, ask to be told one thing you did well and one thing you could do better. Try to seek feedback early in your presentation regarding your efficiency, presentation style, and the like.
- **Be on time.** EM physicians value their time off. Thus, few things upset them more than seeing a colleague show up late for sign-out. Likewise, when you sign out, remember that you are done; unless you want to stick around for something educational, you are expected to go home. There is no need to stay after your shift just to show your face (another reason EM is so popular).
- **Be both effective and efficient.** Again, you don't have all day to work up a patient, so just go for it. At the same time, remember that your evaluation should also be complete enough to ensure that you don't send any sick patients home.

Above all, be nice to your patients. Reassess them; see if there is anything they need; and keep them apprised of what is happening. Not only is this the right thing to do, but it will make your patients appreciate you, and they will mention it to your residents and attendings. Always bear in mind that even if you are tired, grumpy, and bitter, your patient is having a worse day than you are!

CHALLENGES IN THE ED

The ED will provide you with exposure to a highly diverse group of people. Indeed, in the current U.S. health care system, it is the only place where many patients can receive medical treatment. For this reason, overcrowding and long wait times can become major issues. So make it a habit to acknowledge to patients that you know how many hours they had to sit in the waiting room.

KEY FACT

Be thorough and efficient in the ED.

KEY FACT

EM is a "doing" specialty. Be prepared to be moving and working throughout your entire shift, as there is generally little downtime.

In the ED, you will encounter not only interesting medical pathology but also challenging social issues. These encounters will test your ability to gather clinical data in difficult situations as well as your capacity to mold your history-taking skills to each patient. At some point, for example, you will come across patients who are drug seeking, homeless, or victims of abuse. In such cases, the chief complaint you hear may not reflect the reasons these patients are actually in the ED—so taking a carefully tailored and compassionate history will be vital to determining the best course of action. When deciding on a plan of care, you should remember that the emergency physician is often ED patients' only advocate. Also bear in mind that the ED can be a chaotic and stressful environment for physicians and patients alike. Because of this, you may encounter violent patients as well. It is important to remain aware of your environment, predict when extra safety precautions might be necessary, and ask for help early.

KEY PROCEDURES

- Phlebotomy
- Pelvic and rectal examinations
- CPR
- Dressing changes
- IV line placement
- Central line placement
- Arterial line placement
- Arterial blood gas
- Foley placement
- Lumbar puncture
- Intubations
- Chest tube placement
- Suturing
- Incision and drainage
- Splinting
- Paracentesis
- Thoracentesis
- Arthrocentesis

WHAT DO I CARRY IN MY POCKETS?

- ❑ Stethoscope
- ❑ Penlight
- ❑ Pocket drug reference
- ❑ Antibiotic guide
- ❑ Calipers for ECG reading
- ❑ Reflex hammer and tuning fork for neuro examinations (and as a toy to keep your resident occupied)
- ❑ Trauma shears

High-Yield Clinical Topic Checklist

Read about these topics before you start the rotation. Most are discussed in this chapter. A full list of common clerkship topics can be found at the end of this chapter.

- ❑ Angina
- ❑ Acute MI
- ❑ Arrhythmia
- ❑ Appendicitis
- ❑ Ectopic pregnancy
- ❑ Intracranial hemorrhage/acute stroke
- ❑ Syncope
- ❑ Pneumothorax
- ❑ Pulmonary embolism
- ❑ Drug overdose/antidotes
- ❑ Resuscitation
- ❑ Sepsis

Allergy, Immunology, Dermatology

ANAPHYLAXIS

A severe allergic reaction due to reexposure to an allergen after prior sensitization. Etiologies include drugs (penicillin, cephalosporins, ASA, NSAIDs), IV contrast, food, and latex exposure.

Signs and Symptoms

- **Dermatologic: Urticaria,** erythema, pruritus, angioedema.
- **Respiratory:** Nasal congestion, sneezing, coryza, cough, tachypnea, hoarseness, and a sensation of throat tightness may indicate **airway obstruction.**
- **Cardiovascular:** Tachycardia, hypotension.
- **GI:** Vomiting and diarrhea.

Differential

- **Dermatologic:** Angioedema, urticaria.
- **Respiratory:** Asthma, epiglottitis, croup.
- **Psychiatric:** Anxiety.

Workup

Obtain an H&P; diagnosis is clinical.

Treatment

- Bear in mind that an anaphylactic patient may need airway management as well as pharmacotherapy. If the voice sounds muffled or the patient is drooling, the airway is about to close off—so get a tube down there as quickly as possible.
- **Epinephrine:** SQ epinephrine is administered rapidly with an EpiPen. Additional epinephrine may need to be administered in doses of 0.3–0.5 mg subcutaneously. Nebulized epinephrine can ↓ airway edema.
- **β-agonists:** Albuterol (nebulized) to treat bronchospasm.
- **Antihistamines:** Diphenhydramine (Benadryl), an H_1 receptor blocker, to treat the cutaneous effects of anaphylaxis and to provide patient comfort.
- **Methylprednisolone** (Solu-Medrol) 125 mg IV × 1. Although their onset of action is several hours, steroids are of value in preventing recurrent attacks. Up to 20% of anaphylaxis patients have a second reaction within 72 hours without new allergen exposure.

KEY FACT

Remember latex sensitivity as a possible cause of anaphylaxis. It's not all about peanuts and bee stings!

KEY FACT

To understand the role of steroids in treating anaphylaxis, remember that the peanut your patient swallowed is still inside the GI tract, and the epinephrine will eventually wear off!

Q

An 18-year-old girl is brought into the ED by her boyfriend. She has a widespread urticarial rash and is wheezing. Her boyfriend states that her symptoms started while they were having sex. What is the most likely culprit?

Cardiovascular

ACUTE CORONARY SYNDROME (ACS)

Patients presenting to the ED with symptoms compatible with heart disease (eg, pain in the chest, jaw, left arm, or upper abdomen as well as shortness of breath and diaphoresis) must be evaluated for acute coronary syndrome (ACS). ACS develops when blood flow to the myocardium is insufficient, most commonly as a result of a thrombotic event 2° to a ruptured atherosclerotic plaque. ACS can be thought of as falling into 3 categories:

- **Unstable angina:**
  - Angina that deviates from the normal pattern; rest angina lasting > 20 minutes; or new-onset angina that was previously undiagnosed.
  - Angina that ↑ in severity, frequency, or duration.
  - The stenotic lesion in the coronary vessel leads to myocardial hypoxemia but not infarction. Consequently, no cardiac enzymes are released into the bloodstream. An ECG may be normal or may show ischemic changes such as ST-segment depression or T-wave inversion.
- **Non-ST-segment-elevation MI (NSTEMI):**
  - Due to a partially occlusive lesion that leads to ischemia on the epicardial side of the myocardium but infarction of the endocardial side. Infarction leads to detectable release of cardiac enzymes.
  - ECG changes are similar to those seen in unstable angina.
- **ST-segment-elevation MI (STEMI):**
  - Due to a lesion leading to complete occlusion of a coronary vessel. Infarction throughout the entire thickness of the myocardium (ie, transmural infarction) leads to the release of cardiac enzymes.
  - ECG changes are significant for ST-segment elevation (see Figure 3-1). These changes will resolve over days, and Q waves will develop.
  - A new left bundle branch block (LBBB) on ECG is also highly indicative of a STEMI.

KEY POINT

STEMI VS. NSTEMI

- An ST-segment elevation on ECG indicates that the infarction extends through the full thickness of the myocardial wall **(transmural).**
- The absence of ST-segment elevation in the setting of ⊕ cardiac enzymes indicates that the infarction is limited to the **subendocardium.** NSTEMIs are dangerous in that the patient is still at risk for a full-thickness infarct in that area.

SIGNS AND SYMPTOMS

- The "classic" presentation consists of substernal chest pressure and pain that radiates to the lower jaw, left shoulder, or left arm. However, not all patients have these symptoms.
- Nausea, vomiting, dyspnea, and diaphoresis are also seen.
- Hypertension, hypotension, tachycardia, or bradycardia.

DIFFERENTIAL

Etiologies of chest pain include the following (see also the mnemonic TAPUM):

A

A latex condom.

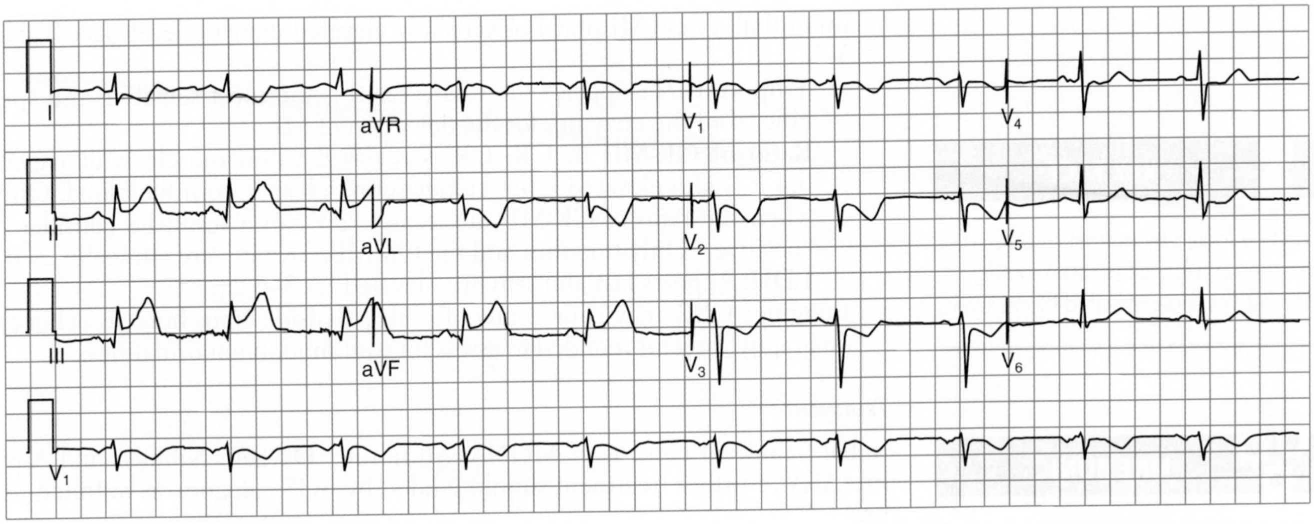

FIGURE 3-1. Myocardial infarction. Leads II, III, and aVF show ST-segment elevations. This is an inferior transmural infarction.

- **Cardiovascular:** Aortic dissection, ACS, pericarditis, cocaine intoxication.
- **Respiratory:** Tension pneumothorax, PE, pneumonia.
- **GI:** Esophagitis, GERD, PUD, cholecystitis.
- **Musculoskeletal:** Costochondritis.
- **Neurologic:** Herpes zoster.

WORKUP

- Twelve-lead ECG:
  - Look for ST-segment elevation or depression, T-wave inversions, and Q waves.
  - Table 3-1 outlines the correlation of lead location with vascular territory.
  - Remember that reciprocal changes can be seen in other leads. For example, ST-segment elevation in leads II, III, and aVF may lead to ST-segment depression in leads I and aVL.
  - Inferior MIs (leads II, III, and aVF) affect the right ventricle, which is preload dependent. Giving nitroglycerin will ↓ preload and worsen the patient's condition.
  - An MI can present as a new LBBB.
- **Cardiac enzymes:** The death of myocardium releases cardiac enzymes into the blood, and these enzymes can be measured. However, bear in

TABLE 3-1. Correlation of ECG Lead Location with Vascular Territory

ECG LEAD	ASSOCIATED VESSEL	LOCATION
II, III, aVF	Right coronary artery (RCA)	Inferior MI
V_1–V_4	Left anterior descending artery	Anterior/septal MI
V_5–V_6, I, aVL	Left circumflex artery	Lateral MI
V_1–V_3 (ST-segment depression)	Depends on dominance; RCA or left circumflex artery	Posterior MI

MNEMONIC

Deadly causes of chest pain—

TAPUM

Tension pneumothorax
Aortic dissection
Pulmonary embolism
Unstable angina
Myocardial infarction

Q

A 67-year-old diabetic woman complains of vague abdominal pain, shortness of breath, and diaphoresis. She states that she thinks she has the flu. Which initial tests should you order?

KEY FACT

Don't be fooled by normal cardiac enzymes. A fresh MI (< 30 minutes) may not yet show elevated blood levels.

MNEMONIC

Initial treatment of ACS–

MONA

Morphine
Oxygen
Nitrates (eg, nitroglycerin)
Aspirin

A

An ECG and cardiac enzymes. Don't be fooled by an atypical presentation of an MI.

mind that a new MI may not yet show elevated enzyme levels (see Table 3-2).

- **Troponin I/T:** Appears the **earliest** and is the **most sensitive and specific** of all the enzymes for the detection of MI.
- **Ratio of CK-MB to CK:** CK is released when muscle is damaged, but it is also elevated if the kidneys don't clear it from the blood. Only when the ratio of CK-MB to CK is > 2.5 can a result be considered "positive." Only troponin and the CK-MB/CK ratio are clinically used.
- **LDH:** Appears **last** and remains elevated for 3–6 days.

- **Imaging:** CXR may show signs of CHF. Bedside transthoracic echocardiography is recommended to assess for wall motion abnormalities.

TREATMENT

Initial treatment consists of **MONA: M**orphine, **O**xygen, **N**itrates, and **A**spirin (ASA). Further treatment should guided by ACS category, as outlined below.

- **STEMI:** All patients with STEMI should receive **invasive therapy,** which consists of percutaneous intervention (PCI), also known as cardiac catheterization.
  - Door-to-balloon time should be kept as low as possible and should not exceed 90 minutes.
  - PCI may be diagnostic and may aid in the definition of coronary anatomy (needed for CABG), or it may be therapeutic by allowing for stent placement.
  - Fibrinolytic therapy (eg, tPA) is appropriate only if a facility lacks PCI capability and the patient presented within 12 hours of symptom onset.
  - If fibrinolytic therapy is administered, consider 2° transport of the patient to a facility with PCI capability as long as the total time from first presentation to balloon remains < 90 minutes.
  - Fibrinolytics are **contraindicated** in patients who have had major surgery in the past 14 days; are severely hypertensive (> 185 mm Hg systolic); or have had brain metastases, a recent GI bleed (< 21 days), a stroke within the past 3 months, or thrombocytopenia.
- **Unstable angina/NSTEMI:** If a patient presents with either unstable angina or NSTEMI, a simple scoring system, the TIMI score (see Table 3-3), can be used to determine if he or she will benefit from invasive therapy or conservative therapy.
  - **Conservative therapy:** Patients with a TIMI score < 3 are candidates for conservative therapy, which consists of the following:
    - **Dual antiplatelet therapy:** In addition to ASA, patients should receive either clopidogrel or a glycoprotein IIb/IIIa inhibitor such as eptifibatide (Integrilin).

TABLE 3-2. Cardiac Enzyme Windows[a]

ENZYME	FIRST DETECTABLE AT	LASTS FOR
Troponin I/T	2 hours	7 days
CK-MB	3 hours	3 days
LDH	24 hours	14 days

[a] Keep in mind that the therapeutic window is only ~ 12 hours. If the patient presents after that, little can be done to reverse the damage.

TABLE 3-3. TIMI Risk Score for Unstable Angina/NSTEMI

CHARACTERISTICS	POINT
History	
Age ≥ 65 years	1
≥ 3 CAD risk factors (premature family history, DM, smoking, hypertension, ↑ cholesterol)	1
Known CAD (stenosis > 50%)	1
ASA use in past 7 days	1
Presentation	
Severe angina (≥ 2 episodes within 24 hours)	1
ST deviation ≥ 0.5 mm	1
+ cardiac marker	1
Risk score—total points[a]	(0–7)

[a] Higher-risk patients (risk score ≥ 3) benefit more from enoxaparin (vs. unfractionated heparin), glycoprotein IIb/IIIa inhibitors, and early angiography.

(Reproduced with permission from Le T et al. *First Aid for the Step 2 CK,* 8th ed. New York: McGraw-Hill, 2012, Table 2.1-10.)

    - **Anticoagulation:** In addition to dual antiplatelet therapy, anticoagulation should be initiated with heparin.
    - **Stress test:** The patient should be admitted and scheduled for a stress test.
  - **Invasive therapy:** If the patient's ischemic symptoms do not resolve on dual antiplatelet therapy and anticoagulation, switch to an invasive therapy approach.
- **Other pathologies:** Treatment of other coronary perfusion pathologies in the ED is as follows:
  - **Variant (Prinzmetal's) angina:** Has the same character as stable angina, but atherosclerosis is minimal. Caused by vasospasm; diagnosis requires angiographic studies. Treat with nitrates and calcium channel blockers (CCBs).
  - **Cocaine chest pain:** Avoid β-blockers, as they may lead to unopposed α-adrenergic activity (peripheral blood vessel constriction), leading the heart to have to pump against a high-resistance circulatory system. Use benzodiazepines in addition to other ACS therapies.

AORTIC DISSECTION

Defined as a **"false lumen"** created 2° to an intimal layer tear, allowing blood to enter the aortic media and subsequently splitting the medial lamellae (see Figure 3-2). **Stanford type A** dissections involve the ascending aorta; **Stanford type B** dissections are distal to the left subclavian artery. Risk factors include the following:

- **Hypertension; coarctation of the aorta.**
- Syphilis, **Marfan's syndrome,** Ehlers-Danlos syndrome.
- Trauma, pregnancy.

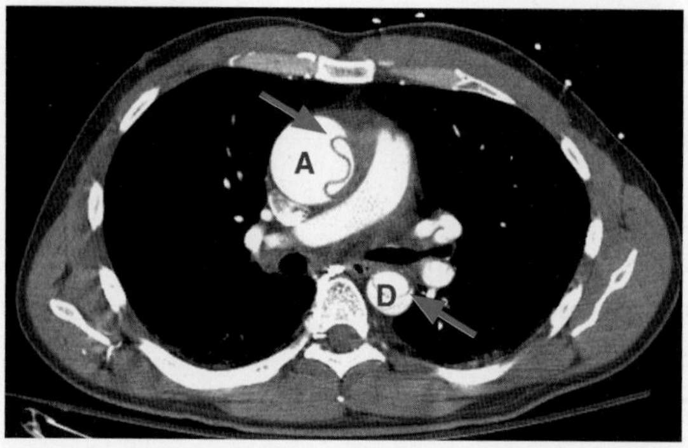

FIGURE 3-2. Aortic dissection. CT angiogram of the chest demonstrates an acute Stanford type A aortic dissection. The intimal flap (arrows) can be seen in the ascending (A) and descending (D) aorta. Note how the larger false lumen is compressing the true lumen in the ascending aorta. (Reproduced with permission from Doherty GM. *Current Diagnosis & Treatment: Surgery,* 13th ed. New York: McGraw-Hill, 2010, Fig. 19-17.)

Signs and Symptoms

- Severe "**tearing**" or "**ripping**" **chest or back pain.**
- Asymmetric or ↓ peripheral pulses.
- Syncope, stroke, shock, MI (dissection may propagate into the coronary vessels). Can rupture into the pericardium and cause cardiac tamponade.

Differential

- **Cardiovascular:** Angina, MI, ruptured thoracic aortic aneurysm.
- **Respiratory:** PE.
- **GI:** Esophageal rupture.

Workup

- ECG to evaluate for LVH and ischemic changes.
- CXR may show mediastinal widening (especially with Stanford type A dissections).
- The study of choice is a CT angiogram (CT with IV contrast), which will show the false lumen. Angiography is the gold standard but takes too long to be of use in an emergent setting.

Treatment

- **Stabilize BP:** For high blood pressure, use IV nitrates and β-blockers.
- **Type A dissections:** Require emergent surgery. If the dissection extends into the carotid arteries, the patient will infarct both cerebral hemispheres. If it extends into the coronary arteries, massive MI will result. Finally, the base of the aorta widens, pulling the leaflets of the aortic valve apart and leading to massive aortic valve incompetence.
- **Type B dissections:** Can be managed medically in stable patients.

KEY FACT

A is bad; B can be managed medically.

ARRHYTHMIA

Asystole

Defined as a "flatline" rhythm that indicates no pulse and no electrical activity of the heart. Remember, you must always check for asystole in 2 separate leads, as a perfectly flat line most likely represents a detached lead.

KEY FACT

Asystole that is perfectly flat is often just a detached lead, so be sure to check 2 separate leads before administering epinephrine!

Signs and Symptoms

- Patients are unconscious and unresponsive.
- Absent pulses; absent heart sounds.

Differential

Detached lead/equipment malfunction; very fine VF.

Treatment

- **Chest compression:** Start compressions immediately (2 inches deep at a rate of about 100 times per minute), and stop only for bag-mask ventilation.
- **Airway management:** Once the patient is intubated, do not interrupt compressions except for rhythm checks as indicated by the team leader.
- **Drugs to give during asystole:** Give 1 mg epinephrine IV q 3–5 min. Forty units of vasopressin IV may also be given initially (recent studies show better survival with vasopressin than with epinephrine). Note that in accordance with ACLS 2010 guidelines, atropine is no longer given.
- Try to address the underlying pathology. You may empirically push glucose, naloxone, calcium gluconate, or sodium bicarbonate. Have the IV fluids wide open.

KEY FACT

Never shock asystole (no matter what you see on TV).

Atrial Fibrillation (AF)

See the Internal Medicine chapter.

Ventricular Fibrillation (VF)/Pulseless Ventricular Tachycardia (VT)

The most common arrhythmia in cardiac arrest patients. Associated with high mortality, so **early defibrillation** is the most important therapy.

KEY FACT

VF is the most common etiology of cardiac arrest.

Signs and Symptoms

Syncope, hypotension, pulselessness.

Differential

- Muscle shivering appears similar to VF on the monitor.
- VT; ventricular premature complexes.

Workup

ECG demonstrates a totally **erratic tracing.**

Treatment

- Initiate CPR until the defibrillator is attached.
- Defibrillate as early as possible. Shocks are no longer stacked (ie, shock only once; then resume CPR). Defibrillation with a biphasic current requires between 120 and 200 J. Biphasic defibrillators have been shown to be superior to monophasic models.
- Immediately continue CPR after the shock is delivered (regardless of what the rhythm is).
- Administer epinephrine 1 mg IV q 3–5 min. Vasopressin 40 U IV × 1 may initially be given in lieu of the initial epinephrine dose.
- After 2 minutes of CPR, reassess rhythm, shock if indicated, and continue CPR if indicated. Continue the 2-minute CPR/defibrillation cycle.

- In addition to asynchronous cardioversion, the following drugs may help reestablish a normal rhythm:
  - **Antiarrhythmics:** Either amiodarone 300-mg IV push (an additional 150-mg IV push may be given after 3–5 minutes) or lidocaine 1.0–1.5 mg/kg IV (an additional 0.50- to 0.75-mg/kg IV push may be given in 3–5 minutes).
  - **Magnesium sulfate** 1–2 g IV for torsades de pointes.

Ventricular Tachycardia (VT)

Consists of a heart rate > 120 bpm that arises distal to the bundle of His. This readily converts to VF. If VT is pulseless (inadequate filling time for the ventricles above certain rates), use the VF algorithm above.

Signs and Symptoms

- Tachycardia, hypotension, tachypnea, palpitations.
- Pallor, diaphoresis.

Differential

AF, atrial flutter, atrial tachycardia with aberrancy, VF.

Workup

- ECG shows a **wide QRS complex and a rate > 120 bpm.**
- Cardiac enzymes; electrolytes.

Treatment

- **If unstable** (eg, hypotensive, unconscious): Immediate **synchronized** cardioversion (shock delivered precisely on the R wave).
- **If stable:**
  - Amiodarone 150-mg IV bolus over 10 minutes.
  - Procainamide 20–30 mg/min (maximum dose 17 mg/kg) may be used in patients with a normal EF.
  - Synchronized cardioversion if medical therapy fails.

KEY FACT

Pulsus paradoxus (a drop of > 10 mm Hg in systolic BP during inspiration) is good to know for the boards but is rarely used as a diagnostic tool in the ED. Get a FAST ultrasound instead.

CARDIAC TAMPONADE

Defined as fluid accumulation in the pericardium that prevents the heart from adequately filling or contracting efficiently, thereby decreasing stroke volume (see Figure 3-3). This can be acute (eg, penetrating trauma to the chest, free wall rupture a few days after an MI) or chronic (eg, pericardial effusion caused by SLE or cancer). In acute situations, only a small amount of blood is needed to cause tamponade physiology, whereas a patient with a chronic effusion can accumulate a significant amount of fluid before hemodynamic changes are seen.

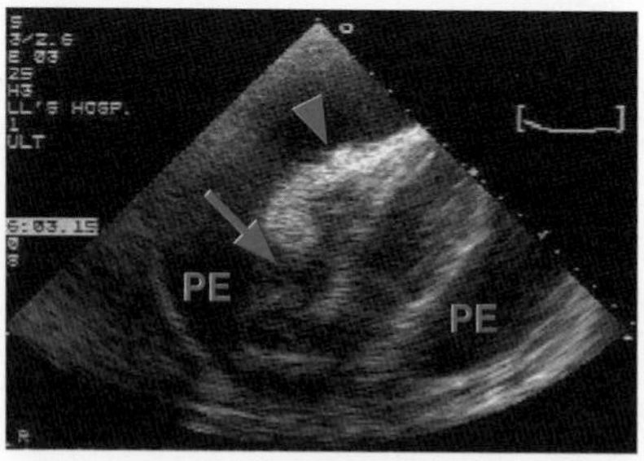

FIGURE 3.3. Cardiac tamponade. Echocardiogram in a patient with cardiac tamponade shows a large pericardial effusion (PE) with right atrial (arrow) and right ventricular (arrowhead) collapse. (Reproduced with permission from Hall JB et al. *Principles of Critical Care,* 3rd ed. New York: McGraw-Hill, 2005, Fig. 28-7A.)

Signs and Symptoms

- Chest pain, dyspnea, fatigue.
- **Beck's triad: Hypotension, JVD, and muffled heart sounds.**
- Electrical alternans on ECG (QRS complexes in the same lead vary in height); tachycardia.

Differential

MI, tension pneumothorax, CHF.

WORKUP

- Echocardiogram if time permits; otherwise obtain a FAST ultrasound.
- CXR may show an enlarged, globular heart (only in patients with chronic effusion; acutely, the pericardium will not have enough time to stretch).
- ECG may show ↓ amplitude and/or electrical alternans.

TREATMENT

- **Pericardiocentesis.**
- Pericardial window may be required.
- Volume expansion with IV fluids.

HYPERTENSIVE URGENCY/EMERGENCY

Note that normal hypertension is not treated in the ED; as a chronic disease, it is best managed by the primary care physician. However, hypertensive urgency/emergency is distinguished as follows:

- **Hypertensive urgency: A BP > 220/> 120 mm Hg** that is asymptomatic (no end-organ damage).
- **Hypertensive emergency:** Any evidence of **end-organ damage** regardless of BP, such as changes in mentation, nausea/vomiting, angina pectoris, elevated creatinine, or blood in the urine.

KEY FACT

The most common cause of hypertensive urgency is noncompliance with medication.

SIGNS AND SYMPTOMS

- **CNS:** Headache, blurred vision, mental status change, nausea/vomiting.
- **Cardiovascular:** Angina, pulmonary edema, dyspnea.

DIFFERENTIAL

- **Cardiovascular:** Angina, abdominal aortic aneurysm, CHF.
- **Neurologic:** Headache (eg, migraine, tension, cluster).
- **Endocrine:** Thyroid storm; pheochromocytoma (very rare, but commonly tested on the boards).
- **Preeclampsia.**

WORKUP

- Cardiovascular, neurologic, ophthalmologic, and abdominal examinations.
- ECG.
- **Labs:**
  - **Blood tests:** CBC, electrolytes, BUN/creatinine.
  - UA to assess for RBCs, protein, and casts.
  - Cardiac enzymes if chest pain is present.
- **Imaging:** CXR and head CT for hemorrhage or edema.

TREATMENT

- The brain autoregulates blood flow and is accustomed to high pressure, so dropping mean arterial pressure (MAP) too quickly will result in hypoperfusion or frank stroke.
  - Therefore, MAP should be ↓ by no more than 25% in the first few **hours** in the setting of hypertensive **emergency.**
  - In hypertensive **urgency**, you should not drop MAP by > 25% **per day.**
- **Oral agents:** β-blockers.

Q

In the movie *Pulp Fiction,* Vincent injects Mia with epinephrine directly into the heart. Although he saves her from a heroin overdose, minutes later she is tachycardic, tachypneic, and hypotensive with chest pain. What structure did Vincent damage?

KEY FACT

Treat the patient, not the numbers on the monitor.

- **IV agents:** Nitroglycerin, nitroprusside, or labetalol.
- In addition to lowering BP to a safe range, treat hypertensive emergency in a manner that is tailored to the end-organ damage it produces. This means that you should treat CHF if the patient has signs of left ventricular failure during the hypertensive emergency.

Gastroenterology

APPENDICITIS

KEY FACT

Appendicitis is the most common surgical emergency. In patients who present with abdominal pain, acute appendicitis must always be in the differential.

Acute appendicitis, or inflammation of the appendix, should **always** be near the top of your differential for an acute abdomen, as approximately 7% of the U.S. population will develop appendicitis at some point in their lives. Appendicitis peaks in the teens to the mid-20s and again in patients in their 60s, with atypical presentations including pregnant patients as well as those with retrocecal appendices. Its etiology can be traced to luminal obstruction of the appendix caused by hyperplasia of lymphoid tissue (55–65%), fecalith (35%), or foreign body (eg, food, carcinoid tumor, parasites). The probable pathophysiology of appendicitis is as follows:

- An obstructed appendix leads to bacterial proliferation, and continuous bacterial proliferation leads to ↑ pressure.
- At some point the appendix will rupture (and the patient will feel better for the moment), but then an abscess will form or the patient may develop frank peritonitis.

SIGNS AND SYMPTOMS

- Patients often present with a history of anorexia (if the patient asks for food, appendicitis is unlikely) as well as with low-grade fever and **abdominal pain.**
- Patients often have a history of dull, vague periumbilical pain of 1–24 hours' duration that localizes to the RLQ at **McBurney's point** (two-thirds of the distance from the umbilicus to the right anterior superior iliac spine).
  - Discomfort progresses to a sharp pain as a result of irritation of parietal peritoneum from the progressively distended appendix.
  - This can be accompanied by rebound, guarding, high fever, hypotension, and a high WBC count. Associated symptoms include nausea, vomiting, and anorexia following the pain.
- Physical examination reveals the following:
  - **Rovsing's sign:** Referred pain in the RLQ elicited by deep palpation in the LLQ. This sign is specific but fairly insensitive.
  - **Iliopsoas sign:** RLQ pain elicited by passive extension of the hip (caused by stretching the iliopsoas tendon, which overlies the appendix). This sign is not sensitive (see Figure 3-4A).
  - **Obturator sign:** RLQ pain elicited by passive internal rotation of the hip. This sign is also insensitive (see Figure 3-4B).
  - A palpable RLQ mass may indicate an abscess.
  - Rectal examination generally elicits pain on the right side.

A

A coronary artery, causing cardiac tamponade and MI at the same time.

DIFFERENTIAL

The differential for lower abdominal pain depends heavily on the age group and sex of the patient. While not complete, the list below can serve as a starting point:

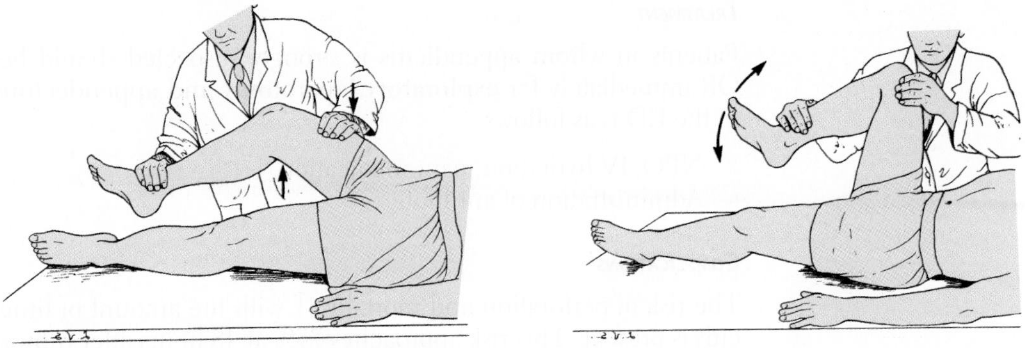

A B

FIGURE 3-4. Iliopsoas (A) and obturator (B) signs. Neither sign is sensitive, but both are quite specific. (Reproduced with permission from Way LW. *Current Surgical Diagnosis & Treatment,* 6th ed. Stamford, CT: Appleton & Lange, 1983.)

- **Children:**
  - Gastroenteritis (look for vomiting/diarrhea).
  - Intussusception ("currant jelly" stool; seen in patients < 2 years of age).
  - DKA (look for Kussmaul breathing, elevated blood glucose, and ketones in urine).
  - Testicular torsion (young boys may be too embarrassed to tell you what really hurts).
- **Teens:**
  - STIs (especially in females, eg, gonorrhea, PID).
  - Ectopic pregnancy (ask for last menstrual period [LMP] and contraception used).
  - Mittelschmerz.
- **Adults:**
  - Refer to the differential for teens.
  - Ruptured ovarian cyst, ovarian torsion.
  - IBD (Crohn's disease, ulcerative colitis).
- **Elderly:**
  - Diverticulitis (common among the elderly).
  - Cystitis.
  - Small bowel obstruction.

KEY FACT

All women of childbearing age with lower abdominal pain should get 2 things: a pregnancy test and a pelvic examination.

WORKUP

The diagnosis of acute appendicitis is based largely on the H&P. Other criteria are as follows:

- **Labs:**
  - CBC shows mild leukocytosis (11,000–15,000/mm^3) with left shift.
  - UA may show RBCs or WBCs.
- **Imaging:**
  - AXR may demonstrate fecalith.
  - Ultrasound may show a noncompressible appendix.
    - Ultrasound is useful for ruling out gynecologic abnormalities in female patients and is also the preferred initial test in children. It will likely be used more frequently in adults given the rising concern over radiation exposure and lifetime cancer risk.
    - If ultrasound is ⊕, it can rule in appendicitis; if ⊖, it **cannot** rule it out.
  - CT is 90–95% sensitive for appendicitis.

KEY FACT

Be sure to obtain a complete medical and surgical history. Patients with an appendectomy are unlikely to have acute appendicitis!

TREATMENT

Patients in whom appendicitis is strongly suspected should be taken to the OR immediately for **exploratory laparotomy and appendectomy.** Treatment in the ED is as follows:

- NPO, IV hydration, pain medication.
- Administration of antibiotics.

COMPLICATIONS

The risk of perforation and mortality ↑ with the amount of time the appendicitis is present. This risk approaches 75% at 48 hours after rupture.

Genitourinary

ECTOPIC PREGNANCY

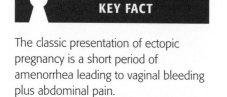

> **KEY FACT**
>
> The classic presentation of ectopic pregnancy is a short period of amenorrhea leading to vaginal bleeding plus abdominal pain.

Lower abdominal pain is a common complaint in the ED. In the female patient population, pregnancy must be ruled out. Should a pregnancy test return ⊕, ectopic pregnancy must be ruled out. Common sites of extrauterine implantation are shown in Figure 3-5. Risk factors include the following:

- A history of STIs or PID
- A prior ectopic pregnancy
- Prior pelvic surgery
- IUD use
- DES exposure (rare)

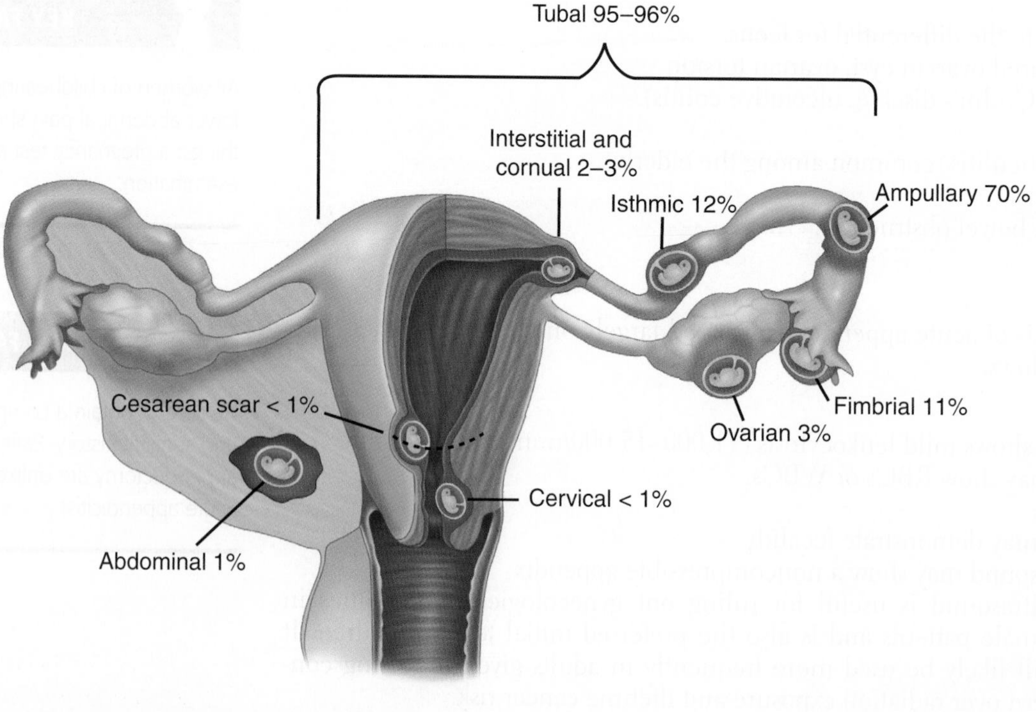

FIGURE 3-5. Sites of implantation of ectopic pregnancy. Note that the most common site is the ampulla. (Reproduced with permission from Cunningham FG et al. *Williams Obstetrics,* 23rd ed. New York: McGraw-Hill, 2010, Fig. 10-1.)

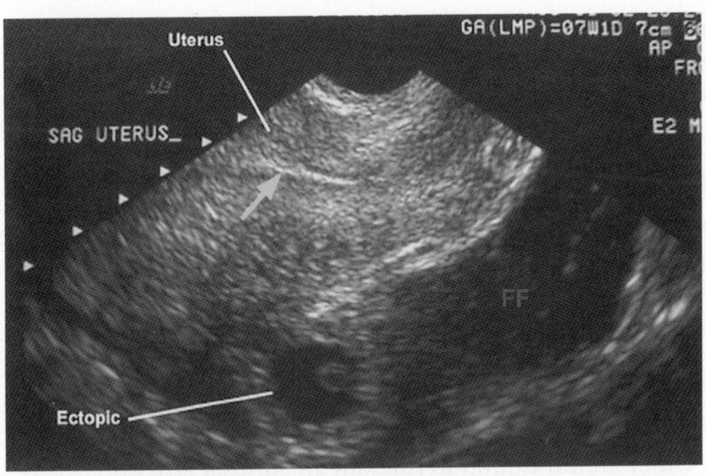

FIGURE 3-6. Ectopic pregnancy on transvaginal ultrasound. Shown are an empty uterus with a normal endometrial stripe (yellow arrow) and a gestational sac containing a yolk sac (ectopic) outside the uterus. Note the associated free fluid (FF). (Reproduced with permission from Stone CK, Humphries RL. *Current Diagnosis & Treatment: Emergency Medicine*, 7th ed. New York: McGraw-Hill, 2011, Fig. 38-4.)

WORKUP

- **Quantitative β-hCG:** In normal pregnancies, a gestational sac can typically be visualized by transvaginal ultrasound when the β-hCG reaches 1800–2000 IU/L. At β-hCG values above this level, nonvisualization of an intrauterine gestational sac is worrisome for ectopic pregnancy. However, β-hCG levels may be abnormally low in ectopic pregnancies. If an ectopic location is suspected, get an ultrasound regardless.
- **Ultrasound:** Look for a noncystic adnexal mass or fluid in the cul-de-sac in the absence of intrauterine gestation (see Figure 3-6).

TREATMENT

- **Medical management** (appropriate only for a patient **without** signs of rupture): **Methotrexate** for unruptured ectopic pregnancies < 3 cm with a β-hCG < 12,000 IU/L.
- **Surgical management:** Choose with the reproductive plans, age, and clinical status of the patient in mind.

PELVIC INFLAMMATORY DISEASE (PID)

A general term describing infection of the uterine lining, fallopian tubes, or ovaries. PID should be high on the differential of any patient who presents with lower abdominal pain accompanied by vaginal discharge. Risk factors include unprotected intercourse, multiple sexual partners, and prior STIs.

SIGNS AND SYMPTOMS

Lower abdominal pain, vaginal discharge, "chandelier sign" (**extreme** cervical motion tenderness).

DIFFERENTIAL

- **Candidiasis:** A cottage cheese–like vaginal discharge that is due to *Candida albicans* (yeast infection); **not** an STI. Risk factors include recent antibiotic exposure and diabetes.

KEY FACT

Always check a β-hCG level on a premenopausal woman with abdominal pain!

KEY FACT

β-hCG should double every 48 hours in normal pregnancy.

Q 1

A 13-year-old girl presents to the ED with nausea and lower abdominal pain. When asked about her LMP, she states that she has not yet reached menarche. What condition must be ruled out?

Q 2

A mother brings her 6-year-old daughter to the ED because of a copious vaginal discharge. She cannot relay any information about the onset of her daughter's symptoms because a neighbor was looking after the child while the mother was away on business. Whom should you consult?

- **Bacterial vaginosis:** Due to bacterial overgrowth; not an STI. Clue cells on wet prep are covered with bacteria. The culprit is often *Gardnerella vaginalis.*

Workup

- Conduct a pelvic examination and obtain swabs of both the vaginal wall and the cervical os. This will allow you to visualize the discharge, tissue changes, and any potential bleeding while also permitting you to take samples for microscopic and culture analysis.
- Assess for adnexal and cervical motion tenderness with your fingers after you remove the speculum.

Treatment

- **PID:** Order an ultrasound to rule out an adnexal abscess.
- **Gonorrhea:** Always treat for chlamydia as well. Give ceftriaxone 250 mg IM × 1 and azithromycin 1 g PO × 1.
- **Chlamydia:** If you diagnose chlamydia only, azithromycin 1 g PO × 1 is sufficient, although some physicians treat for gonorrhea concomitantly.
- In either case, unless the sexual partner is treated as well, you will likely see the patient again in a few weeks. Unfortunately, the partner is technically not your patient, and some states do not allow you to treat him or her, but you are certainly allowed to encourage the patient to get the partner treated.

See the Obstetrics and Gynecology chapter for more details on the diagnosis and treatment of PID.

TESTICULAR TORSION

Twisting of the testicle on its root, usually in the horizontal direction, as a result of a weak connection of the gubernaculum. Most often occurs in young adults and in infants < 1 year of age.

Signs and Symptoms

- Presents with sudden onset of pain in the lower abdomen, inguinal canal, or testicle that is constant, progressive, and unrelieved by changes in position.
- Usually occurs during strenuous activity, but may also occur during sleep.
- The testicle may lie in the "bell-clapper" position—ie, flat on its side (see Figure 3-7).

Differential

- Torsion of the appendix testis or the appendix epididymis.
- Epididymitis, orchitis.
- Hydrocele, varicocele.
- Inguinal hernia, appendicitis, kidney stones.

Workup

- **Doppler ultrasound:** To determine if there is blood flow to the testicle.
- **UA:** Usually normal.

KEY FACT

A word of caution: PID and ectopic pregnancies can be coexisting conditions.

KEY FACT

If there is loss of the cremasteric reflex, think testicular torsion.

KEY FACT

The "blue dot" sign is a tender, often blue nodule found on transillumination of the testes in torsion of the appendix testis or appendix epididymis. If torsion has been ruled out, treat with analgesics and allow the torsed structures to degenerate.

1 A

Pregnancy. It is possible for a girl to get pregnant on her first ovulation and thus fail to experience menstrual bleeding at this time.

2 A

Child Protective Services. An STI in a 6-year-old (in this case gonorrhea) is a result of sexual abuse. However, a vaginal foreign body should be ruled out first.

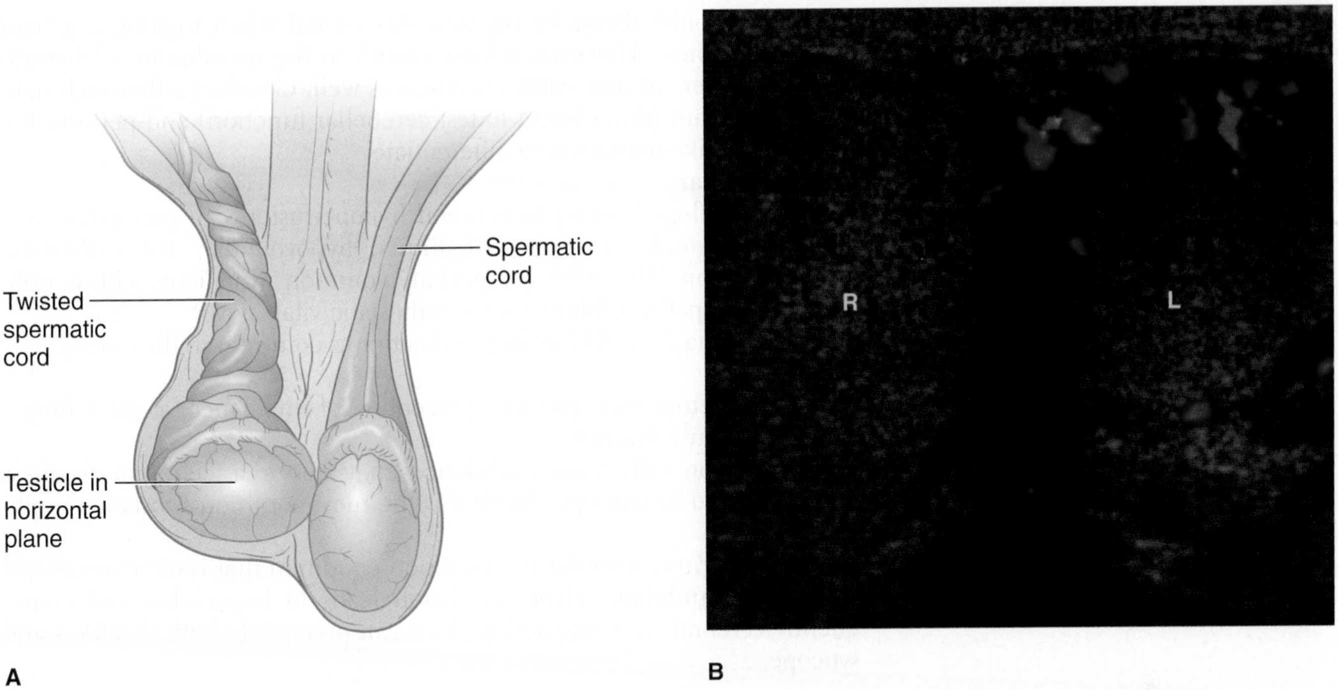

FIGURE 3.7. Testicular torsion. (**A**) The twisted spermatic cord on the right causes the testis to lie horizontally. This is the result of the "bell-clapper" deformity, a failure of the gubernaculum to be fixed posteriorly. (**B**) Doppler ultrasound shows normal blood flow (red and blue) in the left testis (L) and lack of flow on the right (R), consistent with right testicular torsion. (Image A reproduced with permission from Knoop KJ et al. *Atlas of Emergency Medicine,* 3rd ed. New York: McGraw-Hill, 2010, Fig. 8-2. Image B reproduced with permission from USMLERx.com.)

Treatment

- Attempt manual detorsion.
- Request an **immediate** urology consult (after symptom onset, you have < 5 hours to repair).
- Immediate exploratory surgery is warranted ("time is testicle") when ultrasound is equivocal; when there is no alternative diagnosis; and even following manual detorsion to ensure full detorsion and to perform contralateral orchiopexy.

KEY FACT

The direction of rotation during testicular detorsion is like opening a book (ie, right testicle counterclockwise, left testicle clockwise).

Neurology

DIZZINESS/SYNCOPE

A frequent complaint seen in the ED is dizziness and/or syncope. Both have a wide differential that can be narrowed down by means of a thorough history, a good physical examination, and select labs and imaging studies. Both dizziness and syncope are best compartmentalized by system:

- **Neurologic:**
  - Seizures can lead to a syncopal event but generally not dizziness. Ironically, seizure-like activity reported by bystanders is not pathognomonic for seizure, as hypoperfusion of the brain may lead to involuntary muscle movement. A key question to ask is whether the patient experienced postictal confusion.
  - Vasovagal syncope occurs with an overactive vagal response (eg, passing out during your surgery rotation). It can also occur with other vagal stimuli, such as drinking cold water. High vagal tone leads to ↓ cardiac output and precipitates syncope.

    - Stroke should always be on your differential when treating a patient with dizziness. However, a loose otolith in the membranous labyrinth of the inner ear may cause dizziness as well. Conduct a thorough neurologic exam (don't forget to test cerebellar function) and perform the Dix-Hallpike maneuver to differentiate.
- **Cardiovascular:**
    - Any pathology leading to cerebral hypoperfusion can precipitate syncope. Examples include arrhythmia, hypovolemia, and orthostatic hypotension. The latter is especially common in patients with peripheral neuropathy. Obtain a set of orthostatic vital signs.
    - Bradycardia 2° to β-blocking medication is common in the elderly.
- **Metabolic:**
    - Hypoglycemia may lead to a perception of imbalance; a quick fingerstick can rule this out.
    - Intoxication with various substances may lead to a feeling of dizziness and/or lead to syncope. Alcohol is the most common substance implicated.
- **Psychiatric:** Panic disorder is a common condition that is often associated with hyperventilation. Hyperventilation leads to hypocarbia and consequently cerebral vasoconstriction. This can precipitate both dizziness and syncope.

There are a multitude of other, more esoteric causes of dizziness and syncope, such as Ramsay Hunt syndrome, that are best worked up outside the ED once you have ruled out life-threatening conditions. Refer to the Neurology chapter for further details.

INTRACRANIAL HEMORRHAGE

Subarachnoid Hemorrhage (SAH)

SAH typically affects patients 50–60 years of age and has a high mortality rate (35%). Ruptured aneurysms are reported to have a 50% 1-month mortality rate. Etiologies include the following:

- **Ruptured aneurysm (eg, berry, hypertensive): Berry aneurysms** are the **most common cause of SAH** and are associated with polycystic kidney disease and coarctation of the aorta.
- **Other:** AVM; trauma to the circle of Willis (often at the middle cerebral artery).

KEY FACT

SAH classically presents as "the worst headache of my life."

Signs and Symptoms

- **Headache:**
    - Presents with a sudden-onset, intensely painful "thunderclap headache" in the occipital region. May be preceded by "sentinel headaches" in the weeks preceding the hemorrhage.
    - Sometimes associated with fever, nausea, vomiting, and a fluctuating level of consciousness.
- Signs of meningeal irritation (eg, neck stiffness) may also be seen.
- Seizure may result from irritation of the cortex by blood.
- CN III palsy with pupillary involvement may be associated with berry aneurysms of the posterior communicating artery compressing CN III.
- Examination findings can range from normal to neurologic deficits and a depressed level of consciousness.

KEY FACT

If you wish to practice the fundus examination, **never** dilate a patient's eye without informing the rest of the team. It looks just like a blown pupil.

DIFFERENTIAL

Hemorrhagic stroke, trauma, meningitis, first presentation of migraine or cluster headache.

WORKUP

- Emergent **head CT without contrast** to look for blood in the subarachnoid space (see Figure 3-8), especially around the circle of Willis. Fresh blood appears white on noncontrast CT.
- If the head CT is ⊖ but there is any suspicion for SAH, obtain an immediate LP to look for red cells (must be in consecutive tubes to rule out traumatic tap), xanthochromia, and ↑ ICP.
- Four-vessel angiography once SAH has been confirmed to look for an aneurysm.

TREATMENT

Treatment should focus on preventing rebleeding, which is most likely to occur in the first 48 hours after SAH. Measures include the following:

- ↓ ICP by raising the head of the bed.
- Prevent hypo- and hypertension.
- Obtain an immediate neurosurgery consult followed by neuro-ICU admission.
- Secure the airway if necessary.
- **Medications:**
  - CCBs (eg, nimodipine) to prevent vasospasm (see below). Start within 96 hours.
  - Dexamethasone for cerebral edema.
  - Antiseizure medication (generally phenytoin) if the patient seizes (no longer given prophylactically).
- **Surgery:** Surgical treatment involves open or interventional radiologic clipping or coiling of an aneurysm or AVM.

COMPLICATIONS

- **Vasospasm:** Blood is irritating to many tissues in the head. Tissue irritation leads to vasoconstriction. Vasoconstriction leads in turn to hypoperfusion of brain territories, as a result of which the patient may stroke.
- **Neurologic deficits:** Caused by the mass effect of a large AVM or aneurysm impinging on brain parenchyma.
- **Obstructive hydrocephalus:** 2° to intraventricular blood obstructing CSF drainage or interfering with CSF absorption through the arachnoid granulations.

Cerebrovascular Accident (CVA)

See the Neurology chapter.

Epidural Hematoma

Defined as a collection of blood between the dura and skull. Associated with temporal bone fractures due to blunt trauma with resultant tear of the **middle meningeal artery.**

SIGNS AND SYMPTOMS

- Presents with loss of consciousness followed by a lucid interval ranging from several minutes to hours.

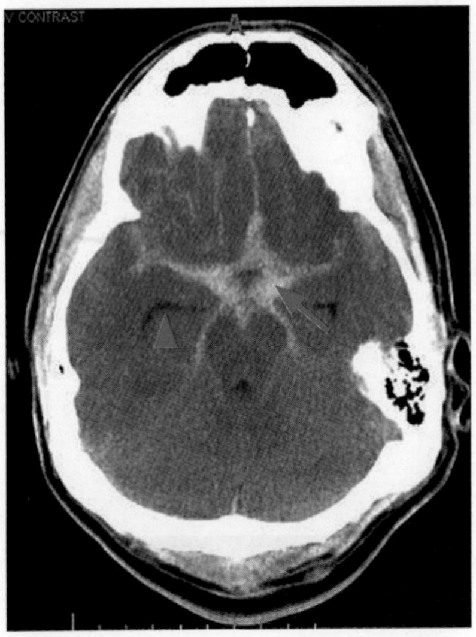

FIGURE 3-8. Subarachnoid hemorrhage. Head CT without contrast shows blood in the basal cisterns of the subarachnoid space (arrow). The dilated temporal horns (arrowhead) suggest developing hydrocephalus, which is often seen with SAH. (Reproduced with permission from Doherty GM. *Current Diagnosis & Treatment: Surgery,* 13th ed. New York: McGraw-Hill, 2010, Fig. 36-22.)

KEY FACT

A low percentage of head CTs will be falsely ⊖ in SAH. If the head CT is ⊖, an LP is needed to rule out SAH.

Q

A 45-year-old woman presents to the ED several hours after a fall in which she sustained blunt trauma to the head with altered consciousness. Her husband reports that shortly after the injury, she had seemed to return to baseline. What is the likely diagnosis and treatment?

- After the lucid interval, there is onset of headache, progressive obtundation, and hemiparesis.
- Ultimately, epidural bleeding may lead to a **"blown pupil,"** in which the pupil becomes fixed and dilated as a result of uncal herniation and compression of CN III.

WORKUP

Head CT shows a **lens-shaped, convex** hyperdensity that is usually limited by the sutures of the cranium where the dura inserts onto the bone.

TREATMENT

Emergent neurosurgical evacuation.

Subdural Hematoma

Defined as a collection of blood between the dura and the brain. Associated with tearing of the bridging veins between the cortex and dural sinuses. Often seen in the elderly and alcoholics, who have significant cortical atrophy that places the bridging veins under tension. Tearing usually occurs as a result of an acceleration-deceleration mechanism.

SIGNS AND SYMPTOMS

- Headache.
- Changes in mental status or new-onset dementia. Changes can be acute (< 24 hours), subacute (24 hours to 2 weeks), or chronic (> 2 weeks).
- Contralateral hemiparesis or other focal deficit (the most common examination finding is nonfocality).
- A remote history of a fall.

WORKUP

- Head CT without contrast shows a **crescent-shaped, concave** fluid collection (see Figure 3-9A), with density depending on the age of the bleed (fresh blood is white but darkens over days). In contrast, epidural hematomas are confined by suture line and result in a convex lens shape (see Figure 3-9B).
- In some cases, a hematocrit line may be observed in which the RBCs have settled down and separated from the plasma.

TREATMENT

- **If symptomatic:** Surgical evacuation.
- **If asymptomatic:** Observation, as subdural blood will frequently regress spontaneously.

Intraparenchymal Hemorrhage

Etiologies include hypertension (usually in the basal ganglia), amyloid angiopathy (seen in the elderly), trauma (coup-contrecoup), and vascular malformations (AVMs, cavernous hemangiomas).

SIGNS AND SYMPTOMS

Lethargy, headache, motor or sensory deficits.

WORKUP

Head CT without contrast to look for an intraparenchymal hemorrhage.

KEY FACT

Acute subdural hematomas have a high mortality rate. By contrast, chronic, asymptomatic subdural hematomas can be managed with observation.

KEY FACT

AVMs are more likely than SAH to produce an intraparenchymal hemorrhage.

A

Epidural hematoma, in which patients are often said to "talk and die." Emergent neurosurgical evacuation is lifesaving.

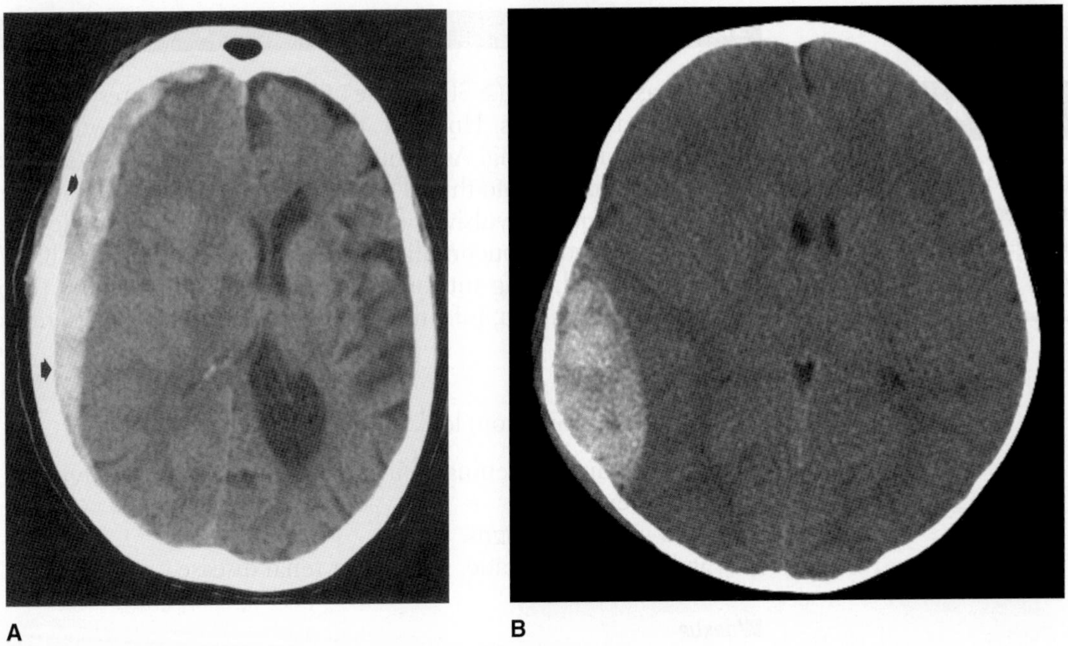

FIGURE 3-9. Acute subdural and epidural hematoma. (A) Noncontrast CT demonstrating an acute right subdural hematoma. Note the characteristic crescentic shape. (B) Noncontrast CT showing an acute right epidural hematoma. Note the characteristic biconvex shape. (Image A reproduced with permission from Chen MY et al. *Basic Radiology,* 1st ed. New York: McGraw-Hill, 2004, Fig. 12-32. Image B reproduced with permission from Doherty GM. *Current Diagnosis & Treatment: Surgery,* 13th ed. New York: McGraw-Hill, 2010, Fig. 36-8.)

TREATMENT

- Raise the head of the bed to ↓ ICP.
- Monitor for and prevent ischemic damage 2° to vasospasm.
- Lowering BP to prevent or reduce bleeding should be done carefully, as it may lead to hypoperfusion.
- Surgical evacuation may be necessary and lifesaving if a mass effect is observed or if the hemorrhage occurs in the posterior fossa, thereby threatening vital brainstem function.

KEY FACT

Look for mass effect and edema on head CT, as they may predict herniation.

NEUROLEPTIC MALIGNANT SYNDROME

Caused by central dopaminergic blockade. Most common in young men who are put on a **typical antipsychotic** for the first time, occurring during the **first 10 days of use.**

SIGNS AND SYMPTOMS

Hyperthermia, altered mental status, autonomic instability, muscular rigidity.

WORKUP

- Look for leukocytosis on CBC.
- Look for ↑ CK.

TREATMENT

- Discontinue the offending agent.
- Give benzodiazepines; consider dantrolene or bromocriptine.

KEY FACT

Neuroleptic malignant syndrome has a 20% mortality rate.

MNEMONIC

Patients with neuroleptic malignant syndrome have—

FEVER

Fever
Encephalopathy
Vitals unstable
Elevated enzymes (CK)
Rigid muscles

STATUS EPILEPTICUS

KEY FACT

Not to state the obvious, but patients with seizure disorders tend to have seizures as well! Be sure to take a careful history.

Defined as prolonged (≥ 30-minute) or repetitive seizures without a return to baseline consciousness. However, this doesn't mean that you have to wait 30 minutes to start treating. As a rule of thumb, if a patient is still seizing when he or she is brought into the ED, consider it a "status." Seizures can be either convulsive or nonconvulsive, a distinction that can be made only by EEG. Etiologies include noncompliance with anticonvulsants, EtOH/benzodiazepine withdrawal, drug intoxication, metabolic disturbances (hyponatremia, hypoglycemia), trauma, infection, and a history of seizure disorders.

SIGNS AND SYMPTOMS

On physical examination, look for the following:

- Signs of trauma, meningeal irritation, or systemic infection.
- Papilledema.
- Focal neurologic signs.
- Evidence of metastatic, hepatic, or renal disease.

WORKUP

- Ensure that the patient has adequate **C**irculation, **A**irway, and **B**reathing—and don't forget to check a blood glucose level!
- **Establish access:** Insert an IV line.
- **Initial workup:** Treatment with anticonvulsants should be instituted immediately. Medications are discussed in Table 3-4 and Figure 3-10 but are generally given in this order: lorazepam (multiple doses) → phenytoin → phenobarbital → midazolam. At the same time, the following measures should be taken:
  - **Check vital signs:**
    - **BP:** To exclude hypertensive encephalopathy and shock.
    - **Temperature:** To exclude hyperthermia.
    - **Pulse:** To exclude life-threatening cardiac arrhythmia with cardiac monitoring.

KEY FACT

Status epilepticus is a medical emergency associated with a 20% mortality rate.

TABLE 3-4. Drug Treatment of Status Epilepticus

DRUG	DOSAGE/ROUTE	ADVANTAGES/DISADVANTAGES/COMPLICATIONS
Lorazepam or diazepam	5 mg IV, multiple doses	Fast acting. Effective half-life is 15 minutes for diazepam and 4 hours for lorazepam. Abrupt respiratory depression or hypotension occurs in 5% of patients, especially when these drugs are given in combination with other sedatives. An additional benefit of benzodiazepines is that they bind to the same receptor as alcohol, thereby treating EtOH withdrawal seizure as well. Seizure recurrence affects 50% of patients; therefore, consider adding a maintenance drug (phenytoin or phenobarbital).
If the seizure is not controlled by benzodiazepines, proceed to phenobarbital.		
Phenobarbital	1000–1500 mg (18 mg/kg), IV slowly (50 mg/min).	Peak brain levels within 30 minutes. Effective as a maintenance drug. Respiratory depression and hypotension are common at higher doses. (Intubation and ventilatory support should be immediately available.)
If the above is ineffective, proceed immediately to general anesthesia.		

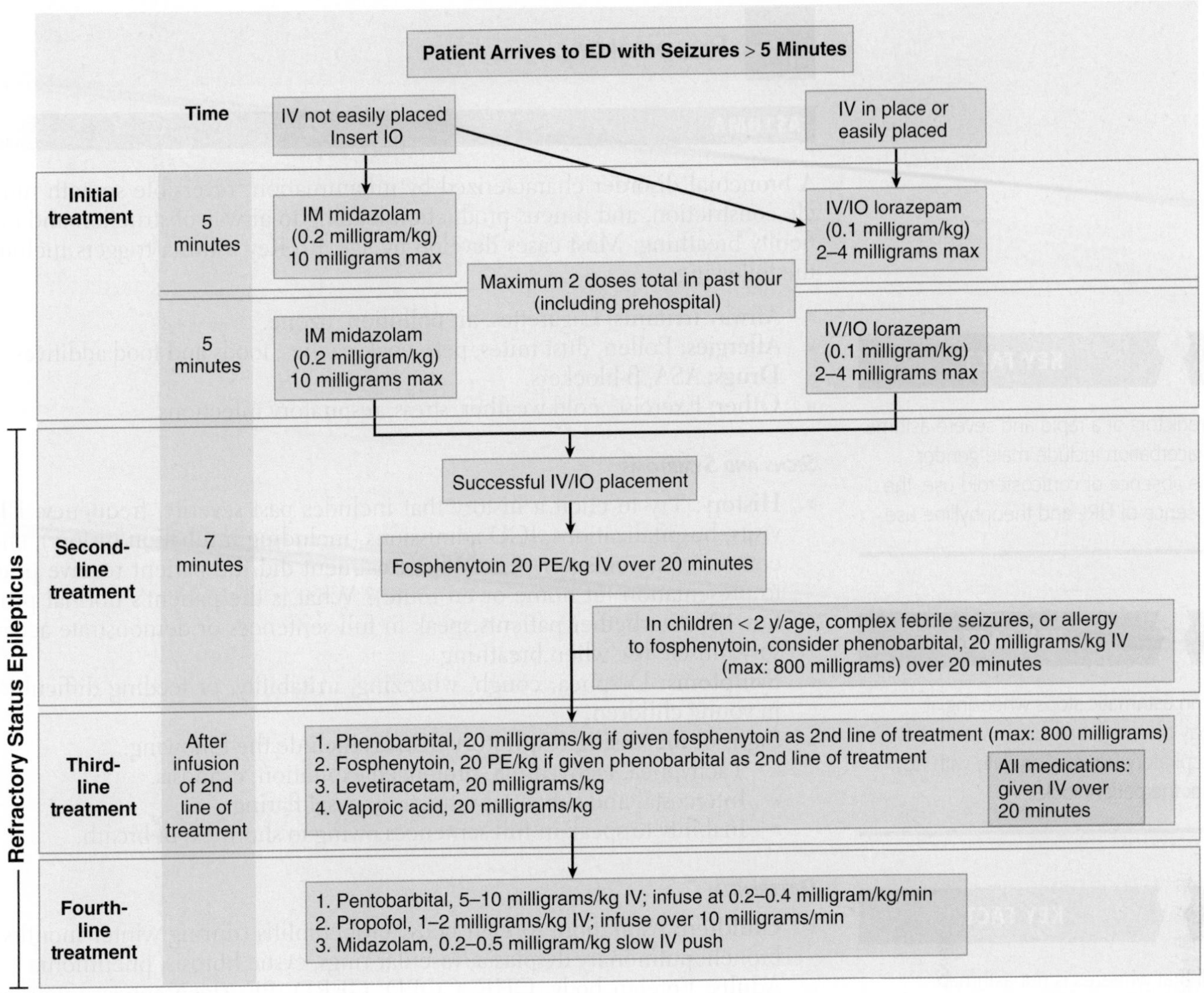

FIGURE 3-10. Algorithm for the management of seizures. (Reproduced with permission from Tintinalli JE et al. *Tintinalli's Emergency Medicine: A Comprehensive Study Guide,* 7th ed. New York: McGraw-Hill, 2011, Fig. 129-3.)

- **Order labs:**
  - CBC, electrolytes, hepatic and renal function tests, calcium, ESR, toxicology, and PT/PTT (in case LP is necessary); serum osmolality.
  - Calculate serum osmolality: 2 (Na^+) + glucose/18 + BUN/2.8 (normal range 270–290); then calculate osmolar gap.
- **Poststabilization:** Once the patient is stabilized, obtain the following:
  - Consider CT to evaluate for head trauma suffered during the seizure.
  - Obtain an LP in the presence of fever, meningeal signs, or **any** clinical suspicion (only after a CT has been done).
  - Once the patient is stabilized, address all 2° injuries (eg, lacerations, fractures).

Treatment

- On admission, attend to cardiopulmonary status (CAB).
- Give thiamine (100 mg) and glucose (50 mL 50% dextrose) IV.
- See Table 3-4 and Figure 3-10 for further treatment guidelines.

KEY FACT

If a woman on INH presents in status epilepticus and is unresponsive to treatment, she should be treated with vitamin B_6.

KEY FACT

If a patient begins to seize while in the ED, just worry about the airway for the first 5 minutes. However, if a patient comes into the ED seizing, treat for status epilepticus right away.

Respiratory

ASTHMA

A bronchial disorder characterized by inflammation, reversible smooth muscle constriction, and mucus production leading to airway obstruction and difficulty breathing. Most cases develop by age 40. Key asthma triggers include the following:

- **Airway irritants:** Cigarettes, air pollution, ozone.
- **Allergies:** Pollen, dust mites, pets, cockroaches, foods and food additives.
- **Drugs:** ASA, β-blockers.
- **Other:** Exercise, cold weather, stress, respiratory infections.

KEY FACT

Predictors of a rapid and severe asthma exacerbation include male gender, the absence of corticosteroid use, the absence of URI, and theophylline use.

Signs and Symptoms

- **History:** Try to elicit a history that includes past severity, frequency, ED visits, hospitalizations, ICU admissions (including intubation history), and courses of steroids per year. What treatment did the patient receive prior to presentation (at home or en route)? What is the patient's normal peak flow? Note whether patients speak in full sentences or demonstrate accessory muscle use when breathing.
- **Symptoms:** Dyspnea, cough, wheezing, irritability, or feeding difficulties in young children.
- **Signs of increasing respiratory distress** include the following:
  - Tachypnea, tachycardia, prolonged expiration, cyanosis.
  - Intercostal and subcostal retraction; nasal flaring.
  - Inability to speak in full sentences owing to shortness of breath.

KEY FACT

If an asthmatic stops wheezing, it may be a sign of ↓ air movement and respiratory failure. Correlate with how sick the patient looks.

Differential

- **Children:** Aspiration, foreign body, bronchiolitis (during winter months), bronchopulmonary dysplasia, vascular rings, cystic fibrosis, pneumonia.
- **Adults:** Foreign body, CHF, COPD, GERD, PE, sleep apnea, pneumonia.

KEY FACT

All that wheezes is not asthma.

Workup

- **Peak expiratory flow (PEF):** < 50% of predicted indicates a severe exacerbation.
- **Pulse oximetry.**
- **ABGs:** Look for hypoxia and respiratory acidosis during acute exacerbations. Be wary of patients with a normal pH and P_{CO_2}, as this may indicate that they are tiring out.

Treatment

- Bronchodilators are the drug of choice in an acute attack. However, the inflammatory (delayed) phase of an asthma attack will be addressed only by corticosteroids. Given that corticosteroids take hours to take effect, administer them early. Other adjunctive therapies for severe asthma exacerbations include SQ epinephrine and IV magnesium.
- Patients with moderate to severe attacks should receive systemic corticosteroids in the ED, such as PO prednisone or IV methylprednisolone (Solu-Medrol). Patients who are ready for discharge should be prescribed a "burst" of prednisone (generally 40–60 mg × 5 days). Treatment with corticosteroids for < 10 days does not require tapering.

KEY FACT

Because steroids target the late inflammatory response in asthma, you should not expect to see symptom improvement for 4–6 hours.

- All patients must get an ambulatory O_2 sat before they can be discharged. Patients do not need to be completely asymptomatic but must be able to manage their asthma at home (nebulizer spacing no closer than q 4 h).

HEMOTHORAX

Blood in the pleural cavity caused by laceration of the lungs or intrathoracic blood vessels. Defined as follows:

- **Simple hemothorax:** < 1500 cc of blood in the pleural cavity.
- **Massive hemothorax:** > 1500 cc of blood.

SIGNS AND SYMPTOMS

- Dyspnea, tachypnea, tachycardia.
- ↓ or absent breath sounds on the affected side; dullness to percussion.
- Signs of hypovolemic shock can be seen if blood loss is severe.

DIFFERENTIAL

- ⊕ **history of trauma:** Consider pneumothorax, hemopneumothorax, tension pneumothorax, and communicating pneumothorax. Keep in mind that trauma may be from an undisclosed source (eg, spousal abuse) or may be iatrogenic (eg, recent lung biopsy, bronchoscopy).
- ⊖ **history of trauma:** Consider other causes of pleural effusions (see the Internal Medicine chapter), chylothorax, and empyema.

WORKUP

CXR shows blunting of the costophrenic angle if > 200 cc of blood is present; there is complete opacification on the affected side in massive hemothorax (≥ 1500 cc).

TREATMENT

- **Simple hemothorax:** Usually self-limited.
  - Tube thoracostomy to control bleeding by apposition of the pleural surfaces.
  - If there is > 1500 cc of drainage from the initial chest tube, > 50% hemothorax, or 200 cc/hr of continued drainage, or if the patient decompensates after initial stabilization, a thoracotomy is needed.
- **Massive hemothorax:** Tube thoracostomy followed by thoracotomy. Patients will most likely need resuscitation with 2 large-bore IVs, IV fluid, and blood products.

> **KEY FACT**
>
> The key determination to make in a hemothorax is whether the patient requires thoracotomy.

PNEUMOTHORAX

A collection of air in the pleural space that can lead to pulmonary collapse. Categorized as follows:

- **1° (spontaneous):** May involve rupture of subpleural apical blebs; most commonly seen in tall, thin young males.
- **2°:** Causes include COPD, asthma, TB, trauma, and *Pneumocystis jiroveci* pneumonia; may also be iatrogenic (thoracentesis, subclavian central line placement, positive-pressure mechanical ventilation, bronchoscopy).

KEY POINT

RESOLUTION OF SMALL PNEUMOTHORACES

You can impress your resident by knowing why small pneumothoraces can be allowed to resolve spontaneously with 100% O_2 delivered by face mask.

- The air in a pneumothorax contains roughly 78% nitrogen. By giving a patient 100% O_2, you ↓ the partial pressure of nitrogen in the patient's blood, thereby establishing a diffusion gradient.
- Of course, you create an O_2 diffusion gradient in the other direction as well, but the O_2 diffuses more slowly and is quickly absorbed by surrounding tissues.

KEY FACT

Don't forget that a patient with pneumothorax may be asymptomatic!

SIGNS AND SYMPTOMS

- Unilateral pleuritic chest pain and dyspnea.
- Tachycardia.
- Respiratory physical examination reveals diminished/absent breath sounds, hyperresonance to percussion, and ↓ tactile fremitus.
- Chest wall crepitus and tenderness.

DIFFERENTIAL

Suspect other deadly causes of chest pain (see the mnemonic **TAPUM** above) as well as pneumonia, pleural effusion, and pericardial tamponade.

WORKUP

CXR shows a visceral pleural line and/or lung retraction from the chest wall (best seen with an end-expiratory film in an upright position).

TREATMENT

- Small pneumothoraces are allowed to resolve spontaneously and may be treated with 100% O_2 by face mask.
- Large, severely symptomatic pneumothoraces are treated with a chest tube and/or pleurodesis.

Tension Pneumothorax

KEY FACT

A CXR of a tension pneumothorax generally represents failure on the part of the treating physician, as the patient should have been diagnosed clinically without the need for imaging. Occasionally, however, a CXR is obtained (see Figure 3-11).

A deadly variant of pneumothorax in which a pulmonary or chest wall defect acts as a one-way valve, drawing air into the pleural space during inspiration but trapping it during expiration. Etiologies include penetrating trauma, infection, CHF, and positive-pressure mechanical ventilation. The pathophysiology of tension pneumothorax involves the following:

- Ipsilateral lung collapse 2° to an ↑ amount of trapped air on the affected side.
- Shift of the mediastinum away from the injured lung.
- Impaired venous return leading to ↓ cardiac output.
- Shock and death occur unless the condition is immediately recognized and treated.

SIGNS AND SYMPTOMS

Suspect tension pneumothorax if you see signs of pneumothorax accompanied by the following:

- Respiratory distress; falling O_2 saturation.
- Hypotension.

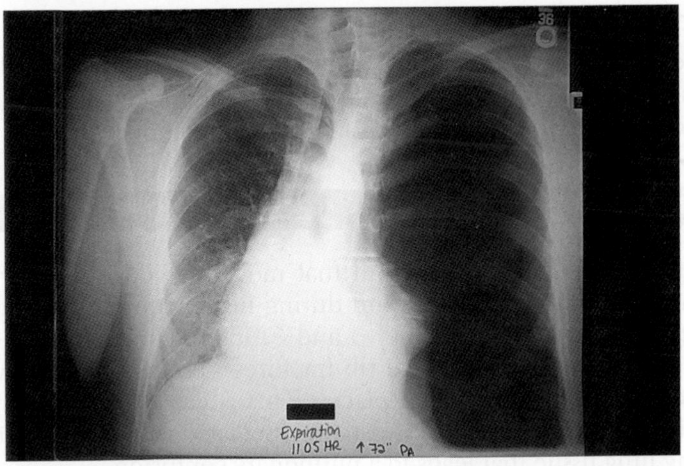

FIGURE 3-11. Tension pneumothorax. Note the hyperlucent left hemithorax, flattening and inferior displacement of the left diaphragm, and rightward shift of the mediastinal structures. These are typical radiographic findings in patients with tension pneumothorax.

- Distended neck veins.
- Tracheal deviation away from the side of the pneumothorax.

Treatment

- **Immediate needle decompression:**
  - Insert a large-bore needle (14 gauge) into the second or third intercostal space at the midclavicular line on the side of the pneumothorax.
  - Don't forget to pull out the needle to allow air to escape. Watch for restoration of hemodynamics to determine the success of the intervention. Sometimes a hissing sound may also signal decompression of the pneumothorax, but this may be difficult to discern in the noisy ED environment.
  - Many patients have too much adipose tissue, so the angiocatheters are not long enough to penetrate into the thoracic cavity. The midaxillary line is an alternative site with less fat. Alternatively, you can find long needles in the central line kits.
- Once decompression is achieved, a chest tube (thoracostomy tube) can be placed.
- Administer IV fluids to ↑ venous return to the heart.

Communicating Pneumothorax (Sucking Chest Wound)

A pneumothorax due to an open defect in the chest wall that allows air to preferentially enter through the defect. This occurs when an open defect, often from a gunshot wound, is greater than two-thirds the diameter of the trachea. The affected lung collapses with inspiration as air enters through the wound, seriously impairing ventilation.

Signs and Symptoms

In addition to respiratory distress, air may be seen or heard bubbling through the wound.

Workup

This is immediately life threatening, and the diagnosis is clinical.

KEY FACT

Watch the movie *Three Kings* for an excellent intrathoracic animation of the pathology of tension pneumothorax.

KEY FACT

Covering a sucking chest wound on 4 sides potentially converts it to a tension pneumothorax, which could be immediately life threatening.

Treatment

Cover the wound with an impermeable dressing on **3 sides.** This allows air to escape during expiration and prevents it from entering during inspiration, effectively converting the defect into a simple pneumothorax.

FLAIL CHEST

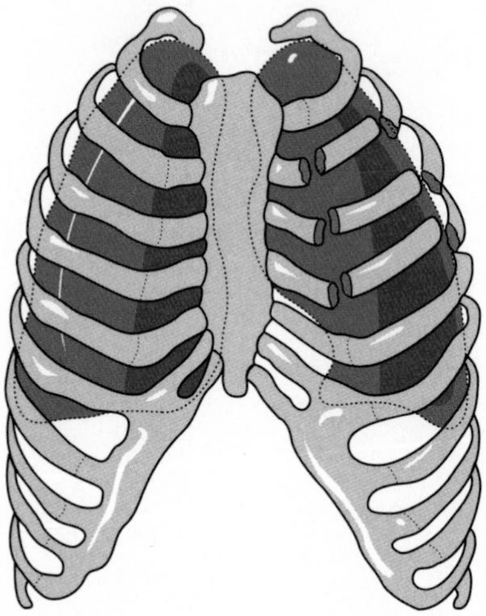

FIGURE 3-12. Flail chest on the left. This segment of the chest wall will be unable to aid in respiration. (Reproduced with permission from Doherty GM. *Current Diagnosis & Treatment: Surgery,* 13th ed. New York: McGraw-Hill, 2010, Fig. 13-6.)

A free-floating segment of chest wall that moves paradoxically during respiration, meaning that it moves inward during inspiration and outward during expiration in accordance with the ⊖ and ⊕ intrapleural pressure. The flail segment is created by consecutive rib fractures (see Figure 3-12), with each having been broken in at least 2 places. This is caused by a mechanism of injury with significant force and is usually associated with significant injury to underlying lung tissue that leads to a pulmonary contusion.

Signs and Symptoms

Respiratory distress; pain associated with rib fractures; paradoxical movement of the flail segment.

Workup

The diagnosis is clinical and is made by seeing or palpating the paradoxical movement of the flail segment. A CXR or chest CT can be obtained to further support the diagnosis and to assess for underlying pulmonary injury.

Treatment

Oxygenation; reexpansion of the lung; analgesia to improve ventilation. Patients are no longer splinted with sandbags.

PULMONARY EMBOLISM (PE)

KEY FACT

Trust your clinical judgment. Even a patient with a low-probability V/Q scan still has a 40% chance of having a PE if clinical suspicion is high.

An occlusion of the pulmonary vasculature, typically by a blood clot. Ninety-five percent of the time, the embolus originates from a DVT above the calf. PE often leads to pulmonary infarction, right heart failure, and tissue hypoxia. Risk factors for DVT and PE include Virchow's triad, which consists of the following:

- **Blood stasis:** Immobility, obesity, CHF, surgery.
- **Venous endothelial injury:** Surgery (especially of the pelvis/lower extremity); trauma; recent fracture.
- **Hypercoagulable states:** Pregnancy or postpartum state, OCP use, coagulation disorders, malignancy, severe burns.

Signs and Symptoms

- Presents with sudden-onset dyspnea and pleuritic chest pain.
- Cough, hemoptysis (rarely), anxiety, syncope, and diaphoresis may be seen.
- Physical examination findings include the following:
  - **Unstable vitals:** Tachycardia, tachypnea, hypotension. Subsequent stabilization of vital signs does not lower the probability of PE.
  - **Right heart failure 2° to PE:** Rales, bulging neck veins, a loud P2.
  - **DVT:** An erythematous, edematous, tender, warm lower extremity with a ⊕ **Homans' sign** (calf pain on forced dorsiflexion, which is neither sensitive nor specific for DVT). Calculate the patient's PERC and Wells scores to assess the pretest probability of a DVT/PE.

TABLE 3-5. Diagnostic Tests for Pulmonary Embolism

Test	Findings/Comments
CXR	Usually normal. **Hampton's hump** (a wedge-shaped infarct) and **Westermark's sign** (↓ vascular markings in an embolized lung zone) are rarely seen.
ECG	Usually sinus tachycardia and/or nonspecific ST-T-wave changes. An **S1Q3T3** pattern is pathognomonic.
ABG	**Respiratory alkalosis** (↑ pH, ↓ Pco_2), $Po_2 < 80$ mm Hg (90% sensitive). Not useful for predicting the absence of PE.
D-dimer	Includes the latex agglutination and ELISA D-dimer tests, the latter being more sensitive. A low D-dimer might help rule out a low-suspicion PE. Neither assay is specific, as D-dimers ↑ in MI, sepsis, and other systemic illnesses. However, the ELISA D-dimer will be ↑ (> 500 ng/mL) in > 90% of patients with a PE.
Pulmonary angiogram	The gold standard. However, the technique is invasive, time consuming, and inherently risky. Not used in acute cases.
V/Q scan	One or more segmental areas of mismatch in the lung (ie, areas that are well ventilated but not perfused) suggest PE. Results are reported as normal or as a low/intermediate/high probability of PE: ▪ A normal result rules out PE. ▪ **High probability:** 85–90% incidence of PE. ▪ **Low probability:** Does not rule out PE (14–31% incidence).
CT angiogram	Helical (spiral) CT (with IV contrast) is sensitive to PE in the proximal pulmonary arteries but less so in the distal segmental arteries. In the ED, this is the study of choice, as it is fast and misses only those PEs that do not kill.
Doppler ultrasound	Helps determine if DVTs are present in the lower extremities.

(Adapted with permission from Tierney LM et al. *Current Medical Diagnosis & Treatment,* 36th ed. Stamford, CT: Appleton & Lange, 1997: 292.)

WORKUP

- Table 3-5 outlines diagnostic tests for PE (see also Figure 3-13).
- Realistically, if PE is suspected, a chest CT with contrast is the single most important study. However, the boards frequently ask about other supportive diagnostic findings.

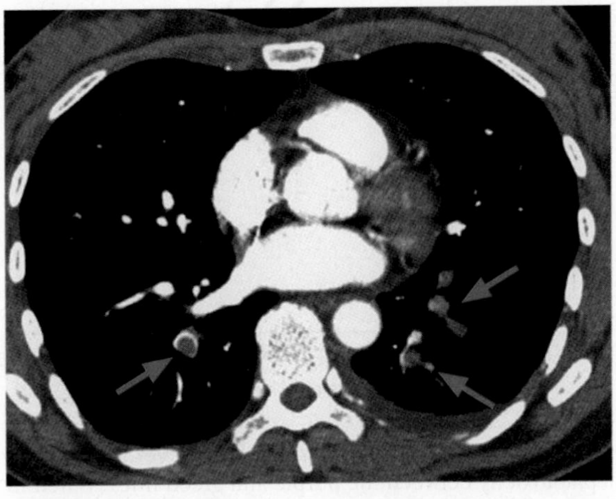

FIGURE 3-13. Pulmonary embolism. CT angiogram of the chest shows multiple filling defects in pulmonary arteries (arrows). (Reproduced with permission from Chen MY et al. *Basic Radiology,* 2nd ed. New York: McGraw-Hill, 2011, Fig. 3-14.)

KEY FACT

The most common CXR finding in PE is a normal CXR. Hampton's hump and Westermark's sign are rarely seen. Think PE in the setting of sudden-onset dyspnea and a clear CXR.

Q

A 67-year-old man with a history of lung cancer collapsed at home and was brought to the ED. Although the patient's ECG shows normal sinus rhythm, a carotid pulse cannot be palpated. What can explain his condition?

TREATMENT

- **Anticoagulation:** Give heparin (for a PTT of 60–90) to prevent clot extension, and then give warfarin (INR goal 2–3) for long-term anticoagulation (usually lasting 3–6 months).
- **Surgical embolectomy:** Seldom successful, and attempted only if the patient is crashing.

Toxicology

Intoxication of several types can be encountered in the ED patient population. Drugs and alcohol are the most common types, but occasionally intentional (suicidal) or accidental ingestions are also seen.

- **Drugs:** The most common presentations are heroin overdose (which presents with respiratory depression/apnea) and cocaine intoxication. Treat heroin overdose with naloxone, and avoid β-blockers in cocaine chest pain.
- **Suicide:** Life-threatening ingestions include acetaminophen (APAP) and TCAs. All patients who prompt concern about a suicide overdose should have an ECG and an APAP and salicylate level. Get a serum APAP level 4 hours after ingestion and compare it to a nomogram (see Figure 3-14); give N-acetylcysteine if indicated. TCA overdose can present with widening of the QRS complex on ECG and is treated with bicarbonate infusion.
- **Toxidromes:** A toxidrome is a constellation of symptoms that is a consequence of the pharmacologic actions of the toxin. In general, there are 7 toxidromes that are commonly seen in the ED; most are due to medication overdoses or substance abuse (see Table 3-6). Table 3-7 lists approaches toward the active removal of toxins from the patient's body.

KEY FACT

Anticholinergic poisoning: "Mad as a hatter, red as a beet, blind as a bat, hot as a hare, dry as a bone."

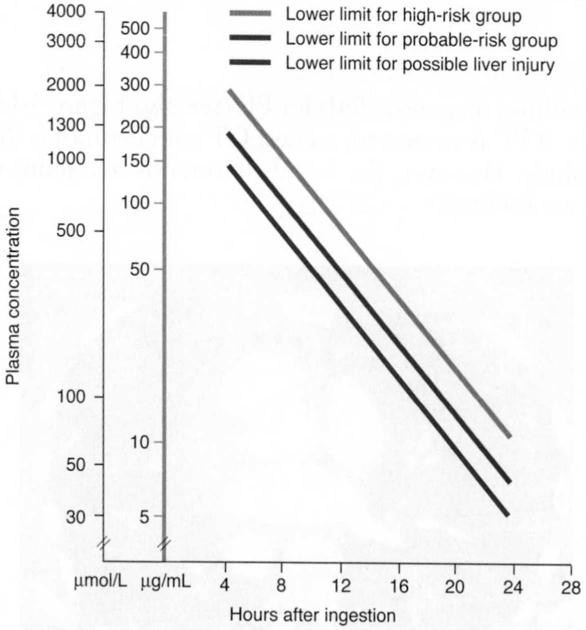

FIGURE 3-14. APAP nomogram predicting the risk of liver injury. Roughly 25% of patients develop hepatotoxicity between the purple and green lines. When in doubt (eg, if the time of ingestion is not known), give N-acetylcysteine.

A

Lung cancer often leads to hypercoagulable states, and a massive PE is a cause of pulseless electrical activity (PEA).

TABLE 3.6. Common Toxidromes

Drug Class	Examples	Vitals	Symptoms	Treatment
Adrenergic/ sympathomimetic	Amphetamines, cocaine, PCP, MDMA, caffeine (in massive doses), ephedrine, bath salts (MDPV)	↑/normal RR ↑ HR ↑ T ↑ BP	Agitation, psychosis, seizures Dilated but reactive pupils Hyperreflexia Diaphoresis, urinary retention Piloerection Emesis, abdominal pain	Haloperidol, benzodiazepines; restraints if needed to ensure patient and staff safety. No antidote is available. Physical restraints may lead to hyperthermia and rhabdomyolysis as a result of continued isometric muscle contractions.
Anticholinergic	Antihistamines, atropine, haloperidol, belladonna, mushrooms, TCAs, scopolamine	Normal RR ↑ HR ↑ T ↑/normal BP	↓ mental status, psychosis, paranoia Delirium, ataxia, agitation, seizures Dilated/slow pupils Dry skin, flushing, ileus, urinary retention Respiratory failure	Cholinesterase inhibitors (eg, neostigmine).
Cholinergic	Black widow spider bites, mushrooms, insecticides (organophosphates)	↑/normal RR ↑/↓ HR Normal T Normal BP	**SLUDGE: S**alivation, **L**acrimation, **U**rination, **D**iarrhea, **GI** complaints, **E**mesis ↓ mental status, coma, confusion Pupillary constriction Seizures, fasciculations, weakness Diaphoresis, respiratory failure	Atropine, pralidoxime. Note that patients exposed to organophosphates may need to be decontaminated. Chemicals on skin/clothes will continue to poison the patient and pose a threat to the ED staff.
Extrapyramidal	Haloperidol, metoclopramide, phenothiazines	–	Tremor, rigidity Opisthotonos, torticollis Dysphonia, oculogyric crisis	Immediate discontinuation of the offending agent. However, some symptoms may be permanent.
Hypermetabolic	Salicylates, some phenols, herbicides	↑ RR ↑ HR ↑ T ↑ BP	Hyperpnea, restlessness Seizures, convulsions Metabolic acidosis, tinnitus (ASA)	Urine alkalinization with $NaHCO_3$ for ASA overdose.
Opioid	Fentanyl, heroin, oxycodone, morphine	↓ RR or apnea ↓ HR ↓/normal T ↓/normal BP	CNS depression Dilated pupils Hypothermia, hypotension Seizures, confusion, lethargy Constipation, urinary retention	Naloxone (Narcan). If the patient responds to naloxone, start a drip (short half-life).
Sedative-hypnotic	Benzodiazepines, barbiturates	↓ RR ↓/normal HR ↓/normal T ↓ BP	CNS depression, ↓ mental status	Flumazenil for benzodiazepine poisoning. Note that the half-life of flumazenil is shorter than that of most benzodiazepines, so the patient may relapse into a toxic state.

TABLE 3-7. Removal of Toxins

Can Be Removed by Dialysis	Cannot Be Absorbed by Charcoal[a]
Barbiturates	Acids
Ethylene glycol	Alcohols
Lithium	Alkalis
Methanol	Hydrocarbons
Salicylates	Iron/lithium
Theophylline	Pesticides
Uremia	Solvents

[a] These substances require whole bowel irrigation.

- **Alcohol:** It's easy to spot an inebriated patient. However, before you put such patients in a hallway bed to let them sober up, you must first rule out hypoglycemia, head trauma, and other causes of mental status changes. In chronic alcoholics, even minor head trauma can lead to a subdural hemorrhage as a result of cortical atrophy and stretching of bridging veins. Thus, if an inebriated patient has a bump or a scratch on his or her head, obtain a CT.
  - There are 2 schools of thought with regard to alcohol intoxication. If you measure serum alcohol levels, you must keep the patient in the ED until they are **legally** sober. If you do not, you can discharge them when they are **clinically** sober.
  - Bear in mind that with chronic abusers, legal sobriety equals withdrawal. Do not let a patient drive home unless he or she is **legally** sober.

Trauma and Shock

RESUSCITATION

The resuscitation of the trauma patient begins during the 1° survey with CAB. Life-threatening injuries are identified and treated, and assessment and resuscitation of vital functions occur. Rapid assessment, diagnosis, and stabilization in the period immediately following trauma—termed the "golden hour"—must occur in order to optimize the patient's prognosis. The **CABDEFs** of resuscitation are as follows (see also mnemonic):

- **Circulation:**
  - Place 2 14- or 16-gauge IVs in the antecubital fossae. Draw blood samples while placing IVs.
  - Assess circulatory status (check vitals, capillary refill, and skin turgor).
  - Give a 1- to 2-L bolus of NS or LR for adults and 20 cc/kg in children. The need for further repletion is indicated by fluid status.
  - Expect to replace blood loss with a 3:1 ratio (ie, replace 1 L of blood with 3 L of crystalloid, as 66% of crystalloid will diffuse out of the vasculature). Monitor your patient's response to treatment.
- **Airway:**
  - Determine if the patient is breathing. Give supplemental O_2 to all trauma patients.
  - If the patient is not breathing, use a chin-lift or jaw-thrust maneuver to open the airway. Assume that all trauma patients have a cervical spine

MNEMONIC

The CABDEFs of resuscitation:

Circulation
Airway (with cervical spine precautions)
Breathing
Disability (neurologic status)
Exposure
Foley

KEY FACT

Intub**EIGHT** below **8** (on the Glasgow Coma Scale). Offer to provide cricoid pressure or inline cervical spine immobilization while the resident/attending is intubating.

injury until proven otherwise. Do not manipulate the neck by putting patients in the sniff position.
  - Clear foreign bodies and insert an oral or nasal airway as necessary. Suction aids in the removal of blood, vomitus, and the like.
  - Patients with apnea, altered mental status, impending airway compromise, closed-head injuries, or failed bag-mask ventilation should have early intubation.
  - A surgical airway or cricothyroidectomy is used for patients who cannot be intubated or in whom there is maxillofacial trauma.
- **Breathing:** Inspect, palpate, and auscultate the chest. If the patient is intubated, make sure breath sounds can be heard bilaterally. Remember that trauma auscultation is not a complete pulmonary examination; listen in the midaxillary line for breath sounds, as they can radiate from the other lung closer to the midline.
- **Disability:**
  - The patient's CNS dysfunction should be rapidly quantified with the Glasgow Coma Scale or with the **AVPU** scale (see mnemonic).
  - Establish pupil size and reactivity, and check for hemotympanum in head trauma patients.
- **Exposure/Environment:**
  - Expose the patient completely so that he or she can be assessed from head to toe during the 2° survey and hooked up to monitors.
  - Be sure to keep the patient warm.
- **Foley:**
  - The urinary catheter is necessary to monitor urinary output. Urine output is an accurate reflection of volume status and renal perfusion.
  - If there is blood at the urethral meatus, **do not** place a Foley. Urethral trauma may be present, in which case the Foley should be placed by urology.

A word of caution: The triad of death in trauma patients includes acidosis, coagulopathy, and hypothermia. Both acidosis and hypothermia ↓ the enzymatic activity of clotting factors. We strip patients down and give them massive amounts of room-temperature IV fluid. Not only do we cause hypothermia, but we also dilute clotting factors. Medical students save lives by giving the patient a warm blanket.

BURNS

Thermal burns are categorized according to depth and surface area in the following manner:

- **Superficial:** Involves the epidermis only. Painful and erythematous without blisters; will heal without a scar.
  - **Superficial partial-thickness burn:** Involves the dermis, sparing the follicles and glands. Characterized by pain, blistering, and erythema; heals in ~ 2 weeks with or without a scar.
  - **Deep partial-thickness burn:** Involves follicles and glands in the dermis. Characterized by pain, blistering, erythema, and charring (due to coagulation necrosis of the upper dermis); heals in 3–4 weeks, leaving a scar.
- **Full thickness:** Involves all skin layers. The burn is painless and waxy white in the case of a chemical burn or completely charred and black in flame injury. Requires skin grafts for healing; leads to significant scarring.

KEY FACT

These 5 things kill quickly: tension pneumothorax, communicating pneumothorax, massive hemothorax, cardiac tamponade, and obstructed airway.

MNEMONIC

Assessing CNS function–

AVPU

Alertness
Verbal responsiveness
Pain responsiveness
Unresponsive

Q 1

A 17-year-old girl is brought in by her parents because she has been "acting weird" ever since returning home from a party. A urine toxicology screen is ⊖, but the patient is fascinated by the unicorns floating on your white coat. What substance did the patient likely ingest?

Q 2

A 12-year-old boy who was in a serious motor vehicle accident urgently needs a blood transfusion. His parents state that they are Jehovah's Witnesses and refuse to give consent. What is the best course of action?

KEY FACT

Although alkali burns result in more local tissue destruction through liquefactive necrosis, acid burns (which cause coagulative necrosis) have a higher mortality rate because they are absorbed systemically.

KEY FACT

Don't be fooled by a small electrical burn. Nonvisible deep destruction may be present.

1 A

LSD (which does not show up on a urine toxicology screen).

2 A

Give the blood transfusion. The life of a child supersedes the religious preferences of the parents.

Workup

- The size of the burn is estimated using the "rule of 9's" (see Figure 3-15) to determine the percentage of total body surface area (TBSA) burned. Get a carbon monoxide and cyanide level to assess the degree of inhalation toxicity.
- Criteria for transfer to a burn unit are as follows:
  - Partial- and full-thickness burns affecting > 10% TBSA in patients < 10 or > 50 years of age.
  - Partial- and full-thickness burns affecting > 20% TBSA in patients between 10 and 50 years of age.
  - Full-thickness burns affecting > 5% TBSA in patients of any age.
  - Electrical or chemical burns.
  - Inhalational injuries.
  - Patients with preexisting medical problems.
  - Burns involving the face, hands, genitalia, perineum, or major joints.

Treatment

- **CAB** is critical:
  - **Circulation:** Fluid resuscitation is critical to the goal of maintaining 1 cc/kg/hr of urine output.
  - **Airway:** Facial burns, singed nose hairs, wheezing, or hoarseness should raise suspicion for smoke inhalation. Early intubation may be needed, as upper airway edema can rapidly progress to complete airway obstruction.
  - **Breathing:** Provide humidified 100% O_2. Be sure that all burned areas have been doused with water, as O_2 can reignite a smoldering burn.

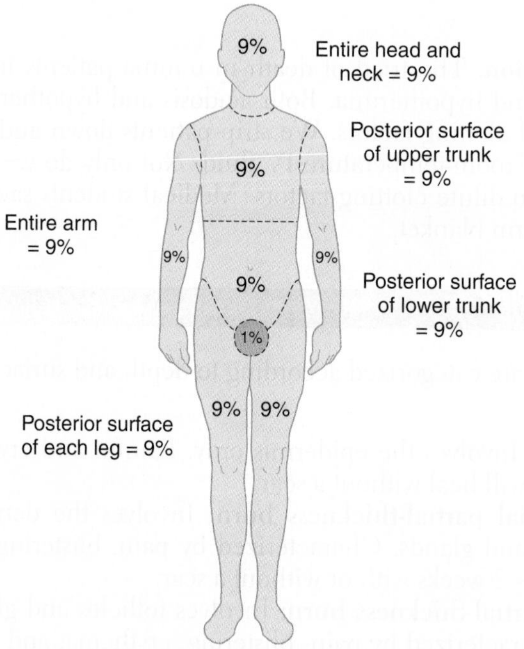

FIGURE 3-15. Estimation of body surface area in burns ("rule of 9's"). (Reproduced with permission from McPhee SJ, Papadakis MA. *Current Medical Diagnosis & Treatment 2012,* 49th ed. New York: McGraw-Hill, 2012, Fig. 37-2.)

- The Parkland formula should be used as a guide for calculating fluid needs over the first 24 hours, and a Foley catheter should be placed to monitor output.
- The patient should be covered with sterile sheets to prevent hypothermia and infection. Lidocaine-soaked blankets are commercially available but result in systemic absorption of the drug (be careful!).
- Provide tetanus prophylaxis.

KEY FACT

The Parkland formula calculates the estimated fluid requirement of a burn victim over the first 24 hours. It is 4 cc/kg/% TBSA burned. Half is replaced over the first 8 hours and half over 16 hours.

HYPOTHERMIA

A core temperature < 35°C (< 95°F). Usually caused by exposure, but patients can be predisposed by conditions such as alcohol ingestion, hypoglycemia, and sepsis.

KEY FACT

A person cannot be pronounced dead until they are warm and dead. Always check core temperatures and resuscitate until the patient's temperature is > 32°C.

Signs and Symptoms

- Shivering.
- Initial tachycardia followed by bradycardia.
- J waves (Osborn waves) on ECG.
- Loss of DTRs.
- Confusion and lethargy.
- Diuresis leading to hypovolemia.
- Slow, shallow respirations.

KEY FACT

Always check the core temperature of a patient with altered mental status to check for hypothermia or heatstroke!

Treatment

- CAB.
- Remove wet or cold clothing.
- Rewarm (except in the setting of frostbite):
  - **Passive external rewarming:** Appropriate for patients with mild hypothermia (32.5°C–35.0°C [90.5°F–95.0°F]). Apply warm clothing in a warm room.
  - **Active external rewarming:** Appropriate for patients with moderate hypothermia (27.5°C–32.5°C [81.5°F–90.5°F]). Apply external heat from sources such as warm blankets, hot water bottles, or immersion in a hot bath.
  - **Active core rewarming:** Appropriate for patients with severe hypothermia (< 27.5°C [81.5°F]) or hemodynamic instability. Involves the following:
    - Warm inhaled O_2.
    - Warm liquid femoral-arterial or cardiopulmonary bypass.

KEY FACT

Leave frostbitten lesions frozen until there is a definitive option for rewarming, such as submerging the area in circulating hot (42°C) water until the extremity is flush. Also offer pain medications such as NSAIDs.

SHOCK

A physiologic state of circulatory failure leading to inadequate tissue perfusion and tissue hypoxia. The cardinal signs of shock are simultaneous tachycardia and hypotension. Subtypes are as follows:

- **Hypovolemic:** The 2 major causes are hemorrhage and dehydration.
- **Distributive:** Think of "misdistribution" of blood due to inappropriately low systemic vascular resistance (SVR). The major causes are septic, neurogenic, and anaphylactic.
- **Cardiac:** Due to inability of the heart to adequately pump blood to the body owing either to intrinsic dysfunction or to extrinsic factors.
  - **Intrinsic heart dysfunction:** Known as cardiogenic shock or CHF.
  - **Extrinsic factors:** Pericardial effusions leading to cardiac tamponade, tension pneumothorax, and massive PE.

Q

EMTs bring a homeless man into the ED in the middle of winter. The man conversed with them initially but lost consciousness the moment they lifted him out of the snow onto the stretcher. Why is this the case?

KEY FACT

Shock can be hypovolemic, distributive, or cardiogenic.

KEY FACT

The hematocrit in acute blood loss is **normal.** But don't be fooled; patients will have tachycardia and in severe cases hypotension.

A

Moving a hypothermic person can push peripheral blood (arms, legs) centrally, dropping the core temperature even further and causing ventricular arrhythmias. Be careful!

Workup/Treatment

- Considering the various etiologies of shock, the evaluation and management of the patient in acute shock involves assessment of volume status, SVR, and cardiac output (see Table 3-8).
- The initial treatment of shock in an emergency is similar to that described for hypovolemic shock below. Remember that the key to treating almost all types of shock is fluid resuscitation. If you do not give fluid to your patient, you are effectively making a diagnosis of cardiogenic shock.

Hypovolemic Shock

Due to any process that depletes intravascular volume. These include the following:

- **Acute blood loss:** Hemorrhage in 1 of 3 compartments: the abdomen, pelvis (retroperitoneum), or thorax. Identifying the source of hemorrhage involves the following measures:
  - FAST abdominal ultrasound.
  - NG tube to evaluate for upper GI bleed.
  - Stool guaiac to rule out a lower GI bleed.
  - Pregnancy test to rule out a ruptured ectopic pregnancy.
  - CXR to rule out an intrathoracic bleed.
  - Pelvic x-ray to rule out pelvic fracture.
- **Dehydration:** Most commonly 2° to protracted diarrhea, vomiting, overdiuresis, or fluid restriction (eg, in elderly patients, who may not be able to drink adequate fluids).
- **Third spacing:** Shifting of intravascular volume into the interstitial space or other compartments. Occurs 2° to burns, trauma, acute pancreatitis, and/or liver disease.

TABLE 3-8. Clinical Presentations of Shock

Type	Condition	SVR	Skin	Neck Veins
Hypovolemic	Hemorrhage	High	Cold, clammy	Flat
	Dehydration	High	Cold, clammy	Flat
	Third spacing	High	Cold, clammy	Flat
Distributive	Septic (early)	Low	Warm	Flat to normal
	Neurogenic	Low	Warm	Flat to normal
	Anaphylactic	Low	Warm	Flat to normal
Cardiac	Cardiogenic	High	Cold, clammy	Distended[a]
	Cardiac compression	High	Cold, clammy	Distended
	Tension pneumothorax	High	Cold, clammy	Distended
Hypoglycemic	Hypoglycemia	High	Cold, clammy	Flat to normal

[a] May be flat if the patient is also hypovolemic.

Signs and Symptoms

Presentation depends on the degree of volume loss (see also Table 3-8).

- **Mild** (10–20% volume loss): The patient feels cold and exhibits orthostatic hypotension, flat neck veins, and pale, cool skin.
- **Moderate** (20–40% volume loss): The patient is thirsty, tachycardic/hypotensive, and oliguric.
- **Severe** (> 40% volume loss): The patient exhibits altered mental status (agitation leading to obtundation), severe hypotension, tachycardia, and tachypnea.
- ↓ central venous pressure and ↑ SVR are also seen.

Treatment

The goal in treating hypovolemic shock is to restore intravascular volume, treat the underlying cause of intravascular depletion, and restore tissue oxygenation. Emergency maneuvers in hypovolemic shock are as follows:

1. Give the patient O_2.
2. Place 2 large-bore (14-gauge) IVs and rapidly deliver 2 L of crystalloid (bolus).
3. Reassess vitals and trend lactate levels. If vitals do not improve or lactate levels do not decline, give 1–2 L of additional crystalloid and reassess. If vitals still have not improved, consider initiating IV pressors, giving steroids (if adrenal crisis is suspected), and delivering blood products.
4. If a peritoneal bleed is identified, the patient must undergo emergent exploratory laparotomy.
5. If a pelvic fracture is identified, a pelvic bleed should be suspected. Binding the pelvis (just tie a sheet around it) can stabilize the fracture and reduce the bleeding. Once stabilized, the patient should have angiography and embolization.
6. If a thoracic bleed is identified, a chest tube should be placed.

KEY FACT

Hemorrhage is the most common cause of shock in the trauma patient.

Cardiogenic Shock

Etiologies include arrhythmias and MI, vascular disease, myocarditis, and cardiomyopathy. There is a spectrum between CHF and frank cardiogenic shock; a lactate level allows you to assess for tissue hypoxia.

Signs and Symptoms

- Tachycardia, hypotension, tachypnea.
- Distended neck veins; peripheral edema.
- Patients may have S_3 with rales.
- ↑ central venous pressure, ↓ pulmonary capillary wedge pressure, ECG abnormalities.

Treatment

Therapy should be directed at the underlying cause and at maintaining adequate BP.

- **Medical management:**
  - **Inotropes:** Dopamine is generally the pressor of choice in cardiogenic shock (↑ contractility).
  - **Vasodilators:** ↓ preload and afterload, leading to ↓ myocardial work.
  - **Diuretics:** ↓ preload.
  - Antiarrhythmics should also be considered.

KEY FACT

Cardiogenic shock is the only form of shock in which fluid resuscitation may actually lead to further failure.

- **Surgical interventions:** Intra-aortic balloon pump (↑ CO, ↓ afterload, ↑ myocardial perfusion).

Septic Shock

Septic shock is 2° to the systemic effects of infection. Its pathophysiology is as follows:

- Toxins from both gram-⊕ and gram-⊖ bacteria as well as systemic inflammatory factors lead to vasodilation of the peripheral circulation and ↑ capillary permeability.
- An as-yet-unidentified myocardial depression factor reduces contractility of the heart, leading to compensatory tachycardia.
- Overall, this results in significantly ↓ SVR, redistribution of cardiac output, and massive fluid loss into the tissue.

SIGNS AND SYMPTOMS

- To meet diagnostic criteria, a patient must fulfill SIRS criteria (see Table 3-9), have a suspected source of infection, and show signs of hemodynamic instability.
- The patient will have hypotension but will be "warm and pink" due to vasodilation.
- Lactic acidosis supports the diagnosis of septic shock.

KEY FACT

Identify and treat the underlying cause of septic shock.

TREATMENT

- A specific treatment protocol exists for the treatment of septic shock in the ED. This "early goal-directed therapy" (EGDT) focuses on increasing cardiac output and ensuring tissue oxygenation (see Figure 3-16).
- Identify and treat the source of infection with IV antibiotics, surgical drainage, and central line removal. Remember the common sources of infection: pneumonia, UTI, and soft tissue infections.
- There is an inverse time correlation between the administration of broad-spectrum antibiotics and the chance for survival. The standard is to give antibiotics within 1 hour of arrival. However, 1 hour is a long time for a patient in septic shock, so the earlier the better.
- The airway must be secured if the patient is unable to do so by him/herself. Aggressive IV fluid resuscitation is key, together with the use of pressors and blood transfusion. Trend the central venous oxygen saturation ($ScvO_2$) and lactate to ensure good O_2 delivery to peripheral tissues.

TABLE 3-9. Criteria for the Diagnosis of SIRS[a]

VARIABLE	FINDING
Temperature	> 38°C (> 100.4°F) or < 36°C (< 96.8°F).
Heart rate	> 90/min.
Respiratory rate	> 20/min or a $Paco_2$ < 32 mm Hg.
WBC count	> 12,000/mm³, < 4000/mm³, or the presence of > 10% bands.

[a] To diagnose SIRS, at least 2 of the above criteria must be met.

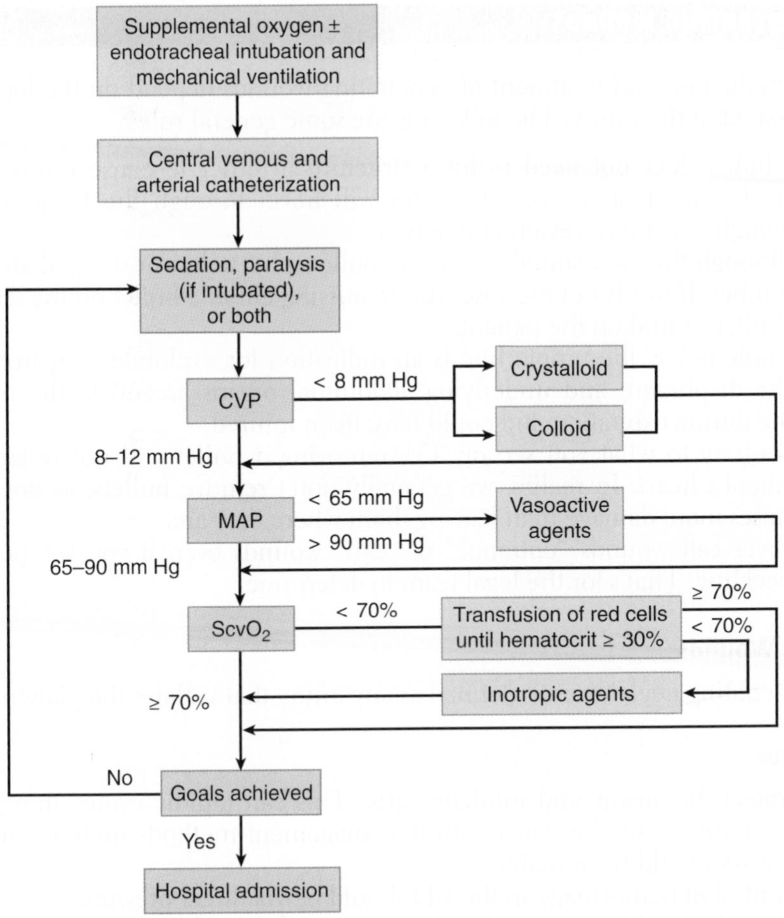

FIGURE 3-16. Early goal-directed therapy in septic shock. (Reproduced with permission from Tintinalli JE et al. *Tintinalli's Emergency Medicine: A Comprehensive Study Guide,* 7th ed. New York: McGraw-Hill, 2011, Fig. 146-3.)

Neurogenic Shock

Due to loss of vascular sympathetic tone, usually 2° to a high cervical spinal injury. Spinal anesthesia can also induce spinal shock.

Signs and Symptoms

- Hypotension; flat neck veins.
- Normal or slow pulse (no reflex tachycardia).
- Warm, dry skin.
- ↓ rectal tone; focal neurologic examination.

Treatment

- First rule out other etiologies of shock.
- Then proceed with IV fluid resuscitation and use vasoconstrictors.
- Give high-dose steroids in the form of a 30-mg/kg bolus of methylprednisolone, followed by 5.4 mg/kg/hr for 23 hours if steroids are initiated within 3 hours of injury, or for 47 hours if steroids are initiated 3–8 hours after injury. Note that steroids have not yet been shown to be of benefit in acute spinal injuries.

KEY FACT

Why should you leave impaled objects in place until a patient goes to the OR? They may be tamponading further blood loss.

KEY FACT

The liver and small bowel are the organs most frequently injured by penetrating trauma.

PENETRATING WOUNDS

The evaluation and treatment of penetrating wounds depend on the location and extent of the injury. The following are some general rules:

- A bullet does not need to hit a structure in order to cause injury. The shock wave that the bullet creates will travel through the tissue and is enough to rupture vessels and nerves.
- Although this may sound simplistic, bullets plus holes must equal an even number. If this is not the case, you're missing either a bullet on the scan or a bullet wound on the patient.
- A hole below the nipple line is an indication for exploratory laparotomy. The diaphragm and underlying abdominal organs ascend to the nipple line during expiration and could have been injured.
- Contrary to what you see on TV, removing a bullet will not restart the patient's heart. In reality, we generally don't remove bullets, as doing so causes more damage than leaving them where they are.
- Never call wounds "entrance" or "exit" wounds even if you see powder speckling. That's for the legal team to determine.

Neck Wounds

A penetrating neck injury is defined as any injury that violates the platysma.

Workup

- Protect the airway and intubate early. This can rapidly evolve into a difficult airway, so alternative airway management methods such as surgical airways should be available.
- Control of hemorrhage in the ED should be via direct pressure.
- Wounds should not be explored, as this may lead to bleeding in a tamponaded wound.
- **Surgery:** Indications for surgical exploration are as follows:
  - Zone 2 injury (between the clavicle and the mandible).
  - Hemodynamic instability despite resuscitation efforts.
  - An expanding hematoma.
  - Subcutaneous emphysema.
  - Tracheal deviation.
  - Voice changes.
- **Radiographic studies:** Films of the neck and a CXR should be ordered to evaluate for soft tissue hematoma, subcutaneous emphysema, and hemopneumothorax. CT imaging with angiography can also be performed in a stable patient to further assess for injury.

Treatment

The evaluation and management of a penetrating neck injury are dictated by zone (see Figure 3-17):

- **Zone 1:** May be evaluated with CT angiogram.
- **Zone 2:** If the platysma is penetrated, the patient should be taken to the OR for exploration. Alternatively, angiography and triple endoscopy can be done.
- **Zone 3:** May be evaluated with CT angiogram, tracheobronchoscopy, and esophagoscopy.

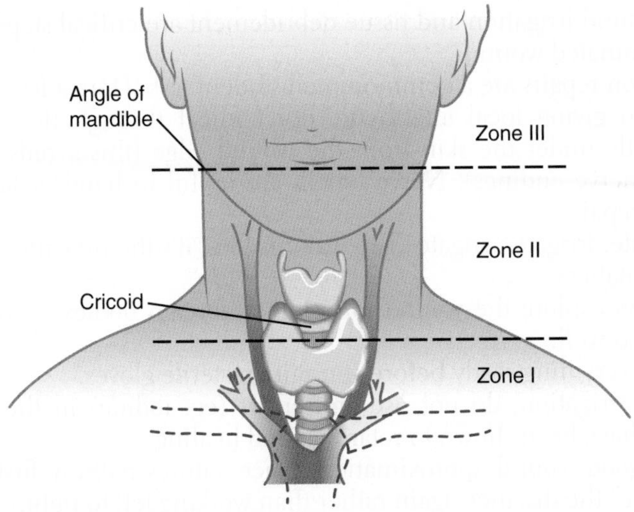

FIGURE 3-17. Zones of the neck. Note that what is commonly referred to as the neck is all zone II. (Reproduced with permission from Doherty GM. *Current Diagnosis & Treatment: Surgery,* 13th ed. New York: McGraw-Hill, 2010, Fig. 13-8.)

Chest Wounds

Workup

One must consider the possibility of aortic disruption, pneumothorax, hemothorax, cardiac tamponade, diaphragmatic tear, and esophageal injury in patients with penetrating thoracic injury.

Treatment

- Intubation and bilateral chest tubes are required for unstable patients with penetrating thoracic injuries.
- If the patient crashes, proceed with thoracotomy in the ED; otherwise it is best performed in the controlled setting of an operating suite.

> **KEY FACT**
>
> If a previously stable chest trauma patient suddenly dies, suspect an air embolism.

Abdominal Wounds

Workup/Treatment

- If the patient is hemodynamically stable with stab wounds or blunt trauma, obtain a CT scan or FAST imaging.
- Otherwise, immediate exploratory laparotomy is indicated for the following:
  - Gunshot wounds
  - Removal of impaled instruments
  - Diaphragmatic injury (known or suspected)
  - Free air in the abdomen

> **KEY FACT**
>
> The spleen is the most commonly injured organ in blunt abdominal trauma. Be suspicious of this if you see left lower rib fractures.

Musculoskeletal Injury

Workup/Treatment

- Check distal perfusion (pulse, capillary refill), sensation, and motor functions both before **and** after treating the patient. Avoid the mistake of anesthetizing first and then trying to assess sensation.
- Give tetanus vaccine if the patient does not know his or her vaccination history or if the last tetanus shot was > 5 years ago.
- Bite wounds are generally not closed (high risk for wound infection).

KEY FACT

When it comes to cleaning a laceration, the only solution to pollution is dilution (irrigate, irrigate, irrigate).

KEY FACT

What does a med student have in common with a sailboat? Top speed is 6 knots/hour.

- Early wound irrigation and tissue debridement are critical steps in treating a contaminated wound.
- Laceration repairs are a common med-student task. Here a few pointers:
  - When giving local anesthetic, don't inject through the skin but go directly under the skin from the wound edge (this avoids the epidermal nerve endings). Nerve blocks are useful in hand or facial laceration repair.
  - Irrigate, irrigate, irrigate. Tap water is fine; it's the pressure of irrigation that matters.
  - Always explore the wound for retained foreign bodies; x-rays can help here as well.
  - Get everything ready **before** you put on sterile gloves.
  - After irrigation, do not use antiseptics (eg, iodine) in the wound, as they have been shown to retard wound healing.
  - For good wound approximation, place sutures halfway first, and then "halve" the distance again rather than working left to right.
  - Pull the sutures tight enough that the wound edges rise up a bit (evert) when they meet. Scar tissue contracts and will even it out.

Common Clerkship Topics

The following is a list of core topics that you are likely to encounter in the course of your EM rotation and on a shelf examination.

- **Allergy, immunology, dermatology:**
  - Anaphylaxis
  - Necrotizing fasciitis
  - Erythema multiforme
  - Stevens-Johnson syndrome
  - Urticaria
- **Cardiovascular:**
  - Abdominal aortic aneurysm (see Surgery)
  - Acute coronary syndrome
  - Aortic dissection
  - Arrhythmia
    - Asystole
    - Atrial fibrillation (see Internal Medicine)
    - Ventricular fibrillation
    - Ventricular tachycardia
  - Cardiac tamponade
  - Congestive heart failure (see Internal Medicine)
  - Hypertensive urgency/emergency
- **Gastrointestinal:**
  - Appendicitis
  - Cholecystitis (see Surgery)
  - Cholelithiasis (see Surgery)
  - Hernia (see Surgery)
  - Obstruction (see Surgery)
- **Genitourinary:**
  - Abnormal uterine bleeding (see Gynecology)
  - Ectopic pregnancy
  - Epididymitis
  - Fournier gangrene
  - Pelvic inflammatory disease (see Gynecology)
  - Sexually transmitted infections (see Gynecology)

  - Testicular torsion
  - Urinary obstruction
  - Urinary tract infection
- **Neurology:**
  - Headaches (see Neurology)
  - Intracranial hemorrhage
    - Subarachnoid hemorrhage
    - Epidural hematoma
    - Subdural hematoma
    - Intraparenchymal hemorrhage
  - Neuroleptic malignant syndrome
  - Status epilepticus
  - Stroke (see Neurology)
    - Hemorrhagic
    - Ischemic
    - Transient ischemic attack
  - Temporal arteritis
- **Respiratory:**
  - Asthma
  - Hemothorax
  - Pneumothorax
    - Tension pneumothorax
    - Communicating pneumothorax (sucking chest wound)
  - Flail chest
  - Pulmonary embolism
- **Toxicology:**
  - Common toxidromes
  - Drug overdose/antidotes
  - Drug withdrawal
- **Trauma and shock:**
  - Resuscitation
  - Burns
  - Hypothermia
  - Shock
    - Hypovolemic shock
    - Cardiogenic shock
    - Septic shock
    - Neurogenic shock
  - Penetrating wounds
    - Neck wounds
    - Chest wounds
    - Abdominal wounds
  - Musculoskeletal injury

CHAPTER 4

INTERNAL MEDICINE

Ward Tips

The internal medicine clerkship, which usually lasts from 8 to 12 weeks, will expose you to a wide variety of disciplines, including cardiology, pulmonology, gastroenterology, endocrinology, nephrology, rheumatology, hematology, oncology, and infectious disease. Both outpatient and inpatient settings are significant to these disciplines. Given the broad scope of internal medicine, this clerkship will provide you with a strong foundation for your other rotations when done early—and when done later, it will help support your existing fund of knowledge.

KEY FACT

Internal medicine addresses clinical issues practitioners face in all specialties.

WHO ARE THE PLAYERS?

Attendings. Consisting of clinical and academic faculty, the attendings are in charge of the ward team and are ultimately responsible for patient care. Attendings are also the source of most of the didactic learning that takes place during attending rounds. Your interaction with attendings will consist primarily of making formal patient presentations in attending rounds and participating in didactic teaching. For this reason, it is crucial that you read up on your patients' problems before attending rounds, especially if you will be presenting a patient.

Residents. Since residents are at least a year ahead of interns, they supervise the ward team and help formulate patients' treatment plans. Residents also serve as a major teaching resource, dispensing clinical pearls on work rounds and bringing in pertinent review articles. Your interaction with the resident will vary depending on his or her style; some residents remain aloof and primarily answer questions, while others are more proactive, giving informal lectures and taking you to patients' bedsides to teach physical findings. Also remember that residents may "pimp" as a means of teaching and assessing your knowledge base. Some may even take the time to give you organized lectures or quote recent trials or studies that are pertinent to patients assigned to the team.

Interns. Interns are the cogs that make the hospital machinery move by providing the bulk of primary patient care. Given that he or she will co-follow your patients, you will probably interact more with your intern than with any other member of your team. For this reason, any questions or management issues you might have with regard to your patients should initially be directed toward the intern. Remember, too, that interns were recently medical students themselves, so they can be an invaluable source of practical information and survival tips. You can use them for feedback on your progress notes and presentation style.

KEY FACT

Try to consult with your intern before rounds to formulate a plan.

Support staff. The medicine team receives additional help from nurses, pharmacists, case managers, social workers, and members of the allied health professions, all of whom may also participate in team rounds. It is critical to maintain positive, respectful working relationships with these staff members. When you are swamped with work or are not sure how to accomplish a task, they can be lifesavers. The pharmacist associated with the team is an excellent source of information regarding medications and dosages to be administered, and he or she can also provide information about what is or is not on the hospital formulary. The case manager and social worker are outstanding resources when it comes to handling the difficult psychosocial issues or needs of your patients.

HOW IS THE DAY SET UP?

Although schedules vary by school and setting, the typical day on a medicine rotation starts at 6:30–7:00 A.M. and usually runs until 4:00–5:00 P.M. on non-call days. Prerounds are usually followed by team rounds and/or attending rounds. Sometimes only new patients are seen with the full team. Morning rounds are then followed by "work time" or the "hour of power." The noon or afternoon conference may be followed by additional work time, teaching sessions, or student lectures. Refer to Chapter 1 for more detail about the daily schedule.

WHAT DO I DO DURING PREROUNDS?

Please refer to "The Schedule—Medicine Wards" in Chapter 1.

HOW DO I EXCEL IN MEDICINE?

Simply learning the material well does not necessarily correlate with doing well on the internal medicine clerkship. You must also push yourself to learn as much about your patient as you can; go beyond your comfort zone to formulate sophisticated differential diagnoses and treatment plans; and strive to learn how to fit in with the different personalities on your team. The following tips should help clarify goals to work toward:

- **Know your patient.** You should know the latest clinical information on your patient, whether it is the most recent lab values, the planned studies of the day, or simply how the patient is feeling. You should then relay this information to the intern so that management plans can be modified accordingly. You should also be sure to keep on top of consults and tests you have ordered. Speak with the consulting service about their recommendations, as consultants can give you valuable information and may even have time to give you short tutorials on your patients' disease processes. Another important part of knowing your patient lies in a daily check of the medication administration record (MAR). This check will allow you to ensure that the antibiotics you ordered were actually administered (which is not always the case) as well as to gauge whether a patient is receiving symptomatic relief. For example, is the patient's pain well controlled, or is he or she asking for additional pain medication? You should also be aware of a patient's social situation so that you can keep the family up to date regarding his or her progress. Finally, be aware of special circumstances to be considered on discharge (eg, getting a hotel room or transportation for a homeless patient).
- **Develop a differential.** The search for the etiology of a patient's problem begins with knowing the differential diagnosis. Therefore, a critical goal of this rotation is to learn the basic differentials of common signs and symptoms. The differential can often be broken down into 3 groups: common etiologies, uncommon etiologies, and etiologies you don't want to miss (because they're either highly treatable or life threatening). Mastering the differentials of common problems will serve you well in any specialty.

> **KEY FACT**
>
> You cannot diagnose what is not in your differential diagnosis.

- **Care about your patients.** Perhaps the single most important thing you can do on any rotation is remain genuinely concerned about your patients. Nothing will elicit more respect from your faculty and team. Don't leave if important work remains to be done or if your patient is crashing.
- **Get along with your team.** It is important to remember that you are part of a team. Although you may be relatively low in the hierarchy, bear in mind that you still have an integral role to play. Also remember that medi-

cal students who make life easier for the team through diligent and efficient work will ultimately be rewarded in their evaluations. It is therefore important that you remain personable and enthusiastic at all times so as to ensure that your team members can work as a cohesive unit. By contrast, encouraging open conflict with others on your team should be avoided at all costs. If you feel uncomfortable with another team member or sense a personality problem developing, it is vital that you do whatever you can to avert a conflict. This may include directly addressing the issue either with the team member in question or with your clerkship director (or whoever else may be in charge of the rotation). Serious rifts within the team are uncommon, but when they do arise, they can have a devastating effect on patient care, team morale, and, ultimately, your development.

- **Be early.** Never underestimate the importance of punctuality. Attendings and residents probably won't take notice when you show up on time, but they are certain to remember if you walk in late.
- **Work independently.** The easier you make your intern's life, the more he or she will appreciate your effort. If you can call the consults, order the lab tests, collect lab and radiology results, and determine if the patient is comfortable, you will go a long way. Expect to be dependent on others at first; this is perfectly normal. But as you gain more experience, you will feel the desire—and have the confidence—to work more independently.
- **Read, read, read.** Keep both a pocket manual and a more complete reference available. Try to read about your patients and their major issues. This will assist you in formulating a plan, save you when the pimping starts, and help you pose intelligent questions. Performing searches for current literature and reading hallmark papers may also be important; you will have to gauge how much you can do in relation to the time constraints you face.
- **Ask for feedback.** Midway through the rotation, ask your attending and resident to set aside some time so that they can give you feedback. "You're doing fine" is **not** a useful response. Be persistent and ask about your weaknesses. This will help you identify areas in which you need improvement while also making your attending and resident aware that you are a responsible student. They may ask you how you think you are doing, so be prepared to explain what you are doing well and in which areas you are trying to improve.

KEY FACT

Remember why you decided to go to medical school in the first place. This is not a 9-to-5 job!

KEY FACT

You should know the latest clinical information on your patient.

If you are sincerely interested in pursuing a career in internal medicine, you will need to take some additional steps. First, let the members of your team know of your interests. If you do so, they may make a special effort to teach and help you. Do not lie, as insincerity is easily detected and is definitely frowned on. Second, the status of your attending becomes crucial; try to schedule (with the help of the course scheduler) at least 1 block of your clerkship with a senior or well-known attending. In a residency application, the person who writes your letter of recommendation can be almost as important as what is actually said about you. Doing well will help ensure a good letter of recommendation from a senior faculty member.

PRESENTATIONS

Work rounds. Presentations during work rounds consist of an oral version of your **SOAP note** (see mnemonic). During these presentations, the team will focus on brevity and efficiency, with emphasis on the assessment and plan (A&P). A well-thought-out A&P takes extra time during prerounds, so start early and discuss your ideas with your intern. Do not be discouraged, however, if your A&P is occasionally in error; remember that you are there to learn, and bear in mind that the team will appreciate the fact that you are trying. In the final analysis, it is better to come up with a well-thought-out plan that is incorrect than to simply say "I don't know" when you are asked about your next move in patient management.

Attending rounds. This is your time in the spotlight, when you really need to shine. So remember that your attending will probably want a lengthier formal oral presentation than the ones you give on work rounds. Also keep in mind that while attendings will primarily want to learn about your patient, they will also be observing your presentation style and will note how well you understand your patient's problems. One key means of demonstrating your knowledge is to include pertinent positives and negatives relating to your patient's condition. This may be difficult at first, especially since it requires an understanding of the presentation of the other possibilities in the differential. Bear in mind, however, that it is okay if you omit something from the history, since the attending will simply ask for additional information if it is important. Don't panic if your attending asks you several additional questions about your patient; instead, make a mental note of the specific tidbits your attending likes to hear so that you can include them in your next presentation. You should also make sure you understand why the attending considers certain pertinent positives or negatives to be relevant to your patient.

Remember, too, that your attending's comments weigh in your final grade. Formal oral patient presentations constitute a large part of how the attending perceives you, so you will want to shine in this arena. Ask the attending how he or she would like you to present the patient. Practice your presentation before attending rounds, even running it by your intern for feedback.

MNEMONIC

SOAP note:

Subjective
Objective
Assessment
Plan

KEY NOTES

Admission notes and SOAP notes are key to your medicine rotation. Please review the sample notes in Chapter 1.

KEY PROCEDURES

Explanations for the basic procedures that follow can be found in any pocket ward manual:

- ❑ Phlebotomy
- ❑ IV line placement
- ❑ Arterial blood gas draw
- ❑ Foley catheter placement

Your resident may also allow you to perform the following advanced procedures on your patient:

- ❑ Thoracentesis
- ❑ Paracentesis
- ❑ Lumbar puncture
- ❑ Musculoskeletal injection
- ❑ Arterial line placement (if in the ICU)

WHAT DO I CARRY IN MY POCKETS?

- ❑ Stethoscope
- ❑ Reflex hammer
- ❑ Patient-tracking smartphone apps and/or index cards and/or patient summary sheets (for recording history, vital signs, and tests)
- ❑ Normal-lab-value reference card
- ❑ Current pharmacopoeia and antibiotic guide (pocketbook or smartphone apps)
- ❑ Penlight

High-Yield Clinical Topic Checklist

Read about these topics before you start the rotation. Most are discussed in this chapter. A full list of common clerkship topics can be found at the end of this chapter.

- ❑ Congestive heart failure
- ❑ Chest pain
- ❑ Hypertension
- ❑ Chronic obstructive pulmonary disease
- ❑ Acute renal failure
- ❑ Abdominal pain
- ❑ Anemia
- ❑ Diabetes
- ❑ Fever of unknown origin
- ❑ Systemic lupus

Cardiology

ATRIAL FIBRILLATION (AF)

AF is the most common arrhythmia besides sinus tachycardia. It is an irregularly irregular rhythm (ie, irregular RR intervals on ECG) that is marked by the absence of P waves prior to each QRS complex. The atrial rate is 400–600 bpm (but there is no organized depolarization of the atria) and induces an irregularly irregular ventricular response rate of 80–160 bpm. AF may be idiopathic, especially in younger patients, but other etiologies are summarized in the mnemonic **PIRATES.** Pertinent epidemiologic data are as follows:

- The risk of developing AF doubles with each decade over the age of 55. By age 80, the prevalence of AF approaches 10%.
- The Framingham Heart Study showed that patients with AF have an ↑ risk of cardiovascular mortality as well as a 3- to 13-fold ↑ in the risk of embolic stroke.

MNEMONIC

Etiologies of AF–

PIRATES

Pulmonary (COPD, pulmonary embolism), **P**heochromocytoma (very rare), **P**ericarditis
Ischemic heart disease and hypertension
Rheumatic heart disease
Anemia, **A**trial myxoma (rare)
Thyrotoxicosis, hypo**T**hyroidism
Ethanol ("holiday heart") and cocaine
Sepsis (especially postoperative)

SIGNS AND SYMPTOMS

- The clinical presentation of AF can vary from asymptomatic to severely symptomatic. Signs and symptoms include the following:
  - Fatigue (most common).
  - Tachypnea, dyspnea.
  - Palpitations, "skipped beats," "racing heart," angina.
  - Lightheadedness, syncope (rare), or alterations in cognitive function (TIAs or stroke).

- A classic irregularly irregular rhythm will be palpated on physical examination. Irregular heartbeats of varying intensity can be heard on cardiac auscultation.

Differential

Paroxysmal atrial contractions, paroxysmal ventricular contractions, multifocal atrial tachycardia, atrial flutter with variable AV conduction.

Workup

- ECG shows a narrow-complex rhythm (QRS < 120 msec), variable RR intervals, and irregular or absent P waves (see Figure 4-1).
- Echocardiogram may show a thrombus in the left atrium but more often will show a dilated left atrium.
- Consider checking TSH levels (hyperthyroidism is a reversible cause of AF).
- Baseline coagulation studies (INR/aPTT) are usually performed prior to the initiation of anticoagulation therapy (determined by the CHADS2 score for those with nonvalvular AF; see Table 4-1).

KEY FACT

A normal echocardiogram (transthoracic, or TTE) has low sensitivity for identifying thrombi. A transesophageal echocardiogram (TEE) is preferred, as it affords better visualization of the left atrial appendage, where thrombi most commonly form.

Treatment

- In those with **new or recent-onset AF** who are **hemodynamically compromised** (as indicated by low blood pressure), emergent cardioversion may be needed.
- **Chronic stable AF: Control ventricular rate** with β-blockers (eg, metoprolol) or with calcium channel blockers (CCBs, eg, diltiazem) to ensure adequate ventricular filling and to maximize cardiac output and **anticoagulate.**
- **Rate vs. rhythm control:**
  - The AFFIRM study, which targeted patients > 65 years of age or with other risk factors for stroke or death, found that rate control and rhythm control were no different for endpoints that included mortality and stroke, with fewer adverse effects observed in the rate control group. Thus, **rate control is now the preferred method** in hemodynamically stable patients.
  - Data from the recent RACE II trial revealed that rate control to a **resting heart rate of < 110 bpm** was as effective as stricter rate control to < 80 bpm.
- **Anticoagulation:** AF ↑ the risk of thromboembolic strokes. This risk is approximately 5% per year in nonvalvular AF and is even higher in valvu-

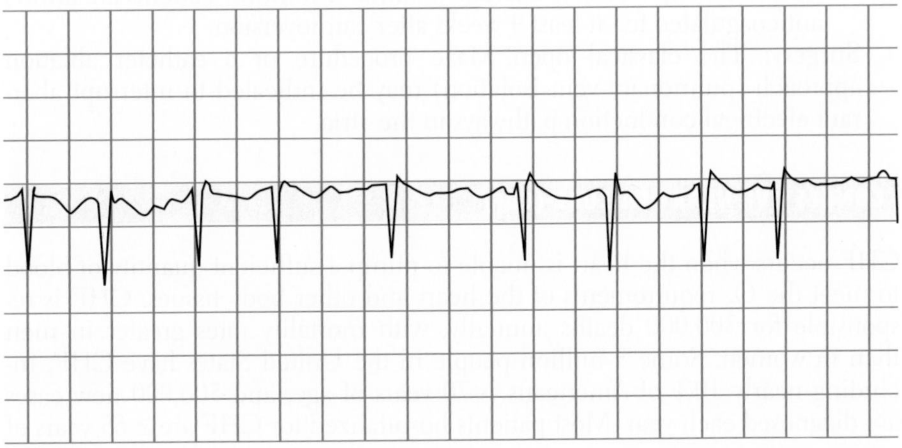

FIGURE 4-1. Atrial fibrillation in V_1. Note the absence of P waves and the irregularly irregular rhythm.

TABLE 4-1. CHADS2 Stroke Risk Score for Patients with Nonvalvular AF

CRITERION	POINTS[a, b]
CHF	1
Hypertension (treated or untreated)	1
Age ≥ 75	1
Diabetes mellitus (DM)	1
Previous stroke or TIA	2

[a] Patients with a total score of 0 are considered low risk for stroke, 1–2 intermediate risk, and > 3 high risk.

[b] Patients with a score ≥ 2 should be anticoagulated with warfarin unless there is a significant contraindication. Those with valvular AF or prior strokes/TIA should also be anticoagulated provided that there are no significant contraindications.

lar AF. The CHADS2 score (see Table 4-1) helps predict the risk of stroke and facilitates the selection of an anticoagulant that will ↓ such risk.
- A CHADS2 score of 0 = ASA. A score of 1 = ASA or warfarin. A score > 2 = warfarin. Stroke risk ↓ by ~ 70% with warfarin administration and by ~ 20% with ASA use compared to placebo. The goal INR is 2–3 with warfarin administration. In deciding which medication to use, one should weigh the benefit of reducing thromboembolic events against the potential bleeding risk.
- New agents that may be used in place of warfarin include direct thrombin inhibitors (eg, dabigatran) and factor Xa inhibitors (eg, apixaban, rivaroxaban). The advantage of these agents is that INR does not have to be measured; their downside lies in the inability to quickly reverse anticoagulation.

- **Cardioversion:**
  - Consider pharmacologic cardioversion (eg, Class III agents such as amiodarone or Class Ia and Ic agents such as procainamide or propafenone) or electrocardioversion to sinus rhythm if this is the first episode of AF or if the patient is refractory to treatment.
  - If the arrhythmia has been present for > 48 hours, the patient must either be anticoagulated with warfarin for 3–4 weeks before cardioversion or undergo TEE to exclude an atrial thrombus. Patients are always anticoagulated for at least 4 weeks after cardioversion.
- **Surgery:** The classical open Maze procedure or a catheter ablation approach (pulmonary vein isolation) may be indicated to interrupt aberrant electrical conduction pathways in the atria.

CONGESTIVE HEART FAILURE (CHF)

KEY FACT

It is important to distinguish systolic from diastolic dysfunction because CHF treatment often depends on the 1° mode of failure. However, both can coexist in the same patient.

CHF occurs when the heart is unable to pump a sufficient quantity of blood to meet the O_2 requirements of the heart and other body tissues. CHF is responsible for 300,000 deaths annually, with mortality rates greater in men than in women. Some 5 million people in the United States have CHF, including nearly 10% of Americans > 70 years of age, and 500,000 new cases are diagnosed each year. Most patients hospitalized for CHF are ≥ 65 years of age.

- Risk factors for developing CHF include MI, hypertension, valvular heart disease (eg, mitral stenosis, endocarditis), pericardial disease, cardiomyopathy, AIDS, alcohol abuse, pulmonary hypertension, and, most commonly, chronic ischemic heart disease.
- CHF can be traced to problems in systolic or diastolic phases (see also Table 4-2).
  - **Systolic dysfunction:** An ejection fraction (EF) < 40% leads to ↑ preload with ↑ left ventricular end-diastolic pressure (LVEDP) in a vain attempt to ↑ systolic contractility and cardiac output. Poor organ perfusion leads to a variety of compensatory mechanisms that are only temporarily effective and eventually result in ↑ myocardial work. In patients with CAD, this ↑ work can lead to cardiac hypertrophy and ventricular dilation and may even precipitate an MI.
  - **Diastolic dysfunction:** ↓ left ventricular compliance with normal contractile function. The ventricle is either unable to relax or unable to passively fill properly (↑ stiffness, ↓ recoil, concentric hypertrophy). There is an ↑ LVEDP, but with normal contractile function; cardiac output remains essentially normal, and the EF is either normal or slightly ↑.

TABLE 4-2. Pathophysiologic Basis of CHF

Etiology	Related Condition
Systolic Dysfunction	
↓ contractility	**Ischemic heart disease:** The most common cause of systolic dysfunction. **Dilated cardiomyopathy:** ↓ contractile functioning in the absence of pressure or volume overload. May be idiopathic or 2°—eg, a drug effect (ethanol, cocaine, heroin, doxorubicin); postmyocarditis; postpartum; or related to HIV, Chagas' disease, anemia, thiamine deficiency, or thyrotoxicosis. **Hypertensive burnout or valvular heart disease:** Both initially cause **diastolic** dysfunction, but after myofibrils stretch, the EF falls, and **systolic** dysfunction results. ↑ **chamber radius** (eg, ventricular dilation due to aortic insufficiency/regurgitation).
↑ afterload	↑ systolic pressure (eg, hypertension); ↑ pumping pressure (eg, aortic stenosis).
Diastolic Dysfunction	
Abnormal active relaxation	**Ischemia.** **Hypertrophic cardiomyopathy:** Due to disorders causing LVH (eg, hypertension, aortic stenosis, hypertrophic obstructive cardiomyopathy [HOCM]).
Abnormal passive filling	**Restrictive cardiomyopathy:** May be idiopathic or due to infiltrative disorders (eg, sarcoidosis, amyloidosis, scleroderma, hemochromatosis, glycogen storage disease) that ↑ ventricular stiffness. The least common cardiomyopathy.

MNEMONIC

CHF exacerbation in previously stable patients—

FAILURE

Forgot medication
Arrhythmia, **A**nemia
Ischemia, **I**nfarction, **I**nfection
Lifestyle (eg, excessive sodium intake, the most common cause)
"**U**pregulation" (↑ cardiac output—eg, pregnancy, hyperthyroidism)
Renal failure with fluid overload
Embolus (pulmonary)

Q

A 75-year-old man presents with worsening shortness of breath, chronic cough, and swollen legs. He is diaphoretic and has an S3, a laterally displaced PMI, cool extremities, and pitting edema to the calves bilaterally. Which critical tests should be run, and what results can be expected?

KEY POINT

ASSESSMENT OF CHF PROGRESSION

- **New York Heart Association (NYHA) functional classification for CHF:**
  - **Class I:** No limitation of activities; no symptoms with normal activities.
  - **Class II:** Slight limitation of activities; patients are comfortable at rest or with mild exertion.
  - **Class III:** Marked limitation of activities; patients are comfortable only at rest.
  - **Class IV:** Patients are confined to complete rest in a bed or chair, as any physical activity brings on discomfort; symptoms are present at rest.
- **Heart failure staging by American College of Cardiology (ACC)/American Heart Association (AHA) Guidelines (2005):**
  - **Stage A:** High risk for developing heart failure, but no structural heart disorder is present. Includes patients with hypertension, CAD, and diabetes. Suggest lifestyle modification (smoking cessation, regular exercise, cessation of alcohol or illicit drug intake), antihypertensive medication, correction of dyslipidemias, and ACEIs/ARBs in appropriate patients (eg, diabetics, those with peripheral vascular disease).
  - **Stage B:** No symptoms of heart failure, but a structural disorder of the heart is present. Includes patients with a history of MI, LVH, low EF, or asymptomatic valvular disease. Treat with ACEIs/ARBs and β-blockers.
  - **Stage C:** Prior or current symptoms of heart failure associated with underlying structural heart disease. Treat with the full range of heart failure drugs (ACEIs/ARBs, β-blockers, and diuretics) and sodium restriction.
  - **Stage D:** Refractory heart failure requiring specialized interventions, such as mechanical circulatory support, continuous inotropes, cardiac transplantation, or hospice care.

Signs and Symptoms

See Table 4-3 for a description of the early and late symptoms of both left-sided and right-sided failure.

Differential

- **Cardiac:** Acute MI, myocarditis, high-output heart failure.
- **Pulmonary:** Pulmonary embolism (PE), pneumonia.

Workup

- **Determine the underlying cause:** CBC, BUN/creatinine, and TSH can rule out severe anemia, renal failure, and thyrotoxicosis, respectively. Obtain an ECG to evaluate for ischemia.
- **Assess severity:**
  - The physical examination is key.
  - CXR (see Figure 4-2) may show cardiomegaly and pulmonary vascular congestion (dilated vessels, interstitial or alveolar edema, Kerley-B lines).
  - Echocardiography provides information on the size and function (eg, the EF) of both ventricles and valves and can also pinpoint an underly-

KEY FACT

An S3 heart sound is present with systolic dysfunction. An S4 is present with hypertension, CAD, and diastolic dysfunction.

A

An ECG may reveal AF or ischemic heart disease; BNP will likely be elevated; and CXR may reveal cardiomegaly, pulmonary vascular congestion (Kerley B lines, cephalization), and/or pleural effusion.

TABLE 4-3. Clinical Presentation of Heart Failure

Type	Early Signs and Symptoms	Late Signs and Symptoms
Left-sided failure	Dyspnea on exertion (DOE) ↓ exercise tolerance	Orthopnea Dyspnea at rest Paroxysmal nocturnal dyspnea Chronic cough Nocturia Pulmonary congestion (crackles, pleural effusion, cardiac wheeze) Tachypnea Diaphoresis Cool extremities Laterally displaced PMI
Right-sided failure	Anorexia (from hepatic congestion) Cyanosis Fatigue Elevated JVP Pulsatile hepatomegaly Peripheral edema	Ascites and ⊕ hepatojugular reflex
Both	Ventricular heave Tachycardia AF Additional heart sounds (S3, S4)	Same

ing cause (eg, ischemia [segmental wall motion abnormalities], valvular disease).

- If concurrent MI is suspected, cardiac catheterization may be indicated.
- ↑ BNP can be used to distinguish dyspnea due to heart failure from other causes of dyspnea.

KEY FACT

The most common cause of right-sided heart failure is left-sided heart failure.

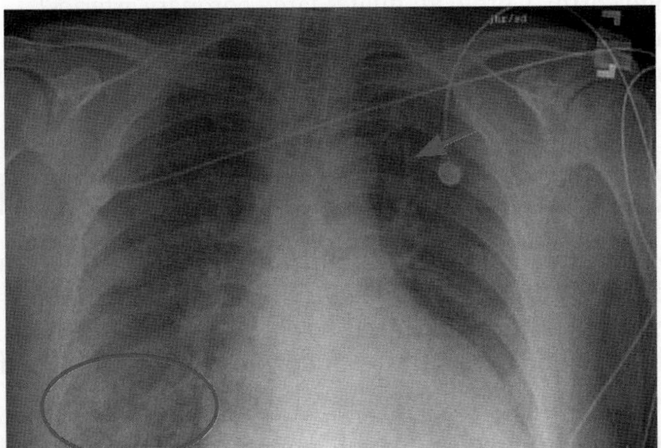

FIGURE 4-2. CXR with evidence of CHF. Frontal CXR demonstrates marked cardiomegaly, engorgement of vessels (arrow), interstitial edema (circle), and left-sided pleural effusion that raise concern for CHF. (Reproduced with permission from Tintinalli JE et al. *Tintinalli's Emergency Medicine: A Comprehensive Study Guide,* 7th ed. New York: McGraw-Hill, 2011, Fig. 57-1.)

KEY POINT

CHF TREATMENT: KEY TRIALS AND OUTCOMES

- **SOLVD trial:** ACEIs (eg, enalapril) were found to ↓ mortality and hospitalization in patients with class II–IV CHF.
- **CHARM trial:** The effect of ARBs on hospitalization and cardiovascular mortality was found to be similar to that of ACEIs.
- **CONSENSUS trial:** In patients with class IV CHF, there was an overall reduction in mortality (27%), NYHA classification (symptoms), heart size, and CHF medication requirement in the enalapril group compared to controls.
- **RALES trial:** Spironolactone ↓ mortality in patients with class III and IV CHF by 30% when given with ACEIs or diuretics +/– digoxin.
- **EPHESUS trial:** Eplerenone was found to confer benefits similar to those of spironolactone along with a ↓ incidence of gynecomastia or impotence.
- **DIG trial:** Digoxin was found to yield symptomatic relief in CHF but had no significant effect on mortality and may ↑ mortality in women.

KEY FACT

Pulmonary congestion in diastolic dysfunction is caused by ↑ hydrostatic pressure. Activation of the renin-angiotensin-aldosterone system is usually not prominent.

- Systems for assessing CHF progression include the NYHA and ACC classifications (see above).

Treatment

- **Systolic dysfunction:**
  - ACEIs, β-blockers (carvedilol, metoprolol succinate), and diuretics are the cornerstones of treatment.
  - Antiarrhythmics (eg, amiodarone) with anticoagulants (eg, warfarin) may be recommended when an arrhythmia is present.
- **Diastolic dysfunction:** Treatment aims to restore the heart's original relaxing and filling properties. Control of hypertension is paramount. Options are as follows:
  - **Diuretics:** ↓ afterload.
  - **CCBs:** Induce bradycardia and facilitate myocardial relaxation.
  - **β-blockers:** Induce mild bradycardia and inhibit coronary remodeling.
  - **Nitroglycerin:** ↓ preload; dilates large coronary arteries.
  - **Antiarrhythmics** should also be used if indicated.
- Nonpharmacologic interventions include weight loss, sodium restriction (< 2 g/day), and fluid restriction (< 1.5 L/day).

KEY FACT

Risk factors for essential (1°) hypertension:

- Age
- DM
- Obesity
- Family history
- Diet (salt, fat, alcohol intake)
- Lifestyle (inactivity, stress)
- Major depression
- Ethnicity—African American > Caucasian = Hispanic > Asian

HYPERTENSION

Hypertension is common in both ambulatory and inpatient internal medicine settings, affecting 50 million patients in the United States and > 40% of all men and women > 65 years of age. It has been estimated that up to one-third of those with high blood pressure go undiagnosed owing to the often "silent," asymptomatic nature of the disease. May be 1° or 2°:

- **1° hypertension:** Some 95% of hypertension cases are 1° ("essential"), which signifies that they have no identifiable 2° cause but have clear, identifiable risk factors.
- **2° hypertension:** The remainder of cases have a 2° cause that is important to diagnose in order to properly treat and potentially cure.

DIFFERENTIAL

The differential diagnosis of 2° hypertension includes the following:

- **Renal:** Renovascular disease (eg, renal artery stenosis from fibromuscular dysplasia in young women, atherosclerotic disease), renal parenchymal disease (polycystic kidney disease, renal cell carcinoma).
- **Drug effects:** OCPs, corticosteroids, COX-2 inhibitors, amphetamines, epoetin alfa (Epogen), lead poisoning.
- **Endocrine disorders:** Cushing's syndrome, hyperaldosteronism, pheochromocytoma, hyperthyroidism, hyperparathyroidism, polycystic ovarian syndrome, acromegaly.
- **Pregnancy:** Gestational hypertension, preeclampsia.
- **Other:** Aortic coarctation, obstructive sleep apnea.

> **MNEMONIC**
>
> ***2° causes of hypertension—***
>
> **Running Doesn't Elevate Our Pressure**
>
> **R**enal
> **D**rugs
> **E**ndocrine
> **O**ther
> **P**regnancy

WORKUP

- Diagnosis is based on the mean of 2 or more seated readings on each of 3 or more encounters. The diagnosis is valid if patients are > 18 years of age, have no acute illness, and have no 2° causes (eg, diabetes, renal failure). See Table 4-4 for the stratification of disease severity.
- The goal of workup is to identify modifiable cardiovascular risk factors; to reveal 2° causes of hypertension (consider if the patient is < 20 or > 50 years of age, has sudden-onset or severe hypertension, has hypertension that is refractory to treatment, or has a suggestive H&P); and to assess for target-organ damage.
- Physical examination should focus on funduscopic, cardiac (listen for murmurs; look for signs of LVH such as left ventricular heave or an S4), vascular, abdominal (pulsatile masses, bruits), and neurologic (TIA/CVA) factors.
- An ECG may also be used to find evidence of LVH.

TREATMENT

- Tables 4-4 and 4-5 outline basic treatment guidelines from the Seventh Report of the Joint National Committee on Prevention, Detection, Evaluation, and Treatment of High Blood Pressure (commonly referred to as the "JNC 7") for patients with classic and complicated hypertension. The goal is to reach a BP < 140/90 mm Hg (unless the patent has diabetes or renal disease, in which case the goal is < 130/80 mm Hg).
- Lifestyle modifications are recommended for all patients and include weight loss, smoking cessation, sodium restriction (≤ 2.6 g/day), exercise, limited alcohol consumption (≤ 2 drinks/day in men; ≤ 1 drink/day in women), and eating a diet high in fruits and vegetables and limited in saturated fat.

TABLE 4-4. Blood Pressure Classification

CLASSIFICATION	SYSTOLIC (mm Hg)	DIASTOLIC (mm Hg)	THERAPEUTIC RECOMMENDATION
Normal	< 120	< 80	–
Prehypertension	120–139	80–89	Lifestyle modification.
Stage I hypertension	140–159	90–99	Thiazide diuretics are first-line treatment.
Stage II hypertension	> 159	> 99	Two-drug combination.

TABLE 4-5. Hypertension Management

Clinical History	Recommendations
Heart failure	Diuretics, β-blockers, ACEIs/ARBs, aldosterone antagonists.
Post-MI	β-blockers, ACEIs, aldosterone antagonists.
High risk for CAD	Diuretics, β-blockers, ACEIs, CCBs.
DM	Diuretics, β-blockers, ACEIs/ARBs, CCBs.
Chronic renal failure	ACEIs/ARBs.
CVA/stroke	Diuretics, ACEIs.
Osteoporosis	Thiazide diuretics.
BPH	α-blockers.

KEY FACT

CCBs are not always first-line treatment for women because the Women's Health Initiative study found that they significantly ↑ the risk of cardiovascular mortality in female patients.

- Thiazide diuretics are effective as first-line therapy for hypertension.
- African Americans may have ↓ nitric oxide levels and may be more sensitive to a high-salt diet than other groups. African American patients should be treated with at least 2 medications if systolic or diastolic BP remains ↑ by > 15 mm Hg.
- Patients with stage II hypertension (≥ 160 mm Hg systolic or ≥ 100 mm Hg diastolic) will likely need a 2-drug combination.
- CCB therapy (amlodipine) +/– ACEIs (perindopril) ↓ the risk of stroke and heart attack in comparison to β-blockers +/– thiazide.

Complications

- **Neurologic:** TIA/CVA, ruptured aneurysms.
- **Retinopathy:** Arteriosclerotic narrowing, AV nicking, ischemic changes ("cotton-wool" spots), hemorrhages, exudates, papilledema, visual acuity loss (if the macula is involved).
- **Cardiac:** CAD, LVH, CHF, MI.
- **Vascular:** Aortic dissection, aortic aneurysm.
- **Renal:** Proteinuria, chronic kidney disease.

CORONARY ARTERY DISEASE (CAD)

CAD (also called coronary heart disease) is a condition in which atherosclerosis of the arteries of the heart results in inadequate cardiac blood flow, producing cardiac ischemia. This can precipitate an MI or promote other chronic changes to the heart, such as CHF. CAD remains one of the most significant health problems in the United States, accounting for roughly one-third of deaths in those > 35 years of age. Subtypes include the following:

- **Angina pectoris:** Chest pain resulting from myocardial ischemia due to a mismatch between O_2 demand and supply to the heart (fundamentally a "demand" problem). Usually occurs with exertion and is associated with atherosclerosis (ie, stable plaques in the coronary arteries that restrict supply when demand ↑).

- **Prinzmetal's (variant) angina:** Chest pain resulting from myocardial ischemia due to coronary vasospasm. Classically seen in young women at rest in the early morning; associated with ST-segment elevations without concomitant cardiac enzyme elevation.
- **Acute coronary syndrome (ACS):**
  - **Unstable angina:** New-onset, accelerating chest pain occurring at rest or with exertion (fundamentally a "supply" problem). The chest pain signals an unstable plaque that can rupture to create an MI. ST-segment elevations may be noted on ECG, but no cardiac enzyme elevations are seen.
  - **Non-ST-elevation MI (NSTEMI):** Similar to unstable angina, except that in NSTEMI there is myocardial necrosis, as evidenced by elevations in troponin and CK-MB. No ST-segment elevations are seen on ECG.
  - **ST-elevation MI (STEMI):** Acute-onset, substernal chest pain that may radiate. Other symptoms (outlined below) may be present. Arrhythmias, valvular regurgitations, hypotension, or new-onset CHF signs may also be seen. ECG reveals ST-segment elevation or LBBB. ST-segment depression in V_1–V_2 may indicate a posterior wall infarct. Troponins and CK-MB are elevated.

Risk factors include age > 65 years, DM, hypertension, dyslipidemia, male gender, a family history of premature CAD (< 50 years of age in men; < 60 years of age in women), smoking, a diet high in saturated fat and low in fruits and vegetables, a sedentary lifestyle (obesity), drugs (eg, cocaine), known CAD (> 50% stenosis), ASA use in the past 7 days, severe angina, ST deviations > 0.5 mm, and ⊕ cardiac enzymes.

Signs and Symptoms

Clinical presentation includes the following:

- Chest pain/tightness/pressure (in angina pectoris, may be relieved by nitrates).
- Shortness of breath.
- Pain in the neck/jaw/back.
- Nausea.
- Diaphoresis.
- Numbness/tingling of the upper extremities.
- Carotid/peripheral bruits suggesting atherosclerosis or hypertension.
- Signs and symptoms consistent with heart failure (see the CHF section for a detailed description of signs and symptoms).

Differential

- **Cardiovascular:** CHF, pericarditis, aortic dissection.
- **Pulmonary:** Pneumonia, PE, pneumothorax.
- **Abdominal:** GERD/PUD, esophageal spasm (also relieved by nitrates), pancreatitis.
- **Musculoskeletal:** Costochondritis, trauma.
- **Psychiatric:** Anxiety, panic disorder.

Workup

- The initial workup for patients with symptoms of CAD includes the following:
  - ECG.
  - Cardiac enzymes (cycle enzymes q 8 h × 3).

KEY POINT: KEY CARDIAC DIAGNOSTIC EXAMINATIONS

- **Exercise electrocardiography:**
  - **Method:** The patient's ECG is monitored during exercise. Exercise often takes the form of a treadmill stress test conducted in accordance with the Bruce protocol, in which treadmill speed and elevation are ↑ every 3 minutes.
  - **Interpretation:** Angina, ST-segment changes on ECG, exercise intolerance, or ↓ systolic BP indicates myocardial ischemia. A ⊕ test should be further evaluated with cardiac catheterization.
- **Myocardial perfusion scintigraphy:**
  - **Method:** Radionuclides (eg, thallium, Tc-MIBI) are injected into the blood. The quantity of radionuclide uptake by the myocardium is directly related to the amount of blood flow.
  - **Interpretation:** Areas of ↓ uptake indicate relative hypoperfusion. With exercise (if patient is exercise tolerant) or drug-induced (if patient is unable to exercise) vasodilation, coronary vessels vasodilate, giving the most blood flow to those vessels without lesions. If no areas of hypoperfusion are observed, the test is ⊖.
  - **Follow-up:** If defects are observed, a resting scan is done to determine if perfusion defects are reversible. Defects that normalize at rest indicate reversible ischemia, whereas fixed defects signify areas of dead tissue (ie, post-MI). Areas of reversible ischemia may be rescued with percutaneous transluminal coronary angioplasty (PTCA) or coronary artery bypass graft (CABG) surgery.
- **Stress echocardiography:**
  - **Method:** A real-time ultrasound of the heart, the echocardiogram ("echo") reveals abnormal wall motion due to ischemia or infarction. A stress echo must be performed with exercise or dobutamine (exercise may be contraindicated in favor of dobutamine because of frailty, ECG abnormality, bundle branch block, and the like).
  - **Interpretation:** Echo confers the additional benefits of assessing left ventricular function and estimating the EF, an important predictor of prognosis. A normal EF is approximately 55–75%.
- **Coronary angiography/cardiac catheterization:**
  - **Method:** An invasive procedure that visualizes the coronary vasculature by injecting dye into the vessels, coronary arteriography is the definitive diagnostic procedure for CAD.
  - **Interpretation:** Stenotic lesions in the vessels will be visualized and quantified with respect to the extent of obstruction (most lesions that lead to symptoms are > 70% stenotic) as well as their location. This procedure also gives an estimate of the EF.
  - **Use:** Catheterization is typically used (1) to confirm the presence and map the extent of CAD, and (2) to define the method of revascularization (PTCA vs. CABG) if indicated.

- If the initial workup is ⊖ but there is moderate risk for CAD according to the Framingham risk score, consider the following:
  - Exercise stress testing.
  - Pharmacologic stress testing.
  - Stress echocardiography (exercise or pharmacologic).
  - Cardiac catheterization.

Treatment

- **Stable angina pectoris:**
  - Acutely, give ASA, O_2, and IV nitrates and/or morphine.
  - β-blockers, CCBs, and ACEIs may also be considered.
  - Chronically, treat with nitrates, ASA, and β-blockers. Short-acting nitrate preparations are used prior to activities that are known to set off angina; long-acting preparations are used if angina is frequent and/or without specific triggers.
  - Risk factor reduction is important as well and includes the following:
    - Lowering of LDL to a goal of < 70 mg/dL.
    - BP control (< 140/< 90 mm Hg).
    - Smoking cessation.
    - Dietary modification to ↑ fruits and vegetables and ↓ red meat intake.
- **Prinzmetal's (variant) angina:**
  - CCBs (diltiazem, verapamil) and nitrates constitute first-line treatment. Statins are often used as well.
  - Nonselective β-blockers should be **avoided** because they promote vasoconstriction.
  - ASA should be used with caution or avoided because of its inhibition of the production of prostacyclin.
  - Risk factor reduction as above.
- **Unstable angina/NSTEMI:**
  - Acutely, treatment is the same as that for angina pectoris.
  - Clopidogrel, heparin, and glycoprotein IIb/IIIa inhibitors should be considered.
  - Risk factor reduction as above.
- **STEMI:**
  - Acutely, give morphine, O_2, nitrates, ASA, β-blockers, and clopidogrel.
  - Consider ACEIs instead of β-blockers if the patient is in heart failure/cardiogenic shock (unless the patient is hypotensive).
  - Cardiac catheterization should be urgently performed (within 90 minutes of arrival if the patient has had symptoms for < 3 hours). If this window has passed, tPA or other thrombolytics may be considered for up to 6 hours.
  - In the long term, give ASA, β-blockers, clopidogrel (if catheterization is done), ACEIs, and statins.
  - Risk factor reduction as above.

SYNCOPE

Syncope is a sudden, transient loss of consciousness and postural tone due to cerebral hypoperfusion. More than 30% of people will experience at least 1 syncopal episode during their lifetimes. Patients usually have lightheadedness preceding the episode. Most people do not even remember falling. Prodromal

KEY FACT

Don't get angina during a possible MI. Instead, get **ABC MNO** (**A**SA, **B**eta blockers, **C**ardiac monitor, **M**orphine, **N**itrates, **O**xygen).

Q

A 70-year-old man presents to the ED with progressive shortness of breath and dyspnea. On examination, he has pulmonary crackles and a prominent mid-diastolic rumble on auscultation of the heart apex. An echocardiogram reveals grade III mitral stenosis. What is the next step in management?

MNEMONIC

Etiologies of syncope–

SVNCOPE

Situational
Vasovagal
Neurogenic
Cardiac
Orthostatic hypotension
Psychiatric
Everything else

symptoms such as diaphoresis, pallor, and abdominal discomfort may also occur. The mnemonic **SVNCOPE** and the descriptions below outline its etiologies.

- **Situational sources:** Include performing the Valsalva maneuver, defecation, coughing, sneezing, micturition, carotid sinus hypersensitivity (syncope with head turning, tight collars, or shaving), and subclavian steal (syncope with arm exercise).
- **Vasovagal responses, or the "common faint":** Usually occurs in young patients; precipitated by an emotional situation. Due to excessive vagal tone.
- **Neurogenic causes:** TIAs of the vertebrobasilar circulation, also known as "drop attacks" (technically not syncope). Very large strokes of the anterior circulation can also lead to loss of consciousness.
- **Cardiac causes:** Include cardiac arrhythmias (eg, bradycardia/tachycardia syndrome), conduction disturbances (eg, second- or third-degree AV heart block, torsades de pointes, ventricular tachycardia, ventricular fibrillation), inflow/outflow obstruction (eg, valvular stenosis, HOCM, PE, pulmonary hypertension), and cardiac ischemia.
- **Orthostatic hypotension:** Caused by hypovolemia from diuretics (furosemide, alcohol), vasodilators (α-blockers, nitrates), or, in patients with DM, autonomic insufficiency. Systolic BP ↓ at least 20 mm Hg, diastolic BP ↓ at least 10 mm Hg, and evidence of cerebral hypoperfusion manifests within 2–5 minutes after the patient changes from a supine to a standing position. Heart rate often ↑ but may stay the same in the case of autonomic failure.
- **Psychiatric:** Psychogenic pseudosyncope.
- **"Everything else":** Includes idiopathic causes as well as nonsyncopal events causing loss of consciousness (eg, drug intoxication, hypoglycemia, hypoxia, seizures/epilepsy).

KEY FACT

An EEG reveals the etiology of syncope in < 1% of cases.

KEY FACT

Don't get faint over syncope. In young patients, vasovagal syncope is common, whereas in older patients orthostasis is a frequent problem.

Workup

- Taking a complete history both from the patient and from a witness (if available) constitutes the most critical part of a syncope workup. Most importantly, try to determine if the event has a cardiac etiology (eg, chest pain, shortness of breath, palpitations).
- It is also important to distinguish syncopal causes of loss of consciousness from nonsyncopal causes. Focus on activity and posture prior to the incident, precipitating factors (exertion or positional changes), whether or not a prodrome occurred, any associated symptoms (incontinence, chest pain, palpitations, neurologic signs), and any medications taken.
- Diagnostic measures include the following:
  - Positional vital signs ("orthostatics") to rule out orthostasis.
  - Electrocardiography to evaluate cardiac conduction (although most are normal).
  - Conducting a tilt-table test to evaluate patients for autonomic insufficiency.
- Additional tests include Holter monitoring (20–50% sensitive for arrhythmias) or continuous-loop event monitoring, echocardiography (for anatomic abnormalities and valvular disease), exercise (stress) testing, cardiac catheterization, and subclavian ultrasound.

A

Balloon valvuloplasty or valve replacement for definitive cure.

Treatment

Treatment is dependent on the cause and includes the following:

- **Subclavian steal:** Patients should be referred to a vascular surgeon.
- **Vasovagal syncope:** Avoidance of triggers in situational syncope. Patients

may benefit from β-blockers and can be treated with anticholinergics (eg, diphenhydramine) or, very rarely, pacemaker placement.
- **Cardiac causes:** If a cardiac condition is present, its treatment is of critical importance.
- **Orthostasis:** Patients should have their volume repleted and underlying conditions (eg, anemia) corrected or offending drugs removed.

VALVULAR HEART DISEASE

Valvular diseases can be divided into 2 general types: stenotic lesions and regurgitant/insufficiency lesions. Most valvular heart disease is detected clinically in the seventh decade of life with the exception of mitral stenosis, which usually presents in the fourth and fifth decades. Causes of valvular disease include the following:

- **Rheumatic fever:** Historically the most common cause of valvular heart disease in adults (usually mitral stenosis or aortic stenosis accompanied by aortic insufficiency). Incidence has ↓ precipitously with treatment of streptococcal infections.
- **Degenerative heart disease:** The leading cause of valvular heart disease; most commonly calcific stenosis (related to atherosclerosis). See Figure 4-3 for an example of calcific aortic stenosis.
- **Congenital abnormalities** (eg, bicuspid aortic valve, congenital heart disease).

Workup/Treatment

- Listen to the murmur. Attempt to describe it in detail. Listen to it with the patient in multiple positions (upright, supine, left lateral decubitus).
- Table 4-6 summarizes the management of major valvular lesions.

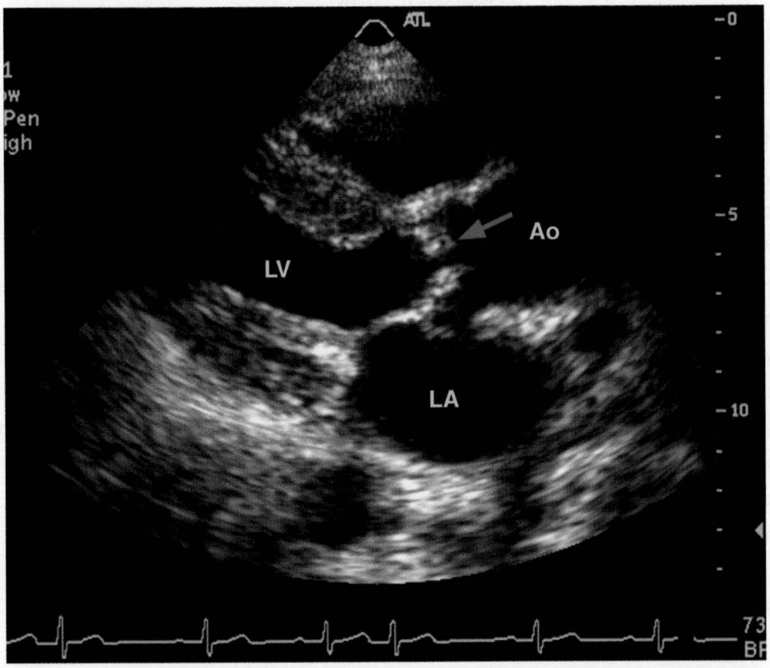

FIGURE 4-3. Aortic stenosis. Transthoracic echocardiogram in a patient with degenerative calcific aortic stenosis shows a thickened aortic valve (red arrow) that is nearly immobile. LV = left ventricle; LA = left atrium; Ao = aorta. (Reproduced with permission from Fuster V et al. *Hurst's The Heart,* 13th ed. New York: McGraw-Hill, 2011, Fig. 18-59.)

TABLE 4-6. Summary of Valvular Heart Diseases

VALVULAR LESION	RISK FACTORS/SETTING	SYMPTOMS/SIGNS	MURMUR	TREATMENT
Aortic outflow obstruction	**Aortic stenosis (AS):** Rheumatic heart disease, congenital stenosis/bicuspid valve, age-related degeneration (eg, calcific sclerosis). **Subvalvular stenosis** (eg, HOCM).	**AS:** The classic triad consists of angina, syncope, and heart failure. Remember them with the **"5-3-2" rule:** 50% mortality rates occur at **5, 3, and 2 years,** respectively, for angina, syncope, and heart failure. May also present with pulsus parvus et tardus (a weak and delayed carotid upstroke), a sustained apical beat, and S4 and soft S2 heart sounds. **HOCM:** Angina, syncope, and sudden death are all possible presentations, although it may also be asymptomatic (and undiagnosed).	**AS:** Midsystolic crescendo-decrescendo (diamond-shaped) murmur heard best at the second right intercostal space; radiation to the carotids with a musical apical component (Gallavardin phenomenon); systolic ejection click. The intensity of the murmur does not necessarily relate to its severity (severe AS = ↓ cardiac output = quieter murmur). **HOCM:** Systolic, diamond-shaped, harsh murmur at the apex and left sternal border, poorly transmitted to the carotids (vs. AS); earlier and longer with ↓ left ventricle size (Valsalva or standing); ↓ with ↑ left ventricle size (squatting).	**AS:** Avoid preload reducers (venodilators) and ⊖ inotropes (β-blockers), since AS is dependent on preload. Gentle diuresis for congestive symptoms. Aortic valve replacement is curative; balloon valvuloplasty (BV) is only palliative (for poor surgical candidates). The critical value for the aortic orifice area is < 1 cm², or a mean pressure gradient > 40 mm Hg. **HOCM: Avoid strenuous exercise** (risk of sudden death). β-blockers may be used to ↓ outflow obstruction. Surgical myomectomy or pacemaker placement.
Aortic insufficiency (AI)	**Valve disease:** Rheumatic heart disease (mixed AS/AI + MS), endocarditis, congenital bicuspid valve. **Root disease:** Hypertension, Ehlers-Danlos syndrome, Marfan's syndrome, collagen vascular disease, vasculitis (Takayasu's, giant cell), aortic dissection, syphilitic aortitis, idiopathic aortic root dilation, subaortic VSD, trauma.	**Acute:** Pulmonary edema +/– hypotension. **Chronic:** Gradual-onset angina (due to reduced diastolic coronary filling); dyspnea, orthopnea, paroxysmal nocturnal dyspnea. **Signs of LVH and left heart failure due to volume overload:** ↑ in stroke volume, widened pulse pressure, laterally displaced PMI. Possible brachial pulsus bisferiens (twin pressure peaks).	1. **High-pitched, blowing diastolic murmur:** Left sternal border; loudest when leaning forward. 2. **Austin Flint murmur:** Low-pitched mid-diastolic rumble (similar to MS, but without opening snap). 3. **Midsystolic murmur at the base** (due to high volume flow).	**Aortic valve replacement is curative.** If this is not possible, treat with afterload reducers (eg, vasodilators such as nifedipine and hydralazine), diuretics, and/or digoxin. In the setting of acute decompensation, use afterload reducers (nitroprusside) and ⊕ inotropes (dobutamine).

TABLE 4-6. Summary of Valvular Heart Diseases *(continued)*

VALVULAR LESION	RISK FACTORS/SETTING	SYMPTOMS/SIGNS	MURMUR	TREATMENT
Mitral stenosis (MS)	Rheumatic heart disease, congenital stenosis, cardiac myxoma, connective tissue disease (SLE).	**Left heart failure symptoms:** Exertional dyspnea, orthopnea, paroxysmal nocturnal dyspnea, pulmonary crackles. **Right heart failure symptoms:** Edema, ascites, hepatosplenomegaly, ↑ JVP, hemoptysis. Often concomitant AF and embolic events. **Signs of left or right heart failure:** ↑ intensity of S1 and P2, right ventricular heave, AF.	Mid-diastolic rumble with opening snap at the apex; no change with inspiration (vs. tricuspid stenosis, which ↑ with inspiration).	Avoid inotropic agents for all grades. Treatment is tailored to the degree of mitral stenosis, determined by mitral valve area: **Grade I (4–6 cm^2):** Sodium restriction, diuretics. **Grade II (1.5–4.0 cm^2):** As with grade I plus BV if there is no improvement. **Grades III/IV (III: 1.0–1.5 cm^2; IV: < 1.0 cm^2):** BV or, for refractory disease, valve replacement.
Mitral valve prolapse (MVP)	Idiopathic (found in 7% of the population, especially in young women or Marfan's syndrome patients). Can progress to mitral regurgitation.	Usually asymptomatic, but may lead to chest pain that is not associated with exertion or dyspnea. Echocardiography to assess severity.	Late systolic murmur with midsystolic click (Barlow's syndrome). Valsalva leads to an earlier and longer murmur.	Generally not necessary to treat unless symptomatic.
Mitral regurgitation (MR)	**Cusp disease:** Rheumatic heart disease, endocarditis, congenital cleft valve, myxomatous degeneration. Chordae tendineae dysfunction (2° to MI, Marfan's syndrome, MVP). Mitral annular expansion (eg, dilated cardiomyopathy).	DOE, orthopnea, paroxysmal nocturnal dyspnea, fatigue. Left heart failure signs; can progress to right heart failure. Laterally displaced PMI with left ventricular heave, S3, AF.	High-pitched, holosystolic murmur at the apex radiating to the axilla; systolic thrill; laterally displaced, hyperdynamic PMI.	**Acute:** Afterload reduction (nitroprusside), inotropic support (dobutamine), or intra-aortic balloon pump (IABP) if the patient is hemodynamically unstable. **Chronic:** Surgical repair or valve replacement if (1) the patient is symptomatic even with normal left ventricular function/size, or (2) the patient is asymptomatic but LVEF is < 50%, or he/she has pulmonary hypertension or new AF.

Pulmonology

CHRONIC OBSTRUCTIVE PULMONARY DISEASE (COPD)

A progressive disease characterized by a ↓ in lung function due to airflow obstruction. In contrast to asthma, COPD is not reversible and is the fourth most common cause of death in the United States. It is generally due to cigarette smoking and is pathologically divided into **chronic bronchitis** and **emphysema** (although most patients exhibit components of both). Distinguished as follows:

- **Chronic bronchitis:** A clinical diagnosis of excessive bronchial secretion with productive cough for at least 3 months per year over 2 consecutive years.
- **Emphysema:** A pathologic diagnosis of terminal airway destruction due to smoking (**centrilobular**) or to an inherited α_1-antitrypsin deficiency (**panacinar**).

KEY FACT

Symptoms of an acute COPD exacerbation include progressive dyspnea, an ↑ in sputum production, a change in the quality of sputum, fever, fatigue, wheeze, and tachypnea.

SIGNS AND SYMPTOMS

- Signs and symptoms of COPD are often absent until the disease is significantly advanced (with loss of > 50% of lung function).
- In both emphysema and bronchitis, patients may present with a barrel chest from high lung volumes, accessory chest muscle use, JVD, end-expiratory wheezing, prolonged expiration, and/or muffled breath sounds.
- Disease-specific presentations are as follows:
  - **Chronic bronchitis:** Patients are described as "blue bloaters" with a severe (usually sterile) productive cough, crackles, early onset of hypercarbia/hypoxia and cyanosis, weight gain, lethargy, peripheral edema due to CHF, and late-onset dyspnea.
  - **Emphysema:** Patients are classically described as "pink puffers" who exhibit ↓ breath sounds, minimal cough, DOE, pursed lips, weight loss, cyanosis (rare), and hypercarbia/hypoxia late in disease.
  - **Acute exacerbation of COPD:** One of the hallmarks of COPD is that the condition may acutely worsen, often necessitating hospital admission. Most exacerbations are caused by respiratory infections. The hallmark manifestations of a COPD exacerbation include progressive dyspnea, an ↑ in sputum production, and a change in sputum quality. Cough, fatigue, fever, tachypnea, and worsening wheezing may also be seen.

KEY FACT

Parenchymal bullae or subpleural blebs are pathognomonic for emphysema.

KEY FACT

In emphysema, the CXR shows hyperinflation, hyperlucency, loss of the capillary-alveolar surface area, a flattened and depressed diaphragm, widened retrosternal airspace, and an ↑ AP diameter.

DIFFERENTIAL

Asthma, bronchiectasis, 1° ciliary dyskinesia, cystic fibrosis (CF), CHF, congenital heart abnormalities, pulmonary hypertension, pneumonia, PE.

KEY FACT

There are no specific findings for chronic bronchitis on CXR or PFTs except those associated with comorbid emphysema.

WORKUP

- Obtain a CXR (see Figure 4-4), PFTs, ABGs, and serum electrolytes.
- Blood and sputum cultures (with Gram stain) are warranted in the presence of fever or ↑ purulent sputum production.
- Spirometry is diagnostic (see Table 4-7).
- For both disorders, an ABG during an acute exacerbation may show hypoxemia with an acute respiratory acidosis (↑ P_{CO_2}; patients with

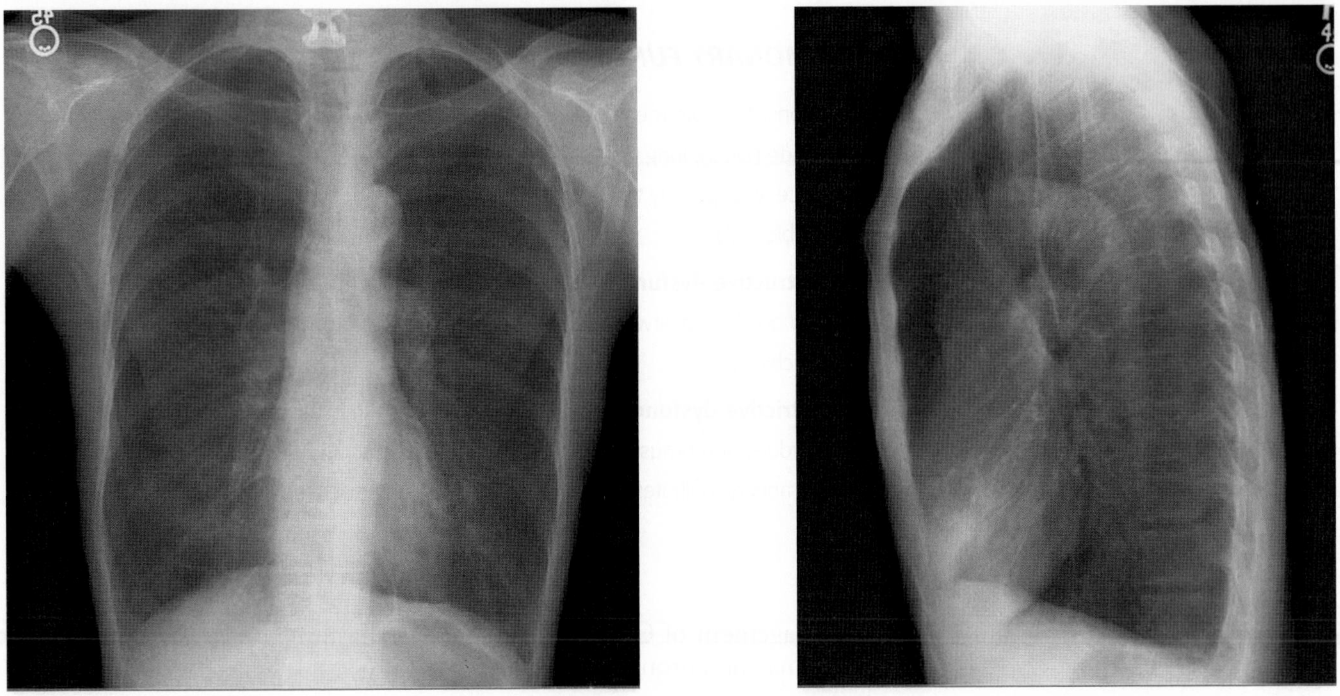

FIGURE 4-4. COPD. PA (A) and lateral (B) radiographs of a patient with emphysema show hyperinflation with large lung volumes, flattening of the diaphragm, and minimal peripheral vascular markings. (Reproduced with permission from USMLERx.com.)

COPD often have a baseline ↑ PCO_2) as well as an ↑ alveolar-arterial (A-a) O_2 gradient.

- Depending on clinical risk factors and presentation, consider ruling out other serious disorders, including PE (D-dimer or chest CT) and cardiac etiologies (ECG).

TABLE 4-7. Pulmonary Function Parameters in Lung Disease

Measurement	Obstructive Disease	Restrictive Disease
	Spirometry	
FEV_1	↓ (< 75% of normal)	Normal
FEV_1/FVC	↓ (< 70% of normal)	↑ or normal
	Lung Volumes	
FVC	↓ or normal	↓
VC	↓ or normal	↓
TLC	↑ or normal	↓
RV	↑	↓ or ↑ or normal

(Adapted with permission from Tierney LM et al. *Current Medical Diagnosis & Treatment,* 36th ed. Stamford, CT: Appleton & Lange, 1997: 239.)

KEY POINT

PULMONARY FUNCTION TESTS (PFTs)

PFTs consist of spirometry with flow volume loops, diffusion capacity for carbon monoxide (DL_{CO}), lung volumes, and ABGs. They are used primarily to detect the presence and quantify the severity of obstructive and restrictive pulmonary disease (see Table 4-7).

- **Obstructive dysfunction:** ↓ expiratory airflow and ↑ air trapping in the lung 2° to obstructed airways. Seen in asthma, chronic bronchitis, emphysema, and bronchiectasis.
- **Restrictive dysfunction:** ↓ lung volume. Seen in extrapulmonary (chest wall disorders, neuromuscular disease, pleural disease) and pulmonary diseases (pulmonary infiltrates and diffuse interstitial lung disease).

TREATMENT

The management of COPD is akin to that of asthma and is similar for both emphysema and chronic bronchitis.

- **Acute exacerbations:**
  - Give supplemental O_2 (with a goal of > 90–92% O_2 saturation), hydration, IV or oral steroids, anticholinergics (eg, ipratropium), and β-agonists (eg, albuterol).
  - No difference has been shown between oral and IV steroids in terms of quality of life, hospital length of stay, PFTs, or treatment failure. However, IV steroids are often used for more severe exacerbations, as patients in severe distress may have difficulty ingesting or absorbing oral medications.
  - Although the optimal dose and duration of steroid treatment have yet to be determined, a moderate dose of steroids (eg, 40 mg of prednisone) is usually given for 7–10 days.
  - Antibiotics have proven useful, especially for moderate to severe exacerbations. A fluoroquinolone or a macrolide is generally used for 3–7 days, depending on symptom improvement and the resistance patterns of the patient population.
- **Chronic management:**
  - Anticholinergics (eg, ipratropium, tiotropium) are preferred; long-acting β-agonists (eg, salmeterol) may also be added.
  - Influenza and pneumococcal vaccines are recommended.
  - Smoking cessation is paramount and is the only treatment measure that can slow the disease process.
  - Mucolytics are often used in chronic bronchitis, but their efficacy has not been conclusively established.
  - As with asthma, prophylactic antibiotics do not seem to be of benefit in preventing exacerbations.
  - Home supplemental O_2 therapy **does prolong life if the patient is hypoxemic** (the cutoff value to indicate this is an $Sao_2 \leq 88\%$, or ≤ 89% if there is evidence of right heart failure or erythrocytosis).
  - PFTs when the patient is stable to assess disease severity.
  - Patients with α_1-antitrypsin deficiency should be given appropriate supplementation.

KEY FACT

Anticholinergics are first-line therapy for COPD.

KEY FACT

Indications for home O_2:

- $Po_2 < 55$ mm Hg or $Sao_2 < 88\%$.
- Po_2 55–59 mm Hg with symptoms of hypoxia (mental status changes, right-sided heart failure from cor pulmonale, polycythemia).

COMPLICATIONS

- **Chronic respiratory failure:** Chronic hypoxemia with a compensated respiratory acidosis (↑ Pco_2).
- **Destruction of pulmonary vasculature:** Leads to pulmonary hypertension and eventually to right heart failure (cor pulmonale).
- Pneumonia.
- Bronchogenic carcinoma.

LUNG CANCER

Solitary pulmonary nodules are discovered in 0.1–0.2% of CXRs. Of these, 60–90% do not represent a malignancy. Approximately half of all lung tumors are metastatic, and half are 1° to the lung. Etiologies are as follows:

- Smoking plays a role in 85% of 1° lung cancers. Nearly 15% of smokers develop lung cancer, with the risk proportional to the number of pack-years smoked (always calculate pack-years).
- Smoking cessation ↓ risk in a time-dependent manner but does not completely return it to baseline.
- Other risk factors include radon exposure, environmental exposure (eg, arsenic, asbestos, uranium, chromium), and a first-generation family history.

SIGNS AND SYMPTOMS

Only 10–25% of patients are asymptomatic at the time of diagnosis. Others present with the following:

- Cough, dyspnea, hemoptysis, chest pain, and constitutional symptoms (fever, chills, weight loss, malaise, and night sweats).
- Physical examination may reveal ↓ breath sounds, crackles, ↑ fremitus with postobstructive pneumonitis, and pleural effusion (with ↓ fremitus).
- May present with dermatomyositis, anemia, DIC, eosinophilia, clubbing, thrombocytosis, or acanthosis nigricans. Specific syndromes may be associated with cancer subtypes (see Table 4-8).

DIFFERENTIAL

TB and other granulomatous diseases; fungal disease (aspergillosis, histoplasmosis); lung abscess; metastasis, carcinoid, or benign tumor.

WORKUP

The workup and management of a single pulmonary nodule should proceed as follows (see also Table 4-9):

- Assess age and risk factors for lung cancer or metastasis (eg, smoking, asbestos exposure, family history, previous diagnosis of malignancy).
- CXR, CBC with differential, electrolytes, LFTs, calcium.
- CXR may show hilar and peripheral nodules/masses, atelectasis, infiltrates, or pleural effusion (see Figure 4-5).
- Chest CT can better characterize involvement of the parenchyma, pleura, and mediastinum.
- Important radiologic factors to evaluate include nodule size, calcifications, and borders.
- Additional workup should proceed according to probability of malignancy:
  - **Low probability of malignancy:** Follow with CT scans.
  - **Nodules ≥ 1 cm with intermediate probability of malignancy:** Assess with FDG-PET. A ⊖ scan can then be followed by CT scans.

KEY FACT

Lung cancer is the leading cause of cancer-related death in the United States for both men and women.

KEY FACT

Is it a nodule or a mass? Distinguish them as follows:

- A pulmonary **nodule** is considered to be < 3 cm in diameter.
- A pulmonary **mass** is considered to be > 3 cm in diameter.

Q

A 67-year-old woman with a 60-pack-year smoking history presents with hemoptysis. CXR reveals a centrally located pulmonary mass. What is the most likely type of cancer, and how can this diagnosis best be confirmed?

TABLE 4-8. Malignant Pulmonary Lesions

Lesion Type/Incidence	Most Common Location	Risk Factors	Related Conditions	Five-Year Survival
		Small Cell Lung Cancer (SCLC) (15–25%)		
N/A	Central hilum.	Strong association with smoking (99%).	Cushing's syndrome, SIADH, hypercalcemia, ectopic ACTH, peripheral neuropathy, Lambert-Eaton syndrome, SVC syndrome.	5–10%.
		Non–Small Cell Lung Cancer (NSCLC) (60–70%)		
Squamous cell carcinoma (20%)	Central or in main bronchus.	Strong association with smoking (> 90%).	Hypercalcemia from PTH-related peptide (PTHrP), hypertrophic pulmonary osteoarthropathy (HPO), SVC syndrome.	Varies with stage.[a]
Adenocarcinoma (60%)	Peripheral subpleural, 67%; central, 33%; bronchoalveolar subtype in airways.	Weak association with smoking; the most common type in nonsmokers. Ras gene mutations (30%).	HPO, thrombophlebitis.	Varies with stage.[a]
Large cell carcinoma (20%)	Peripheral.	Moderate association with smoking.	Gynecomastia, galactorrhea, HPO.	Varies with stage.[a]
Mesothelioma (3–5%)	Pleural based.	Asbestos exposure 20–40 years prior (80%).	Pleural effusion.	20%.
Carcinoid of the lung (6%)	Subsegmental bronchi.	All groups except African Americans.	Tachycardia, flushing, bronchial constriction, diarrhea, Cushing's syndrome.	60–95%.
Metastasis (most commonly colon, breast, renal, osteosarcoma, melanoma) (2–8%)	Random (may be vascular or lymphatic in distribution).	—	—	Varies by 1° site.

[a] Five-year survival is stage dependent: I = 50–60%; II = 30–50%; III = 5–10%; IV = < 5%.

A

Squamous cell carcinoma of the lung is the most common type of lung cancer, and 98% of cases are related to smoking. Bronchoscopy is used for brushing and biopsy of the suspicious lesion.

- **High probability of malignancy or rapidly growing:** Biopsy and/or remove.
- When a nodule is found incidentally on CT, the Fleischner guidelines (see Table 4-9) can be used to determine the frequency and duration of serial CT scans based on the patient's risk of lung cancer.
- For malignancy, a histologic diagnosis from fine-needle aspiration (FNA), bronchoscopy with biopsy, lymph node biopsy, thoracentesis, mediastinoscopy, or thoracotomy is necessary, as the treatment and prognosis for SCLC and NSCLC differ.

TABLE 4-9. Fleischner Guidelines for a Solitary Pulmonary Nodule

Nodule Size	Low-Risk Patients	High-Risk Patients
< 4 mm	No follow-up.	CT at 12 months (no further follow-up if unchanged).
4–6 mm	CT again at 12 months (no further follow-up if unchanged).	CT at 6–12 months and then again at 18–24 months if no changes are seen.
6–8 mm	CT at 6–12 months and then again at 18–24 months if no changes are seen.	CT at 3–6 months and then at 9–12 months and 24 months if no changes are seen.
> 8 mm	CT at 3, 9, and 24 months; contrast CT, PET, and biopsy should be considered.	CT at 3, 9, and 24 months; contrast CT, PET, and biopsy should be considered.

Treatment

Treatment depends on the type and extent of the lung cancer and includes surgery, chemotherapy, and radiation therapy.

- NSCLC: Surgical resection followed by radiation/chemotherapy. Early-stage NSCLC is curable.
- SCLC: Generally nonresectable owing to early nodal metastasis, but usually responsive to combination and radiation therapy; recurrence is common.

Complications

Complications include those outlined in the mnemonic **SPHERE.**

MNEMONIC

SPHERE *of lung cancer complications:*

Superior vena cava syndrome
Pancoast's tumor (a peripheral lung tumor that may result in shoulder/arm pain, shoulder/arm/hand muscular atrophy, and/or Horner's syndrome)
Horner's syndrome
Endocrine (paraneoplastic–SIADH, ACTH secreting, PTHrP secreting)
Recurrent laryngeal symptoms (hoarseness)
Effusions (pleural or pericardial)

CHRONIC COUGH

Defined as a cough that is present for > 3 weeks. For nonsmokers, the prevalence is 14–23%; for smokers, prevalence ↑ with the number of packs

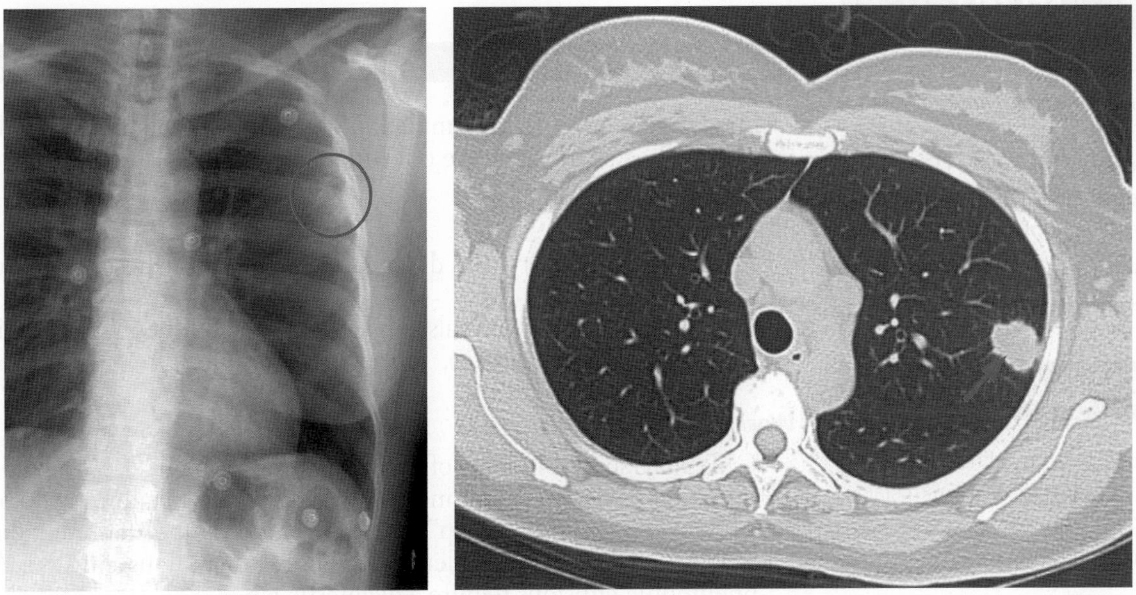

A B

FIGURE 4-5. Lung cancer. (**A**) CXR of a patient with weight loss shows a left upper lobe peripheral nodule (circle). (**B**) CT confirms the presence of a peripheral nodule (arrow), which proved at biopsy to be 1° adenocarcinoma of the lung. (Reproduced with permission from USMLERx.com.)

smoked, from 25% with half a pack per day to 50% in those who smoke > 2 packs per day. Chronic cough may have > 1 etiology.

- Some 90% of cases are caused by the 5 most common etiologies: smoking, postnasal drip, asthma, GERD, and chronic bronchitis.
- Other causes include medication (eg, ACEIs), airway hyperresponsiveness 2° to URI, malignancy, TB, aspiration, foreign bodies, occupational irritants, psychogenic factors, CHF, and irritation of cough receptors in the ear.

KEY FACT

Wheezing may be absent in "cough-variant asthma."

Signs and Symptoms

Presentation varies according to the etiology:

- **Asthma related:** Coughing that worsens at night, a family history of atopy, wheezing, worsening around specific irritants (eg, pollen, smoke, temperature).
- **GERD:** Sour mouth, heartburn, or worsened symptoms while supine.
- **Postnasal drip:** Mucus draining from the nose or down the throat and, on examination, cobblestone mucosa.
- **Malignancy:** Constitutional symptoms such as fever, chills, unintentional weight loss, malaise, fatigue, and night sweats.
- **Chronic bronchitis:** Cough for 3 months for at least 2 years. Usually associated with smoking.

MNEMONIC

Common causes of chronic cough—

GASP-Cough

GERD
Asthma
Smoking
Postnasal drip
Chronic bronchitis

Workup/Treatment

- Workup should proceed in a stepwise manner to rule out the various causes:
  - Treat postnasal drip with a combination antihistamine-decongestant; if symptoms persist, consider adding a steroid and/or obtaining a CT of the sinuses.
  - Evaluate and treat for asthma (see the Pediatrics chapter); avoid suspected irritants (eg, medications, allergies) or triggers.
  - If postnasal drip and asthma are ruled out, treat for GERD with H_2 blockers or PPIs; perform a CXR and consider endoscopy or 24-hour pH monitoring if refractory.
- If all of the above are ⊖, consider bronchoscopy.

PLEURAL EFFUSION

Defined as an abnormal accumulation of fluid in the pleural space. It is normally classified as **transudative** or **exudative.**

KEY FACT

Light's criteria for an exudative effusion:

- Pleural fluid protein/serum protein > 0.5.
- Pleural fluid LDH/serum LDH > 0.6 (or pleural fluid LDH > two-thirds the upper limit of normal serum LDH).

Signs and Symptoms

- Frequently presents with dyspnea and pleuritic chest pain, but often asymptomatic.
- Physical examination reveals ↓ breath sounds, dullness to percussion, and ↓ fremitus (see Table 4-10).

KEY FACT

Signs of "complicated" effusion include a pus-like appearance, a ⊕ Gram stain, low pH (< 7.3), low glucose (< 60 mg/dL), and high LDH (> 1000 IU/L).

Workup

- CXR may show blunting of the costophrenic angles (see Figure 4-6). A decubitus CXR can determine whether the fluid is free flowing or loculated.
- Thoracentesis ("pleural tap") or open biopsy is the definitive diagnostic test. A needle biopsy of pleura diagnoses tuberculous effusion. All parapneumonic effusions require a diagnostic tap.

KEY POINT

TRANSUDATIVE VS. EXUDATIVE EFFUSION

- **Transudative effusion:**
  - **Mechanism:** ↑ hydrostatic pressure and/or ↓ oncotic pressure, with intact capillaries leading to protein-poor pleural fluid that is an ultrafiltrate of plasma.
  - **Causes:** "Systemic" conditions such as CHF, cirrhosis, nephrotic syndrome, peritoneal dialysis, SVC obstruction, myxedema, protein-losing enteropathy, and PE.
- **Exudative effusion:**
  - **Mechanism:** Inflammation resulting in leaky capillaries, leading to a protein-rich fluid.
  - **Causes:** "Localized" conditions such as bacterial infection (pneumonia-associated ["parapneumonic"] effusion and empyema), neoplasm, PE with infarction, TB, viral infection, collagen vascular disease, pancreatitis, hemothorax, sarcoidosis, uremia, asbestosis, pericardial disease, chylothorax, and iatrogenic factors (eg, traumatic pleural tap).

KEY POINT

PLEURAL FLUID APPEARANCE

- **Bloody:** Neoplasm, TB, traumatic tap, pulmonary infarction, hemothorax.
- **Low glucose:** Neoplasm, TB, empyema, RA (extremely low glucose).
- **Lymphocytic:** Viral infection, TB, malignancy.
- **Milky (triglyceride rich):** Chylothorax.

KEY POINT

RECOMMENDATIONS FOR PLEURAL FLUID ANALYSIS

- **CBC with differential:** Evaluate for signs of infection or trauma (eg, ↑ RBCs).
- **Protein and LDH ratios (Light's criteria):**
  - Ratio of pleural fluid protein to serum protein > 0.5.
  - Ratio of pleural fluid LDH to serum LDH > 0.6 (or pleural fluid LDH more than two-thirds the upper limit of normal serum LDH).
  - Both are suggestive of an exudate as opposed to a transudate.
- **Amylase:** High amylase supports esophageal rupture, pancreatic pleural effusion, or malignancy.
- **pH:** If < 7.3, suggests empyema, rheumatoid pleurisy, tuberculous pleurisy, or malignancy (normal pH is 7.6).
- **Glucose:** If < 60 mg/dL, suggests bacterial infection, rheumatoid pleuritis, or malignancy.
- **Gram stain:** To look for bacteria.
- **Cytology:** To reveal malignant cells.

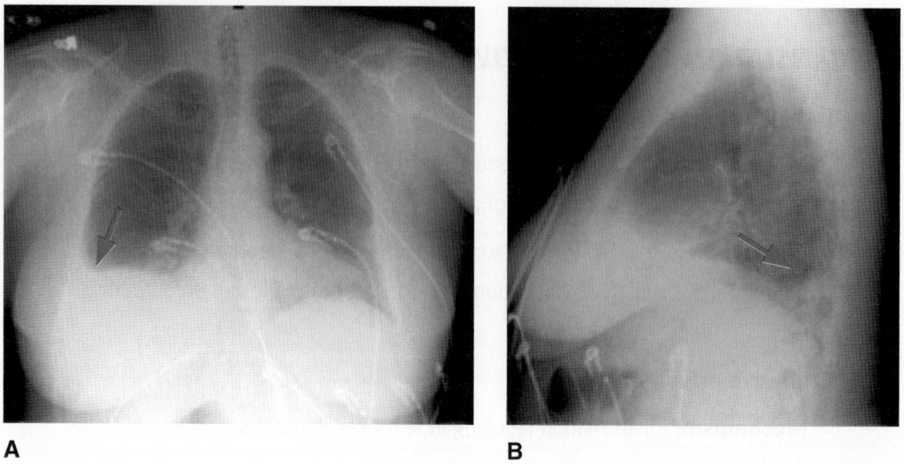

FIGURE 4-6. Pleural effusion. PA (**A**) and lateral (**B**) CXRs show blunting of the right costophrenic sulcus (arrows). (Reproduced with permission from USMLERx.com.)

TREATMENT

- **Transudative effusion:**
  - Address the underlying condition.
  - Perform a therapeutic lung tap when massive effusion leads to dyspnea.
- **Exudative effusion:**
  - **Malignant:** Consider pleurodesis (injection of an irritant such as talc into the pleural cavity to scar the 2 pleural layers together) in symptomatic patients who are unresponsive to chemotherapy and radiation therapy. Therapeutic thoracentesis, pleuroperitoneal shunting, and surgical pleurectomy are alternatives.
  - **Parapneumonic:** Consider drainage via a chest tube for a "complicated" parapneumonic effusion or an empyema.
  - **Hemothorax:** Place a chest tube to control bleeding by the apposition of pleural surfaces, determine the amount of blood loss, and assess the risk of infection and late fibrothorax.

> **KEY FACT**
>
> *Streptococcus pneumoniae* is the most common cause of CAP.

> **KEY FACT**
>
> Elderly patients with CAP and those with underlying COPD or DM may have minimal signs on examination. Your level of suspicion should remain high.

PNEUMONIA

Pneumonia is defined by infection of the bronchoalveolar unit with an associated inflammatory exudate. Community-acquired pneumonia (CAP) causes the greatest number of deaths of any infectious disease in the United States. Causes include the following:

TABLE 4-10. Pulmonary Diagnostic Tips

PHYSICAL FINDING	PLEURAL EFFUSION	PNEUMONIA	PNEUMOTHORAX
Breath sounds	↓	↓ vesicular but ↑ bronchial	↓
Adventitial sounds	None	Egophony ("E" → "A"), bronchophony, whispered pectoriloquy	None
Percussion	Dull	Dull	Hyperresonant
Tactile fremitus	↓	↑	↓

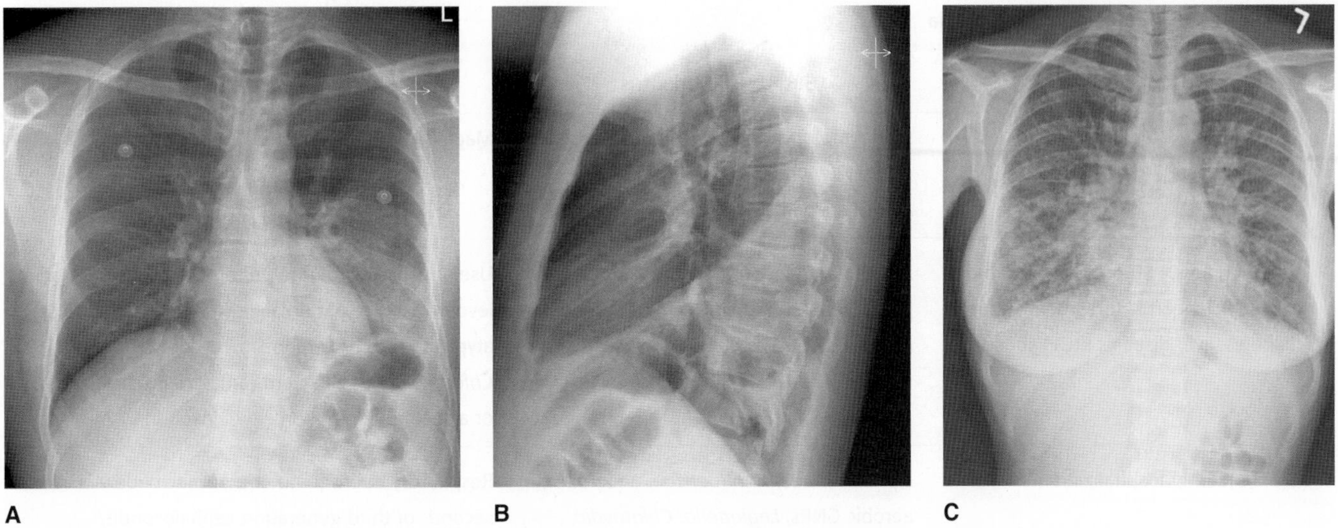

FIGURE 4-7. Pneumonia on CXR. PA (A) and lateral (B) CXRs in a patient with pneumococcal pneumonia show a lobar pneumonia pattern in the left lower lobe. (C) Contrast with the "atypical" appearance of bilateral, ill-defined opacities in a case of *Legionella* pneumonia. (Images A and B reproduced with permission from USMLERx.com. Image C reproduced with permission from Tintinalli JE et al. *Tintinalli's Emergency Medicine: A Comprehensive Study Guide*, 7th ed. New York: McGraw-Hill, 2011, Fig. 68-3.)

- **"Typical" infectious pneumonia:** Bacteria from the nasopharynx.
- **"Atypical" infectious pneumonia:** Organisms inhaled from the environment (eg, bacteria such as *Mycoplasma*, *Legionella*, and *Chlamydia* as well as viruses and fungi). Often difficult to visualize on Gram stain, and not susceptible to antibiotics that act on the cell wall (eg, β-lactams).
- **Other:** For persistent, recurrent infections, consider underlying lung injury, obstruction (eg, bronchogenic carcinoma, lymphoma, Wegener's granulomatosis, TB, *Nocardia*, *Coxiella burnetii*, *Aspergillus*), or ↓ immune status.

Signs and Symptoms

- **Classic "typical" symptoms:** Productive cough (purulent yellow or green sputum), hemoptysis, tachypnea, dyspnea, fever/chills, night sweats, pleuritic chest pain.
- **Atypical pneumonia:** Classic symptoms may be the same as those above, or patients may present with a more gradual onset of symptoms, including dry cough, myalgias, headaches, sore throat, and pharyngitis.
- Physical examination reveals bronchial breath sounds, bronchophony, dullness to percussion, whispered pectoriloquy, egophony, ↑ fremitus, and possible crackles or wheezes (see Table 4-10).

Workup

- **CBC:** Demonstrates leukocytosis and left shift (an immature form of WBCs is present) with bands.
- **CXR:** Shows lobar consolidation or patchy or diffuse infiltrates (see Figure 4-7).
- **Sputum Gram stain and culture and blood culture:** Identify the pathogenic organism, the organism's susceptibility to antibiotics, and the presence of bacteremia. Evidence does not support routine sputum or blood culture in patients with CAP.
- **ABGs and pulse oximetry:** Poor O_2 saturation and acid-base disturbances may be seen in severe cases.
- **Other:** Urine antigens for *Legionella* and pneumococcus can be helpful.

KEY FACT

Classic disease-specific clues to pneumonia:

- Rust-colored sputum: pneumococcus
- "Currant jelly" sputum: *Klebsiella*
- Cold agglutinins: *Mycoplasma*
- GI symptoms: *Legionella*
- CD4 < 200 and/or ↑ LDH: *Pneumocystis jiroveci* pneumonia (PCP)

KEY FACT

A good sputum sample has many PMNs and few epithelial cells. Otherwise, suspect contamination by oral flora.

Q

An 80-year-old man presents with cough, pleuritic chest pain, and confusion. He is febrile with dullness to percussion, ↑ fremitus, and bronchial breath sounds in his lower right lung field. His WBC count is elevated, and his CXR shows right lobe consolidation. What is the best initial treatment strategy?

TABLE 4-11. Treatment of Pneumonia

Demographics	Suspected Pathogens	Initial Coverage (Nonviral)
Outpatient CAP, age < 60, otherwise healthy	*S pneumoniae, Mycoplasma pneumoniae, Chlamydia pneumoniae, Haemophilus influenzae,* viruses.	Macrolide or doxycycline.
CAP with age > 60 or with comorbidity (eg, COPD, heart failure, renal failure, diabetes, liver disease, EtOH abuse)	*S pneumoniae, H influenzae,* aerobic gram-⊖ rods (GNRs–*E coli, Enterobacter, Klebsiella*), *S aureus, Legionella,* viruses.	Use a respiratory fluoroquinolone (eg, moxifloxacin, levofloxacin) or a macrolide (for coverage against atypicals such as *Legionella, Mycoplasma,* or *Chlamydia*) + a β-lactam (amoxicillin/clavulanate) or a second-generation cephalosporin.
CAP requiring hospitalization	*S pneumoniae, H influenzae,* anaerobes, aerobic GNRs, *Legionella, Chlamydia.*	Respiratory fluoroquinolone or macrolide + a second- or third-generation cephalosporin/β-lactam.
Severe CAP requiring hospitalization	*S pneumoniae, H influenzae,* anaerobes, aerobic GNRs, *Legionella, M pneumoniae, Pseudomonas.*	Macrolide, third-generation cephalosporin with antipseudomonal activity (ceftazidime). Consider vancomycin if MRSA is a possibility.
Health care–associated pneumonia (ie, patient hospitalized > 48 hours or in a long-term care facility > 14 days)	GNRs, including *Pseudomonas, S aureus, Legionella,* and mixed flora.	Aminoglycoside and a third-generation antipseudomonal cephalosporin.

MNEMONIC

To determine whether to admit for pneumonia, assess–

CURB-65

Confusion (MMSE or disoriented to person/place/time)
Urea (BUN > 20 mg/dL)
Respiratory rate (> 30 bpm)
Blood pressure (< 90 mm Hg systolic or < 60 mm Hg diastolic)
> **65** years of age

Treatment

- **Outpatient treatment:** Initial treatment should consist of empiric oral antibiotics and should be based on the suspected etiology (see Table 4-11).
- **Inpatient treatment:**
  - The **CURB-65** score (see mnemonic), which assesses mental status, renal function, respiratory status, BP, and age, can be used to determine whether a patient should be admitted for CAP.
  - Hospitalization should also be considered for those with significant comorbidities, immunosuppression, aspiration, malnutrition, alcohol abuse, sepsis, hypoxemia, or multilobar involvement.
  - Any patient admitted to the hospital likely warrants IV antibiotics (see Table 4-11). However, patients who have been afebrile for > 24 hours can be switched to an oral antibiotic. Once oral antibiotics are tolerated, some physicians will have the patient finish the course of treatment (7–14 days total) on an outpatient basis. Others may elect to ensure that the patient remains afebrile before discharge.
  - While the patient is in the hospital, encourage incentive spirometry, chest physical therapy, hydration, and ambulation to loosen consolidation and improve aeration.

A

The patient likely has bacterial pneumonia. Pending the results of Gram stain and cultures, he should be admitted and given antimicrobial therapy for CAP. This could be a fluoroquinolone such as levofloxacin or a combination of a β-lactam and a macrolide (eg, ceftriaxone + azithromycin).

KEY POINT

INDICATIONS FOR PNEUMOCOCCAL VACCINATION

The CDC National Immunization Program recommends that the following adults receive pneumococcal vaccination:

- **Patients ≥ 65 years of age.**
- **Patients 19–64 years of age who:**
  - Have chronic or systemic illness (eg, heart disease, diabetes, cirrhosis, COPD, asthma, pulmonary fibrosis, alcoholism, CSF leak).
  - Are smokers.
  - Have invasive pneumococcal disease.
  - Are residents of nursing homes or long-term care facilities.
  - Have ↓ immune function (eg, AIDS, lymphoma, leukemia, asplenia, sickle cell, nephrotic syndrome, steroid therapy, radiation therapy, transplant patients).

COMPLICATIONS

- Some 30% of pneumococcal pneumonia patients exhibit bacteremia.
- Patients are at an ↑ risk for MI and stroke.

Nephrology

ACUTE RENAL FAILURE (ARF)

Defined as an abrupt ↓ in renal function leading to the retention of creatinine and BUN, often accompanied by oliguria (urine output 100–400 mL/day) or anuria (urine output < 100 mL/day). Clinical manifestations are nonspecific and include malaise, fatigue, anorexia, oliguria, nausea/vomiting, and hypertension. ARF is categorized as prerenal, intrinsic, and postrenal. A summary of the etiologies, distinguishing features, and treatment of each of these subtypes can be found in Figure 4-8. The BUN/Cr ratio and fractional excretion of sodium (Fe_{Na}) are important ways to distinguish prerenal from intrinsic renal failure (see Figure 4-8):

$$Fe_{Na} = (\text{urine Na/plasma Na}) \,/\, (\text{urine creatinine/plasma creatinine}) \times 100\%$$

Note that Fe_{urea} can be used if a patient is on a diuretic such as furosemide, as Fe_{Na} would be misleading (falsely elevated) in this circumstance.

The RIFLE criteria (**R**isk, **I**njury, **F**ailure, **L**oss, **E**SRD) can be used to classify the severity of kidney injury on the basis of urine output or serum creatinine level (see Table 4-12). Mortality risk ↑ as the patient progresses on this classification scheme.

KEY FACT

A RIFLE in your kidneys can cause a multitude of problems, including volume overload, metabolic acidosis, hyperkalemia, hyperphosphatemia, and postobstructive diuresis.

COMPLICATIONS

- **Volume overload** leads to CHF and hypertension. Pay careful attention to fluid balance and optimize hemodynamics (mean arterial pressure, cardiac output).

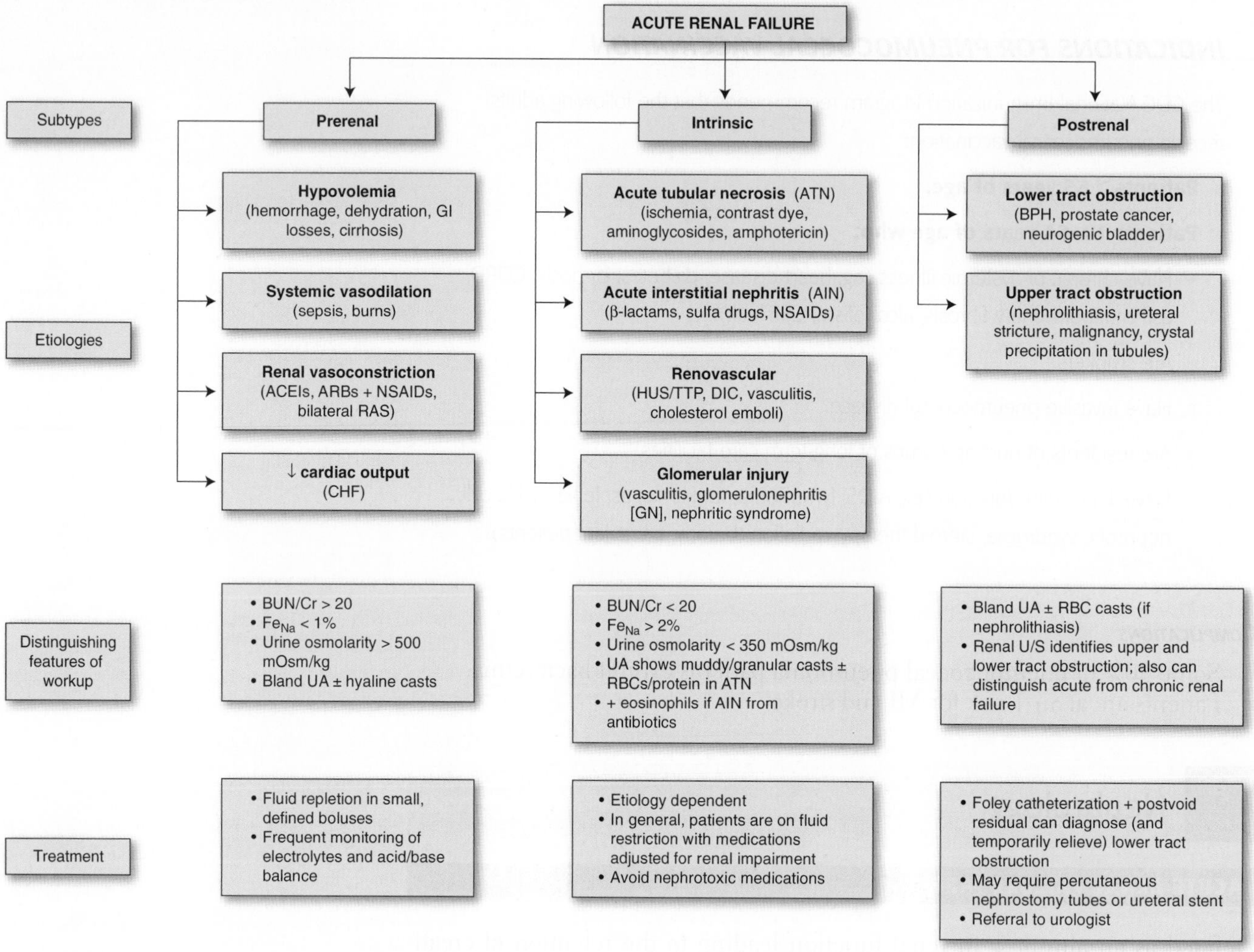

FIGURE 4-8. Summary of acute renal failure.

TABLE 4-12. RIFLE Criteria for the Classification of Kidney Injury

Classification	GFR	Urine Output
Risk	Creatinine ↑ by 50%. GFR ↓ by 25%.	< 0.5 mL/kg/hr for 6 hours.
Injury	Creatinine is doubled. GFR ↓ by 50%.	< 0.5 mL/kg/hr for 12 hours.
Failure	Creatinine is tripled (or a creatinine level of ≥ 4 mg/dL or an acute rise of 0.5 mg/dL). GFR ↓ by 75%.	< 0.3 mL/kg/hr for 1 day or anuria for 12 hours.
Loss	Persistent ARF for a duration of > 4 weeks.	
ESRD	Complete loss of kidney function lasting > 3 months.	

- **Metabolic acidosis:** Replace bicarbonate if HCO_3^- is ≤ 16 or serum pH is < 7.2.
- **Hyperkalemia and hyperphosphatemia** are common and can usually be treated with dietary restriction (K ≤ 40 mEq/day, PO_4 < 800 mg/day).
- After relief of obstruction, **postobstructive diuresis** can lead to inappropriate loss of fluid and electrolytes, which must often be replaced.
- Notably, ARF is an independent risk factor for mortality in hospitalized patients.

KEY FACT

A fluid challenge (0.5–1.0 L NS) can help distinguish prerenal from intrinsic ARF in non-volume-overloaded, oliguric patients.

CHRONIC KIDNEY DISEASE (CKD)

Defined as 3 or more months of ↓ GFR (< 60 mL/min/1.73 m^2) and/or kidney damage (abnormal pathology, blood/urine tests, or imaging). CKD is a growing problem, affecting 16.8% of the U.S. population and a disproportionately higher number of African Americans. CKD is classified into 5 stages on the basis of GFR (see Table 4-13). It has many etiologies, among the most common of which are diabetes, hypertension, glomerulonephritis, and adult polycystic kidney disease.

Signs and Symptoms

CKD is initially asymptomatic and can be detected only by a rise in serum creatinine. As GFR declines, the following symptoms develop, usually around stage 3 or 4, as a result of the retention of solutes and nitrogenous waste (also indicated by ↑ BUN):

- **General:** Anorexia, nausea/vomiting, fatigue, pruritus, a metallic taste in the mouth, fetor uremicus (breath smelling of urine/ammonia), uremic frost (white urea crystals on the skin).
- **Cardiovascular:** Hypertension, often with resultant LVH; pericarditis, accelerated atherosclerosis, volume overload, CHF, hyperlipidemia.
- **Neurologic:** Peripheral neuropathy, encephalopathy (↓ attention and memory), seizures, stupor, coma.
- **Hematologic:** Anemia (due to ↓ production of erythropoietin by the kidneys), iron deficiency (anemia of chronic disease).
- **Metabolic:** Hyperkalemia, metabolic acidosis, ↑ PO_4, ↓ Ca^{++} (due to vitamin D_3 deficiency and binding with excess PO_4), 2° hyperparathyroidism leading to osteoporosis.

TABLE 4-13. Stages and Management Goals of Chronic Kidney Disease

Stage	GFR	Goals
1 (normal or ↑ GFR)	≥ 90	Diagnose and treat underlying conditions (particularly if reversible); cardiovascular risk reduction.
2 (mild)	60–89	Estimate progression; determine if the patient is likely to need renal replacement therapy (RRT).
3 (moderate)	30–59	Monitor for and treat any complications.
4 (severe)	15–29	Continue to monitor and treat complications; prepare for RRT.
5 (ESRD)	< 15	RRT; dialysis (hemo- or peritoneal dialysis) is often used as a bridge to transplantation if the patient is on a waiting list for cadaveric renal transplantation.

WORKUP

- Where possible, diagnose and treat the underlying etiology.
- Obtain frequent lab work to monitor for signs of uremia and worsening kidney function. Labs should include serum creatinine, BUN, PO_4, Ca^{++}, albumin, K^+, HCO_3^-, hemoglobin, PTH to assess for hyperparathyroidism, UA, and a first-morning urine spot protein/creatinine ratio to evaluate for proteinuria.

TREATMENT

- **General:**
  - Avoid nephrotoxic drugs (NSAIDs, aminoglycosides, contrast); provide early referral to a nephrologist.
  - Avoid blood draws on 1 arm and avoid subclavian lines to preserve vasculature for future access (eg, AV fistula).
- **Cardiovascular:**
  - ACEIs/ARBs for hypertension with a BP goal of < 130/80 mm Hg (have been shown to ↓ the progression of CKD).
  - Sodium restriction and/or loop diuretics to prevent volume overload.
  - Statins to lower LDL cholesterol (with a goal LDL of < 100 mg/dL, although some recommend < 70 mg/dL).
- **Hematologic:** Administer weekly injections of an erythropoietin analog (epoetin or darbepoetin) only if hemoglobin is < 12 mg/dL in females or < 13.5 mg/dL in males. Give iron supplementation if anemia is found to be due to iron deficiency as evidenced in iron studies.
- **Metabolic:** Dietary restriction (Na, K, PO_4, Mg); Kayexalate as needed for hyperkalemia; bicarbonate or citrate if HCO_3^- is < 22; oral PO_4 binders (calcium carbonate taken with meals) and calcitriol (1,25-OH vitamin D) for renal osteodystrophy.
- **Renal replacement therapy (preparation starts in stage 4 kidney disease):**
  - Includes hemodialysis, peritoneal dialysis, and renal transplantation (either living-donor or cadaveric).
  - Peritoneal dialysis affords patients the opportunity to receive dialysis at home rather than having to go to a center, and it is also considered more physiologic than hemodialysis. However, infection is a concern, and medical personnel are not present as often as they are in a hemodialysis center to observe whether other interventions are needed.
  - If available, renal transplantation is the treatment of choice and has been shown to ↓ mortality and ↑ quality of life. However, lifelong immunosuppression, with its numerous complications, is required.

MNEMONIC

Indications for dialysis–

AEIOU

Acidosis unresponsive to medical therapy
Electrolyte abnormalities (K > 6.5 mEq/L)
Ingestions (methanol, ethylene glycol)
Overload (fluid)
Uremic symptoms (eg, pericarditis, encephalopathy)

(Note that creatinine level is **not** an indication for dialysis.)

GLOMERULAR DISEASE

Glomerular disease encompasses a broad differential of disorders that all lead to injury to the glomerulus, impaired GFR, and the appearance of protein and/or blood cells in the urine. The 2 general categories are **nephrotic** and **nephritic syndromes** (see Table 4-14).

Nephrotic Syndrome

- Characterized by severe proteinuria (> 3.5 g/day), generalized edema, hypoalbuminemia, and hyperlipidemia. Hypercoagulability may result from an imbalance of clotting factors in the coagulation cascade due to an overall ↓ in anticoagulation proteins, especially antithrombin 3 (lost in urine), and to ↑ hepatic synthesis of procoagulant proteins such as fibrinogen.

TABLE 4-14. Summary of Renal Syndromes

Syndrome	Common Etiologies	Uncommon Etiologies
Nephrotic syndrome	Minimal change disease, focal segmental glomerulosclerosis, diabetic nephropathy.	Membranous glomerulonephritis (GN)—75% of cases are idiopathic, but 2° causes include SLE, penicillamine, gold, NSAIDs, HBV, HCV, syphilis, and malignancy. Renal amyloidosis, SLE WHO Class V.
Nephritic syndrome	Postinfectious GN; IgA nephropathy; rapidly progressive, ANCA-associated, pauci-immune GN; SLE.	Membranoproliferative GN, HCV, cryoglobulinemia, Goodpasture's syndrome, vasculitides, TTP, HUS, hereditary nephritis (Alport's syndrome).

- **Signs/Sx:** Presents with generalized edema (puffy eyes in the morning, pitting edema in the legs, pleural effusions, ascites) and foamy urine. Also associated with an ↑ risk of thromboembolism as well an ↑ risk of infection (especially from encapsulated organisms) due to loss of immunoglobulins.
- **Workup:** UA reveals proteinuria; a 24-hour urine collection is preferred (the protein-to-creatinine ratio can be used as well). Serum studies reveal hyperlipidemia (↑ LDL cholesterol) and an albumin level < 3 g/dL. A renal biopsy may be useful.
- **Tx:** Etiology dependent, but protein and salt restriction, diuretics, anticoagulants, and antihyperlipidemics are indicated. Steroids may be necessary for severe disease.

Nephritic Syndrome

- **Signs/Sx:** Presents with tea-colored urine, ↓ urine output, hypertension, and edema in dependent areas (including the periorbital and scrotal regions), although edema is not as significant as in nephrotic syndrome. The signs and symptoms of nephritic syndrome can be remembered using the mnemonic **PHAROH.**
- **Workup:** UA reveals hematuria and some degree of proteinuria; serum studies show ↓ GFR with elevated BUN and creatinine. Complement, ANA, ANCA, and anti-GBM antibodies should be measured. A ⊕ antistreptolysin O (ASO) titer indicates postinfectious GN.
- **Tx:** Etiology dependent, but hypertension, fluid congestion, and uremia should generally be treated with salt and water restriction. Diuretics, dialysis, steroids, and stronger immunosuppressants may be administered as necessary.

HYPONATREMIA

Hyponatremia is, in general, an excess of body water in relation to serum sodium, with serum sodium < 135 mEq/L. It is believed to be the most common electrolyte disorder and has numerous etiologies, prominent among which are inappropriate volume status and inability to suppress ADH (see Figure 4-9 and Table 4-15).

Signs and Symptoms

- Mild hyponatremia may be asymptomatic, especially when it is chronic. When hyponatremia is acute or of increasing severity, clinical manifestations are primarily neurologic; an acutely ↓ plasma osmolality gradient favors water movement into cells, leading to cerebral edema.

MNEMONIC

Presentation of nephritic syndrome—

PHAROH

Proteinuria (usually minimal compared to nephrotic syndrome)
Hematuria
Azotemia (↑ BUN)
RBC casts
Oliguria
Hypertension

KEY FACT

You don't need to look like a prune to be hyponatremic. Cirrhosis and CHF can also cause hyponatremia, all the while being hypervolemic.

Q

A 65-year-old woman with CHF presents with difficulty breathing and mental status changes. She has pulmonary crackles bilaterally and soft heart sounds. CXR shows pulmonary edema, and ECG reveals LVH. Her breathing, but not mental status, improves with diuresis. What lab abnormality may be causing her symptoms?

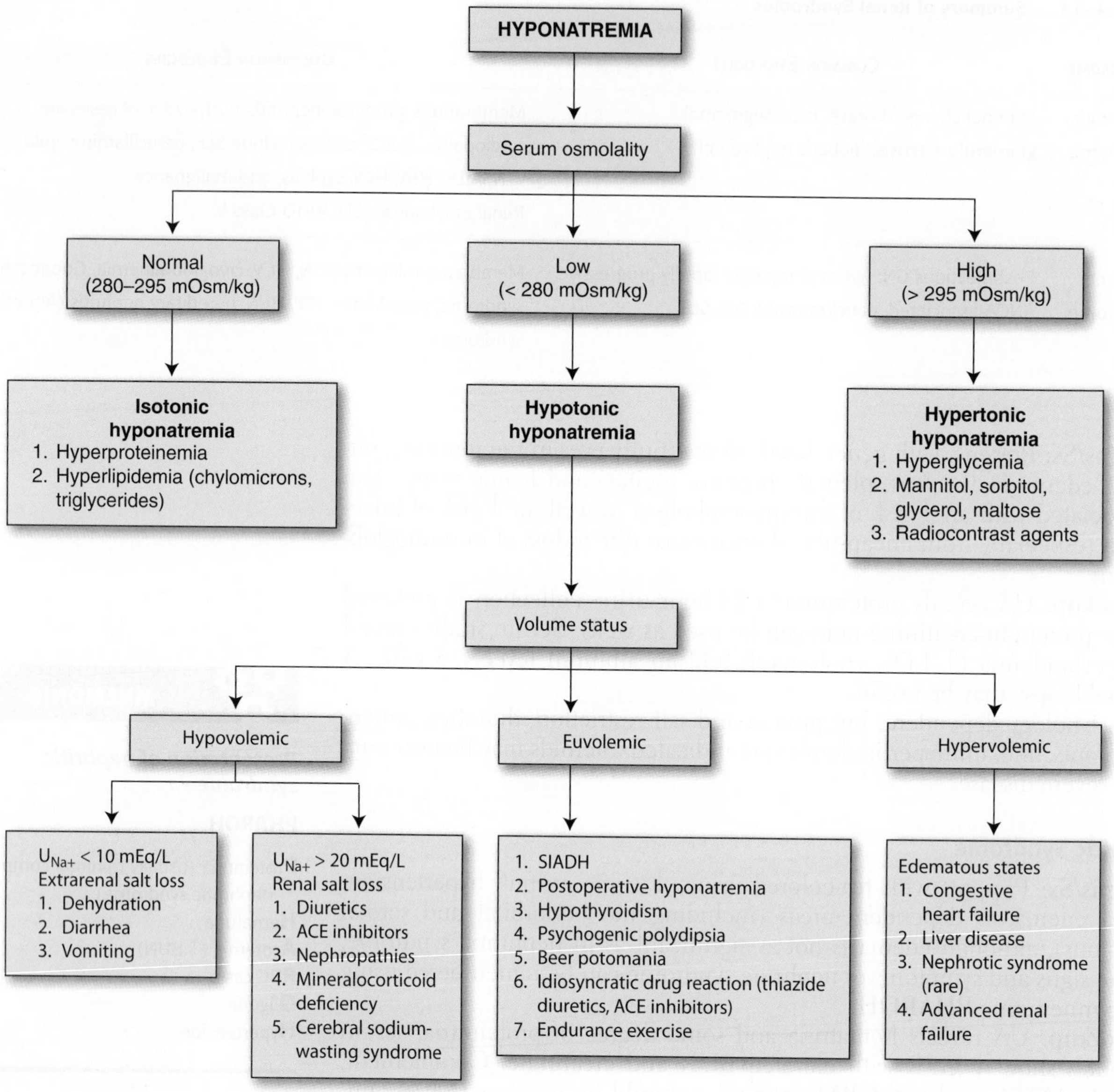

FIGURE 4-9. Workup of hyponatremia. (Reproduced with permission from Tierney LM et al. *Current Medical Diagnosis & Treatment*, 41st ed. New York: McGraw-Hill, 2002: 893.)

- **Plasma osmolality < 240 mOsm/kg:** Confusion, muscle cramps and twitching, nausea, lethargy, headache, seizures.
- **Serum sodium < 120 mEq/L:** Status epilepticus, stupor, and coma may ensue.

A

Hyponatremia in the setting of hypervolemia from CHF.

WORKUP

Plasma and urine osmolality, plasma and urine electrolytes, and urine volume must be measured. These labs can then be used to categorize the type of hyponatremia (see Figure 4-9).

TREATMENT

- The underlying etiology should be addressed, with specific treatment methods varying according to volemic status:
  - **Hypovolemic:** Replete volume with NS.
  - **Euvolemic/hypervolemic:** Salt and water restriction.

TABLE 4-15. Classification of Hyponatremia by Volume Status and ADH Level

Type	Cause
Volume Status	
Hypovolemic	GI or renal losses.
Euvolemic	SIADH.
Hypervolemic	Cirrhosis, CHF.
ADH Secretion Etiology	
Volume depletion	GI or renal losses.
↓ tissue perfusion	Cirrhosis, CHF.
1° ADH secretion	SIADH.

- Symptomatic patients may initially need rapid correction of sodium levels (2 mEq/L/hr) for the first few hours until symptoms resolve. In general, however, hyponatremia should be treated at a measured pace, with no more than 10–12 mEq/L corrected for the first day and 18 mEq/L over the first 2 days.

KEY FACT

Overly rapid correction of hyponatremia may result in the dreaded complication of central pontine myelinolysis.

NEPHROLITHIASIS

Nephrolithiasis (kidney stone formation) most commonly occurs in men, with a peak age of onset in the 20s and 30s. Stones usually result from an imbalance of salts and minerals that are normally found in the urinary tract. Table 4-16 outlines stone types in terms of composition and etiology.

KEY FACT

There's no "Y" in UTI. *Proteus* infections causing UTI are much more common causes of kidney stones in women than in men.

Signs and Symptoms

- **Classic symptoms:** Progressive, severe flank pain that radiates to the inguinal region. Patients often writhe in bed from colicky pain. Physical examination often reveals CVA tenderness.

TABLE 4-16. Etiology of Kidney Stones by Composition

Stone Composition	Etiology
Calcium phosphate/oxalate (most common)	High-oxalate diets, hyperparathyroidism, sarcoidosis.
Struvite/magnesium ammonium phosphate	More common in females, as they are often due to UTIs with urease-producing organisms (eg, *Proteus*).
Cystine	Hereditary cystinuria.
Uric acid (radiolucent)	Gout, chemotherapy.
Indinavir	HIV treatment (note that indinavir stones are undetectable on CT, as they are radiolucent by this modality).

KEY FACT

Magnesium, phosphorus, calcium, and ammonia are the most common elements found in stones.

KEY FACT

Risk factors for nephrolithiasis:

- Family history
- Age 20–40
- Diet (high protein, low fluids)
- Medications
- Immobility
- Ileostomy
- Liver disease
- Renal disease (medullary sponge kidney, RTA, PKD)

- **Associated symptoms:** Hematuria, nausea, vomiting, dysuria, tenesmus, and oliguria (in the setting of obstruction of the bladder or urethra or, less commonly, bilateral obstruction of the ureters); ↑ risk of UTIs proximal to the stone.

DIFFERENTIAL

Renal infarct, lumbar disk disease, aortic dissection, renal malignancy, pyelonephritis, trauma, glomerulonephritis.

WORKUP

- UA with culture to evaluate pH and the presence of bacteria, blood, and crystals. Urine pH is < 5.5 in uric acid stones, whereas struvite stones have a urine pH > 6.5.
- CT without contrast is often the first imaging choice, as it can identify all types of stones and can also help differentiate the various causes of flank pain. Uric acid stones are radiolucent and do not show up on CT.
- Renal ultrasound can identify hydronephrosis if obstruction is suspected; it is also a good choice for pregnant women to **minimize radiation.**
- AXR will detect 90% of stones (see Figure 4-10) but will miss uric acid stones, which are radiolucent.

TREATMENT

- Treatment varies by stone type, but all patients should have adequate fluid intake to ↑ urine output to > 2.5 L/day.
- Analgesia is an important part of treatment and often requires IV medications (ketorolac is an effective IV NSAID that is often used to avoid narcotics).
- Some 80% of small stones **(those < 4 mm)** will pass spontaneously, although this may be painful.

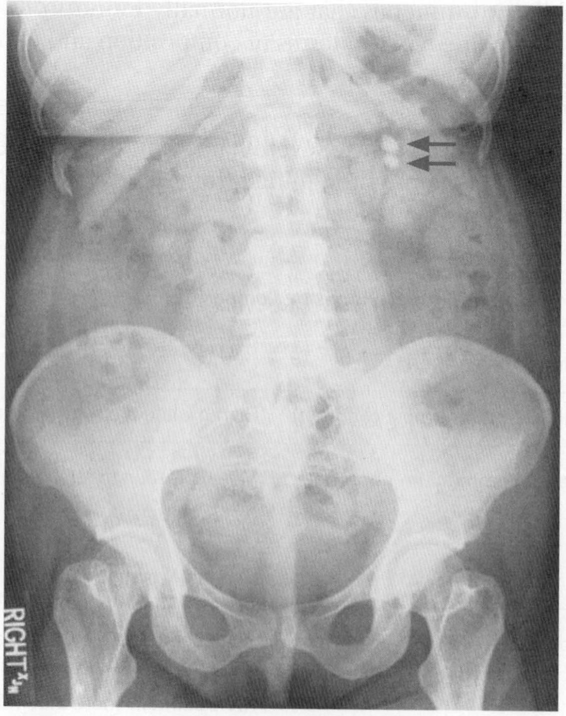

FIGURE 4-10. Kidney stone. Two radiodense renal calculi (arrows) can be seen in the left mid-kidney. (Reproduced with permission from Chen MY et al. *Basic Radiology,* 2nd ed. New York: McGraw-Hill, Fig. 9-27.)

- Stones > 5 mm require more invasive procedures, such as extracorporeal shock-wave lithotripsy, retrograde ureteroscopy (for midureteral stones), or percutaneous nephrolithotomy. If a stone is > 5 mm or if signs of infection are seen, a urology consult is warranted.
- Even with treatment, recurrence is common (10% per year).

Prevention

- Preventive measures include the following:
  - ↑ fluid intake.
  - Dietary restriction (low protein, nitrogen, and sodium; minimizing oxalate-containing foods).
  - Maintenance of adequate calcium intake.
  - Administration of thiazides (which ↓ urinary calcium excretion).
- For uric acid stones, urine should be alkalinized with potassium citrate, and allopurinol should be considered.

Gastroenterology

APPROACH TO ABDOMINAL PAIN

Visceral pain and **parietal** pain present with different qualities and can help localize the source of abdominal pain to various anatomic locations. The location of the pain can also indicate not only the organs involved but also the possible pathophysiologic processes that might be occurring.

- **Visceral pain** involves distention of a hollow organ or viscus and is dull and crampy, poorly localized, and vague.
- **Parietal pain** involves the parietal peritoneum, is sharp and stabbing, and is well localized (see Table 4-17).

Workup

- When evaluating abdominal pain, consider narrowing the differential by assessing the pain in terms of quality, location, and physical examination findings.
- Key findings pointing to an emergency include absent bowel sounds (eg, pancreatitis, bowel ischemia, ileus, acute abdomen), high-pitched bowel sounds (eg, obstruction), rebound tenderness, abdominal rigidity, involuntary guarding, and pulsatile masses. Attention should also be heightened when patients have point tenderness, a ⊕ Murphy's sign, or palpable masses.

Treatment

Treatment is etiology specific.

CIRRHOSIS

Defined as the irreversible destruction of normal hepatic architecture with characteristic diffuse fibrosis and regenerative nodules. The most common cause in the United States is alcohol abuse; the most common etiology worldwide is viral hepatitis. Other etiologies are as follows:

- **Metabolic diseases:** Wilson's disease, hemochromatosis, α_1-antitrypsin deficiency.
- **Drugs and toxins:** INH, methyldopa, acetaminophen, methotrexate, carbon tetrachloride.

KEY FACT

Diagnosing RLQ pain can stress out anyone. Look to the appendix and reproductive organs, particularly in younger patients, although intestinal causes and kidney stones are also possibilities. And don't miss a Meckel's!

Q

A 38-year-old man with a recent history of bloody diarrhea and progressive abdominal pain is brought to the ED. He begins to have nausea and vomiting as well. Examination reveals "tinkling" bowel sounds. What is his likely condition and its possible etiology?

TABLE 4-17. Characterization of Abdominal Pain by Location

Location	Organs Affected	Possible Disease Entities
Right upper	Liver, gallbladder, kidney, small bowel	Hepatitis, cholelithiasis, choledocholithiasis, cholecystitis, biliary colic, 1° sclerosing cholangitis, 1° biliary cirrhosis, pyelonephritis, hepatic tumors/abscesses, right lower lobe pneumonia.
Epigastric	Stomach, abdominal aorta, pancreas	MI, pericarditis (pain ↓ when sitting forward), PUD, perforated ulcer, gastritis, pancreatitis, abdominal aortic aneurysm.
Left upper	Spleen, kidney, small bowel	Splenomegaly, splenic infarct, splenic rupture, pyelonephritis, pneumonia, MI, pericarditis, perforated ulcer.
Periumbilical	Abdominal aorta, small bowel, appendix	Abdominal aortic aneurysm or dissection, ischemic bowel (abrupt, episodic pain out of proportion to examination that worsens with food intake–"intestinal angina"), small bowel obstruction (crampy, episodic pain that worsens with food and/or vomiting that ↑ with any PO intake), umbilical hernia, appendicitis, gastroenteritis.
Right lower	Appendix, ovary, fallopian tubes, kidney, ureter, intestines, testes	Nephrolithiasis (flank pain), pyelonephritis, appendicitis, Meckel's diverticulum, right-sided diverticulitis, IBD or other forms of colitis, ovarian cyst, PID, tubo-ovarian abscess (TOA), ectopic pregnancy, ovulatory pain (mittelschmerz).
Suprapubic	Bladder, uterus, ovaries, fallopian tubes	UTI, bladder or cervical cancer, PID, bladder outlet obstruction, endometriosis.
Left lower	Ovary, fallopian tubes, kidney, ureter, intestines, testes	Nephrolithiasis, pyelonephritis, left-sided diverticulitis, IBD or other forms of colitis, ovarian cyst, PID, TOA, ectopic pregnancy, ovulatory pain (mittelschmerz).

- **Biliary diseases:** 1° biliary cirrhosis or chronic biliary obstruction.
- **Other:** Cardiac cirrhosis or impaired venous drainage of the liver (eg, IVC or hepatic vein [Budd-Chiari] occlusion).

KEY FACT

A former alcoholic presents with confusion and has a flapping tremor of the wrists with extension (asterixis). This patient likely has hepatic encephalopathy.

Signs and Symptoms

- Presents with fatigue, malaise, and peripheral edema.
- Physical examination reveals stigmata of liver disease, summarized in Figure 4-11.
- **Hepatic encephalopathy:** The etiology remains unclear, although serum ammonia levels are ↑. With more severe forms, asterixis, confusion, and coma are evident.
- **Hepatorenal and hepatopulmonary syndromes:**
  - Hepatorenal syndrome is marked by liver disease along with oliguria, low Fe_{Na}, and failure of the azotemia to respond to fluid bolus.
  - Hepatopulmonary syndrome is characterized by liver disease along with dyspnea, platypnea (an ↑ in dyspnea when the patient is in an upright position compared to supine), hypoxemia, and/or orthodeoxia (a ↓ in Sao_2 > 5% when the patient is moved from a supine to an upright position).

A

The patient likely has bowel obstruction, potentially from Crohn's disease.

Differential

Nephrotic syndrome, CHF, constrictive pericarditis, abdominal malignancy, peritoneal TB.

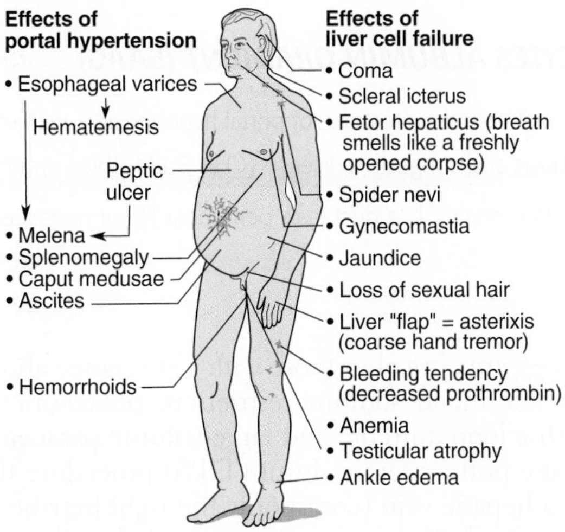

FIGURE 4-11. Signs and symptoms of cirrhosis and portal hypertension. (Adapted with permission from Chandrasoma P, Taylor CE. *Concise Pathology*, 3rd ed. Stamford, CT: Appleton & Lange, 1998: 654.)

Workup

- Cirrhosis severity is defined by the Child-Pugh criteria (see Table 4-18) and the Model for End-Stage Liver Disease (MELD) score.
- Other laboratory studies include ammonia (↑), BUN (↓ owing to a fall in protein production), sodium (hyponatremia), CBC (anemia, thrombocytopenia), and transaminases/alkaline phosphatase (↑).
- Additional tests are etiology dependent and include ANA, anti–smooth muscle antibody, anti-LKM (presence indicates autoimmune hepatitis), ceruloplasmin (↓ serum level indicates Wilson's disease), α-fetoprotein (↑ in hepatocellular carcinoma), iron studies (↑↑↑ ferritin and TIBC indicate hemochromatosis), and serum electrophoresis (absence of α-globulin indicates α_1-antitrypsin deficiency).
- RUQ ultrasound may show fatty infiltration of liver consistent with nonalcoholic fatty liver disease.
- The serum-ascites albumin gradient (SAAG), derived from paracentesis, is an excellent general test but is invasive.

TABLE 4-18. Child-Pugh Criteria for the Classification of Cirrhosis[a]

Factor	Points: 1	Points: 2	Points: 3
Serum bilirubin (mmol/L) [mg/dL]	< 34 [< 2.0]	34–51 [2.0–3.0]	> 51 [> 3.0]
Serum albumin (g/L) [g/dL]	> 35 [> 3.5]	30–35 [3.0–3.5]	< 30 [< 3.0]
Ascites	None	Easily controlled	Poorly controlled
Neurologic changes	None	Minimal	Advanced coma
INR	< 1.7	1.7–2.3	> 2.3

[a] The Child-Pugh score is calculated by adding the scores of the 5 factors (range 5–15). The Child-Pugh class is A (a score of 5–6), B (7–9), or C (≥ 10).

(Reproduced with permission from Braunwald E et al. *Harrison's Principles of Internal Medicine,* 15th ed. New York: McGraw-Hill, 2001: 1711.)

KEY FACT

Albumin, PT, and bilirubin are tests of liver function. AST, ALT, and alkaline phosphatase are ↑ when there is hepatocellular injury or cholestasis.

KEY FACT

In general, "decompensation" indicates cirrhosis with Child-Pugh class B, and this level is the accepted criterion for applying for liver transplantation. The timing of liver transplantation is based on the MELD score.

KEY POINT

SERUM-ASCITES ALBUMIN GRADIENT (SAAG)

- **SAAG ≥ 1.1:** Indicates the presence of portal hypertension, with etiologies including cirrhosis and congestive disease (CHF, Budd-Chiari syndrome).
- **SAAG < 1.1:** Pancreatitis, bile duct leak, peritoneal TB, or metastases.

TREATMENT

- Lifestyle changes are critical in those with a substance abuse history.
- For ascites, recommend sodium restriction, potassium-sparing diuretics combined with a loop diuretic, and large-volume paracentesis. A transjugular intrahepatic portosystemic shunt (TIPS) procedure that connects the portal vein to a hepatic vein (commonly the right hepatic vein) is effective for refractory ascites but can precipitate encephalopathy.
- Esophageal varices can be treated with nonselective β-blockers (usually nadolol) to prevent initial bleeding. Bleeding varices are a medical emergency and can be treated with IV vasopressin (with nitroglycerin), IV somatostatin, endoscopic sclerotherapy or band ligation, and balloon tamponade.
- Management of hepatic encephalopathy includes protein restriction, lactulose (to promote ammonia excretion with 3 bowel movements a day), and neomycin (to inhibit ammonia-producing bacteria in the colon).
- Consider liver transplantation for refractory disease. There is currently a sobriety requirement period that EtOH abuse patients must fulfill before they are eligible for transplantation (6 months is the period most widely used).

KEY FACT

Here's a TIP(S): Connect the portal vein to a hepatic vein rather than the IVC for refractory ascites, but be prepared for some confusion!

HEPATITIS

Acute or chronic inflammation of the liver is considered hepatitis. The most common causes include hepatitis viruses and alcohol abuse. Autoimmune/granulomatous and drug-induced hepatitis are rarer entities. Viral etiologies are distinguished as follows:

- **HAV/HEV:** Spread by fecal-oral contact. Acute rather than chronic; do not cause cirrhosis.
- **HBV/HCV:** Spread by blood or other body fluids (eg, IV drug use—HBV and HCV; sexual contact—HBV). Can become chronic, causing cirrhosis.

KEY FACT

The major risk factors for viral hepatitis are IV drug use (HBV, HCV), unprotected sexual intercourse (HBV), and overseas travel (HAV, HEV).

SIGNS AND SYMPTOMS

- **Acute hepatitis:** Often starts with a viral prodrome (malaise, fatigue, URI symptoms, nausea, vomiting, joint pain) followed by fever and diarrhea.
- **Chronic hepatitis:** Presents with symptoms of chronic liver disease and cirrhosis.
- Physical examination reveals jaundice, scleral icterus, hepatomegaly, splenomegaly, lymphadenopathy, and RUQ tenderness.

DIFFERENTIAL

Systemic shock with liver hypoperfusion, neoplasm (hepatocellular carcinoma or metastatic liver lesions), abscess, toxoplasmosis, rickettsial diseases, biliary obstruction, systemic viral illnesses (eg, mononucleosis).

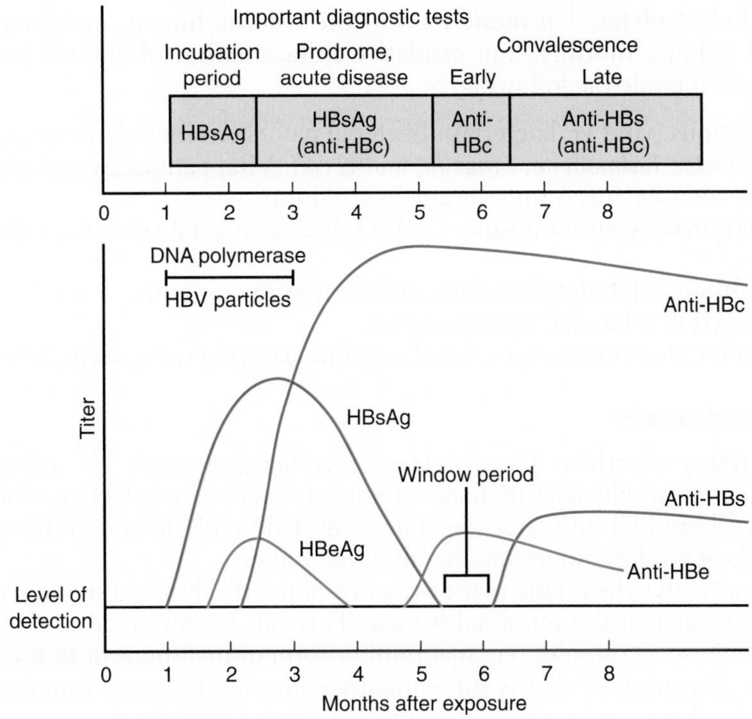

FIGURE 4-12. **Serum antibody and antigen levels in HBV.**

Workup

- **Acute hepatitis:** CBC and LFTs; viral serology if HBV is suspected (see Figure 4-12).
- **Chronic hepatitis:** Hepatitis virus serology, liver biopsy, transaminases (must be ↑ for > 6 months). ↑ alkaline phosphatase and, in severe cases, ↑ PT may also be observed.

Treatment

- **Acute hepatitis:**
  - Supportive, including rest and assessment of sick contacts.
  - For HBV/HCV, consider α-interferon.
  - Steroids can be used for severe alcoholic hepatitis.
- **Chronic hepatitis:**
  - α_{2b}-interferon (or pegylated interferon) and lamivudine.
  - α-interferon + ribavirin for chronic HCV. Viral RNA is assayed to assess treatment response.
  - Several new drugs have been approved by the FDA for the treatment of chronic HCV:
    - **Boceprevir:** Combined with α_{2b}-interferon, has shown improved viral response in chronic HCV genotype 1.
    - **Telaprevir:** Combined with pegylated interferon and ribavirin, may induce sustained virologic response at 24 weeks' posttreatment.

DIARRHEA

Diarrhea is the excretion of > 250 g of stool per day. **Acute diarrhea** is usually infectious, often has a sudden onset, and lasts < 3 weeks. **Chronic diarrhea** has a broader differential, often waxes and wanes, and generally persists for > 3 weeks. The basic mechanisms of diarrhea can include ↑ **secretion of wa-**

KEY FACT

Roughly 15–20% of alcoholics develop hepatitis. An AST/ALT ratio > 2:1 points to alcoholic hepatitis.

KEY FACT

Some 30% of HCV-infected patients have comorbid major depression, making interferon treatment more difficult.

Q

An otherwise healthy 20-year-old woman presents to her physician with persistent diarrhea of 3 days' duration. She notes that the diarrhea is bloody. On examination, she is febrile and tachycardic but otherwise normal. Which important history questions would greatly aid in diagnosis?

KEY FACT

Give me a **Y-E-S-S-C!** ***Y****ersinia,* ***E*** *coli,* ***S****almonella,* ***S****higella,* and ***C****ampylobacter* are the most common causes of infectious diarrhea.

KEY FACT

Diarrhea is technically defined as the excretion of > 250 g of stool daily, but patients may consider the term to have different meanings. Obtain a clear history!

KEY FACT

If a patient who was recently treated with clindamycin presents with watery, foul-smelling diarrhea, think *C difficile* colitis and initiate treatment with oral metronidazole or vancomycin.

A

Ask about sick contacts, travel history, antibiotic use, previous history of diarrhea, food diary, and comorbidities.

ter and electrolytes, ↑ osmotic load in the colonic lumen, malabsorption, altered colonic motility, and **exudative inflammation of colonic mucosa.** Etiologies include the following:

- **Infectious (viral vs. bacterial):** Bacterial pathogens include *Yersinia, Campylobacter, Salmonella, Shigella,* and *E coli.* Viral pathogens include norovirus and rotavirus (primarily affects children).
- **Inflammatory/autoimmune:** Crohn's disease, ulcerative colitis, celiac disease.
- **Antibiotic related:** *Clostridium difficile* is most common.
- **HIV/AIDS related:** *Cryptosporidium.*
- **Other:** Other medications, small intestine bacterial overgrowth, IBS.

Signs and Symptoms

- **Secretory diarrhea:** Occurs when secretagogues such as endogenous endocrine products (VIPomas, serotonin), endotoxins/infection (cholera), and GI luminal substances (eg, bile acids, fatty acids, laxatives) stimulate ↑ levels of fluid transport into the intestinal lumen.
- **Osmotic diarrhea:** Due to the presence of poorly absorbed substances that retain water in the intestinal lumen. This can be attributed to the ingestion of excess osmoles (eg, mannitol or sorbitol ingestion) or to the ingestion of a substrate that is subsequently converted to excess osmoles. Can also be due to an enzyme deficiency (eg, lactase deficiency).
- **Malabsorptive diarrhea:** Due to the inability to digest or absorb a particular nutrient, which can in turn be attributable to bacterial overgrowth, pancreatic enzyme deficiency, or altered motility/anatomy (eg, celiac disease).

Workup

- Obtain a complete history, including recent **sick contacts, recent travel, immune status,** and **antibiotic use.**
- **Acute diarrhea:** Does not require laboratory investigation unless the patient has a high fever, bloody diarrhea, or diarrhea lasting > 4–5 days.
  - If studies are warranted, check for fecal leukocytes (Wright's stain), bacterial culture, *C difficile* toxin, and ova/parasites.
  - Consider sigmoidoscopy or colonoscopy in patients with severe proctitis, bloody diarrhea, or possible *C difficile* colitis.
- **Chronic diarrhea:** Differentiate osmotic from secretory forms (see also Figure 4-13):
  - Secretory diarrhea may be watery, whereas osmotic diarrhea may be greasy or bulky.
  - Osmotic diarrhea will improve with fasting, but secretory diarrhea will not.
  - A stool osmotic gap > 50 mOsm/kg H_2O suggests an osmotic diarrhea.
- The differential diagnosis for colitis includes ischemia as well as inflammatory or infectious causes.

Treatment

- **Acute diarrhea:**
  - Oral or IV fluids and electrolyte replacement.
  - Antidiarrheal agents (eg, loperamide or bismuth salicylate) may improve symptoms but are contraindicated in patients with bloody diarrhea, high fever, or systemic toxicity (eg, *E coli* O157:H7, *Salmonella*).
  - Antibiotic use is controversial in that it is beneficial for treating certain organisms (eg, *C difficile*) but possibly harmful for others (*Salmonella*

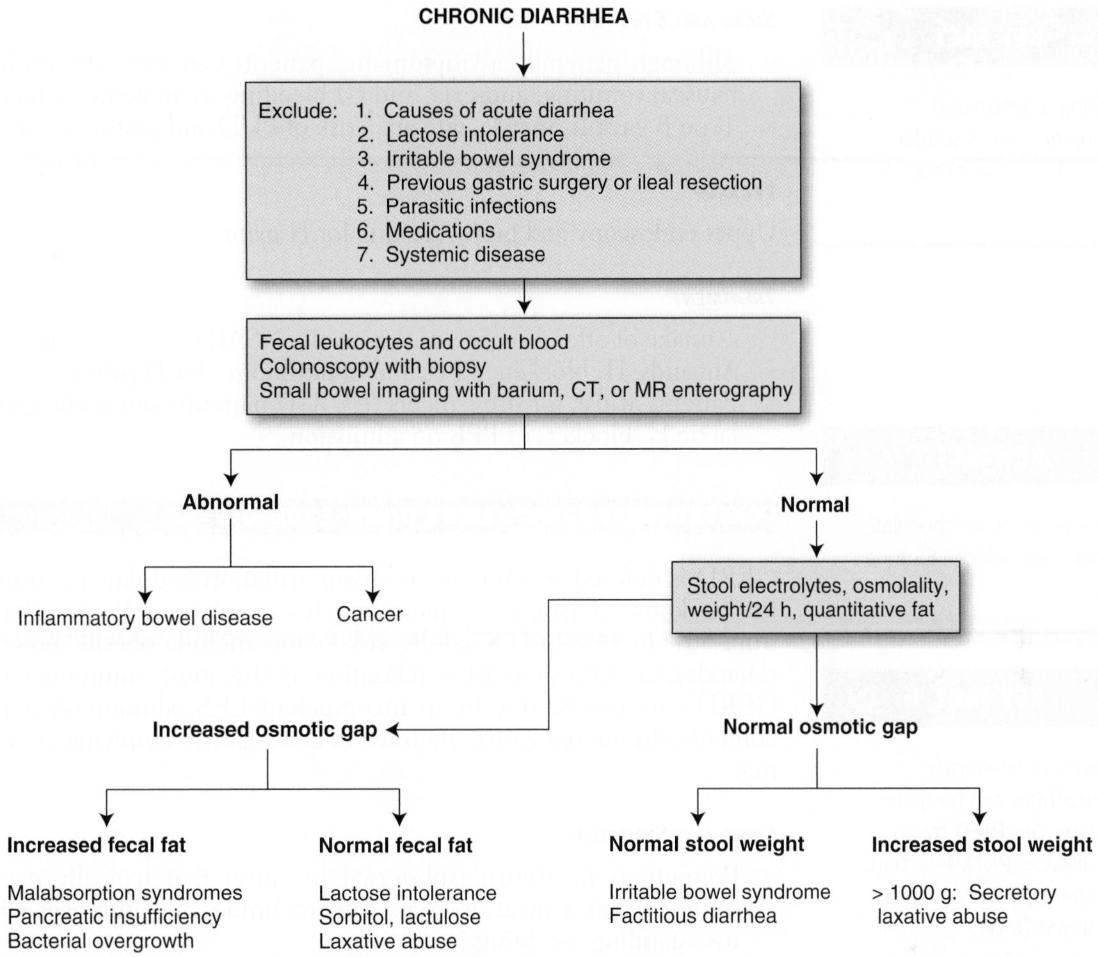

FIGURE 4-13. Decision diagram for the diagnosis of causes of chronic diarrhea. (Reproduced with permission from McPhee SJ et al. *Current Medical Diagnosis & Treatment 2012.* New York: McGraw-Hill, 2012, Fig. 15-2.)

and *E coli* O157:H7). Treat patients with antibiotics if there is a high likelihood of **bacteremia** (especially immunosuppressed patients).

- **Chronic diarrhea:**
  - Treat underlying causes and avoid dietary substances contributing to diarrhea. Consider antibiotics to treat bacterial overgrowth.
  - Loperamide, opioids, clonidine, octreotide, cholestyramine, and enzyme supplements can also be tried.

> **KEY FACT**
>
> In patients who have been traveling, think about parasites. In patients who have eaten shellfish, consider *Vibrio* and norovirus. In patients who have eaten undercooked poultry, think about *Campylobacter* and *Salmonella*.

GASTRITIS

Gastritis, or inflammation of the gastric mucosa, can be divided into **acute** and **chronic** types. Causes include the following:

- **Acute "stress" gastritis (superficial lesions that evolve rapidly):** NSAID use, alcohol, and stress from severe illness (eg, Curling's ulcers in burn patients).
- **Chronic "nonerosive" gastritis:** Has 2 subtypes:
  - **Type A:** Fundal gastritis 2° to autoantibodies to parietal cells. Accounts for 10% of chronic gastritis cases and is often comorbid with pernicious anemia, thyroiditis, and other autoimmune disorders.
  - **Type B:** Antral gastritis caused by NSAIDs (the most common cause), *H pylori*, CMV, and HSV. Accounts for 90% of chronic gastritis cases.

KEY FACT

Not all vomiting is associated with preceding nausea. A sudden presentation is known as precipitate vomiting.

KEY FACT

Alcohol, caffeine, nicotine, chocolate, and fatty foods can reduce LES tone and ↑ reflux.

KEY FACT

The implications of seemingly innocuous heartburn can be quite serious, so don't **G**et **PIED** by **G**allbladder disease, **P**UD, **I**nfection, **E**sophageal spasm/**E**sophagitis, or **D**ying heart tissue (MI).

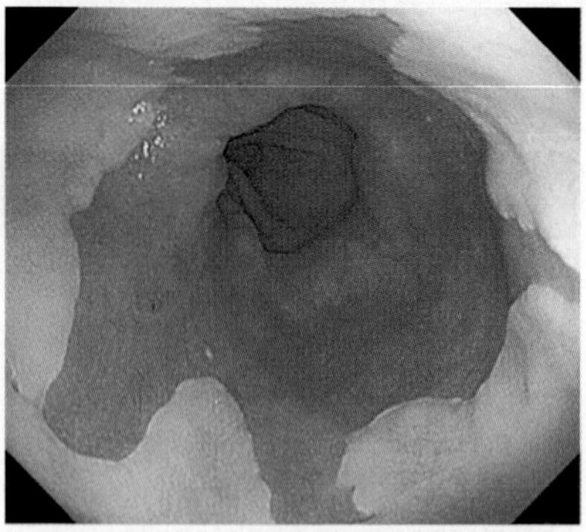

FIGURE 4-14. Barrett's esophagus. Note the pink "tongues" that are characteristic of Barrett's. (Reproduced with permission from Longo DL et al. *Harrison's Principles of Internal Medicine,* 18th ed. New York: McGraw-Hill, 2012, Fig. 291-3A.)

KEY FACT

On an upper GI radiographic series, esophageal spasm classically resembles a corkscrew.

Signs and Symptoms

- Although generally asymptomatic, patients can present with indigestion, nausea, vomiting, anorexia, and GI bleeding (hematemesis, melena).
- Type B gastritis may lead to an ↑ risk of PUD and gastric cancer.

Workup

Upper endoscopy and biopsy; testing for *H pylori.*

Treatment

- ↓ intake of offending agents (especially NSAIDs and alcohol).
- Antacids, H_2 blockers, PPIs, and/or antibiotics for *H pylori.*
- Patients at risk for stress ulcers (eg, ICU patients) should be given prophylactic H_2 blockers or PPIs on admission.

GASTROESOPHAGEAL REFLUX DISEASE (GERD)

GERD is defined as symptomatic tissue irritation and damage resulting from the backflow of gastric contents into the esophagus. Its prevalence ranges from 36% to 44% in U.S. adults; risk factors include obesity, pregnancy, and scleroderma. Transient LES relaxation is the most common etiology, but GERD can also be due to an incompetent LES, abnormally acidic gastric contents, disordered gastric motility, delayed gastric emptying, and hiatal hernia.

Signs and Symptoms

- Presents as heartburn (substernal burning) that typically occurs 30–90 minutes after a meal, worsens with reclining, and improves with antacid use, standing, or sitting.
- Other symptoms include sour taste ("water brash"), regurgitation, dysphagia, epigastric pain, halitosis, morning cough, laryngitis, chronic cough, and wheezing/dyspnea (which can mimic or exacerbate asthma).

Differential

- PUD, infectious (CMV/candidal) or chemical esophagitis, gallbladder disease, achalasia, esophageal spasm (most common in adults).
- CAD and pericarditis.

Workup

- Physical examination is typically normal unless GERD is 2° to systemic disease (eg, scleroderma).
- Upper endoscopy should be performed in patients with longstanding symptoms or to identify and grade esophagitis or Barrett's esophagus (see Figure 4-14).
- Esophageal manometry and 24-hour pH monitoring.
- Obtain an AXR, a CXR, and a barium swallow (of limited use, but can help diagnose hiatal hernia and possibly motility problems).
- Can often be treated empirically, with further testing conducted only if treatment fails.

Treatment

- **Lifestyle modification:** Weight loss, head-of-bed elevation, avoidance of late meals.
- **Pharmacologic management:** H_2 blockers, PPIs, promotility agents.

- **Surgical intervention:** For severe hiatal hernia or congenital cases; Nissen fundoplication is the most common intervention (since the advent of PPIs, this is performed very infrequently).
- Upper endoscopy with biopsy is useful in monitoring for Barrett's esophagus and esophageal adenocarcinoma.

Complications

Esophageal ulceration, esophageal stricture, aspiration of gastric contents, upper GI bleeding, Barrett's esophagus, adenocarcinoma of the esophagus.

PEPTIC ULCER DISEASE (PUD)

Peptic ulcers are breaks that occur in the gastric or duodenal mucosa (and in some cases the submucosa). Duodenal ulcers are 5 times more common than gastric ulcers; however, gastric ulcers are associated with an ↑ risk of gastric cancer, whereas duodenal ulcers carry only a minimal risk. The lifetime incidence of PUD is 5–10%. Duodenal ulcers are associated with excess gastric acid production; gastric ulcers are associated with impaired mucosal defenses, usually without acid hypersecretion. The 3 major causes of PUD are as follows:

- NSAID use.
- Chronic *H pylori* infection (plays a causative role in > 90% of duodenal ulcers as well as in 60–70% of gastric ulcers).
- Acid hypersecretory states such as Zollinger-Ellison syndrome.

Signs and Symptoms

- PUD usually presents with chronic or periodic burning/dull/aching epigastric pain.
  - Pain from duodenal ulcers can be alleviated with food and antacids but usually recurs roughly 3 hours later.
  - Pain from gastric ulcers can worsen with food intake, leading to weight loss.
- Less common symptoms include nausea, hematemesis with "coffee-ground" or bright red emesis, blood in the stool/melena, early satiety, or pain radiating to the back.

Differential

- GERD, perforation, gastric cancer, gastritis, nonulcer dyspepsia, esophageal rupture, Zollinger-Ellison syndrome.
- Pancreatitis (acute or chronic), cholecystitis, choledocholithiasis, IBS.
- Ureteral colic.
- CAD, angina, MI, aortic aneurysm.

Workup

- Physical examination reveals epigastric tenderness and, if active bleeding is present, a ⊕ stool guaiac. A "succussion splash" (the sound of air and fluid in a distended stomach) can also be heard as a result of gastric outlet obstruction roughly 3 hours after eating.
- Upper endoscopy and concurrent biopsy of the lesion can be used to rule out active bleeding and determine the presence of malignancy.
- *H pylori* can be detected by endoscopic biopsy with a direct rapid urease test (*Campylobacter*-like organism or CLO test), urease breath tests, or

KEY FACT

Barrett's esophagus is columnar metaplasia of the distal esophagus 2° to chronic acid irritation. It is associated with an ↑ risk of esophageal adenocarcinoma.

KEY FACT

Some 10% of gastric ulcers are found to harbor adenocarcinoma on biopsy. Gastric ulcers thus require more scrupulous follow-up than do duodenal ulcers.

KEY FACT

Rule out Zollinger-Ellison syndrome in GERD or PUD that is refractory to treatment. Serum gastrin is usually > 1000 pg/mL. Patients also have a paradoxical rise in serum gastrin with secretin stimulation.

Q

A 47-year-old woman with chronic back pain presents to her physician with epigastric pain that has lasted > 1 month. She notes that eating makes her pain worse. Aside from mild epigastric tenderness, her physical examination is unremarkable. What is a likely etiology for her abdominal pain?

KEY FACT

The most common source of hemorrhage in PUD is erosion into the gastroduodenal artery.

KEY FACT

PUD **P**erforates into the **P**eritoneal space and **P**enetrates into adjacent organs.

KEY FACT

Some 50–94% of IBS patients who seek medical care suffer from concurrent psychiatric disorders such as major depression or generalized anxiety.

A

PUD (likely a gastric ulcer because eating makes her pain worse) induced by chronic NSAID use to help control her back pain.

serum IgG (which is less expensive but less sensitive, indicating only exposure, not active infection); all have a sensitivity of > 90%.
- Barium contrast upper GI series.

TREATMENT

- Treatment has 3 major goals: protecting the mucosa, decreasing acid production, and eradicating *H pylori* infection if present.
- All exacerbating agents (NSAIDs, nicotine, alcohol) should be discontinued.
- Antacids, H_2 blockers (eg, cimetidine, ranitidine, famotidine), PPIs (eg, omeprazole, lansoprazole), and sucralfate are used to promote healing.
- The 1° treatment regimens for *H pylori* elimination are quadruple or triple therapies consisting of a combination of an antacid (a PPI or an H_2 blocker), bismuth salicylate, and antibiotics (metronidazole, amoxicillin, clarithromycin).
- All patients with symptomatic gastric ulcers for > 2 months despite therapy must undergo endoscopy with biopsy to rule out gastric adenocarcinoma.
- Refractory cases (rare) may require a surgical procedure such as vagotomy (proximal gastric vagotomy is preferred) or a highly selective truncal vagotomy with antrectomy.

COMPLICATIONS

Hemorrhage, gastric outlet obstruction, perforation (usually anterior ulcers), intractable disease, MALT lymphomas.

IRRITABLE BOWEL SYNDROME (IBS)

A functional disorder characterized by continuous or recurring symptoms of abdominal pain and irregular bowel habits. Patients most commonly present in their teens and 20s, but since the syndrome is chronic, they can present at any age. Some 22 million people in the United States are affected, with a two- to threefold ↑ prevalence in females. The etiology is unknown but may involve a disruption in normal colonic motility and altered neurologic perceptions. GI inflammation and alterations in natural GI flora may also play a role.

SIGNS AND SYMPTOMS

- Commonly presents as follows:
  - Abdominal pain that is relieved by a bowel movement.
  - A change in frequency.
  - A change in consistency.
- Alternates between constipation and diarrhea. Generally, one or the other state predominates.

DIFFERENTIAL

IBD, mesenteric ischemia, diverticulitis, PUD, celiac disease, colonic neoplasia, infectious or pseudomembranous colitis, gynecologic disorders, thyroid disorders.

WORKUP

- Physical examination is often unremarkable except for mild abdominal tenderness.
- Obtain CBC, electrolytes, TSH, ESR, stool cultures, abdominal films, contrast CT, and barium contrast studies to rule out other conditions.
- Manometry may be used to assess sphincter function.

Treatment

- Initiate lifestyle changes such as ↑ fiber intake and ↓ consumption of gas-producing foods (eg, legumes).
- Provide psychological assurance.
- Pharmacologic therapy may include antidiarrheals (eg, loperamide), antispasmodics, anticholinergics (eg, dicyclomine and hyoscyamine), and antidepressants.
- Other medications include cholestyramine (for diarrhea-predominant IBS) and alosetron (a 5-HT_3 antagonist for women with severe, chronic or diarrhea-predominant IBS). The availability of alosetron is limited owing to reports of ischemic colitis.

Hematology

ANEMIA

Defined as a ↓ in the number of total RBCs, a ↓ in hemoglobin, or a ↓ in hematocrit. Etiologies are numerous (see Figure 4-15) but can be distinguished according to the following general mechanisms:

- ↓ RBC production (macrocytic, microcytic, normocytic).
- ↑ RBC destruction (eg, hemolysis, which can be due to intra- or extracorpuscular factors and may occur intra- or extravascularly).
- ↑ blood loss. Chronic loss can lead to a production problem through iron deficiency.

The first mechanism has a ↓ reticulocyte count, whereas the second and third mechanisms are characterized by an ↑ reticulocyte count.

Signs and Symptoms

- Usually asymptomatic, but may present with fatigue, dyspnea, dizziness, and/or exertional angina.
- Mildly anemic patients will have a normal physical examination, but those with moderate to severe anemia can have pallor of the skin and conjunctiva, a flattened jugular vein, tachycardia, and a systolic flow murmur.
- In anemia, physical manifestations depend on the etiology and include the following:
  - **B_{12} deficiency:** Peripheral neuropathy with loss of position and vibratory sense.
  - **Blood loss** (eg, heavy menstruation, malignancy).
  - **Sickle cell disease:** Pain crisis, acute chest.
  - **Hypothyroidism:** Menorrhagia, dry and coarse skin and hair, personality change, loss of lateral eyebrows, periorbital edema.
  - **Severe iron deficiency:** Angular cheilitis, atrophic glossitis, ↑ bilirubin, ↑ platelet count, weak nails, koilonychia.
  - **Chronic diseases** (eg, renal or liver disease).

Workup

- CBC, iron studies (iron saturation and serum ferritin; see Table 4-19), serum B_{12}, serum folate, reticulocyte count, and peripheral blood smear (see Figure 4-16).
- Coombs' test, PT/PTT, haptoglobin, D-dimer, fibrinogen, and LDH to determine whether there is hemolysis and to differentiate between hemolytic anemias if present.

KEY FACT

Anemia found on testing rarely requires blood transfusion except in cases of acute, severe blood loss or marked symptoms.

KEY FACT

Be aware of folate deficiency 2° to medications (eg, methotrexate, TMP-SMX, sulfa drugs).

KEY FACT

Anemia **H**as to **S**uck your **B**lood: **H**ypothyroidism, **S**ickle cell disease/**S**evere iron deficiency, **B**lood loss/**B**$_{12}$ deficiency.

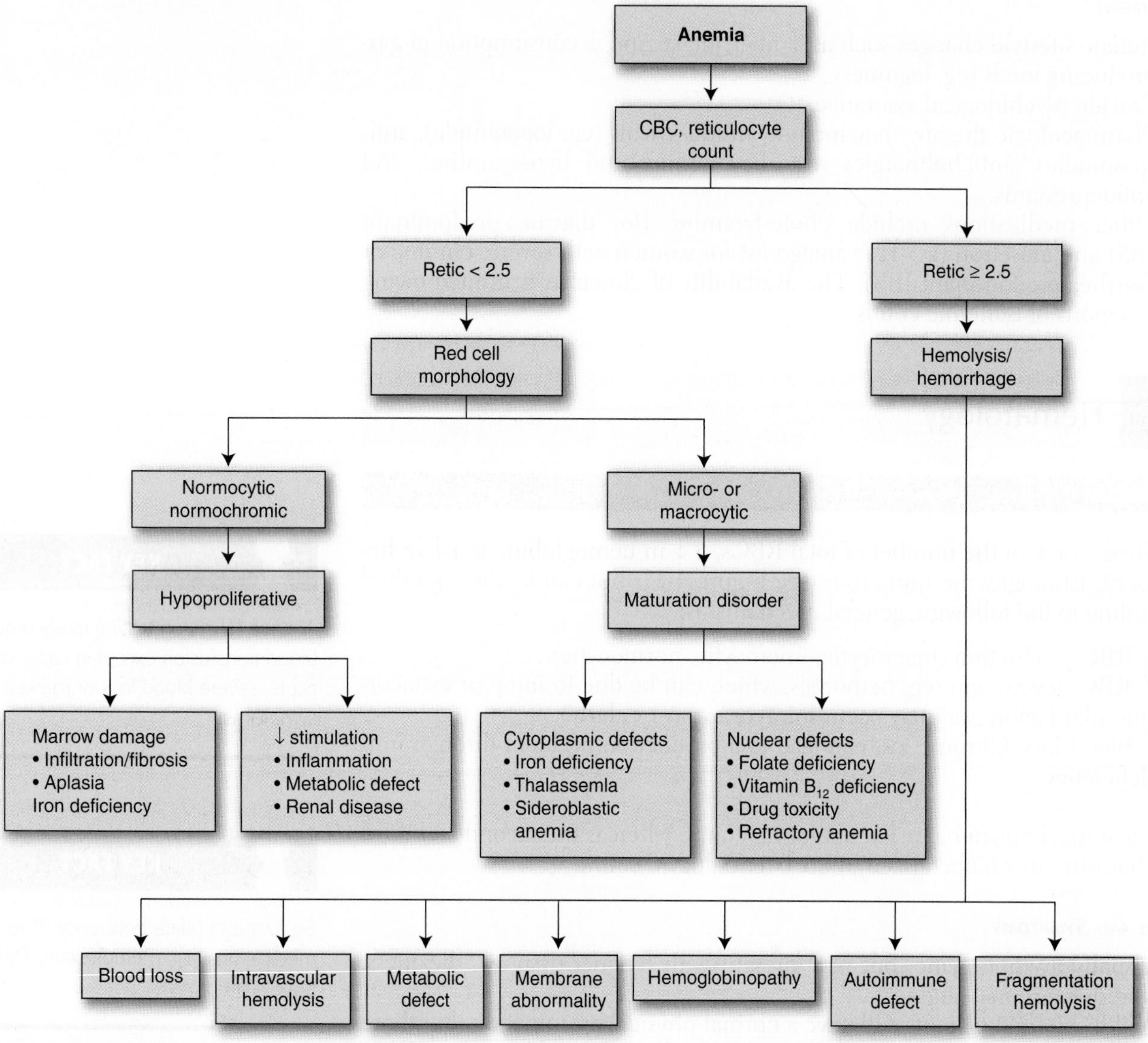

FIGURE 4-15. Physiologic classification of anemia. (Reproduced with permission from Longo DL et al. *Harrison's Principles of Internal Medicine,* 18th ed. New York: McGraw-Hill, 2012, Fig. 57-17.)

TABLE 4-19. Iron Studies in Microcytic Anemia

Disorder	Serum Iron	Serum Ferritin	TIBC	Percent Saturation	Hemoglobin Electrophoresis Pattern
Iron deficiency anemia	↓	↓	↑	↓	Normal
Anemia of chronic disease	↓	↑	↓	↓	Normal
α-thalassemia	Normal	Normal	Normal	Normal	Normal for 1- and 2-gene deletions; abnormal for 4-gene deletions
β-thalassemia	Normal	Normal	Normal	Normal	↓ A1, ↑ A2, ↑ F

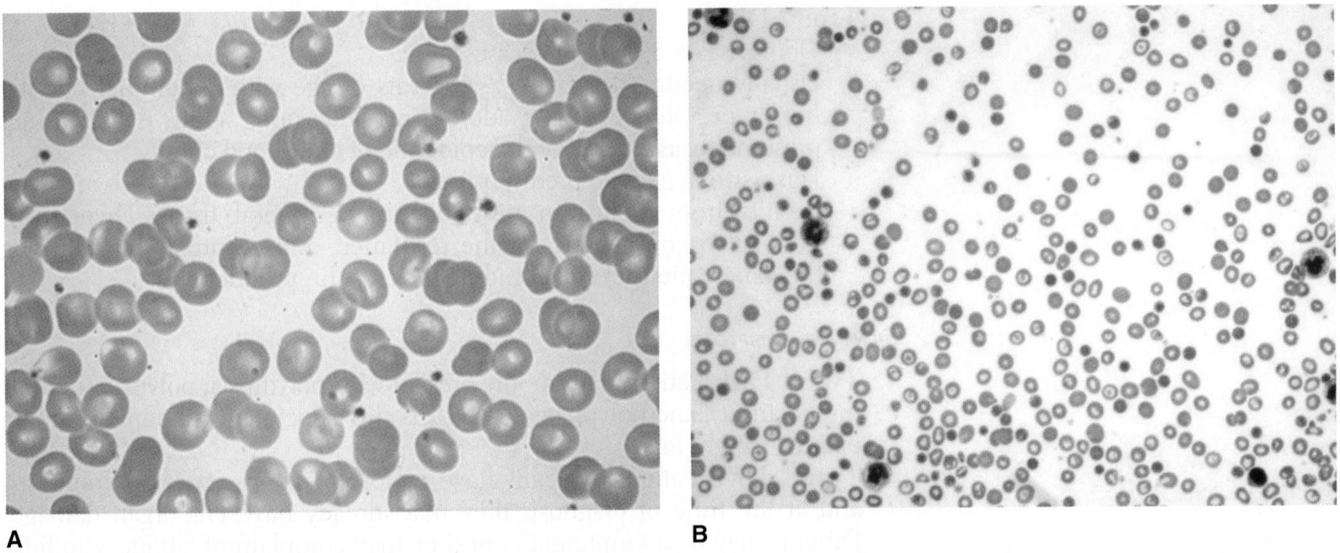

FIGURE 4-16. **Iron deficiency anemia.** Compare the normal blood smear (A) with that showing severe iron deficiency anemia (B). Note the variations in shape and size (poikilocytosis and anisocytosis, respectively) in the smear on the right. (Image A reproduced with permission from Longo DL et al. *Harrison's Principles of Internal Medicine,* 18th ed. New York: McGraw-Hill, 2012, Fig. 115-1A. Image B reproduced with permission from USMLERx.com.)

- Other lab tests are etiology specific and include TSH (for hypothyroidism), fecal occult blood (GI bleed), LFTs (liver disease), BUN and creatinine (renal disease), and SPEP or UPEP (multiple myeloma).
- Bone marrow biopsy is indicated if the patient presents with pancytopenia, macrocytic anemia with an unknown etiology, or a myelophthisic process (infiltration of the marrow space).

TREATMENT

Treatment depends on etiology.

KEY FACT

A Schilling test can help determine whether the cause of B_{12} deficiency is inadequate diet, lack of intrinsic factor (pernicious anemia), bacterial overgrowth, or a terminal ileal disease.

Endocrinology

DIABETES MELLITUS (DM)

Although DM is occasionally diagnosed on admission when it presents as diabetic ketoacidosis (DKA) or as hyperosmolar hyperglycemic nonketotic coma (HHNK), it is most often seen as a chronic medical issue. DM is a metabolic syndrome of abnormal hyperglycemia 2° to ↓ insulin or abnormal insulin resistance coupled with inadequate levels of insulin secretion to compensate. It can be classified into 2 types:

- **Type 1 DM:**
  - Caused by autoimmune destruction of pancreatic β-islet cells (anti-GAD and anti-insulin antibody), resulting in insulin deficiency.
  - Accounts for 10% of cases and is most commonly diagnosed in juveniles.
  - Not associated with obesity.
  - Strongly associated with HLA-DR3 and -DR4, but has a weak genetic predisposition.
  - Characterized by a lack of insulin, thus necessitating exogenous insulin.

Q

A 23-year-old woman presents with nausea/vomiting, mental status changes, and extreme thirst. She is hypovolemic, diaphoretic, and tachycardic and is found to have Kussmaul respirations and diffuse abdominal tenderness. What lab abnormalities are most likely to be found?

- **Type 2 DM:**
  - Comprises > 85% of DM cases.
  - Usually occurs in patients > 40 years of age with abdominal obesity, but its prevalence among adolescents and young adults is increasing, presumably as a result of the epidemic of childhood obesity.
  - Has a strong genetic predisposition.
  - Results from ↑ insulin resistance in peripheral tissues, hyperinsulinemia to compensate for the resistance, and eventual "burnout" by the pancreatic islet cells, leading to ↓ insulin production.

SIGNS AND SYMPTOMS

- **Type 1 DM:** Patients commonly present with polydipsia, polyuria (including nocturia), and polyphagia. Type 1 is also associated with rapid or unexplained weight loss.
- **Type 2 DM:** Patients typically have a more insidious onset of symptoms, and at the time of diagnosis they may already have end-organ damage. Patients may be asymptomatic, or they may complain of fatigue, candidal infections, poor wound healing, or blurred vision due to a change in the hydration status of the lens.

DIFFERENTIAL

- Other pancreatic disease (eg, chronic pancreatitis, hemochromatosis, CF).
- Hormonal abnormalities (eg, glucagonoma, Cushing's syndrome, acromegaly).
- Medications (eg, corticosteroids, thiazide diuretics, phenytoin).
- Gestational DM, stress, diabetes insipidus (central or nephrogenic), surreptitious insulin administration.

KEY FACT

C-peptide is **low** in type 1 DM and **present** in type 2 DM. The C-peptide test measures endogenous insulin production.

WORKUP

Lab testing is necessary to make a definitive diagnosis according to National Diabetes Data Group (NDDG) and World Health Organization (WHO) criteria. This includes the following:

- **Serum and urine glucose and ketones.**
- ↑ **HbA_{1c}:** Used to diagnose DM as well as to monitor the efficacy of and compliance with therapy over the preceding 3 months.

KEY POINT

DIAGNOSTIC CRITERIA FOR DIABETES

- **Prediabetes:** Blood glucose 100–125 mg/dL or 140–199 mg/dL after a 2-hour glucose tolerance test with 75-g challenge.
- **DM:**
  - Two of the following values met on 2 occasions (either the same test or 2 different tests):
    - A 2-hour glucose tolerance test > 200 mg/dL (the diagnostic gold standard).
    - A fasting (8-hour) serum glucose > 126 mg/dL.
    - Classic symptoms (polyuria, polydipsia, or unexplained weight loss) and random glucose > 200 mg/dL.
  - An HbA_{1c} > 6.5% is also considered diagnostic.

A

The patient likely has new-onset type 1 DM, so her labs will show markedly elevated glucose and low potassium. She should be started immediately on IV fluids and insulin and should be given glucose and potassium as her condition stabilizes.

TREATMENT

- **Type 1 DM:**
  - A regular regimen of insulin injections (see Figure 4-17). Insulin may be given through daily SQ injections or through an insulin pump, which delivers a continuous, predetermined dosage of insulin, supplemented by bolus insulin injections at mealtimes.
  - Vigilant monitoring of blood glucose at home, as tight glycemic control of glucose reduces end-organ damage.
  - Careful monitoring for end-organ damage.
- **Type 2 DM:** Lifestyle modification (weight loss, diet, and exercise) is first-line treatment to ↑ insulin sensitivity in target tissues. If glucose levels fail to normalize, start on oral hypoglycemic therapy (before resorting to insulin injections).
  - **Metformin:** First-line therapy; ↑ peripheral uptake of glucose and inhibits hepatic gluconeogenesis. Also results in weight loss. The most serious side effect is lactic acidosis (rare).
  - **Sulfonylureas (eg, glyburide, glipizide, tolbutamide):** ↑ pancreatic secretion of insulin. Side effects include weight gain and hypoglycemia.
  - **Glitazones:** ↑ insulin sensitivity in the muscle and liver.
  - **Acarbose:** ↓ intestinal absorption of carbohydrates by inhibiting the breakdown of oligosaccharides. A major side effect is postprandial GI discomfort.
  - **Incretins:** Glucagon-like peptide–1 (GLP-1) and gastric inhibitory peptide (GIP) (synthetic analog: exenatide) are released by the body when a meal is eaten. They stimulate glucose-dependent insulin secretion from beta islet cells of the pancreas. Dipeptidyl peptidase–IV (DPP-IV) breaks down GLP-1, so DPP-IV inhibitors (eg, sitagliptin) act along the same pathway.
- **DM in pregnancy:** For patients with chronic DM who become pregnant, **insulin** is usually used for control even in those who were previously on an oral hypoglycemic. ACEIs/ARBs must be discontinued and replaced in pregnancy owing to their teratogenic effects. Refer to the Obstetrics/Gynecology chapter for further information on the diagnosis and management of gestational diabetes.

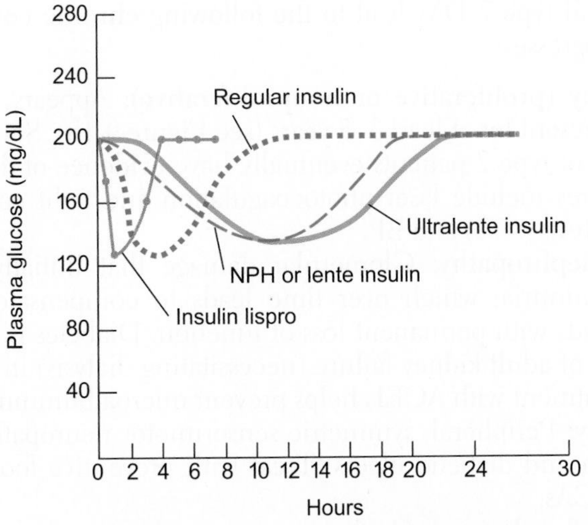

FIGURE 4-17. Effects of various insulins in a fasting diabetic patient. (Reproduced with permission from Tierney LM et al. *Current Medical Diagnosis & Treatment,* 41st ed. New York: McGraw-Hill, 2002: 1220.)

> **KEY FACT**
>
> You've never **met gli**stening candy you don't want to eat. Use **metformin** and **glipizides** as first-line therapies to combat type 2 DM.

> **KEY FACT**
>
> In the Somogyi effect, nocturnal hypoglycemia leads to ↑ morning glucose as a result of the release of counterregulatory hormones. Treat by decreasing rather than increasing nighttime insulin.

PREVENTION

- **Outpatient diabetes management** includes encouraging a regular diet and exercise; monitoring HbA_{1c} every 3–4 months (goal < 7%); a yearly spot microalbumin-to-creatinine ratio to monitor kidney function (goal < 30 μg/mg); regular BP monitoring (goal < 130/80 mm Hg); yearly lipid monitoring (goal LDL < 100, TG < 150, HDL > 40); low-dose ASA for patients > 40 years of age with other cardiac risk factors; a yearly dilated retinal examination; and a podiatric examination yearly or as needed.
- Regardless of serum cholesterol level, statin therapy ↓ the risk of major vascular events.

COMPLICATIONS

Acute complications of DM are as follows:

- **Type 1 DM: DKA/hyperglycemia-induced crisis.** Lack of insulin causes the liver to turn fat into ketone bodies, a fuel used primarily by the brain.
  - Precipitated by the **"5 I's"**: **I**nfections, **I**schemia (MI), **I**atrogenic (alcohol, corticosteroids, thiazide diuretics), **I**ntra-abdominal processes (pancreatitis, cholecystitis), and **I**nsulin deficiency (failure to take enough insulin).
  - **Signs/Sx:** Patients often present with abdominal pain, vomiting, Kussmaul respirations (a rhythmic, gasping, and very deep breathing pattern also known as "air hunger"), and a fruity/acetone breath odor. Patients are severely dehydrated with many electrolyte abnormalities (eg, hypokalemia, hypophosphatemia, ↑ anion-gap metabolic acidosis), and if not rapidly treated, they may also develop somnolence, stupor, coma, and death. (Note that patients may have normal or elevated serum potassium levels but depleted total body potassium.)
  - **Tx:** Aggressive IV fluids, potassium, and insulin to correct electrolyte abnormalities; treatment of the initiating event.
- **Type 2 DM:** HHNK coma.
  - Precipitated by acute stress and dehydration.
  - **Signs/Sx:** Presents as profound dehydration, mental status changes, and an extremely high plasma glucose level (> 600 mg/dL) without ketoacidosis. May be fatal.
  - **Tx:** IV fluids, insulin, and aggressive electrolyte replacement.

Both type 1 and type 2 DM lead to the following **chronic complications** as the disease progresses:

- **Retinopathy (proliferative or nonproliferative):** Appears when diabetes has been present for at least 3–5 years (see Figure 4-18). Some 98% of type 1 and 80% of type 2 patients eventually have evidence of disease. Preventive measures include laser photocoagulation and tight control of blood glucose (HbA_{1c} < 7%) and BP.
- **Diabetic nephropathy:** Glomerular damage that initially manifests as microalbuminuria, which over time leads to compensatory hyperfiltration and ends with permanent loss of function. Diabetes is the most common cause of adult kidney failure (necessitating dialysis) in the developed world. Treatment with ACEIs helps prevent microalbuminuria.
- **Neuropathy:** Peripheral, symmetric sensorimotor neuropathy resulting in foot trauma and diabetic ulcers. Treat with preventive foot care, analgesics, and TCAs.
- **Macrovascular damage:** Cardiovascular, cerebrovascular, and peripheral vascular disease. Cardiovascular disease is the most common cause of death in diabetic patients.

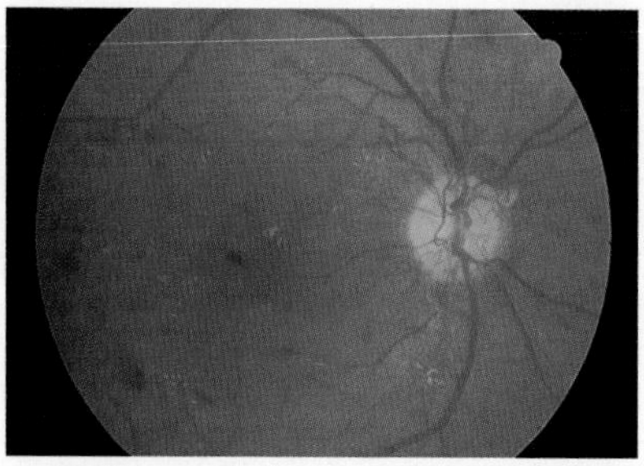

FIGURE 4-18. Diabetic retinopathy. Note the scattered hemorrhages, yellow exudates, and neovascularization. (Reproduced with permission from Longo DL et al. *Harrison's Principles of Internal Medicine,* 18th ed. New York: McGraw-Hill, 2012, Fig. 344-9.)

KEY FACT

The dawn phenomenon is early-morning hyperglycemia caused by ↓ effectiveness of insulin at that time.

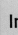

Infectious Disease

FEVER OF UNKNOWN ORIGIN (FUO)

FUO is one of the more vexing dilemmas in internal medicine. It is defined as a fever of at least 38.3°C (101°F) for at least 3 weeks with an undetermined source after 1 week of workup in the hospital. In adults, infections and cancer account for > 60% of cases. Broadly, FUO can be divided into 4 etiologic categories, outlined in Table 4-20.

> **KEY FACT**
>
> In some 10–15% of cases of FUO, no cause is identified.

Workup

- Obtain a complete history and physical; rule out sepsis.
- Obtain a CBC with differential, ESR, LFTs, and multiple blood cultures.
- Imaging studies may include CXR, CT, and MRI.
- Additional tests, depending on suspicion, include echocardiography (eg, TEE), bone marrow biopsy, skin biopsy, lymph node biopsy, liver biopsy, and exploratory laparotomy.

> **KEY FACT**
>
> Don't use steroids in FUO unless infection has been ruled out and an autoimmune cause is probable. Be aware that steroids can mask the symptoms of a neoplasm as well.

Treatment

- Start broad-spectrum antibiotics empirically in severely ill patients, but discontinue if the fever does not abate.
- Avoid empiric steroids except for vasculitis.
- Additional details on the management of FUO in children can be found in the Pediatrics chapter.

HUMAN IMMUNODEFICIENCY VIRUS (HIV)/ACQUIRED IMMUNODEFICIENCY SYNDROME (AIDS)

HIV affects 5 million new patients annually worldwide, with > 40 million people currently infected and 20 million fatalities attributed to AIDS since 1981. In the United States, symptomatic disease most commonly presents around age 30. HIV is more prevalent in males than in females, but as transmission via heterosexual contact ↑, the incidence in women is rising. HIV is spread almost exclusively through the transmission of body fluids. Risk factors for HIV infection include the following:

- Unprotected anal, oral, and vaginal sex.
- Needle sharing and accidental sticks (or mucocutaneous exposure).
- Multiple transfusions of blood (and blood products).
- Infants of HIV-⊕ mothers are also at risk.

> **KEY FACT**
>
> Hepatitis B is 50–100 times more infectious than HIV.

TABLE 4-20. Etiologies of FUO

Category	Examples
Infection	TB, endocarditis (HACEK organisms), abscess.
Neoplasm	Leukemias, lymphomas, hepatocellular carcinoma, renal cell carcinoma.
Autoimmune disease	Still's disease, temporal arteritis, RA, SLE, polyarteritis nodosa.
Miscellaneous	Drug fever, cirrhosis, hyperthyroidism, sarcoidosis, Addison's disease, Whipple's disease, PE, IBD, factitious fever.

KEY POINT

CRITERIA FOR THE DIAGNOSIS OF AIDS

AIDS is defined as either a CD4 count of < 200 cells/mm³ or the presence of an AIDS-defining illness.

- **AIDS-defining illnesses** include CMV infection, *Mycobacterium avium–intracellulare,* progressive multifocal leukoencephalopathy (PML), HSV esophagitis or recurrent oral/genital lesions, candidal esophagitis, AIDS wasting syndrome (cachexia), invasive fungal infection, toxoplasmosis, PCP, Kaposi's sarcoma, lymphoma (CNS), TB, and pneumococcal pneumonia.
- **Additional opportunistic infections** include candidal vaginitis, VZV reactivation, oral hairy leukoplakia, and chronic diarrhea from *Cryptosporidium, Microspora,* and *Isospora.*

SIGNS AND SYMPTOMS

- Many HIV-infected individuals are initially asymptomatic.
- Some 50–60% of HIV-infected patients may present with flulike symptoms (fever, malaise, rash, headache, sore throat, generalized lymphadenopathy) during acute seroconversion.

WORKUP

- **Serum screening:** ELISA testing is used for screening, and Western blot is used for confirmatory testing. Further testing involves HIV viral load (the number of viral RNA copies per milliliter of blood) and CD4 count.
- **Infectious screens:** PPD; VDRL; antibodies against CMV, toxoplasmosis, HBV, HAV, and HCV.
- Additional tests include CBC, electrolytes, LFTs, creatinine, CXR, Pap smear, and a pregnancy test for women (if indicated).

TREATMENT

Treatment depends primarily on CD4 count and viral load.

- Begin highly active antiretroviral therapy (HAART) if the CD4 count is < 500 cells/mm³ or if the patient has an AIDS-defining illness. The optimal timing of treatment initiation is still controversial.
- Treatment regimens usually include a protease inhibitor (eg, saquinavir, ritonavir, indinavir) and 2 nucleoside analogs (eg, AZT, ddI, 3TC, D4T).
- Once-daily and reduced-pill regimens are becoming available for patients for whom adherence is an issue. Patients should not be treated with HAART if adherence is an issue. Ninety percent adherence is probably more likely to induce new resistance patterns than 20% adherence.
- 1° prophylaxis of various opportunistic infections is indicated if CD4 counts fall below particular levels or if symptoms are present (see Table 4-21). Prophylaxis can be discontinued when the CD4 count ↑ adequately.

TABLE 4-21. Preventable Opportunistic Infections Associated with AIDS

Organism	Indications for Prophylaxis	Prophylactic Medication
PCP	CD4 < 200 or oral candidiasis.	TMP-SMX (Bactrim); dapsone (second line).
S pneumoniae	CD4 ≤ 200.	Pneumococcal vaccine.
Toxoplasma gondii	CD4 < 100 and IgG to *Toxoplasma.*	TMP-SMX.
Mycobacterium avium–intracellulare	CD4 < 50.	Azithromycin.
Histoplasma capsulatum	CD4 < 150 in endemic areas.	Itraconazole.
Mycobacterium tuberculosis (TB)	Skin test > 5 mm, active TB contact, or prior ⊕ skin test without treatment.	INH only for latent disease; multidrug cocktail for active disease.
Influenza virus	All patients (yearly).	Influenza vaccine.
VZV	Significant exposure without a history of disease or vaccination.	VZV vaccination for preexposure prevention. For postexposure therapy, administer VZV immune globulin within 96 hours of exposure.
HBV	Any susceptible anti-HBcAg-⊖ patients.	HBV vaccine.
HAV	Any susceptible anti-HAV-⊖ patients.	HAV vaccine.

Complications

Most patients recover from the initial retroviral syndrome and enter the latency phase, during which they are asymptomatic despite high levels of viral replication. Eventually the patient's immune system cannot control the infection, at which point CD4 counts fall, and AIDS and opportunistic infections ensue (see above).

KEY POINT

HIV TESTING PROTOCOL

- The **ELISA** test is a general HIV screening measure that detects the presence of anti-HIV antibodies in the bloodstream. The test has high sensitivity but moderate specificity, leading to numerous false ⊕s.
- Those with a ⊕ ELISA test must have a follow-up **Western blot** to confirm HIV infection.

KEY FACT

TB is a reportable disease according to local and state health departments.

KEY FACT

Although the most common extrapulmonary site of TB infection is the kidney, TB can affect nearly every organ system.

KEY FACT

CXR findings in pulmonary TB:

- **1°:** Enlarged, calcified mediastinal lymph nodes and calcified pulmonary granulomas (Ghon complex) in the apical and posterior areas of the upper lobes of the lungs.
- **Reactivation:** Apical pleural scarring; cavitary lesions.

TUBERCULOSIS (TB)

After declining in the 1980s, infection with *Mycobacterium tuberculosis* is once again increasing in prevalence, with a growing number of drug-resistant strains. TB primarily affects the lungs but may involve other organ systems, with presentations ranging from cough to meningismus. Worldwide, it is responsible for more infectious disease deaths than any other single agent, and one-third of the world's population are carriers. Spread is via infectious airborne droplets that lead to 1° and then 2° phases of infection. Risk factors include the following:

- Immunosuppression (eg, HIV, solid organ transplantation, TNF inhibitors, carcinoma), alcoholism, preexisting lung disease (eg, silicosis), diabetes, CKD/dialysis, old age, homelessness, malnourishment/low body weight, and crowded living conditions with poor ventilation (eg, military barracks).
- Immigrants from Africa, Latin America, Asia, and Caribbean countries as well as persons with known exposure to infected patients are also at ↑ risk.

Signs and Symptoms

- Symptoms of active pulmonary TB include productive cough, hemoptysis, weakness, anorexia, weight loss, malaise, night sweats, and fever. Symptoms can resemble those of bacterial pneumonia.
- Physical examination may reveal inspiratory rales and dullness to percussion with ↓ fremitus if effusions are present.
- Extrapulmonary manifestations include cervical lymphadenopathy and Pott's disease (spinal spread).

Differential

Pneumonia (bacterial, fungal, viral), other atypical mycobacterial infections, HIV infection, HIV-related opportunistic infections (eg, PCP), lung abscess, lung cancer, sarcoidosis, URI.

Workup

- Presumptively diagnosed with CXR (see Figure 4-19) and a ⊕ acid-fast stain of the sputum. Culture of *M tuberculosis* from sputum may take several weeks given its slow incubation period.
- A ⊕ PPD test is indicative only of previous exposure to *M tuberculosis* and may not be present in immunocompromised individuals (eg, HIV-infected patients) who have TB.

KEY POINT

PPD TESTING FOR TB

PPD is injected intradermally on the volar surface of the arm. The transverse length of induration is measured at 48–72 hours. BCG vaccination typically renders a patient PPD ⊕ for at least 1 year. The size of induration that indicates a ⊕ test for particular populations is as follows:

- $>$ **5 mm:** HIV or risk factors, close TB contacts, CXR evidence of TB.
- $>$ **10 mm:** Indigent/homeless, immigrants from developing nations, IV drug users, those with chronic illness, residents of health and correctional institutions.
- $>$ **15 mm:** All others.

A ⊖ reaction with ⊖ controls implies anergy from immunosuppression, old age, or malnutrition and thus does not rule out TB.

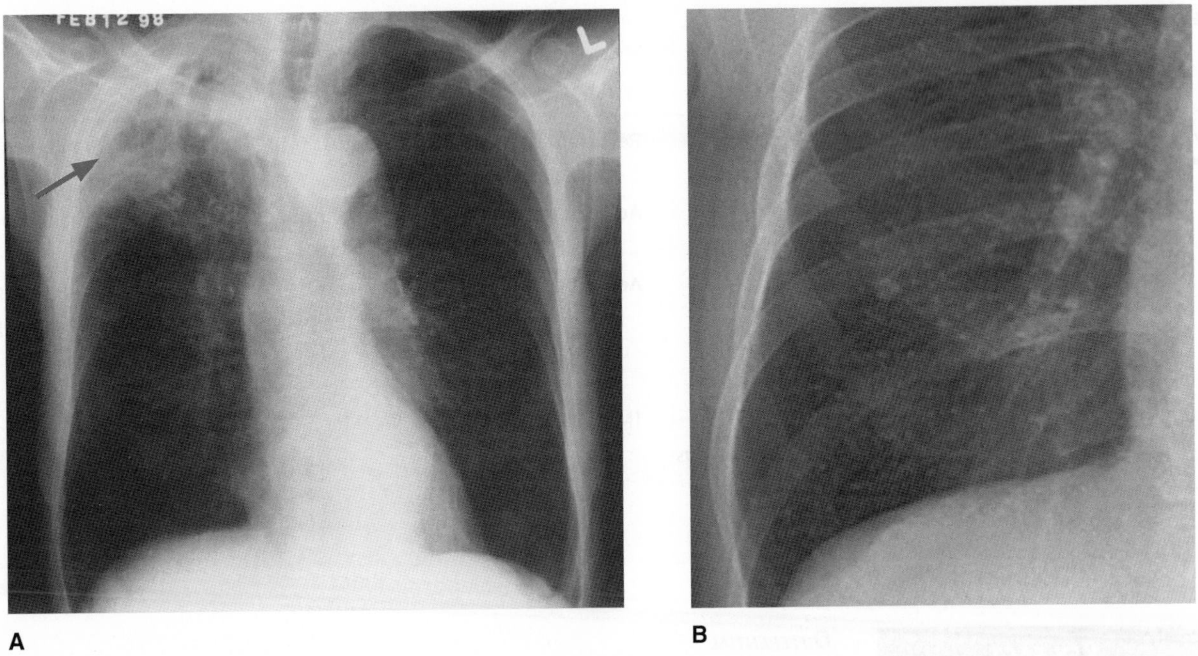

FIGURE 4-19. Pulmonary TB. (**A**) Right apical opacity with areas of cavitation (arrow) is seen in an elderly man with reactivation TB. (**B**) Coned-in view of a CXR in a young male with miliary TB shows innumerable 1- to 2-mm pulmonary nodules. (Image A reproduced with permission from Halter JB et al. *Hazzard's Geriatric Medicine and Gerontology,* 6th ed. New York: McGraw-Hill, 2009, Fig. 126-7. Image B reproduced with permission from USMLERx.com.)

Treatment

- For active TB, antimycobacterial therapy should be instituted immediately and the patient should be isolated.
- Vitamin B_6 (pyridoxine) is commonly given with INH to prevent the common side effect of peripheral neuritis.
- For outpatients, directly observed therapy may be necessary to ensure adherence and prevent drug resistance.
- Respiratory isolation should be instituted when active TB is suspected.
- Prophylactic treatment for HIV-⊕ and HIV-⊖ patients < 35 years of age who show conversion to a ⊕ PPD but have no symptoms of active pulmonary TB on CXR include INH therapy for 9 months. Many physicians forgo INH prophylaxis in patients > 35 years of age because the risk of INH-induced liver toxicity ↑ with age.

KEY FACT

TB multidrug treatment regimens:

- **Induction phase:** INH + pyrazinamide + rifampin + ethambutol × 8 weeks.
- **Standard full course:** INH + rifampin × 9 months.

URINARY TRACT INFECTION (UTI)

UTIs are most commonly caused by ascending infections and occur 30 times more frequently in women than in men (due to a short urethra). UTIs in men are usually due to congenital abnormalities or, in elderly men, to prostatic enlargement. Risk factors also include sexual intercourse, diaphragm and/or spermicide use, urinary tract instrumentation (eg, Foley catheters), DM, and immunosuppression. Common microbial causes are listed in Table 4-22.

Signs and Symptoms

- Presents with dysuria, suprapubic pain, nocturia, and ↑ frequency and urgency. These symptoms may be absent in elderly patients, who may be asymptomatic or may instead present with delirium.
- Patients with pyelonephritis can have fever, chills, flank pain, and CVA tenderness.

MNEMONIC

UTI agents–

SEEKS PP

S *saprophyticus*
E *coli*
E*nterobacter*
K*lebsiella*
S*erratia*
P*roteus*
P*seudomonas*

TABLE 4-22. GU Tract Infections

Condition	Common Organisms	Treatment
UTI/pyelonephritis	*E coli* (50–80%), *Staphylococcus saprophyticus* (10–30%), *Klebsiella pneumoniae* (8–10%), *Proteus mirabilis*	**Recurrent UTI unrelated to coitus:** TMP-SMX, cephalexin, or nitrofurantoin × 3–7 days. May be continued for 6 months for prophylaxis. **Acute, uncomplicated pyelonephritis (outpatient):** A fluoroquinolone or amoxicillin/clavulanate × 7 days. **Acute, uncomplicated pyelonephritis (inpatient):** An IV fluoroquinolone or ampicillin/sulbactam until the patient is afebrile for 24–48 hours; then PO ciprofloxacin × 14 days.
Uncomplicated UTI	*E coli* (30–60%), *Proteus* (10%), *Klebsiella, Serratia* spp., *Pseudomonas aeruginosa, Enterococcus faecalis, Enterobacter* spp.	TMP-SMX or ciprofloxacin. Treat for 3–7 days.

KEY FACT

Treat asymptomatic bacteriuria in pregnant patients or those with chronic pyelonephritis. Do not treat asymptomatic bacteriuria in patients with indwelling catheters.

KEY FACT

Chronic complicated UTIs show ↓ responsiveness to antibiotics and may result from structural abnormalities/changes or functional disorders, pregnancy, DM, AIDS, indwelling catheters, or renal obstruction.

KEY FACT

Severe sepsis starting from a UTI must be considered in any elderly patient with altered mental status.

DIFFERENTIAL

- **Common:** Vaginitis, vulvar HSV lesions, allergic reactions, nephrolithiasis, TOA, infected ovarian cyst, appendicitis, epidural abscess, diskitis, vertebral osteomyelitis.
- **Rare:** Bladder cancer, mycobacterial infection.

WORKUP

- **UA:** ⊕ leukocyte esterase and nitrites, ↑ urine pH (if *Proteus* is present), and hematuria. Microscopic examination will show pyuria (> 2–5 WBCs/hpf) and possibly WBC casts (in pyelonephritis). Nitrites are the most specific test.
- **Culture:** The diagnostic gold standard is > 100,000 colony-forming units of bacteria per milliliter of clean-catch urine.
- CT imaging may be helpful in delineating the extent of disease.

TREATMENT

Treatment is initially empiric (see Table 4-22).

SEPSIS

Septic shock (see Figure 4-20) and multiorgan dysfunction are the most common causes of death in patients with sepsis; thus, rapid diagnosis is critical. Knowledge of relevant nomenclature is also necessary:

- **Bacteremia:** Refers to the presence of bacteria in the blood.
- **Systemic inflammatory response syndrome (SIRS):** Presents with fever/hypothermia, tachypnea, tachycardia, and leukocytosis/leukopenia.
- **Sepsis:** Defined as suspected or proven infection plus SIRS.
- **Severe sepsis:** Sepsis with organ dysfunction (hypotension, hypoxemia, oliguria, metabolic acidosis, thrombocytopenia, or mental status changes).
- **Septic shock:** Severe sepsis with hypotension despite adequate fluid resuscitation (see the Emergency Medicine chapter for more details).

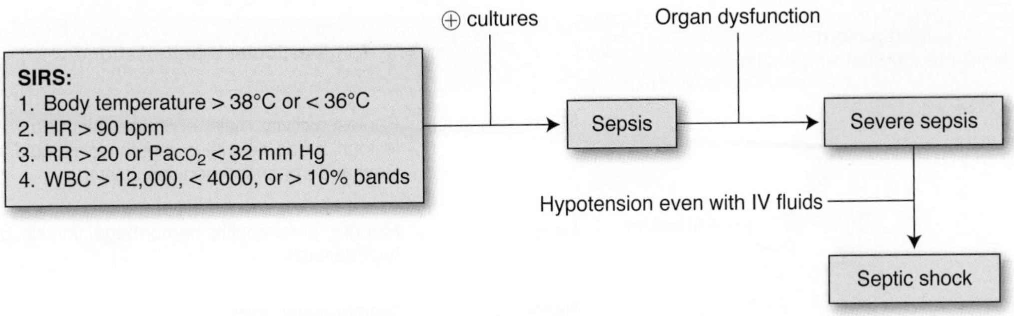

FIGURE 4-20. Progression of SIRS to septic shock. As the clinical condition worsens, the patient progresses from SIRS to sepsis, then to severe sepsis, and finally to septic shock.

Signs and Symptoms

With SIRS, 2 of the following criteria must be met:

- A body temperature > 38°C (> 100.4°F) or < 36°C (< 96.8°F).
- A heart rate > 90 bpm.
- Tachypnea as manifested by a respiratory rate > 20 breaths per minute or hyperventilation as indicated by a $Paco_2$ < 32 mm Hg.
- An alteration in the WBC count, such as a count > 12,000/mm^3, a count < 4000/mm^3, or the presence of > 10% immature neutrophils ("bands").

Workup

Directed at finding a source of infection—blood and urine cultures, CXR, stool for *C difficile*.

Treatment

- Therapy should ideally be provided early and includes **aggressive fluid resuscitation, lung-protective ventilation, broad-spectrum antibiotics,** possibly **steroids (controversial),** and possibly **activated protein C.**
- Broad-spectrum antibiotics should be aimed at covering organisms such as MRSA, penicillin-resistant pneumococci, fungi, and gram-⊕ bacteria but should be adjusted once an organism and its drug sensitivities are determined.

Rheumatology

SYSTEMIC LUPUS ERYTHEMATOSUS (SLE)

SLE is an inflammatory autoimmune disorder that primarily strikes young women, having a female-to-male ratio of 8:1. It is a multisystem disease that is characterized by recurrent exacerbations ("flares") and remissions due to autoantibody formation and immune complex deposition. There is a familial concordance and a correlation with HLA-DR2 and -DR3. African American women are at especially high risk.

Signs and Symptoms

SLE is one of the "great imitator" diseases, with famously protean manifestations as outlined in the mnemonic **SOAP BRAIN MD** and in Figure 4-21.

KEY FACT

Some 90% of SLE patients are women of childbearing age.

KEY FACT

The presence of antiphospholipid antibody (including lupus anticoagulant and anticardiolipin antibody) ↑ the risk of stillbirth and abortion in pregnancy.

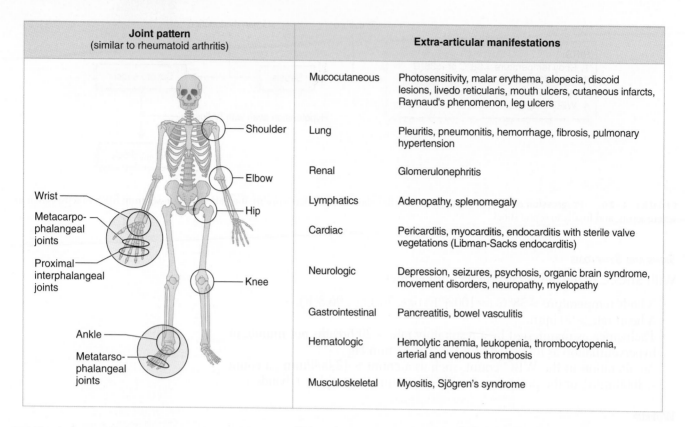

Joint pattern (similar to rheumatoid arthritis)

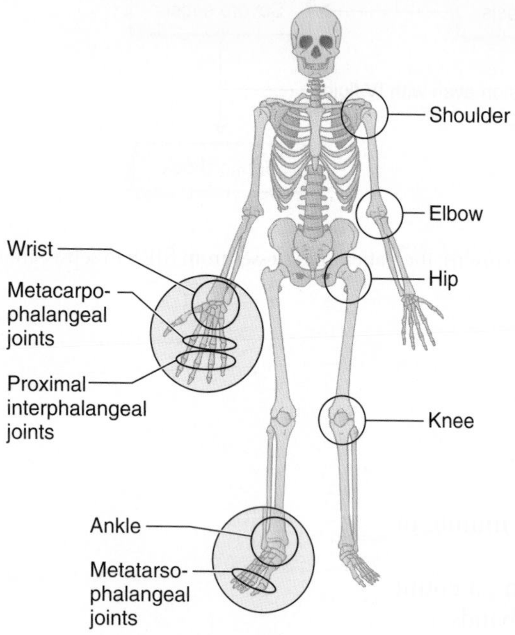

Extra-articular manifestations

Mucocutaneous	Photosensitivity, malar erythema, alopecia, discoid lesions, livedo reticularis, mouth ulcers, cutaneous infarcts, Raynaud's phenomenon, leg ulcers
Lung	Pleuritis, pneumonitis, hemorrhage, fibrosis, pulmonary hypertension
Renal	Glomerulonephritis
Lymphatics	Adenopathy, splenomegaly
Cardiac	Pericarditis, myocarditis, endocarditis with sterile valve vegetations (Libman-Sacks endocarditis)
Neurologic	Depression, seizures, psychosis, organic brain syndrome, movement disorders, neuropathy, myelopathy
Gastrointestinal	Pancreatitis, bowel vasculitis
Hematologic	Hemolytic anemia, leukopenia, thrombocytopenia, arterial and venous thrombosis
Musculoskeletal	Myositis, Sjögren's syndrome

FIGURE 4-21. Manifestations of SLE. (Reproduced with permission from Stobo JD et al. *The Principles and Practice of Medicine,* 23rd ed. Stamford, CT: Appleton & Lange, 1996: 198.)

MNEMONIC

Systemic manifestations of SLE—

SOAP BRAIN MD

Serositis (pleuritis, pericarditis, myocarditis)
Oral aphthous ulcers
Arthritis (especially small joints of hand/wrist)
Photosensitivity
Blood abnormalities (hemolytic anemia, thrombocytopenia, leukopenia, lymphopenia)
Renal disease (proteinuria or urinary cellular casts)
ANA ⊕
Immunologic abnormalities (⊕ anti-dsDNA, ⊕ anti-Sm, antiphospholipid)
Neurologic abnormalities (lupus cerebritis; seizures or psychosis)
Malar rash (photosensitive butterfly-shaped rash on face)
Discoid rash

Differential

- Drug-induced lupus (a complication of hydralazine, procainamide, quinidine, and others) and mixed connective tissue disease (MCTD) can present with multisystem involvement and autoantibodies.
- Discoid lupus presents with the characteristic skin manifestations without systemic involvement.
- Also consider epilepsy, dermatitis, MS, psychiatric disorders, porphyria, and ITP.

Workup

- The American Rheumatism Association criteria for SLE (1997) require that patients fulfill at least 4 of the manifestations outlined in the **SOAP BRAIN MD** mnemonic.
- Because of the variable presentation of SLE, it may take several years before a formal diagnosis can be made. Recently revised criteria suggest the identification of 3 manifestations, with confirmatory antibody screening testing as a second step.
- Antibody tests are the best screening tool for this disease and other autoimmune disorders (see Table 4-23). Most patients with SLE will have a ⊕ ANA; however, many other disorders are ANA ⊕ as well.
- Other tests routinely performed are complement system levels (↓ during flares), electrolytes, CBC, and renal function measures (serum creatinine, spot urine protein/creatinine ratios).

TABLE 4-23. Common Autoantibodies and Associated Conditions

Serum Test	Related Conditions and Prevalence of Findings
RF	RA (80%), SLE (15–35%), Sjögren's syndrome (75–95%), MCTD (50–60%). **RF may also be detected in the setting of viral infection, syphilis, TB, sarcoidosis, and malignancy.**
Anti–cyclic citrullinated peptide 2 (CCP2)	RA (often precedes diagnosis by several years).
ANA	Drug-induced lupus (100%), SLE (99%), scleroderma (97%), Sjögren's syndrome (96%), MCTD (93%), polymyositis/dermatomyositis (78%), RA (40%). **ANA may also be detected in 5% of healthy adults.**
Anti-dsDNA	Very specific for SLE (60%), and titers parallel disease activity (especially renal disease).
Antihistone	Drug-induced lupus (90%), SLE (50%).
Anti-Sm	Very specific for SLE (20–30%).
Anti-Ro (anti-SSA)	Sjögren's syndrome (75%), SLE (40%; ↑ risk of neonatal SLE).
Anti-La (anti-SSB)	Sjögren's syndrome (40%), SLE (10–15%; ↑ risk of neonatal SLE).
Antiphospholipid (anticardiolipin or anti-β2 glycoprotein 1 and antiprothrombin)	1° antiphospholipid syndrome or 2° disease (eg, SLE).
Anticentromeric	Scleroderma (22–36%).
Anti-topo-I (anti-Scl-70)	Scleroderma (22–40%).
Anti-Jo 1	Polymyositis/dermatomyositis (30%).
Anti–thyroid peroxidase	Hashimoto's thyroiditis.
Anti–smooth muscle	Autoimmune hepatitis.
Antimitochondrial	1° biliary cirrhosis.
c-ANCA/antiproteinase	Wegener's granulomatosis (90%).
p-ANCA/anti-MPO	Wegener's granulomatosis (10%). **Also detected in crescentic GN, microscopic polyangiitis, and Churg-Strauss syndrome.**
Anti-GBM	Goodpasture's syndrome.
Antitransglutaminase	Celiac disease.
Complement C3/C4 (↓ levels)	SLE, cryoglobulinemia. **Also detected in GN.**
HLA-B27	Ankylosing spondylitis (50–95%), reactive arthritis (Reiter's syndrome) (50–80%), psoriatic arthritis (50–80%), IBD-associated arthritis (50–80%).

TREATMENT

There is no single treatment for SLE, as treatment depends largely on the systemic manifestations of the disease. Patients are initially treated with NSAIDs, which effectively treat serositis and arthritis.

- Steroids are used for flares.
- Disease-modifying antirheumatic drugs (DMARDs) are used preventively to ↓ the incidence of flares and ↓ the need for steroids. Hydroxychloroquine (Plaquenil), methotrexate, cyclophosphamide, and azathioprine are used in progressive or refractory cases. Hydroxychloroquine is especially effective in treating arthritis, skin disease, and fatigue.
- Cyclophosphamide (Cytoxan) and mycophenolate (CellCept) with steroids are effective for lupus nephritis.
- Pregnant women with prior fetal loss and the presence of antiphospholipid antibodies should receive low-dose heparin.
- Drug-induced lupus resolves when the offending medication is discontinued.

COMPLICATIONS

Survival with treatment ranges from 90% to 95% at 2 years and up to 75% at 20 years; mortality results from end-organ damage (especially renal failure) and opportunistic infections 2° to immunosuppression.

General Medicine

OUTPATIENT SCREENING

Table 4-24 summarizes suggested outpatient screening measures in the United States.

TABLE 4-24. Outpatient Screening Measures

METHOD	INTERVAL/AGE RANGE	RECOMMENDING ORGANIZATION[a]
	COLON CANCER	
Flexible sigmoidoscopy	Every 3–5 years in patients > 50 years of age.	ACS
Fecal occult blood testing	Yearly in patients > 50 years of age.	USPSTF
Digital rectal examination (DRE)	Yearly in patients > 40 years of age.	ACS
Colonoscopy	Every 10 years in patients > 50 years of age.	ACG
	PROSTATE AND BREAST CANCER	
Prostate DRE	Not currently recommended for men.	USPSTF
PSA testing	Not currently recommended for men.	USPSTF

TABLE 4-24. Outpatient Screening Measures *(continued)*

Method	Interval/Age Range	Recommending Organization[a]
	Prostate and Breast Cancer *(continued)*	
Breast self-examination	Not currently recommended for women.	USPSTF
Clinician breast examination	No evidence to recommend for or against this for women.	USPSTF
Mammography	Every 12–24 months for patients ≥ 50 years of age (or beginning at > 40 years of age for those with a family history of breast cancer).	USPSTF
	Gynecologic Cancer	
Pap smear	Yearly for sexually active patients or those 18–65 years of age; every 3 years after 3 normal smears.	USPSTF
Pelvic examination	Every 1–3 years in patients 20–40 years of age; yearly in patients ≥ 40 years of age.	USPSTF
HPV testing	No current recommendation for or against for women, but there is currently insufficient evidence to use as a 1° test for the screening of cervical cancer.	USPSTF
	Lung Cancer	
CXR (controversial)	No current sufficient evidence to recommend for or against screening.	USPSTF
Noncontrast CT (under study)	There is evidence that noncontrast CT screening in high-risk patients confers a mortality benefit. However, no current organizations are recommending it at this point.	–
	STIs (high-risk patients)	
Gonorrhea culture	All sexually active women at ↑ risk.	USPSTF
Chlamydia culture	All sexually active women < 25 years of age and > 25 years of age at ↑ risk.	USPSTF
Syphilis (RPR/VDRL)	All patients at ↑ risk of infection.	USPSTF
HIV serology	All patients at ↑ risk of infection.	USPSTF
	TB (high-risk immunosuppressed patients, immigrants)	
PPD	Yearly.	CDC
	CAD	
Total serum cholesterol	Every 5 years in men ≥ 35 years of age and women > 45 years of age.	USPSTF

[a] ACS = American Cancer Society, ACG = American College of Gastroenterology (2000), CDC = Centers for Disease Control and Prevention, USPSTF = U.S. Preventive Services Task Force (1996).

Common Clerkship Topics

Because internal medicine covers so many domains, you should set achievable goals in your bid to attain a solid fund of knowledge. The following is a list of core topics that you are likely to encounter in the course of your medicine rotation and on a shelf examination.

- **Cardiology:**
  - Coronary artery disease/acute coronary syndrome (eg, angina pectoris, unstable angina, Prinzmetal's angina; see Emergency Medicine)
  - Acute myocardial infarction (see Emergency Medicine)
  - Arrhythmias (eg, bradyarrhythmias, tachyarrhythmias, atrial fibrillation)
  - Cardiomyopathies
  - Congestive heart failure
  - Hypertension
  - Infective endocarditis, myocarditis, and pericarditis
  - Syncope
  - Valvular heart disease
- **Pulmonology:**
  - Acute respiratory failure
  - Asthma (see Emergency Medicine)
  - Chronic cough
  - Chronic obstructive pulmonary disease
  - Interstitial lung disease
  - Lung cancer
  - Pleural effusion
  - Pneumonia
  - Pneumothorax (see Emergency Medicine)
  - Pulmonary embolism (see Emergency Medicine)
  - Pulmonary nodules and masses
- **Nephrology:**
  - Acid-base disturbances
  - Acute renal failure
  - Chronic renal failure and uremia
  - Electrolyte disorders (eg, hyponatremia and hypernatremia, hypo- and hyperkalemia)
  - Glomerular disease
  - Nephrolithiasis
- **Gastroenterology:**
  - Abdominal pain
  - Diarrhea
  - Disorders of swallowing (eg, achalasia, esophageal cancer)
  - Gastritis
  - Gastroesophageal reflux disease
  - Gastrointestinal bleeding (see Surgery)
  - Gastrointestinal cancer
  - Hepatic disease (eg, cirrhosis, hepatic encephalopathy, hepatitis, portal hypertension)
  - Inflammatory bowel disease (eg, Crohn's disease, ulcerative colitis; see Surgery)
  - Irritable bowel syndrome
  - Malabsorption
  - Pancreatitis (see Surgery)
  - Peptic ulcer disease

- **Hematology:**
  - Anemia, including hemolytic anemias
  - Coagulation disorders (eg, excessive bleeding and hypercoagulable states)
  - Neutropenic fever
- **Oncology:**
  - Breast cancer
  - Leukemias
  - Lymphadenopathy
  - Lymphomas
  - Paraneoplastic syndromes
  - Prostate cancer
- **Endocrinology:**
  - Adrenal disorders (eg, hyperaldosteronism, hypoaldosteronism, Addison's disease, Cushing's disease), diabetes insipidus (central and nephrogenic)
  - Diabetes mellitus (types 1 and 2), including diabetic ketoacidosis
  - Gonadal disorders (eg, testicular feminization, 5α-reductase deficiency)
  - Hyper- and hypocalcemia
  - Hyperlipidemias (eg, familial hypercholesterolemia)
  - Nutritional disorders (eg, osteomalacia, scurvy, pellagra, beriberi)
  - Pituitary disorders (eg, acromegaly)
  - Thyroid disorders (eg, Graves' disease, Hashimoto's thyroiditis)
- **Infectious disease:**
  - Animal-borne diseases (eg, Lyme disease, rabies, malaria)
  - CNS infections (eg, meningitis, encephalitis; see Neurology)
  - Fever of unknown origin
  - HIV and AIDS
  - Intra-abdominal infections (eg, spontaneous bacterial peritonitis)
  - Respiratory tract infections (eg, pneumonia, URI)
  - Sexually transmitted infections (eg, chlamydia, syphilis, gonorrhea, HSV)
  - Tuberculosis
  - Urinary tract infection
- **Rheumatology:**
  - Fibromyalgia
  - Gout and pseudogout
  - Osteoarthritis
  - Rheumatoid arthritis
  - Sarcoidosis
  - Septic arthritis
  - Seronegative spondyloarthropathies (eg, ankylosing spondylitis)
  - Systemic lupus erythematosus
  - Vasculitis (eg, polyarteritis nodosa, temporal arteritis)
- **General medicine:**
  - Health maintenance issues
  - Medical ethics issues
  - Outpatient management
  - Outpatient screening

CHAPTER 5

NEUROLOGY

Ward Tips

KEY FACT

Where is the lesion? Use the history and physical examination to determine the location of the lesion.

Welcome to your neurology rotation! In this highly academic and scientific field, you will discover one of the things neurologists love most to do: talk, talk, and talk about neurology. So get ready for lengthy rounds in which you'll discuss detailed differentials, neuroscience, and the latest research while simultaneously attempting to answer the ever-present question, "Where's the lesion?" Of course, you won't be expected to learn all of neurology in a few weeks—so, as is the case in many other rotations, your questions will be more important than your answers.

HOW DO I EXCEL IN NEUROLOGY?

Neurology rotations differ notably from site to site, so the first thing you need to find out is how your responsibilities will be divided among inpatient wards, outpatient clinics, consult-liaison, and neurosurgery. Inpatient neurology tends to be like medicine: You get to manage patients with neurologic diseases who frequently have active medical issues as well. For this reason, you'll need to know your medicine while managing patients on the neurology wards. Day-to-day activities include following labs and neuro examinations, writing notes, and playing a supportive role in management. The workload tends to depend on the number of students per team, the presence of interns, the number of admissions, and the inpatient census. To make the most out of this rotation, don't hesitate to ask your residents/attendings on the first day: What is the evaluative process? What are my responsibilities? Whom can I ask for help? What is the call schedule? For more details on how the day is often set up, refer to Chapter 1.

One of your primary goals during this rotation should be to learn how to conduct and present a complete screening neurologic examination. In addition, you should plan to read about your patients and understand the neuroanatomy, pathophysiology, and treatment involved in their care. **Always** try to trace the neuroanatomic pathways that might underlie your patient's symptoms so that you can better localize the lesion. See the Neuroanatomy section below for review.

Patients on this rotation tend to be admitted for ischemic strokes and hemorrhages, status epilepticus, meningitis and encephalitis, Guillain-Barré syndrome (GBS), myasthenic crises, and acute changes in mental status of unknown etiology, with some variation from hospital to hospital. Trauma and tumor patients are often managed by neurosurgery. Outpatient clinics are a great place to see a spectrum of common and uncommon nonacute diseases, such as peripheral neuropathies, MS, migraine, and movement disorders. If you have a particular area of interest, such as neuromuscular disorders, you may want to find out if you can spend a few afternoons each week seeing patients in clinic and observing electrophysiologic testing. In general, you are encouraged to seek out the full range of interesting experiences neurology offers. Your residents and attending will likely be impressed by your initiative, and you will benefit from the experience.

Other ground rules, as always, are to be prompt and courteous, take good care of your patients, try to know them better than anyone else, read about their diseases, ask questions, give clear presentations, and demonstrate your interest in the subject. Focus on the basics by reviewing neuroanatomy and studying disease presentation, workup, and treatment. You shouldn't be expected to understand obscure diseases or to track down remote articles (unless your patient happens to have a rare and interesting condition), but if you find yourself researching a case out of genuine interest, your residents and fellow students might appreciate seeing a report or an article that you have uncovered. At the very least, your residents will notice your effort and quite possibly learn from you. You may also want to develop a list of course objectives that fit your future aspirations—perhaps focusing on the execution of the neuro examination and on a basic understanding of the common neurologic diseases.

There are many tools that a prepared medical student should bring on the neurology wards, but there is no need to have exploding white coat pockets. Three key tools that every medical student should carry on the neurology rotation are a penlight, a stethoscope, and a reflex hammer. If you have a bit more room, you can carry an eye chart, a tuning fork, and safety pins for pain sensation testing. Your tuning fork can do double duty and can be used for cold-temperature sensation if you run out of pins, as the same neurologic pathway is involved in pain and temperature sensation. There is no need to purchase an ophthalmoscope for your neurology rotation, as many outpatient clinic rooms will already be equipped with one. On the wards, however, it may be useful to bring your own.

KEY NOTES

Neurology admission notes are like medicine notes, with a few key distinctions:

- Indicate the handedness of the patient (eg, "46-year-old RH [right-handed] male").
- Take a full medical history as well as a neurologic history, including a history of seizures, cerebrovascular accidents (CVAs), transient ischemic attacks (TIAs), diabetes mellitus (DM), myocardial infarctions (MIs), and other indicators of peripheral vascular disease.
- When you are documenting the neuro examination, remember that while the admission history and physical (H&P) is expected to include the full examination, progress notes can be more brief. An example of a brief physical/neuro examination with commonly used abbreviations is shown below. When presenting your patient, remember that neurologists expect information to be presented in a certain order. Please refer to the example below for the suggested order.
- The assessment and plan (A&P) is a good place to organize and summarize. In it, you should include important symptoms and findings; localize the lesions to an anatomic location; and, finally, give an organized differential diagnosis by likelihood. This process, more than anything else, will make you shine as a student of neurology.

> **KEY FACT**
>
> Don't forget to report imaging studies and lumbar puncture (LP) results. LP results often have a significant impact on decisions you make about the A&P.

KEY PROCEDURES

The main procedure involved in inpatient neurology is the LP, known to your patients as the dreaded "spinal tap." Make sure your resident knows that you are interested in doing LPs. See a video demonstration of LP at the *New England Journal of Medicine*'s Video in Clinical Medicine series at www.nejm.org. Contraindications to performing an LP include a suspected intracranial mass lesion, local infection near where the LP will be performed (skin/muscle/spinal cord), a spinal cord mass, and coagulopathy. Remember, too, that the patient must give informed consent for an LP (although this is not always possible in cases with altered mental status), and you must write a pro-

> **KEY FACT**
>
> Before attempting an LP, always rule out the possibility of herniation. Any patient who presents with altered mental status, immunosuppression, or focal neurologic deficits should have a head CT to rule out mass lesion.

cedure note documenting the indication for the procedure and a summary (see Chapter 1 for a sample procedure note). You should also find a good and enthusiastic teacher and ask for plenty of supervision early on. Attempting a difficult LP alone can be a nightmare both for you and for the patient!

Key:

A&O × 3 = alert and oriented to person, place, and time

APD = afferent pupillary defect

BP = blood pressure

CN = cranial nerves

EOMI = extraocular movements intact

HEENT = head, eyes, ears, nose, and throat

LAD = lymphadenopathy

LLE = left lower extremity

LUE = left upper extremity

MSE = mental status examination

NAD = no acute distress

O/P = oropharynx

P = pulse

PERRL = pupils equal, round, and reactive to light

RA = room air

RAM = rapid alternating movements

RLE = right lower extremity

RR = respiratory rate

RUE = right upper extremity

T = temperature

VS = vital signs

SAMPLE NEUROLOGY PHYSICAL EXAM

GENERAL EXAM:

Gen: Well-developed, well-nourished, pleasant male in NAD.

VS: T 37.2, P 59, BP 167/89, RR 18, 98% O_2 sat on RA.

Skin: Anicteric, no rashes, no bruises.

HEENT: Head normocephalic. Ears symmetric with no gross deformity. No epistaxis. O/P normal with moist mucous membranes, no lesions, and no bleeding.

Neck: Stiff neck, ⊕ Brudzinski, ⊕ meningismus. No LAD or swollen glands.

Lungs/Cardiac/Abd/Ext: Include pertinent ⊕s and ⊖s.

NEURO EXAM:

MSE: The patient is A&O × 3. The patient is able to recall recent and remote events.

Follows simple and complex commands.

Able to perform 7-digit span without difficulty.

Memory: 3/3 registration; 0/3 → 2/3 with prompts at 5 minutes.

Speech: Patient can name, repeat, and follow instructions and is fluent. No dysarthria.

CN:

I: Not tested.

II: Vision intact with no APD; visual fields are full to confrontation independently. Fundi normal; no papilledema, exudates, or hemorrhages.

III, IV, and VI: PERRL directly and consensually and to accommodation. EOMI with smooth pursuits; no nystagmus noted on any direction of gaze.

V: Facial sensation normal to touch in all V_1–V_3 divisions. Masseter strength normal bilaterally. No pain with palpation of the temples. Normal temporal artery pulsations bilaterally.

VII: Facial appearance symmetric at rest. No asymmetry on grimace.

VIII: Hearing normal to finger bilaterally.

IX and X: Soft palate elevation symmetric and normal.

XI: Shoulder shrug performed with normal strength and is symmetric. No sternocleidomastoid weakness.

XII: No tongue atrophy or fasciculations. Tongue protrudes midline.

Motor: Normal muscle tone and bulk in arms and legs.

No fasciculations or tremor at rest. No spasticity. No pronator drift.

Strength 5/5 throughout LUE and LLE; 5/5 RUE and RLE.

Sensory: Grossly intact to light touch, vibration, and pinprick throughout bilateral extremities. Proprioception normal in fingers and toes. Romberg test ⊖.

Coordination: RAM: normal with RUE and LUE.

Normal finger-to-nose and heel-to-shin without dysmetria.

Gait: Normal stance and stride, normal arm swing, normal tandem gait, can walk on heels and tiptoes.

Reflexes: +2 biceps, brachioradialis, patellar, Achilles bilaterally. Toes are downgoing bilaterally.

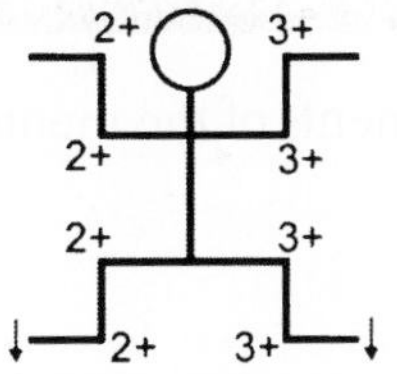

High-Yield Clinical Topic Checklist

The most important things to learn on your neurology rotation are the screening and complete neurologic examinations as well as the workup and management of common neurologic problems such as headache, seizure, meningitis, and stroke. Toward these goals, you should focus on the H&P, the development of differentials, and the recognition of emergency conditions. This is also a good time to learn about the indications for and interpretation of investigational studies, especially CT, MRI, LP, and, perhaps, EEG, EMG, and nerve conduction studies. The following is a list of 12 high-yield topics that are used extremely frequently on most neuro rotations.

- ❑ **The complete neurologic examination:** Mental status, cranial nerves, motor, sensory, gait and coordination, reflexes.
- ❑ **Key neuroanatomy.**
- ❑ **Imaging basics:** CT/CTA, MRI/MRA, contrast imaging.
- ❑ **LP:** Indications, procedural skills, interpreting results, when an LP is contraindicated.
- ❑ **Stroke:** Clinical features, risk factors, acute stroke treatments, prevention.
- ❑ **Coma:** Assessing a comatose patient, use of the Glasgow Coma Scale, primitive brainstem reflexes, etiologies.
- ❑ **Delirium and dementia.**
- ❑ **Headache:** Migraine, cluster, tension, 2° headaches.
- ❑ **Low back pain, spinal cord injuries:** Cord compression, cord lesions.
- ❑ **Movement disorders:** Parkinson's disease, Huntington's disease.
- ❑ **Seizures:** Partial (focal), generalized, absence, tonic-clonic, status epilepticus.
- ❑ **Weakness:** Upper motor neuron vs. lower motor neuron; anatomic localization and diagnosis.

KEY FACT

Create a systematic approach!

The Complete Neurologic Examination

Don't expect to master the neuro examination in just a few weeks. Instead, spend time creating a systematic approach toward the examination and learning to feel comfortable with its components. Perhaps the best approach is to carefully observe the examinations (and notes) of your residents and attendings, taking note of how (and why) they choose to abbreviate or focus their examinations. Tables 5-1 through 5-5 provide information on a complete examination.

SCREENING EXAMINATION FOR MENTAL STATUS

Table 5-1 outlines the components of the mental status examination.

TABLE 5-1. Mental Status Examination

What You're Looking For	What You're Doing
	Level of Consciousness
Alertness	Observe—are the eyes open? Does the patient appear drowsy?
Orientation	Can the patient answer the following: ▪ What's your name? ▪ Where are you? ▪ What is the day of the week/month/year? Patients are "A&O × 3" if they know their name, the date, and their location.
Response to voice	Call the patient's name; ask to open eyes.
Response to pain	Try sternal rub or pinching extremities, and watch response for purposefulness in obtunded patients.
	Attention
Ability to focus on a task	Ask the patient to list the months of the year forward and backward, serially subtract 7 from 100 (or 3 from 20), or spell the word *world* backwards.
	Language
Comprehension of spoken word	Ask the patient to close his or her eyes, show 3 fingers, and touch the right ear with the left thumb.
Comprehension of written word	Hold up a card reading, "Close your eyes."
Repetition of phrases	Have the patient repeat sentences such as "No ifs, ands, or buts."
Fluency of speech	Is speech intelligible, fluent, and grammatical? Can the patient write a complete sentence?
Naming	Try pointing to a watch and its parts to elicit "watch, band, crystal."
	Mood, Insight, Thought Process, Content
Look for signs of depression, other psychiatric disturbance, and denial	Ask the patient, "How are your spirits?" "Do you know why you are here in the hospital?"

TABLE 5-1. Mental Status Examination *(continued)*

What You're Looking For	What You're Doing
Memory	
Registration	List 3 words (eg, *cat, pencil, banana*) and ask the patient to repeat them.
Short term	Three minutes later, ask the patient to recall 3 items. Offer prompts if the patient is unable to do so (such as "a kind of animal," "used to write," "a kind of fruit"); you can also try current events.
Long term	Ask for birth date and about historical events.
Higher Cognitive Function	
Fund of knowledge	Ask for names of current/past presidents.
Calculations	Try simple addition and division (how many quarters in $2.50).
Abstractions	Ask the patient to interpret a proverb such as "A rolling stone gathers no moss." Be aware of cultural differences.
Constructions	Ask the patient to copy sketches (square, cube) and to draw a clock (analog).
Praxis	Ask the patient to act out combing of the hair or brushing of teeth.

SCREENING EXAMINATION FOR CRANIAL NERVES

Table 5-2 delineates the elements that make up the cranial nerve examination.

SCREENING EXAMINATION FOR MOTOR NERVES

Tips for a motor nerve screening examination include the following (see also Tables 5-3 through 5-5):

- Check tone in all 4 extremities.
  - ↑ tone refers either to spasticity or to rigidity. *Spasticity* is a velocity-dependent state in which the muscles are in a persistent state of ↑ involuntary reflex activity in response to a stretch. By contrast, the term *rigidity* is used to describe an involuntary ↑ in the resistance of a muscle to a passive stretch that is uniform throughout the range of motion (ROM) of the muscles being stretched and is **not** velocity dependent.
  - Rigidity and spasticity are often confused and can be difficult to distinguish, but they are 2 separate and distinct phenomena. In rigidity, DTRs are not hyperactive as they are in spasticity. Both rigidity and spasticity imply an upper motor neuron (UMN), or central, process.
- Check strength throughout the major muscle groups in the upper and lower extremities using the standardized grading scale (see Table 5-4). Use the strength of finger extension, index finger abduction, big toe dorsiflexion, and plantar flexion to look for subtle distal weakness.
- Subtle weakness can also be evaluated with the pronator drift. Check pronator drift by asking the patient to extend both arms with palms up and eyes closed. Weakness manifests as pronation and/or downward drift. Corticospinal tract weakness will also lead to a ⊕ "orbit sign." Ask the patient

KEY FACT

Cranial nerve testing:

- The pupillary reflex tests CN II and III.
- The corneal reflex tests CN V and VII.
- The vestibulo-ocular reflex tests oculomotor nuclei (CN VI, IV, and III) and the inner ear apparatus.
- The gag reflex tests CN IX and X.

KEY FACT

Central neurologic lesions lead to lower facial weakness only. Peripheral lesions lead to weakness of both the upper and lower face. Hint: Look for wrinkles in the forehead; a patient with a peripheral lesion will **lack** wrinkles when asked to raise their eyebrows.

TABLE 5-2. Cranial Nerve Examination

What You're Looking For	What You're Doing
	Optic Nerve
Visual acuity	Use the Snellen eye chart.
Visual fields	Test by confrontation if the patient cooperates; estimate by visual threat otherwise.
Ocular fundi	Look for papilledema, retinal hemorrhages, retinopathy, and/or optic atrophy.
Afferent pupillary defect	Using the "swinging flashlight test," look for dilation of the pupil on direct application of light, but consensual constriction when a stimulus is applied to the contralateral eye.
	Oculomotor Nerve
Pupillary function	Check baseline size, shape, and symmetry; direct and consensual constriction (using penlight); and accommodation.
Levator palpebrae function	Check for elevation of the eyelid and ptosis.
Superior rectus, inferior rectus, inferior oblique function	Examine extraocular movements (EOM)—elevate, depress, and elevate the adducted eye, respectively.
	Trochlear Nerve
Superior oblique function	EOM (depress the adducted eye).
	Abducens Nerve
Lateral rectus function	EOM (abduction).
Assessment of EOM	Ask the patient to follow a target in the shape of the letter *H* and look for full movement and coordination.
	Trigeminal Nerve
Motor: Temporalis, masseter muscles	Palpate muscles as the patient clenches teeth.
Sensory: V_1, V_2, V_3	Check sensation to the forehead, cheek, and jaw.
Reflex: Corneal blink	Touch the cornea with a cotton thread or tissue.
	Facial Nerve
Motor to facial muscles (also checked in motor response to corneal reflex)	Check raised eyebrows, tightly squinted eyes, smile, and puffed-out cheeks for asymmetry.
	Vestibulocochlear Nerve
Auditory function	Grossly test hearing by rubbing fingers together by each ear or scratching a pillow. Also consider doing Weber and Rinne tests.
Vestibular function	Check for nystagmus and a history of vertigo. Caloric testing can be done on comatose patients.

TABLE 5-2. Cranial Nerve Examination *(continued)*

What You're Looking For	What You're Doing
Glossopharyngeal Nerve	
Sensory: Palate, pharynx, gag reflex	Stroking the back of the throat to test for gag reflex is often avoided in conscious patients, as it may lead to vomiting.
Vagus Nerve	
Motor: Palate, pharynx, vocal cords	Check the voice for hoarseness and articulation; check palatal elevation, uvular position, and gag reflex.
Spinal Accessory Nerve	
Motor: Trapezius	Have the patient shrug the shoulder against resistance.
Motor: Sternocleidomastoid	Have the patient turn the head to the side against resistance.
Hypoglossal Nerve	
Motor: Tongue	Examine the tongue in the mouth for position, atrophy, and fasciculations; have the patient protrude the tongue and move it from side to side while checking for asymmetry.

TABLE 5-3. Motor Nerve Examination

What You're Looking For	What You're Doing
Appearance	
Bulk (atrophy, hypertrophy), fasciculations, spasms, spontaneous motion.	Observing.
Tone	
Rigidity: ↑ tone in full ROM, not dependent on rate or location; may be constant (lead-pipe rigidity) or fluctuating (cogwheel rigidity).	Passively move wrists, elbows, ankles, and knees; remind the patient to relax, shake gently, move evenly through ROM, and then move abruptly (note pattern of resistance).
Spasticity: ↑ tone in most arm flexors and leg extensors that ↑ as rate of motion ↑; noted more at initiation of motion than at continuation.	Same.
Flaccidity: ↓ tone; joints tend to flop and hyperextend like a rag doll.	Same.
Paratonia: ↑ tone in response to passive movement of muscles; associated with frontal lobe dysfunction and dementias.	Passively move different muscle groups and look for an ↑ in tone.

(continues)

TABLE 5-3. Motor Nerve Examination *(continued)*

What You're Looking For	What You're Doing
	Strength
Identify the pattern of weakness (or absence of weakness).	History (weakness, clumsiness); screening examination (see below). Perform confrontational testing to quantify strength/weakness.
Explore the extent of weakness and elucidate possible etiologies.	Focused motor examination based on information given in history and screen. Also use functional testing (see the entry on gait below).
Examination tips.	Give the patient mechanical advantage (start with the joint in midposition) and apply force to overcome the patient's strength, not to match it.
	Reflexes
DTRs (jaw, biceps, brachioradialis, triceps, finger flexors, patellar, thigh adductors, ankle jerk).	Ask the patient to relax and position the limbs and alternate from side to side for comparison. Watch for clonus and spreading of the reflex, and record briskness (see Table 5-5 for grading).
Superficial reflexes (abdominal, cremasteric).	Pay attention to symmetry!
Pathologic reflexes (Babinski, frontal release).	For Babinski (plantar response), stroke the lateral plantar surface of the foot with a key and look for the direction of big toe motion (dorsiflexion = Babinski's sign).
	Coordination
Point-to-point testing.	**Finger-to-nose test:** Have the patient touch his nose and then your finger; repeat. **Heel-to-shin test:** Have the patient run the heel up and down the opposite shin from knee to foot.
Rapid alternating movements (strength and coordination).	Index finger tapping on the thumb; foot tapping on the ground.
	Gait
Normal gait. Important for testing power of the lower extremities; functional testing is more sensitive than manual testing.	Is gait balanced and coordinated with feet no wider than shoulders and arms swinging?
Test for tandem gait.	Can the patient walk in a line heel to toe?
Test for distal weakness.	Have the patient walk on toes (plantar flexion) and on heels (dorsiflexion of ankles).
Test for proximal weakness.	Have the patient hop on 1 foot or try a knee bend (standing on 1 foot). Can the patient get out of the chair without using arms?

TABLE 5-4. Muscle Strength Grading

SCORE	STRENGTH
0	No movement.
1	Flicker of contraction.
2	Full ROM with gravity eliminated (eg, arm on table; squeeze hand).
3	Full ROM against gravity (eg, arm hanging on side; flex elbow).
4	Full ROM against gravity and some resistance.
5	Full power against resistance.

to make fists and revolve them around each other as if boxing a punching bag. The strong hand will orbit around the weak arm.
- Evaluate for a UMN pattern vs. a lower motor neuron (LMN) pattern:
  - A UMN pattern includes weakness of the deltoid, triceps, wrist extensor, finger extensors, iliopsoas, hamstrings, and dorsiflexors. Patterns of LMN involvement are less specific and tend to vary depending on the lesion.
  - UMN implies brain or spinal cord, whereas LMN implies nerve roots, plexus, or peripheral nerves.

KEY FACT

Ptosis is caused by a lesion in the sympathetic nerves (above T1) that innervate the smooth muscle of the eyelid or a CN III palsy or dysfunction of the neuromuscular junction.

SCREENING EXAMINATION FOR SENSATION

Consists of the following (see also Table 5-6):

- Check pain (or temperature) sensation in the hands and feet. This assesses small fibers and the anterolateral sensory tract.
- Check vibration (or joint position sense) in the hands and feet. This assesses large fibers and posterior columns.

KEY FACT

DTRs and nerve roots tested:
- Biceps = C5, C6
- Brachioradialis = C5, C6
- Triceps = C6, C7
- Patella = L2–L4
- Achilles = S1

TABLE 5-5. DTR Grading

SCORE	STRENGTH
0	Absent.
1	Hypoactive.
2	Normal.
3	Hyperactive with spread across a joint.
4	Hyperactive with clonus.

KEY FACT

Be familiar with dermatomal patterns:
- T4 = nipple
- T7 = xiphoid process
- T10 = umbilicus
- L1 = inguinal ligament
- S2–S4 = genital/anal zones

TABLE 5-6. Sensory Examination

WHAT YOU'RE LOOKING FOR	WHAT YOU'RE DOING
SENSORY MODALITIES	
Pain	Pricking with a safety pin or a cotton swab stick broken in half.
Temperature	Touching with a cool tuning fork.
Vibration	Touching a buzzing tuning fork to bone and joint.
Joint position sense	Moving the patient's finger or toe up or down. **Romberg test:** Have the patient stand with feet together and eyes closed for 10 seconds. If the patient is okay with the eyes open but not with the eyes closed, the test is ⊕.
Light touch	Lightly touching the patient with finger or cotton.
HIGHER SENSORY FUNCTION	
Graphesthesia: The ability to recognize numbers by touch.	Ask the patient to close his or her eyes; then write a number in the patient's palm and ask to identify it.
Point localization: The ability to localize sensory input.	Quickly touch the patient; then ask to identify location.
Extinction: The ability to recognize 2 bilateral stimuli.	Touch the same areas bilaterally and ask the patient to identify the location of the stimulus.

KEY FACT

When testing position sense, grip the digit on the sides rather than top and bottom to avoid influencing the patient's sensation as you move the digit.

- Check light touch on the arms and legs to look for asymmetry:
  - Sensory loss in the distribution of a single nerve implies mononeuropathy.
  - Sensory loss in the distribution of a nerve root may imply radiculopathy.
  - Sensory loss that is concentric with a distal gradient (stocking/glove) implies peripheral neuropathy.
  - Sensory levels on the trunk (eg, sensory loss from the umbilicus down) imply a cord lesion.
  - Sensory loss that is patchy and involves 1 limb may imply plexopathy.

Key Neuroanatomy

Success on your neurology rotation requires a thorough understanding of the basic principles of neuroanatomy, not only of the cerebral cortex but also of the deeper structures of the brain and brainstem as well as the anatomy of the spinal cord. Before you begin your clerkship, be sure to review the sensory and motor homunculus (see Figure 5-1), as this will be critical to understanding the symptoms of patients with stroke or focal brain lesions. Also review the major vascular territories of the brain, cerebellum, and brainstem as well as the syndromes associated with specific ischemic or hemorrhagic injuries.

Finally, while imaging studies will likely easily identify the location of the patient's lesion, your aim should be to pinpoint the location of the lesion based

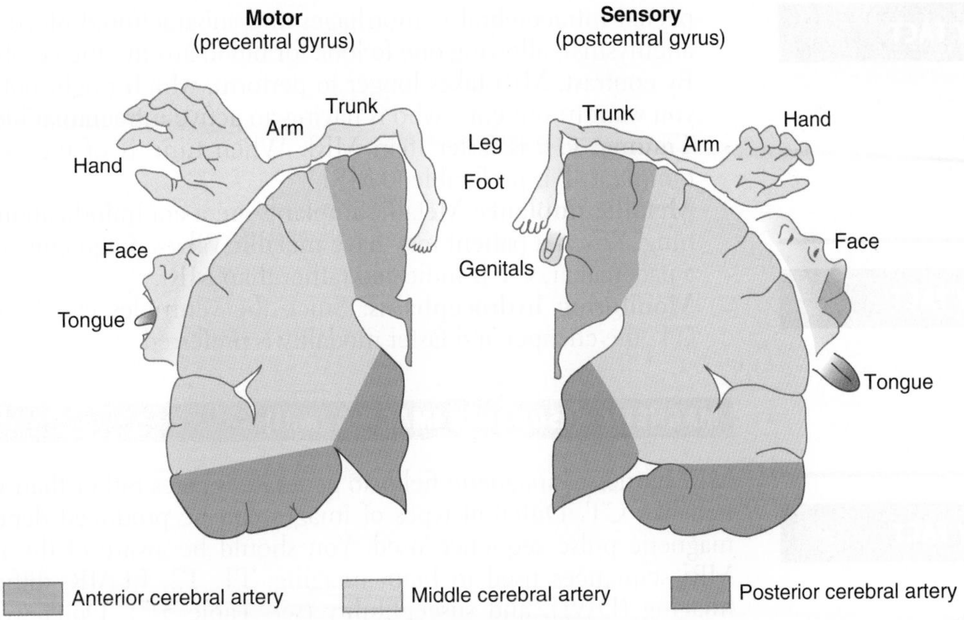

FIGURE 5-1. Sensory and motor homunculus. The homunculus shows a pictorial representation of the innervation of the primary sensory and motor cortices. (Reproduced with permission from Waxman SG. *Clinical Neuroanatomy,* 26th ed. New York: McGraw-Hill, 2010, Fig. 12-6.)

on your examination findings and your neuroanatomy knowledge. See the Neurology portion of the Top-Rated Review Resources section for suggested texts to help you refresh your neuroanatomical knowledge.

Imaging Basics

After you have conducted a complete neurologic examination, you should theoretically be able to localize a lesion in the nervous system. However, modern neurology increasingly relies on imaging for confirmation and diagnostic purposes. You will thus be a step ahead if you familiarize yourself with the basic imaging modalities used in neurology before you start your rotation.

The 2 modalities used most in neurology are CT and MRI. Both modalities have their advantages and disadvantages, and each is indicated under different circumstances. Always identify what type of image you are looking at before trying to interpret it; otherwise, you may run into some trouble.

COMPUTED TOMOGRAPHY (CT)

CT scans can be thought of as 3-dimensional radiographs, where the densities of tissues determine their CT appearance. Dense structures like the skull and metal appear white, while on the other extreme air is black. The intracranial contents appear as shades of gray. For example, CSF is darker than white matter, which is darker than gray matter. The contrast resolution of CT is inferior to that of MRI. Even so, there are specific circumstances in which CT is preferred:

- **Suspected skull fracture:** Because CT uses x-rays for imaging, fractures are easily discerned. CT is usually preferred over MRI for skull fractures.
- **Suspected intracranial bleeds:** Acute bleeds appear whiter than brain on CT scans within 20 minutes of their onset. CT is especially useful in sus-

> **KEY FACT**
>
> **CT:**
> Bone = white
> CSF = gray
> Air = black

KEY FACT

T1:
Bone marrow = white
Bone cortex = no signal
CSF = black

KEY FACT

T2:
Bone = gray
CSF = white

KEY FACT

DWI:
Ischemic areas = white

pected intracerebral hemorrhages and subarachnoid bleeds (eg, ruptured aneurysms), allowing one to look for blood around the cerebral peduncles. By contrast, MRI takes longer to perform, which might not be something you want in someone who is having an active intracranial bleed.

- **Trauma:** CT is faster than MRI. When time is of the essence, as in a trauma, CT is preferable to MRI.
- **Metallic implants:** Metallic implants are a contraindication to MRI scanning. When a patient may have metallic valves, fragments (eg, trauma), or a pacemaker, CT is indicated rather than MRI.
- **Monitoring hydrocephalus:** Since the ventricles can be easily seen by CT, the cheaper and faster modality is preferred.

MAGNETIC RESONANCE IMAGING (MRI)

MRI harnesses magnetic fields to generate images rather than ionizing radiation like CT. Different types of images can be produced depending on the magnetic pulse sequence used. You should be aware of the major types of MRI sequences used in brain imaging: T1, T2, FLAIR, diffusion-weighted imaging (DWI), and susceptibility (see Table 5-7). Don't worry about the physics underlying these sequences; instead, try to be able to recognize the sequences and know what each can tell you.

TABLE 5-7. MRI Sequences

Sequence	Appearance	Uses	Notes
T1	Gray matter = dark. White matter = light. CSF = black. Classically, very bright areas on a T1 image will contain a high degree of protein, fat, subacute blood, or contrast agent.	Studying the anatomy of the brain.	The spatial extent of pathology is often underestimated by T1 imaging. Gadolinium enhancement can be used to ↑ the conspicuity of certain pathologic processes.
T2	Gray matter = light. White matter = dark. CSF = white.	The study of choice for identifying pathology. Pathology appears white owing to edema and water accumulation in the area of pathology.	Both edema and CSF have a large water component, and therefore both appear white.
FLAIR	Gray matter = light. White matter = dark. CSF = black.	The best modality for identifying both acute and chronic pathology.	Similar to a T2 image except that the bright CSF has been nulled, making pathology easier to recognize.
Diffusion	Ischemic areas = white.	Used in suspected cases of acute stroke.	Reveals ischemic areas within minutes of onset.
Susceptibility	Blood = black.	Useful in traumatic brain injury as well as in stroke and hemorrhage.	Exquisitely sensitive to venous blood, hemorrhage (including microhemorrhage not seen on CT), and iron accumulation.

CONTRAST

CT and MRI studies will often be ordered with contrast. IV contrast can elucidate vascular anatomy and suggest the presence of any occlusions. If the blood-brain barrier is interrupted, contrast will "leak" out of the vessels and into the brain. This tells the clinician about the severity or acuity of the condition and can also ↑ the contrast resolution and sensitivity of a study. Contrast is particularly helpful when assessing for inflammation, neoplasm, or infection. It is not helpful for hemorrhagic stroke. Iodinated contrast agents are used for CT contrast; gadolinium is used for MRI contrast.

In a small subset of the population, severe contrast reactions may occur, so it is important to obtain a history of any prior reactions to contrast during CTs. In addition, it is now known that gadolinium can on rare occasions cause a progressive debilitating syndrome called nephrogenic systemic fibrosis (NSF). This syndrome clinically resembles scleroderma and eosinophilic fasciitis, and it affects patients with a history of renal insufficiency. Although relatively uncommon, the syndrome has caused hospitals to pay closer attention to the routine use of gadolinium in MRI studies, particularly for patients with acute or chronic renal insufficiency.

KEY FACT

An LP is performed between L4 and L5 (the level of the iliac crests).

KEY FACT

In bacterial meningitis, think of bacteria as being made of protein and consuming glucose (high CSF protein, low CSF glucose), causing an acute inflammatory reaction (PMNs).

Lumbar Puncture (LP) Results

As you read through this chapter, you will notice that in many cases an LP may be ordered to narrow the differential. Table 5-8 provides CSF profiles for the various neurologic diseases you may encounter.

TABLE 5-8. CSF Profiles

Profile	RBCs (per mm³)	WBCs (per mm³)	Glucose (mg/dL)	Protein (mg/dL)	Opening Pressure (cm H_2O)	Appearance	Gamma Globulin (% protein)
Normal	< 10	< 5	~ 2/3 of serum	15–45	10–20	Clear	3–12
Bacterial meningitis	↔	↑ (PMN)	↓	↑	↑	Cloudy	↔ or ↑
Viral meningitis	↔	↑ (mono)	↔	↔ or ↑	↔ or ↑	Most often clear	↔ or ↑
SAH	↑↑	↑	↔	↑	↔ or ↑	Yellow/red	↔ or ↑
GBS	↔	↔	↔	↑↑	↔	Clear or yellow (high protein)	↔
MS	↔	↔ or ↑	↔	↔	↔	Clear	↑↑

Stroke

Stroke is a clinical syndrome defined by the acute onset of a focal neurologic deficit resulting from a disturbance in blood flow. This disturbance can be either ischemic (85%) or hemorrhagic (15%). A neurologic deficit that does not resolve symptomatically is referred to as a **cerebrovascular accident (CVA).** If the deficit reverses within 24 hours, the event is redesignated a **TIA.** However, TIA symptoms generally reverse in roughly 1 hour. TIAs also significantly ↑ the risk of future stroke, especially within 48 hours of the TIA. The etiologies of **ischemic stroke** include the following:

- **Embolic:**
  - **Atrial fibrillation (AF):** The most common cause of cardioembolic stroke. Patients with AF have a five- to sixfold greater risk of stroke than the general population.
  - **Other cardiac causes:** Include embolism of mural thrombi, thrombi from diseased or prosthetic valves, other arrhythmias, endocarditis (septic, fungal, or marantic emboli), and paradoxic (venous) emboli in patients with right-to-left shunt in the heart (from ASD or patent foramen ovale).
- **Thrombotic:**
  - **Large vessel atherothrombosis** (internal and common carotids, basilar and vertebral arteries): Accounts for 35% of all strokes and roughly 40% of ischemic strokes. Symptoms are typically maximal at onset and may slowly improve.
  - **Small vessel atherothrombosis:** Lacunar infarcts (the source of 20% of all strokes) occur in regions supplied by small perforating vessels deep in the brain and result from either atherosclerotic or hypertensive occlusion. They commonly occur in the basal ganglia, brainstem, and internal capsules (due to small vessel disease).
- **Other:** Less common causes of ischemic stroke include the following:
  - **Hematologic disorders,** including **hypercoagulable** states such as sickle cell disease, polycythemia, thrombocytosis, leukocytosis, malignancy, hereditary coagulopathies, and collagen vascular disease.
  - Fibromuscular dysplasia (young females), inflammatory diseases, arterial dissection, migraine, venous thrombosis.

KEY FACT

Ischemic strokes are much more common than hemorrhagic strokes.

Hemorrhagic strokes are most often caused by hypertensive rupture of small vessels, AVMs, hemorrhagic conversion of ischemic strokes, amyloid angiopathy, cocaine use, and/or bleeding diatheses.

Signs and Symptoms

- Presentation depends on the location of the stroke; different **vascular** territories will have different presentations (see Table 5-9).

KEY POINT

RISK FACTORS FOR STROKE

- **Nonmodifiable:** Age, male gender, ethnicity (African American, Hispanic, Asian), genetics.
- **Modifiable:** Hypertension, DM, smoking, heavy alcohol intake, cocaine use, obesity, hypercholesterolemia, carotid stenosis, AF.

TABLE 5-9. Stroke Sites and Resulting Neurologic Deficits

Vessel[a]	Region Supplied	Neurologic Deficit
Anterior Circulation		
MCA	Lateral cerebral hemisphere; deep subcortical structures.	Combined deficits of superior/inferior divisions; may see coma and ↑ ICP.
Superior division	Motor/sensory cortex of the face, arm, and hand; Broca's area.	Contralateral hemiparesis of the face, arm, and hand; expressive aphasia if dominant hemisphere.
Inferior division	Parietal lobe (visual radiations, Wernicke's area), macular visual cortex.	Homonymous hemianopia, receptive aphasia (dominant), impaired cortical sensory functions, gaze preference, apraxias, and neglect (nondominant).
ACA	Parasagittal cerebral cortex.	Contralateral leg paresis and sensory loss.
Ophthalmic artery	Retina.	Monocular blindness.
Posterior Circulation		
PCA	Occipital lobe, thalamus, rostral midbrain, medial temporal lobes.	Contralateral homonymous hemianopia, memory or sensory disturbances.
Basilar	Ventral midbrain, brainstem, posterior limb of internal capsule, cerebellum, PCA distribution.	Coma or depressed level of consciousness, cranial nerve palsies, apnea, cardiovascular instability, locked-in state.
Deep Circulation		
Lenticulostriate, paramedian, thalamoperforate, circumferential arteries	Basal ganglia, pons, thalamus, internal capsule, cerebellum.	There are many "lacunar" syndromes, including pure motor or sensory deficits, ataxic hemiparesis, and "dysarthria–clumsy hand" syndrome.

[a] MCA = middle cerebral artery; ACA = anterior cerebral artery; PCA = posterior cerebral artery.

- The time course varies for thrombotic, embolic, and hemorrhagic strokes.
  - **Thrombotic:** Evolve in minutes to hours and may follow a TIA.
  - **Embolic:** Often present with the full deficit acutely and do not evolve.
  - **Hemorrhagic:** Onset can include headache and/or altered mental status; deficits may not strictly follow vascular territories and may progressively worsen as a result of hematoma expansion and edema surrounding the bleed.
- Examination may reveal signs of arrhythmias (eg, AF) and atherosclerotic disease (carotid and/or subclavian bruits). Remember, however, that the presence of bruits is not very sensitive for carotid stenosis.

Differential

Todd's paralysis (postictal), subdural or epidural hematoma, brain abscess, brain tumor, MS, complicated migraine headache, metabolic abnormalities, neurosyphilis, conversion disorder.

Q

A 64-year-old woman with a history of AF, hypertension, and hyperlipidemia is found by her caretaker to be unresponsive with left facial droop. She is rushed the ED for evaluation of acute stroke. The caretaker is asked when she last saw the patient at her baseline neurologic function. Why is this question important?

WORKUP

The goal of workup is twofold: (1) to urgently determine whether the stroke is ischemic or hemorrhagic, and (2) if the stroke is ischemic, to ascertain whether it can be reversed within a 4.5-hour window using tPA both to salvage ischemic brain and to prevent further ischemia. Concurrently, one must localize the lesion, rule out other lesions, and determine the etiology. Tests include the following:

- **Imaging:**
  - CT without contrast to distinguish ischemic from hemorrhagic stroke (see Figure 5-2). Note that ischemic strokes, which appear on CT scan as a loss of gray-white differentiation or as a hypodensity, are generally not visible for at least 3–6 hours after symptom onset.
  - MRI to identify early ischemic changes (use DWI and ADC to identify acute infarcts; if present on DWI and absent on ADC, the infarct may be chronic) as well as to identify neoplasms and adequately image the brainstem and posterior fossa.

KEY POINT

GUIDELINES ON WHEN TO INSTITUTE tPA THERAPY

- **Indications for tPA therapy:**
  - Age > 18.
  - A clinical diagnosis of ischemic stroke.
  - Symptom onset within **4.5 hours.**
- **Absolute contraindications to IV tPA therapy:**
  - Current intracranial or subarachnoid hemorrhage.
  - Intracranial surgery, head trauma, or stroke within the last 3 months.
  - Active internal bleeding or known bleeding diathesis such as:
    - Platelet count < 100,000/mL.
    - Heparin within 48 hours with elevated PTT.
    - Current or recent use of oral anticoagulants with elevated PT.
  - Systolic BP > 185 or diastolic BP > 110 mm Hg despite aggressive treatment.
  - A history of intracranial hemorrhage, AVM, or aneurysm.
- **Relative contraindications to IV tPA therapy:**
  - Major surgery or trauma within the last 14 days.
  - A history of GI or urinary bleeding within the last 21 days.
  - Recent LP or arterial puncture at a noncompressible site.
  - Blood glucose < 50 or > 400 mg/dL.
  - Seizures present at the onset of stroke.
  - MI within 3 months.
  - Use of dabigatran within 48 hours.
  - For treatment from 3 to 4.5 hours, the risk/benefit ratio is unclear for patients with any of the following: NIH stroke scale > 25, age > 80, a history of both diabetes and prior stroke, and use of oral anticoagulation regardless of INR.

A

The time since the patient was last seen to have normal neurologic function is critical in the decision regarding whether to treat ischemic stroke with tPA. In the absence of other contraindications, tPA is considered in patients with symptom onset within 4.5 hours.

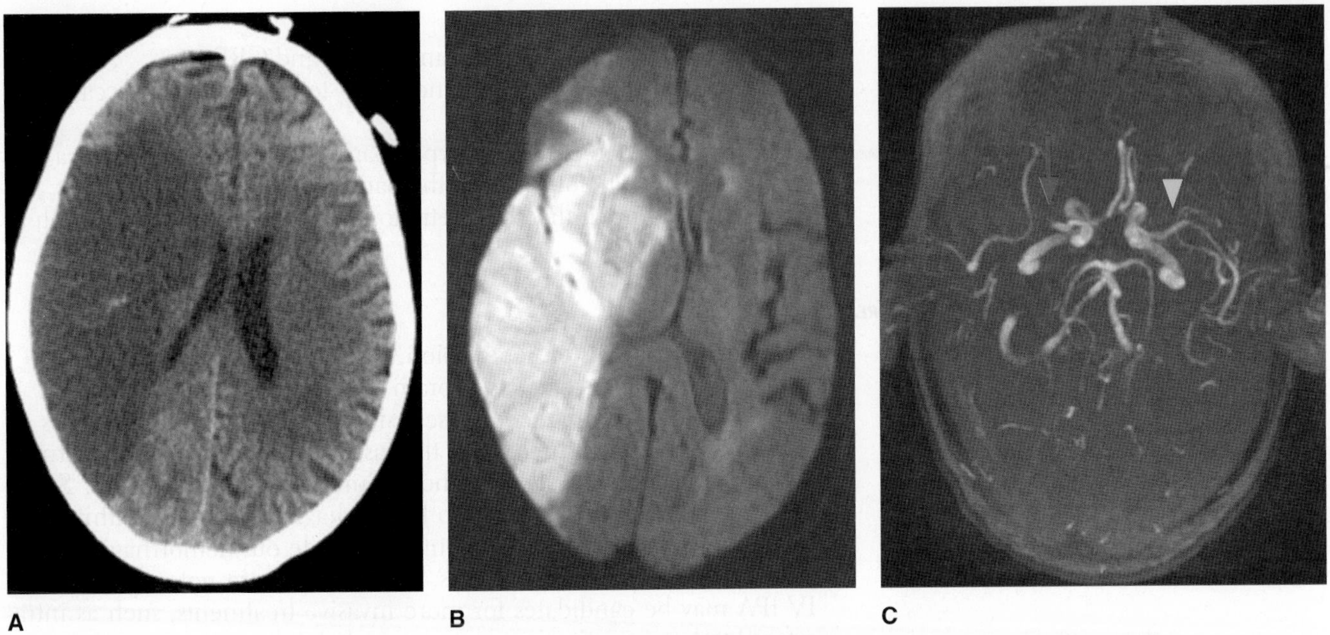

FIGURE 5-2. Acute ischemic stroke. Acute left hemiparesis in a 62-year-old woman. (**A**) Noncontrast head CT with loss of gray and white matter differentiation and asymmetrically decreased size of the right lateral ventricle in a right MCA distribution (indicating mass effect). (**B**) Diffusion-weighted MRI with reduced diffusion in the same distribution, consistent with an acute infarct; **diffusion-weighted sequences are the most sensitive modality for diagnosing an acute ischemic infarct.** (**C**) MRA shows the cause: an abrupt occlusion of the proximal right MCA (arrow). Compare with the normal left MCA (arrowhead). (Reproduced with permission from USMLERx.com.)

- Vascular studies include carotid Doppler ultrasound (extracranial only), magnetic resonance angiography (MRA), and CT angiography (CTA) or catheter angiography.
- Echocardiography to investigate whether there is a cardiac thrombus as a source of embolic stroke, if there are any wall motion abnormalities, and if there is a patent foramen ovale present. Transesophageal echocardiography (TEE) is most sensitive for mural thrombi, but transthoracic echocardiography (TTE) is most commonly performed.

KEY POINT

AVOIDING THE "HYPOS" AND "HYPERS" IN STROKE TREATMENT

- In treating stroke, avoid:
  - **Hypo**tension
  - **Hypo**xemia
  - **Hypo-/hyper**glycemia
  - **Hyper**thermia
- Maintain systolic BP approximately 20 mm Hg above normal to ensure adequate cerebral perfusion (permissive hypertension), and do not lower unless it is > 220/130 mm Hg or in cases where the patient is a candidate for tPA therapy.
- Tightly controlled blood sugars and euthermia have been shown to preserve penumbra (tissue surrounding the infarct).

> **KEY FACT**
>
> For stroke patients, especially those with new stroke or age < 50, consider B_{12}/folate, ESR, RPR, CRP, TSH, a lipid panel, HbA_{1c}, urine toxicology, and a hypercoagulable workup.

- **Labs:**
  - CBC, coagulation panel, lipid panel, ESR, and CRP.
  - TSH, RPR, B_{12}/folate, glucose, and HbA_{1c} to investigate other causes of acute neurologic symptoms.
  - Blood cultures; screening for hypercoagulable states (if there is a history of bleeding or clotting, or if the patient is < 50 years of age).
- **Other tests:** ECG or cardiac telemetry to evaluate for arrhythmias such as AF or for MI.

Treatment

- **Acute treatment:** Focus on reperfusion, neuroprotection, and salvage.
  - Watch for symptoms or signs of brain swelling, ↑ ICP, or herniation.
  - Revascularize thrombotic disease using IV tPA within 4.5 hours of ischemic onset (measured from the last time the patient is confirmed to have been "well"). The 4.5-hour time limit is an absolute. Some people who receive tPA undergo hemorrhagic conversion within their infarct and may suffer a worse outcome. Rule out hemorrhagic stroke, and screen for contraindications. Patients who are not candidates for IV tPA may be candidates for more invasive treatments, such as intra-arterial tPA or investigational mechanical clot disruption.
  - ASA is associated with ↓ morbidity and mortality in acute ischemic stroke presenting ≤ 48 hours from onset.
- **Prevention and long-term treatment:** Manage modifiable risk factors, especially hypertension, DM, and hypercholesterolemia.
  - **Cardioembolic:** Heparin and warfarin therapy can prevent further embolization; target an INR of 2–3 for warfarin therapy. The CHADS2 score (see Table 4-1 from the Internal Medicine chapter) is used to predict the risk of cardioembolic disease in patients with AF.
  - **Lacunar:** Antiplatelet agents such as ASA, clopidogrel (Plavix), or dipyridamole/ASA; BP control.
  - **Carotid stenosis:** Carotid endarterectomy is appropriate in the setting of symptomatic/asymptomatic stenosis > 70%. Do not perform with 100% blockage.

Aphasias

Aphasia is a general term used to describe language disorders. Aphasias generally result from insults (eg, strokes, tumors, abscesses) to the language centers in the "dominant hemisphere." The left hemisphere is dominant in 90% of right-handed people and in 50% of left-handed people. Just as the job of the motor cortex is to move the body, the job of the language centers is to name. Therefore, a patient with a naming deficit of any kind is said to have an aphasia.

> **KEY FACT**
>
> Aphasia is a problem with language and usually results from a **cortical** lesion. Dysarthria is a problem with articulation that usually involves a **subcortical** lesion such as an internal capsule or brainstem lesion.

- To characterize an aphasia, assess the patient's language abilities in 3 domains: **production, comprehension,** and **repetition.** Reading and writing are other aspects of language you may want to evaluate.
- There are 8 main types of aphasias, 6 of which are described here (see Table 5-10). The 2 principal aphasias with which you should be familiar are Broca's and Wernicke's (see Figure 5-3).

TABLE 5-10. Summary of Aphasias

Type	Fluency	Comprehension	Repetition	Naming	Reading	Writing	Lesion Localization
Broca's	↓	Normal	↓	↓	↓	↓	Posterior inferior frontal gyrus
Wernicke's	Normal	↓	↓	↓	↓	↓	Posterior superior temporal lobe
Conduction	Normal	Normal	↓	↓	Normal	↓	Arcuate fasciculus
Global	↓	↓	↓	↓	↓	↓	Large portion of dominant hemisphere
Transcortical motor	↓	Normal	Normal	Mildly ↓	Normal	↓	ACA/MCA border zone
Transcortical sensory	Normal	↓	Normal	↓	↓	↓	PCA/MCA border zone

BROCA'S APHASIA

Broca's aphasia is an expressive aphasia; it is a disorder of language production and repetition with intact comprehension. It is often 2° to a superior MCA stroke.

Signs and Symptoms

- Speech is nonfluent, with ↓ rate, short phrase length, and impaired articulation.
- Repetition is impaired, but comprehension is intact. Patients are noticeably frustrated with their speech because they are aware of their deficit.
- Associated features include arm and face hemiparesis, hemisensory loss, and apraxia of oral muscles due to the proximity of Broca's area (the posterior inferior frontal gyrus) to the motor and sensory strips (the pre- and postcentral gyri, respectively).

KEY FACT

Broca's is **B**roken speech. For example: "Read paper. Book new. Good time."

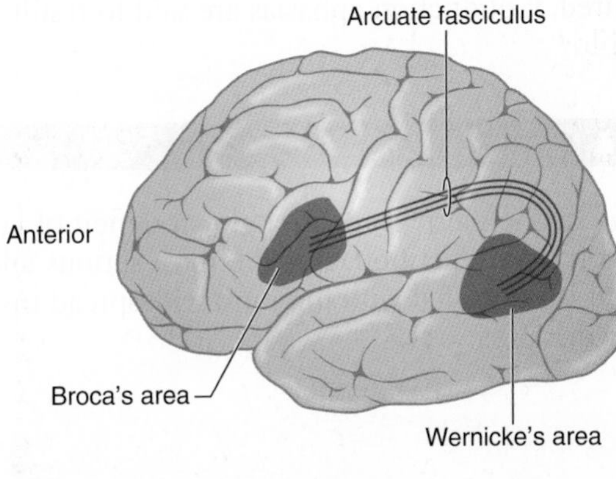

FIGURE 5-3. Broca's and Wernicke's areas. Broca's and Wernicke's areas are the 2 major language centers in the brain. The arcuate fasciculus connects these areas. Injury to the arcuate fasciculus results in language repetition errors.

TREATMENT

Treat the underlying pathology; begin speech therapy (has varying outcomes with an intermediate prognosis).

> **KEY FACT**
>
> **W**ernicke's is **W**ordy but makes no sense. For example: "I know that poodle blubbered and he wants to get you parker and I take care of her as you like before."

WERNICKE'S APHASIA

Wernicke's aphasia is a receptive aphasia; it is a disorder of language comprehension and repetition without a deficit in language production. The lesion is often in the left posterior superior temporal lobe and is often 2° to a left inferior MCA stroke.

SIGNS AND SYMPTOMS

- Speech is fluent but empty of meaning.
- Comprehension, naming, and repetition are impaired, with frequent use of marked neologisms (made-up words) and paraphasic errors (word substitutions).
- No notable hemiparesis or dysarthria is present.
- Patients are often unaware of their deficit because they lack comprehension.

> **KEY FACT**
>
> Wernicke-Korsakoff encephalopathy results from thiamine deficiency, often 2° to alcoholism. A lesion in the mammillary bodies leads to confabulations and anterograde amnesia.

TREATMENT

Treat the underlying pathology; begin speech therapy (even though it is not as successful as in Broca's aphasia).

TRANSCORTICAL APHASIAS

Transcortical motor aphasia and transcortical sensory aphasia are marked by impaired language motor output (production deficit) and impaired language comprehension ("sensory"), respectively. Both are distinct from Broca's and Wernicke's in that repetition remains intact.

CONDUCTION APHASIA

A conduction aphasia is a subtle aphasia that can be easily missed because both language production and comprehension remain intact, but language repetition is impaired. Conduction aphasias are said to result from damage to the arcuate fasciculus.

GLOBAL APHASIA

A global aphasia is, as the name implies, a global deficit of language production, comprehension, and repetition. It is the most serious and devastating of all the aphasias and is associated with the most widespread insult to the brain. It also carries the worst prognosis.

Coma

Defined as a profound suppression of responses to external and internal stimuli caused either by catastrophic structural injury to the CNS or by diffuse metabolic dysfunction. Coma is distinct from "brain death" in that patients with coma may have preserved cranial nerve reflexes and detectable brain activity on EEG. The severity of coma is measured by the Glasgow Coma Scale (GCS) (see Table 5-11). Coma etiology is the best predictor of coma outcomes; whereas coma 2° to drug overdose is associated with 5–10% mortality, coma 2° to anoxia carries a 90% mortality rate. In addition, the younger the patient, the better the prognosis.

The reticular activating system is necessary for consciousness. This structure extends from the brainstem, through the thalamus bilaterally, and to the cerebral hemispheres bilaterally. Bilateral hemispheric insults, bilateral thalamic insults, or brainstem insults lead to coma. Etiologies can be broken down as follows:

- **Supratentorial processes:** Hemorrhage, infarction, abscesses, and tumors. Must be recognized in order to prevent potential herniation.
- **Infratentorial lesions:** Hemorrhage, vertebrobasilar strokes, and tumors of the brainstem or cerebellum. Infratentorial masses require prompt evacuation due to impending compression/damage to the brainstem.
- **Metabolic causes:** Electrolyte or endocrine disturbances; ethanol, drugs, or toxins.
- **Miscellaneous:** Infectious or inflammatory disease; subarachnoid blood; generalized seizure activity or postictal states; anoxia 2° to cardiac arrest, respiratory arrest, carbon monoxide poisoning, or asphyxia.

KEY FACT

GCS scoring: Think "**4**-Eyes," the roman numeral **V** (**V**erbal) for **5,** and the rest adds up to **15.**

Signs and Symptoms

The physical examination should check for vital signs, trauma, nuchal rigidity, and funduscopic changes. However, the patient's presentation will vary with the etiology of the coma (see Table 5-12).

TABLE 5-11. Glasgow Coma Scale

Variable	Response	Score
Eye opening	Spontaneous	4
	To verbal command	3
	To pain	2
	None	1
Verbal responsiveness	Oriented	5
	Confused	4
	Inappropriate words	3
	Incomprehensible words	2
	None	1
Motor response	Obeys	6
	Localizes	5
	Withdraws (pain)	4
	Flexion (pain)	3
	Extension (pain)	2
	None	1
		TOTAL

TABLE 5-12. Presentation of Coma Based on Etiology

Initial Presentation	Etiology
Sudden onset	Brainstem infarctions, SAH.
Initially focal but rapidly progressive	Intracerebral hemorrhage.
Subacute	Tumor, abscess, subdural hematoma.
Focal neurologic deficits	Structural lesions.
No focal signs	Diffuse processes such as metabolic or drug intoxication.

KEY FACT

Determining coma etiology is critical because it is the best predictor of outcomes.

KEY FACT

Reactive pupils in a patient with absent oculocephalic reflexes cannot be truly localized and point to a toxic/metabolic insult.

MNEMONIC

Normal eye deviations (fast phase) to caloric stimulation–

COWS

Cold
Opposite
Warm
Same

Differential

- Locked-in states (central pontine myelinolysis, brainstem stroke, advanced ALS).
- Persistent vegetative state.
- Trauma with diffuse cortical injury or hypoxic ischemic injury.
- Nonconvulsive status epilepticus.

Workup

- The absence or asymmetry of **primitive brainstem reflexes** can help localize the lesion and elucidate coma etiology.
  - **Pupil size:** Are pupils symmetric? A "blown pupil" may be a sign of ipsilateral uncal herniation.
  - **Pupillary light reflex:** A normal pupillary light reflex is said to occur when the pupils constrict symmetrically to light shone into either eye.
  - **Corneal reflex:** Normally, both eyes blink in response to corneal irritation (usually with a Q-tip or a cotton swab).
  - **Oculocephalic reflex (or "doll's eye" reflex):** The **vestibulo-ocular reflex (VOR)** is a reflex eye movement that stabilizes images on the retina during head movement by producing an eye movement in the direction opposite to head movement, thereby preserving the image on the center of the visual field. For example, when the head moves to the right, the eyes move to the left and vice versa. The VOR does not depend on visual input and works even in total darkness or when the eyes are closed.
- **Hot/cold-water calorics:** Infusion of cold water into an ear will inactivate the ipsilateral semicircular canal, and thus the eyes will move toward the cold-water infusion followed by nystagmus in the opposite direction (fast-phase opposite). If the eyes look slowly toward the stimulus side with no fast-phase correction, the brainstem is intact and the lesion is in the cerebral hemispheres. If there is no movement of the eyes, then the lesion involves the brainstem.
- Test passive muscle tone, DTRs, the Babinski reflex, and ankle clonus.
- Look for unusual **respiratory patterns:**
  - **Cheyne-Stokes:** A crescendo-decrescendo pattern due to bilateral hemispheric dysfunction.
  - **Central neurogenic hyperventilation:** Rapid deep breathing due to midbrain damage.
  - **Apneustic breathing:** Prolonged inspiration with subsequent apnea due to pontine dysfunction.
  - **Ataxic breathing:** Irregular breathing due to medullary dysfunction.

- **Labs:** Check glucose and electrolytes, LFTs, BUN, creatinine, PT/PTT, CBC, ABGs, and blood cultures (if sepsis is suspected). In addition, a toxicology screen (for alcohol and drugs of abuse) and an LP (if CNS infection is suspected) should be ordered.
- **Imaging:**
  - A CT scan is indicated, particularly if a structural lesion, trauma, or SAH is suspected.
  - Remember "**stick, scan, and wave**"—include LP, MRI, and EEG in the coma workup in addition to the evaluation of metabolic disturbances.

Treatment

- **Stabilize the patient:** Attend to **ABCs**—**A**irway, **B**reathing, and **C**irculation.
- **Reverse the reversible:** Administer **DON'T: D**extrose, **O**xygen, **N**aloxone, and **T**hiamine.
- **Prevent further damage:** This requires recognition of the progressive and/or treatable etiologies of coma. Some things to look for include the following:
  - Signs of herniation can be managed by decreasing ICP and/or by surgical decompression.
  - Patients with signs of possible meningitis, including fever and nuchal rigidity, should receive IV antibiotics immediately and an LP within 4 hours.
  - Signs of SAH warrant emergent CT and LP.
  - Seizure activity should be treated if verified by clinical findings (shaking, gaze deviation) or EEG.
  - Trauma may suggest cervical spine injury and may warrant cervical x-rays and/or a CT.
- **Investigate further:** Management can shift to the treatment of metabolic disturbances and further investigation.

KEY FACT

Dextrose is administered to coma patients because a common cause of coma is severe hypoglycemia.

Delirium and Dementia

Differentiating delirium and dementia can be challenging. Although both conditions reflect a so-called alteration of mental status and a global ↓ in cognition, delirium and dementia differ in terms of their etiologies, their time course, and the cognitive domains affected. Delirium and dementia are compared in the paragraphs that follow and in Table 5-13.

DELIRIUM

Delirium is defined by the Confusion Assessment Method (CAM) as an acute change in mental status **and** symptoms that fluctuate over minutes and hours **and** inattention combined with **either** altered level of consciousness **or** disorganized thinking. All human beings, even medical students, are at risk for delirium; younger and healthier people have higher reserve, allowing them to sustain more insults before delirium sets in. The elderly are at particular risk for delirium 2° to medical illness, polypharmacy, and preexisting dementia. Other predisposing factors include unfamiliar surroundings, sleep deprivation, sensory deprivation, and sensory overload. The more common etiologies are outlined in Table 5-14.

MNEMONIC

Causes of delirium–

MOVE, STUPID

Metabolic
Oxygen
Vascular
Endocrine/**E**lectrolytes
Seizures
Tumor/**T**rauma/**T**emperature
Uremia
Psychogenic
Infection/**I**ntoxication
Drugs/**D**egenerative diseases

TABLE 5-13. Dementia vs. Delirium

Variable	Dementia	Delirium
Hallmark feature	Memory loss.	Fluctuating orientation.
Level of arousal	Normal.	Stupor or agitation.
Development	Slow and insidious.	Rapid.
Reversibility	Often irreversible.	Frequently reversible.
Other comments	Dementia predisposes a patient to delirium.	Brain damage predisposes; most common in children and the elderly. Fluctuates; duration is brief.

Signs and Symptoms

- Waxing and waning consciousness and perceptual disturbances (hallucinations, delusions, agitation, persecutory thoughts) are common.
- Anxiety, paranoia, or combativeness may be present. Symptoms often worsen at night, a phenomenon known as "sundowning." However, some patients may have ↓ responsiveness known as "quiet delirium," which may go unnoticed if the team is monitoring only for agitated patients.
- Also characterized by ↓ attention span, ↓ short-term memory, and reversed sleep-wake cycles.

TABLE 5-14. Common Causes of Delirium

Type of Insult	Examples
Metabolic	Hepatic encephalopathy, thiamine deficiency, hypoglycemia.
Oxygen	Hypoxia/hypercarbia.
Vascular	MI, anemia.
Endocrine/**E**lectrolytes	Hyponatremia, hypercalcemia, fluid imbalance, hyper-/hypothyroidism.
Seizures	Ictal/postictal.
Tumor/**T**rauma/**T**emperature	–
Uremia	Acute renal failure, dehydration.
Psychogenic	–
Infection	UTI, pneumonia, meningitis, sepsis.
Intoxication	Alcohol, benzodiazepines, carbon monoxide, barbiturates, hallucinogens, opioids.
Drugs/**D**egenerative diseases	–

WORKUP

- Perform a thorough H&P, particularly for fevers, chills, nausea, vomiting, bowel movements, nutrition, medications (eg, narcotics, antipsychotics, benzodiazepines), substance use (eg, alcohol, illicit drugs), pain, and recent illnesses. Pay particular attention to signs of infection or dehydration on physical examination. Check vital signs and perform a complete neurologic examination.
- Consider chronic medical conditions that may make the patient more susceptible to delirium (including dementia!).
- Obtain electrolytes (including calcium), a CBC with differential (to rule out infection), a UA (to rule out UTI), and a urine toxicology screen.
- Also obtain an ABG (to rule out hypoxia) and LFTs (to rule out hepatic encephalopathy), and consider TFTs, RPR or VDRL, LP (to rule out meningitis/encephalitis), and serum B_{12} and folate (to rule out vitamin deficiencies and malnutrition).
- Imaging studies may include CXR (to rule out pneumonia, TB, and CHF). CT and MRI should be performed if (1) head trauma or CNS pathology is suspected **after** lab work is done and is found to be noncontributory to a medical diagnosis, or (2) there is a high index of suspicion of anatomic CNS pathology (eg, if the patient has an abnormal neurologic examination in addition to the mental status examination).
- Other tests include EEG (to rule out seizures), ECG (to rule out MI), and LP (especially if the patient is febrile with or without meningismus).

TREATMENT

- Treat the underlying cause of delirium.
- Normalize fluid and electrolyte status, and provide an appropriate sensory environment (windows and light).
- Use nonsedating antipsychotics (eg, haloperidol) for agitation (except in alcohol withdrawal).
- Avoid benzodiazepines for sedation, as they will worsen most patients' symptoms (except in the setting of alcohol or benzodiazepine withdrawal, when benzodiazepines are clearly indicated).

DEMENTIA

A chronic, progressive, global decline in multiple cognitive areas, especially memory loss. Other cognitive deficits include aphasia (language disturbance), apraxia (inability to execute commands), agnosia (disruption of recognition), and disturbances in executive function (eg, abstraction). Alzheimer's disease accounts for 70–80% of all cases; other etiologies are outlined in the mnemonic **DEMENTIAS:**

- **D**egenerative diseases: Alzheimer's, Parkinson's, Huntington's, Pick's, Lewy body disease.
- **E**ndocrine: Thyroid, parathyroid, pituitary-adrenal axis.
- **M**etabolic: Alcohol, fluid electrolytes, vitamin B_{12}, glucose, hepatic/renal disease, Wilson's disease.
- **E**xogenous: Heavy metals, carbon monoxide, drugs.
- **N**eoplasm.
- **T**rauma: Subdural hematoma.
- **I**nfection: Meningitis, encephalitis, abscess, endocarditis, HIV, syphilis, prions, Lyme disease.
- **A**ffective disorders: Pseudodementia 2° to depression.
- **S**troke/Structure: Multi-infarct (vascular) dementia, ischemia, vasculitis, normal pressure hydrocephalus.

MNEMONIC

The 5 A's of dementia:

Amnesia
Aphasia
Agnosia
Apraxia
Abstract thought disturbances

KEY FACT

Be careful not to mistake inattentiveness or depression for cognitive decline.

WORKUP

- **Conduct a thorough H&P:** Talk to family members about the time line of symptom progression. How long have there been problems? Are there other symptoms, such as tremor, rigidity, staring episodes, loss of consciousness, or excessive somnolence?
- **Labs/imaging:**
  - Obtain a CBC, electrolytes (including calcium), glucose, BUN/creatinine, LFTs, TFTs, B_{12} levels, and RPR or VDRL.
  - Neuroimaging (CT or MRI) is also indicated to rule out other etiologies and to identify specific patterns of brain atrophy consistent with a particular dementia type—eg, frontotemporal vs. vascular dementia.
  - Consider an LP, ESR, folate, HIV, CXR, UA, 24-hour urine for heavy metals, and a urine toxicology screen.

> **KEY FACT**
>
> Slowly progressive cognitive decline is characteristic of Alzheimer's dementia, whereas patients with a stepwise decline in function more commonly have vascular dementia.

TREATMENT

- Prevent further insult to the brain by avoiding toxic agents, normalizing diet, and treating any underlying disease that may be exacerbating the dementia.
- Avoid benzodiazepines, as they will often exacerbate disinhibition and confusion.
- Low-dose atypical antipsychotics (eg, quetiapine, risperidone) may be used for agitation.
- Treat any associated depression.
- Support for the caregiver is essential.

ALZHEIMER'S DISEASE (AD)

Risk factors for AD include **age**, female gender, a ⊕ family history, Down syndrome, ApoE4 homozygosity, and low educational level. Pathology includes neurofibrillary tangles, neuritic plaques with amyloid deposition, amyloid angiopathy, and neuronal loss. Survival is approximately 5–10 years from the onset of symptoms, and death is usually 2° to aspiration pneumonia or other infections.

SIGNS AND SYMPTOMS

- Anterograde amnesia is the first sign of AD.
- Subsequent cognitive deficits include aphasias, acalculia, depression, agitation, and apraxia.

WORKUP

- AD is a clinical diagnosis of exclusion that can be definitively diagnosed only on autopsy.
- Neurobehavioral and neuropsychological tests can be ordered to identify specific cognitive deficits.
- PET is increasingly being used to determine specific patterns of hypometabolism that may be highly sensitive and specific for diagnosing AD.

> **KEY FACT**
>
> Medicare now partially covers PET scans for AD.

TREATMENT

- **Anticholinesterase inhibitors** (rivastigmine, galantamine, donepezil) are first-line therapy. Tacrine can cause hepatotoxicity.
- Memantine is an NMDA antagonist that has been shown to be neuroprotective against excitotoxicity.
- Vitamin E (α-tocopherol) and selegiline, both of which are antioxidants, may slow cognitive decline.

> **KEY FACT**
>
> In patients with AD, life expectancy from the time of diagnosis is approximately half that of age-matched controls.

Dizziness

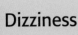

Equilibrium is maintained through the input of visual, vestibular, and proprioceptive sensory systems and through processing by the cerebellum and brainstem. Dizziness is a vague term that may signify a number of phenomena, including the following (see also Table 5-15):

- **Vertigo:** A false sense of motion, often accompanied by a spinning sensation.
- **Presyncope:** A feeling of imminent loss of consciousness.
- **Lightheadedness:** A feeling of weakness accompanied by variable symptoms.
- **Disequilibrium:** A sensation of imbalance with no illusion of movement.

KEY FACT

When interviewing a patient, it is important to identify true vertigo: "Did it feel as if everything was spinning around you?" vs. "Did you feel weak and lightheaded?"

Signs and Symptoms

- Dizziness manifests clinically as vertigo or ataxia (incoordination without weakness of voluntary movement of the eyes, speech, gait, trunk, or extremities).
- Peripheral and central vertigo are compared and further discussed in Tables 5-16 and 5-17. The brainstem signs cited in Table 5-16 refer to signs such as ataxia, dysarthria, cranial nerve abnormalities, and motor system dysfunction.

Workup

- Through the history, determine what the patient actually means by "dizziness," paying particular attention to the duration of the "dizzy spells"

TABLE 5-15. Etiologies of Dizziness

Etiology	Sensation	Causes
		Vertigo
Peripheral labyrinthine or vestibular dysfunction	Illusion of movement	**Benign paroxysmal positional vertigo (BPPV):** Responsible for 50% of cases of peripheral disequilibrium. Characterized by brief spells of vertigo triggered by changes in head position; caused by loose debris (otoliths) within the inner ear. **Ménière's disease:** Intermittent vertigo from dilation and periodic rupture of the inner ear endolymphatic compartment. Hearing loss and tinnitus are also common. **Other:** Acoustic neuroma (vestibular schwannoma), viral labyrinthitis.
Central neurologic lesion	Illusion of movement	Brainstem or cerebellar processes such as stroke, tumor, or MS.
		Other
Presyncope	A feeling of impending loss of consciousness	Hypotension, MI, vasovagal reaction, cardiac conduction abnormalities, valvular disease.
Lightheadedness	Variable	Anxiety, depression, psychosis, hyperventilation, hypochondriasis.
Disequilibrium	A feeling of imbalance without an illusion of movement	Peripheral neuropathies, Parkinson's disease, ataxias.

TABLE 5-16. Central vs. Peripheral Vertigo

Manifestation	Peripheral	Central
Illusion of movement	Often intermittent; severe.	Often constant; usually less severe.
Nystagmus	Unidirectional or rotatory, never vertical.	Unidirectional or bidirectional; may be vertical.
Hearing loss or tinnitus	Often present.	Rarely present.
Brainstem signs	Absent.	Often present.

KEY FACT

Vertical nystagmus is pathognomonic for a central lesion.

KEY FACT

Other tests for disequilibrium include TFTs, a B_{12} level, and CSF for cells, IgG index, and oligoclonal bands (WBCs in a CSF sample indicate infection, while an elevated IgG index and oligoclonal bands can point to MS).

(seconds vs. minutes vs. hours) and precipitating events such as movement. Patients will often report dizziness after feeling faint, lightheaded, or ataxic, so it is important to carefully listen to the patient's description of symptoms and ask questions to elucidate differences between these symptoms.

- Rule out other cranial nerve deficits, motor weakness, orthostasis, cardiac arrhythmia, and ear canal occlusions.
- Perform the Dix-Hallpike maneuver for BPPV (see below).
- Test for cerebellar dysfunction; perform the Romberg test and observe the patient's stance and gait. Test for dysmetria, checking finger-to-nose and heel-to-shin coordination; these should be unimpaired in peripheral processes.
- Test for nystagmus, paying close attention to direction and character. BPPV is usually torsional nystagmus toward the affected side.
- If necessary, obtain an audiogram, brainstem auditory evoked responses, and an electronystagmogram to distinguish peripheral from central vertigo.
- Obtain an MRI if the patient shows signs of central involvement or if a peripheral disturbance cannot be explained by a benign etiology.

Treatment

- Use antihistamines (especially meclizine), anticholinergics such as scopolamine, benzodiazepines, or sympathomimetics to treat benign conditions such as BPPV and Ménière's disease. Ménière's may also respond to diuretics.

TABLE 5-17. Central vs. Peripheral Causes of Dizziness

Peripheral	Acute Central	Chronic Central
BPPV	Drug intoxication	MS
Ménière's disease	Wernicke's encephalopathy	Cerebellar degeneration
Acute peripheral vestibulopathy	Vertebrobasilar ischemia/infarction	Hypothyroidism
Otosclerosis	Inflammatory disorders	Wilson's disease
Cerebellopontine-angle tumor	Cerebellar/brainstem hemorrhage	Creutzfeldt-Jakob disease
Vestibulopathy/acoustic neuropathy	Demyelinating/MS	Posterior fossa masses
Perilymphatic fistula		Ataxia-telangiectasia

KEY POINT

THE DIX-HALLPIKE MANEUVER

- In the Dix-Hallpike maneuver, vertigo is elicited with a change in the patient's head position. The patient is brought from a sitting to a supine position, with the head turned 45 degrees to 1 side and extended about 20 degrees backward.
- Once the patient is supine, his or her eyes are typically observed for about 30 seconds. If no nystagmus ensues, the patient is brought back to a sitting position. Following an additional delay of about 30 seconds, the other side is tested. A ⊕ Dix-Hallpike test consists of a burst of rotatory nystagmus and can provide clear evidence of a peripheral lesion.

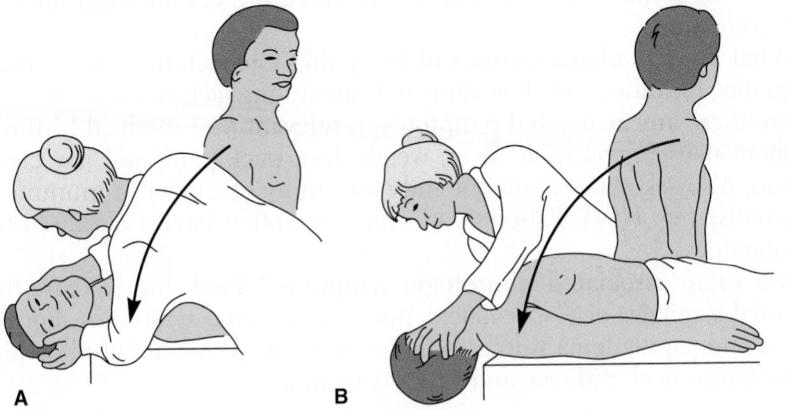

(Reproduced with permission from Lalwani AK. *Current Diagnosis & Treatment in Otolaryngology—Head and Neck Surgery*, 2nd ed. New York: McGraw-Hill, 2007, Fig. 56-1.)

- The Epley maneuver can be used to treat BPPV, although the condition usually subsides spontaneously in weeks to months.
- Discontinue vestibulotoxic drugs such as quinidine, alcohol, and ASA. Tobacco and high-salt diets should be avoided in Ménière's.
- Treat the underlying disorder if known (eg, thiamine deficiency, hypothyroidism).

Headache

1° headache is generally classified into 3 categories: migraine, tension, and cluster. However, headache may also be the presenting symptom of serious neurologic disease and should therefore be taken seriously, as it is your job to differentiate between benign and life-threatening causes. Etiologies include the following:

- **Acute:** SAH, epidural and subdural hematoma, hemorrhagic stroke, meningitis, acutely elevated ICP, hypertensive encephalopathy, post-LP (spinal headache), ocular disease (glaucoma, iritis), new migraine headache, cerebral venous thrombosis, posterior reversible encephalopathy.

- **Subacute:** Temporal arteritis, intracranial tumor, subdural hematoma, pseudotumor cerebri, trigeminal/glossopharyngeal neuralgia, postherpetic neuralgia, hypertension.
- **Chronic/episodic:** Migraine, cluster headache, tension headache, sinusitis, dental disease, neck pain.

WORKUP

There are 4 important questions you should ask with regard to headache:

- **Is this a new or an old headache?** Is it qualitatively different from headaches the patient has had in the past? Is it the "worst headache of my life"? Any new, severe headache warrants an **emergent workup.** In contrast, headache that is chronic or characteristic does not usually warrant diagnostic workup in the absence of abnormal neurologic findings or fever. CT with contrast or MRI may be warranted if there are focal findings on examination.
- **What are the characteristics of the pain?** Characterize onset, duration, quality, location, and alleviating and aggravating factors.
- **Are there any associated symptoms or relevant past medical history?** Ask about nausea, vomiting, fever, weight loss, neck pain, and jaw claudication. Also ask about a present and past history of cancer or immune compromise (eg, HIV). Patients with migraines often have a family history of migraines.
- **Are there associated neurologic symptoms?** Look for ⊕ (paresthesias, visual stigmata) or ⊖ (weakness, numbness, ataxia) symptoms. Focal deficits and papilledema warrant immediate workup. Ask about photophobia, dizziness, neck stiffness, and a history of auras.

KEY FACT

Recent-onset headaches require immediate workup! For those associated with neurologic deficits, order a CT or an MRI. For acute symptoms, perform an LP to rule out meningitis or SAH.

MIGRAINE HEADACHE

Migraines afflict up to 18% of women (most commonly beginning before age 30) and 6% of men and tend to run in families. The etiology is not fully understood; vascular abnormalities (eg, intracranial vasoconstriction, extracranial vasodilation) may be 2° to a disorder of serotonergic neurotransmission.

SIGNS AND SYMPTOMS

- A throbbing headache lasting between 2 and 20 hours. Headache is usually unilateral but may also be bilateral. In addition, it is generally frontal and retro-orbital but may also be occipital.
- Often precipitated by identifiable triggers, including the intake of certain foods (eg, chocolate, caffeine), skipping meals, sleep deprivation, stress, menses, OCP use, and bright light.
- Associated with nausea and vomiting, photophobia, and noise sensitivity (see Figure 5-4A).
- **"Classic migraines"** are preceded by a visual aura in the form of either scintillating scotomas (bright light or flashing lights, often in a zigzag pattern, moving across the visual field) or field cuts.
- **"Common migraines"** are not associated with these symptoms and can be bilateral and periorbital.

KEY FACT

If a visual aura is present, it occurs roughly 10–30 minutes before the onset of a migraine headache.

TREATMENT

- Counsel patients to avoid known triggers, regulate sleep and dietary patterns, and exercise regularly.
- **Pharmacotherapy** includes the following:
  - **Abortive therapy:** ASA/NSAIDs, sumatriptan and other triptans, antiemetics, ergots (partial 5-HT_1 agonists), and, rarely, opiates (although

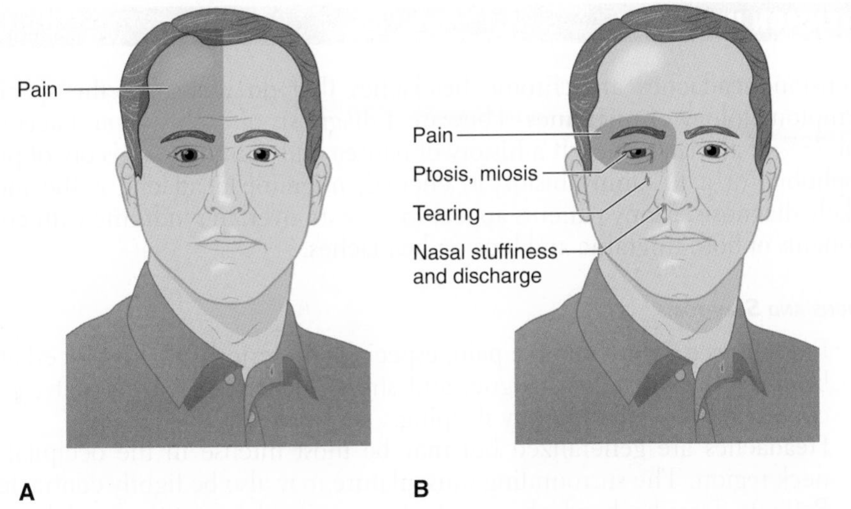

FIGURE 5-4. Distribution of pain in headache. **(A) Migraine headache.** Pain in migraine headache is most commonly hemicranial. Pain can also be holocephalic, bifrontal, or unilateral frontal. **(B) Cluster headache.** Pain is commonly associated with ipsilateral conjunctival injection, tearing, nasal stuffiness, and Horner's syndrome. (Reproduced with permission from Aminoff MJ et al. *Clinical Neurology,* 3rd ed. Stamford, CT: Appleton & Lange, 1996: 91–92.)

opiates should be avoided if possible). Triptans are contraindicated in patients with CAD (as they cause vasoconstriction) or in those with complicated migraine headaches (eg, basilar migraines) that include focal neurologic symptoms.

- **Prophylactic therapy:** Propranolol (β-blockers), verapamil (calcium channel blockers [CCBs]), amitriptyline (TCAs), and topiramate (anticonvulsants). Narcotics should not be used prophylactically.

> **KEY FACT**
>
> Abortive therapy is used to end a migraine headache once it has started. Prophylactic therapy is used for patients with severe and frequent migraines.

CLUSTER HEADACHE

Cluster headaches affect approximately 1% of the population and are seen more often in men than in women. They are much less common than migraines. The average age of onset is 25. Cluster headache may be precipitated by alcohol intake or vasodilator use.

Signs and Symptoms

- A brief, severe, unilateral periorbital headache lasting 30 minutes to 3 hours (see Figure 5-4B). May present as "stabbing" eye pain that awakens the patient from sleep.
- Attacks tend to occur in clusters (hence the name), affecting the same part of the head and taking place at the same time of day (usually at night) and the same time of the year.
- Associated symptoms include ipsilateral tearing of the eye and conjunctival injection, Horner's syndrome, and nasal stuffiness.

Treatment

- **Abortive therapy:** High-flow (100%) O_2, sumatriptan, ergots, intranasal lidocaine, corticosteroids, lithium.
- **Prophylactic therapy:** CCBs, valproic acid, prednisone, topiramate, methysergide.

TENSION HEADACHE

Tension headaches are chronic headaches that do not share the specific symptomatology of migraines. They are a diagnosis of exclusion and account for 75% of all headaches. If a history of nausea and vomiting, a history of photophobia, or a ⊕ family history is elicited, migraine headache is the more likely diagnosis. Many patients appear to have an overlap syndrome with components of both migraine and tension headaches.

> **KEY FACT**
>
> Differential diagnosis of headache:
> - **Migraine:** Often associated with an aura, nausea, and photophobia.
> - **Cluster:** Sharp, unilateral periorbital pain with autonomic phenomena.
> - **Tension:** Bandlike pain.

Signs and Symptoms

- Presents as a tight, bandlike pain, especially posteriorly, that is exacerbated by noise, bright lights, fatigue, and stress. Associated with anxiety, poor concentration, and difficulty sleeping.
- Headaches are generalized but may be most intense in the occipital or neck region. The surrounding musculature may also be tightly contracted.
- Patients describe headache onset as occurring later in the workday—as distinguished from migraines, which can occur on awakening.
- No focal neurologic signs.
- A diagnosis of exclusion. Other causes of headache must first be considered.

Treatment

- Relaxation, massage, hot baths, regular diet, exercise, and avoidance of exacerbating factors may alleviate symptoms.
- Abortive medications are generally restricted to NSAIDs, although triptans and ergots may be considered. Analgesic overuse should be avoided, as it can precipitate an analgesic rebound headache syndrome. Analgesic rebound headaches are seen in 1% of the population, primarily in middle-aged women with underlying migraines.
- Prophylactic therapy is uncommon.
- Headache diaries are helpful in isolating triggers and evaluating treatment trials.

TRIGEMINAL NEURALGIA (TN)

A neuropathic disorder causing episodes of intense pain in the distribution of the trigeminal nerve. Although its etiology is still not well defined, a possible framework involves compression or irritation of the trigeminal nerve near its connection with the pons causing injury to the myelin sheath, leading to erratic hyperfunctioning of the nerve. Aneurysms of the superior cerebellar artery, tumors, or arachnoid cysts may cause nerve compression. TN is sometimes associated with MS, especially in younger women.

Signs and Symptoms

- Presents with paroxysmal episodes of severe pain in the jaw, forehead, and scalp and around the eyes and lips. Often triggered by movement of the face such as speaking, chewing, or brushing teeth. Episodes can occur up to hundreds of times a day.
- Symptoms are usually unilateral.
- Allodynia of the face (an exaggerated response to otherwise non-noxious stimuli) may also be noted.

Treatment

- Although there is no cure, medications can be of benefit.
  - Anticonvulsants (carbamazepine, phenytoin, topiramate) are first-line therapy.
  - Gabapentin, also an anticonvulsant, is often used in the treatment of neuropathic pain states (eg, TN, postherpetic neuralgia). TCAs such as nortriptyline are also used for neuropathic pain.
  - Botox injections into the nerve may be of benefit.
- If medication fails, surgery or gamma knife may be attempted.

Q

A patient presents with horizontal diplopia accompanied by an inability to abduct the right eye on lateral gaze. CT reveals an area of acute hemorrhage. Given the presentation, is the lesion supratentorial or infratentorial?

PSEUDOTUMOR CEREBRI

Also known as idiopathic intracranial hypertension. The pathogenesis of the disease remains unknown, but it is classically seen in obese women of child-bearing age (those 20–45 years of age). Patients with pseudotumor cerebri have chronically elevated ICP, leading to papilledema. The main potentially permanent morbidity is vision loss resulting from decompensation of papilledema and progressive optic atrophy. It can also occur 2° to medications such as tetracyclines, excess vitamin A or other retinoids, or steroid taper.

Signs and Symptoms

- Findings resulting from ↑ ICP are as follows:
  - **Headache** (the most common presenting complaint); nausea/vomiting. May have morning predominance or a postural component (worse when flat).
  - **Pulse tinnitus:** A rhythmic or "rushing" sound heard in 1 or both ears that may be exacerbated by bending movements.
  - **Horizontal diplopia:** A false-localizing sixth-nerve palsy. Other than this, patients should have no localizing signs.
- Findings resulting from papilledema include the following:
  - Transient visual dimming or blackouts, progressive peripheral vision loss, and blurring and distortion (ie, metamorphopsia) of central vision.
  - Pain behind the eye or pain on eye movements.
  - Bilaterally swollen, edematous optic nerves consistent with papilledema on funduscopic examination.
- Acute and chronic papilledema can be clinically distinguished as follows:
  - **Acute:** Flame hemorrhages, venous engorgement, and hard exudates.
  - **Chronic:** Optic disk pallor.

Workup

- LP (preferably in the lateral decubitus position) shows a high opening pressure (ie, > 250 mm of water).
- CT/MRI reveals normal to small ventricles.

Treatment

- **Pharmacologic:**
  - **Diuretics:** Carbonic anhydrase inhibitors (eg, acetazolamide).
  - **Corticosteroids:** In severe cases, a short course of high-dose steroids can be used to combat vision loss.
  - **Hormonal:** Cessation of OCPs.

A

Traction on CN VI may result from ↑ ICP, leading to stretching of the nerve along the skull base. Thus, a supratentorial hemorrhage may cause a sixth-nerve palsy (although a sixth-nerve palsy would usually suggest a brainstem lesion, ie, a false-localizing lesion).

KEY FACT

Malignancies that commonly metastasize to the brain include breast, lung, renal, bladder, melanoma, germ cell, and testicular cancer.

- **Procedural:**
  - Large-volume therapeutic LP.
  - Lumboperitoneal or ventriculoperitoneal CSF shunts and optic nerve sheath fenestration should be considered as last resorts.
- **Long term:** Weight loss; dietary changes (eg, a low-sodium diet).

Intracranial Neoplasms

Intracranial neoplasms may be 1° (30%) or metastatic (70%).

- **1°:** Of all 1° brain tumors, 40% are benign and often affect those > 65 years of age. The most frequently reported 1° tumors include meningiomas and glioblastoma multiforme (GBM) in adults (see Figure 5-5) and medulloblastomas and astrocytomas in children. These rarely spread beyond the CNS.
- **Metastatic:** Metastatic tumors to the brain most commonly arise from breast, lung, kidney, and GI tract neoplasms or from melanoma. They most often appear at the gray-white junction and are characterized by rapid growth, edema, invasiveness, necrosis, and neovascularization. One should suspect metastatic disease and seek a 1° source when multiple discrete neoplastic nodules appear in the brain simultaneously.

Signs and Symptoms

- Symptoms usually develop gradually and are due to local growth and resulting mass effect, cerebral edema, ventricular obstruction, and ↑ ICP.
- Patients often complain of persistent vomiting and headache or focal neurologic deficits.
- Other common symptoms include personality changes, lethargy, intellectual decline, aphasias, seizures, and mood swings.

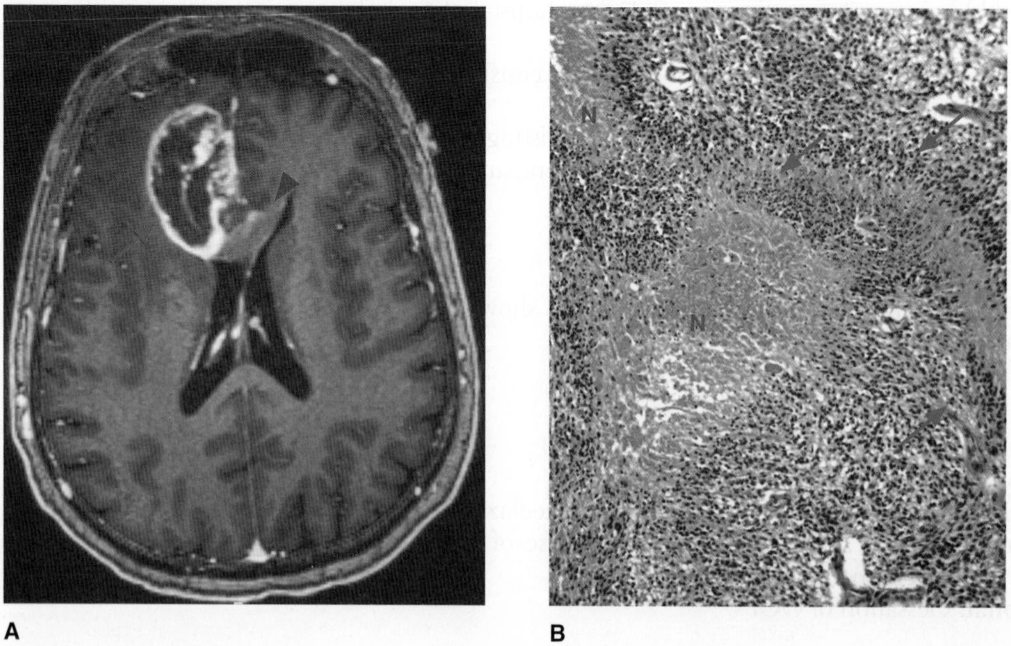

FIGURE 5-5. Glioblastoma multiforme. (**A**) Contrast-enhanced axial T1-weighted MRI image of a 45-year-old male with new-onset seizures shows a heterogeneous enhancing mass in the right frontal lobe (arrow) with associated mass effect (arrowhead). (**B**) Histology demonstrates necrosis (N) surrounded by pseudopalisading (arrows) of malignant astrocytes. (Reproduced with permission from USMLERx.com.)

- Only 30% of patients present with headache. When present, headache is typically dull and steady, worse in the morning, associated with nausea and vomiting, and exacerbated by coughing, changing position, or exertion.

> **KEY FACT**
>
> Two-thirds of 1° brain tumors in adults are supratentorial. Only one-third are supratentorial in children. Most CNS tumors are not 1° lesions but are metastases from the breast, lung, kidney, and other cancers.

WORKUP

- CT with contrast and MRI with gadolinium to localize and determine the extent of the lesion (see Figure 5-5).
- Certain metastatic brain tumors—eg, those from thyroid cancer, melanoma, renal tumors, and choriocarcinoma—tend to bleed. Breast and lung metastases do not tend to bleed; however, they may be found in conjunction with brain hemorrhages owing to these tumors' frequency in the population.
- Histologic diagnosis may be obtained via stereotactic biopsy or during surgical tumor debulking, although the most likely diagnosis may be evident from tumor morphology and location on imaging studies.

TREATMENT

- Observation, radiation therapy, chemotherapy, or surgical resection, depending on tumor type (see Table 5-18).
- GBM tumors are poorly responsive and require palliative care.
- Corticosteroids can be used to reduce vasogenic edema.

TABLE 5-18. Common 1° Neoplasms

Tumor	Presentation	Treatment
Astrocytoma	Presents with headache and ↑ ICP. May cause unilateral paralysis in CN V–VII and CN X. Has a slow, protracted course. The prognosis is much better than that of GBM.	Resection if possible; radiation.
GBM (grade IV astrocytoma)	The most common 1° brain tumor. Often presents with headache and ↑ ICP. Progresses rapidly. Has a poor prognosis (< 1 year from the time of diagnosis).	Surgical removal and resection. Radiation and chemotherapy have variable results. Palliative care.
Meningioma	Originates from the dura mater or arachnoid. Has a good prognosis. Incidence ↑ with age.	Observation if asymptomatic; surgical resection in the presence of symptoms; radiation for unresectable tumors.
Acoustic neuroma (schwannoma)	Presents with ipsilateral hearing loss, tinnitus, vertigo, and signs of cerebellar dysfunction. Derived from Schwann cells.	Surgical removal.
Medulloblastoma	Common in children. Arises from the fourth ventricle and leads to ↑ ICP. Highly malignant; may seed the subarachnoid space.	Surgical resection; radiation, chemotherapy.
Ependymoma	Common in children. May arise from the ependyma of a ventricle (commonly the fourth) or the spinal cord; may lead to hydrocephalus.	Surgical resection, radiation.

MNEMONIC

To remember the major symptoms of Parkinson's disease, think–

TRAP

Tremor
Rigidity
Akinesis
Postural instability

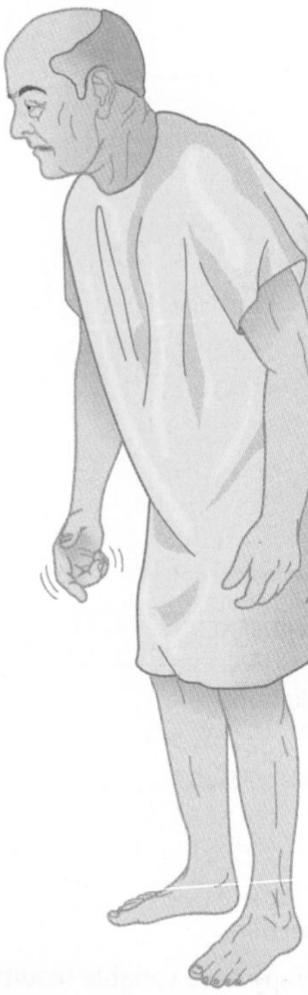

FIGURE 5-6. Patient with parkinsonism in typical flexed posture. Note the masklike facies and resting hand tremor. (Reproduced with permission from Aminoff MJ et al. *Clinical Neurology,* 3rd ed. Stamford, CT: Appleton & Lange, 1996: 220.)

Movement Disorders

PARKINSON'S DISEASE

Parkinson's disease is a hypokinetic syndrome caused by the idiopathic depletion of dopamine in the substantia nigra and nigrostriatal tract. The usual age of onset is roughly 60 years, and life expectancy is approximately 9 years from the time of diagnosis. Other insults that can cause a parkinsonian syndrome include neuroleptic (eg, antipsychotic) and metoclopramide use, postencephalitis, toxic exposures (manganese, MPTP, carbon disulfide), bihemispheric ischemia, and trauma.

Signs and Symptoms

- The "**Parkinson's tetrad**" consists of the following (see also Figure 5-6):
  - **Resting tremor:** A coarse "pill-rolling" tremor that can affect the extremities, trunk, and head; one of the earliest signs. Typically has an asymmetric onset. Improves or resolves with action (movement).
  - **Rigidity:** Resistance to passive motion; "cogwheeling."
  - **Bradykinesia:** Includes difficulty initiating movement and slow execution. A festinating gait (a wide leg stance with short accelerating steps) without arm swing is also common.
  - **Postural instability:** Stooping, impaired righting reflex, freezing, falls, retropulsion.
- Other signs include masked facies, memory loss/mild dementia, micrographia, and a soft voice.

Differential

- "**Parkinson's-plus**" **syndromes** (Parkinson's symptoms plus additional neurologic symptoms): Include progressive supranuclear palsy, corticobasal ganglionic degeneration, Lewy body dementia, and Shy-Drager syndrome.
- **Parkinsonism:** Extrapyramidal side effects of medications such as antipsychotics and antiemetics can present in a manner similar to Parkinson's disease.
- **Other:** Essential tremor, depression, normal pressure hydrocephalus, and Wilson's disease can also present with tremors, psychomotor slowing, and instability.

Treatment

See Table 5-19.

HUNTINGTON'S DISEASE

Huntington's disease is a hyperkinetic autosomal dominant disorder involving multiple abnormal CAG triplet repeats (< 29 is normal) in the huntingtin gene on chromosome 4p. The number of repeats expands in subsequent generations, leading to earlier expression and more severe disease. Life expectancy is 20 years from the time of diagnosis.

Signs and Symptoms

Presents at 30–50 years of age with gradual onset of symptoms:

- **Chorea:** Early motor symptoms of stiffness and rigidity give way to prominent choreiform activity. Patients are highly aware of their movements.

KEY POINT

ESSENTIAL TREMOR VS. PARKINSON'S DISEASE

- **Essential tremor:**
  - Characterized by a postural/intention tremor that resolves at rest. Fifty percent of patients have a ⊕ family history.
  - Alcohol reduces the tremor; tremor can affect the voice.
  - Treated with propranolol or primidone.
- **Parkinson's disease:**
  - Characterized by a **resting tremor** that resolves of improves with action.
  - Other Parkinson's symptoms (eg, bradykinesia, cogwheeling) are also present.
  - Treated with benztropine (effective only for tremor symptoms) or carbidopa/levodopa.

- **Altered behavior:** Irritability, moodiness, antisocial behavior, schizophreniform illness, depression, suicidality.
- **Dementia.**

DIFFERENTIAL

Senile chorea, hemiballismus, Wilson's disease, Parkinson's disease.

WORKUP

- A clinical diagnosis; however, CT/MRI reveal cerebral atrophy, especially of the caudate and putamen.
- Genetic testing to determine the number of CAG repeats. Also important is genetic counseling for offspring, with attention given to the social aspects of the disease.

TREATMENT

There is no cure, so treatment is symptomatic:

- Reserpine to minimize unwanted movements.
- Haloperidol for treatment of psychosis; antidepressants for depression; benzodiazepines for anxiety.

TABLE 5-19. Treatment Options for Parkinson's Disease

MECHANISM	TREATMENT
Dopaminergic	Levodopa and carbidopa (dopamine analogs) are the mainstays of therapy. Marked response to carbidopa-levodopa is an important supportive feature in making the diagnosis of Parkinson's disease. Entacapone (a catechol-*O*-methyltransferase [COMT] inhibitor) ↑ the availability of levodopa to the brain and may ↓ motor fluctuation. Bromocriptine and pramipexole are dopamine agonists. Amantadine promotes dopamine release.
Anticholinergic	Benztropine improves tremor and rigidity.
Surgical	Surgical pallidotomy or chronic deep brain stimulation may be tried for refractory cases.

Seizures

Cortical events characterized by excessive or hypersynchronous discharge by cortical neurons. The etiology is multifactorial, depending on a fine balance between (1) seizure threshold, (2) the presence of an epileptogenic focus, and (3) a precipitating factor or provocative event. A change in any of these factors can ↑ the frequency of seizures. For example, a 1° nervous system disorder may produce an epileptogenic focus that has a lower seizure threshold than "healthy tissue." Alternatively, systemic diseases or disturbances can lead to an altered seizure threshold. Some definitions related to seizures are essential:

- **Partial (focal) seizures** are seizures arising from a discrete region of 1 cerebral hemisphere; they can be categorized as simple or complex. Simple seizures do not involve a loss of consciousness; complex seizures cause an alteration of consciousness.
- **Generalized seizures** are seizures involving both cerebral hemispheres, with alteration of consciousness.

Workup/Treatment

The evaluation and treatment of a patient with a recent history of seizure should seek to answer the following questions:

- **Did the patient actually have a seizure?** A syncopal event with postsyncopal convulsion can easily be confused with a seizure.
  - Distinguish pseudoseizures (psychogenic) from true seizures (electrical). Serum prolactin levels are usually ↑ after true tonic-clonic seizures but are unaffected by pseudoseizures (and may also be unaffected by partial seizures). However, prolactin levels remain elevated only in the first half-hour following seizure activity. One should take care not to overinterpret prolactin levels, as they can also ↑ after a syncopal event.
  - In taking a history from the patient and from observers, ask about possible prodromes, onset, course, and postseizure period (see Table 5-20).
- **Was the seizure provoked by a systemic process?**
  - Non-neurologic etiologies include **hypoglycemia or hyperglycemia, hyponatremia, hypocalcemia, hyperosmolar states, hepatic enceph-**

KEY FACT

Tonic-clonic movements do not exclude syncope.

TABLE 5-20. Seizure vs. Syncope

Variable	Seizure	Syncope
Onset	Sudden onset with or without preceding aura. Focal sensory or motor phenomena. Sensation of fear, smell, memory.	Progressive lightheadedness; dimming of vision, faintness.
Course	Sudden loss of consciousness with tonic-clonic activity. May last 1–2 minutes. Tongue laceration, head trauma, and bowel/urinary incontinence may be seen.	Gradual loss of consciousness, limp or with jerking. Rarely lasts > 14 seconds. Less commonly injured.
Postspell	Postictal confusion and disorientation.	Typically immediate return to lucidity.

alopathy, uremia, porphyria, **drug overdose** (especially cocaine, antidepressants, neuroleptics, methylxanthines, and lidocaine), **drug withdrawal** (especially alcohol and other sedatives), eclampsia, hyperthermia, hypertensive encephalopathy, and cerebral hypoperfusion.
  - Workup should focus first on reversible causes and provocative factors.
- **Was the seizure caused by an underlying neurologic disorder?** Seizures with focal onset (or focal postictal deficit) suggest focal CNS pathology. Seizures may be the presenting sign of a tumor, stroke, AVM, infection, or hemorrhage, or they may represent the delayed presentation of a developmental abnormality.
  - Patients without a known cause for their seizures should undergo neurologic evaluation, particularly for treatable causes (see Table 5-21).
  - The history should include past seizures; birth, childhood, and recent trauma; and developmental delays.
- **Is anticonvulsant therapy indicated?** Patients with a first seizure are frequently not treated when the underlying cause is unknown. However, one-third of idiopathic seizures will recur. Recurrence rates are higher in patients with abnormal EEGs or MRIs, with abnormal examinations, or with irreversible predisposing factors (see Figure 5-7).

KEY FACT

Epilepsy is defined as a predisposition to recurrent, unprovoked seizures. Not everyone with seizures has epilepsy!

KEY FACT

Most seizures are self-limited and last < 2 minutes. Prolonged or repetitive seizures are called status epilepticus and constitute a medical emergency.

PARTIAL (FOCAL) SEIZURES

Focal seizures arise from a discrete region in 1 cerebral hemisphere. Such seizures may, however, generalize to involve both hemispheres. Partial seizures are divided into simple and complex seizures (see Table 5-22).

Signs and Symptoms

Table 5-22 outlines the clinical presentation of partial seizures.

Differential

TIAs, panic attacks, pseudoseizures, syncope.

Workup

- Perform a detailed neurologic examination.
- Obtain a CBC, electrolytes, calcium, glucose, ABGs, LFTs, a renal panel, RPR, ESR, and a toxicology screen to rule out systemic causes.

KEY FACT

Determining the etiology of a seizure is key to guiding treatment and elucidating the prognosis. In a patient with a known seizure disorder, consider subtherapeutic levels of medications or a new factor, such as infection or trauma.

KEY FACT

Todd's paralysis is often confused with acute stroke and can be differentiated by MRI (DWI).

TABLE 5-21. Common Etiologies of Seizure by Age

Infants	Children (2–10)	Adolescents (11–17)	Adults (18–35)	Adults (35+)
Perinatal injury/ischemia Infection Metabolic disturbance Congenital/genetic disorders	Idiopathic Infection Trauma Febrile seizure	Idiopathic Trauma Drug withdrawal AVM	Trauma Alcoholism Brain tumor Drug withdrawal	Trauma Stroke Metabolic disorders Alcoholism Brain tumor

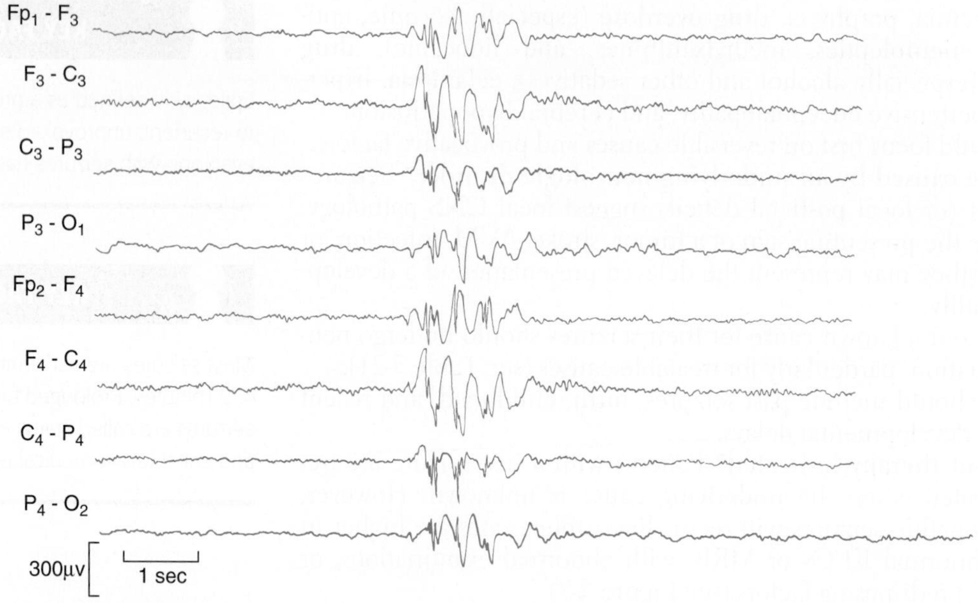

FIGURE 5-7. EEG in idiopathic seizures. Note the burst of generalized epileptiform activity on a relatively normal background. (Reproduced with permission from Aminoff MJ et al. *Clinical Neurology,* 3rd ed. Stamford, CT: Appleton & Lange, 1996: 241.)

- An EEG is often ordered to look for epileptiform waveforms and to confirm epileptic seizures.
- Rule out a mass by MRI or CT with contrast. MRI is more sensitive and specific in seizure evaluations.

KEY FACT

The side effects of phenytoin include gingival hyperplasia, hirsutism, and ↓ vitamin B_{12} levels.

Treatment

- **Treat the underlying cause** if it is known.
- Give antiepileptics (see Table 5-23).
- For intractable temporal lobe seizures, surgical options include anterior temporal lobectomy or vagal nerve stimulator.

TABLE 5-22. Partial Seizure Syndromes

Seizure Type	Clinical Presentation	Consciousness
Simple partial	Depends on the region of the cortex that is affected. Seizure foci in the motor or sensory areas (the frontal or parietal lobes, respectively) may lead to phenomena such as twitching of the face or tingling of the hand. Involvement of the insular cortex can lead to autonomic phenomena such as alterations in BP, changes in heart rate, and bronchoconstriction.	**No alteration in consciousness.**
Complex partial	Classically involve the temporal lobe, frontal lobe, and occipital lobe, in descending order of frequency. Involvement of the temporal lobe or medial frontal lobe leads to effects such as memories (déjà vu), feelings of fear, and automatisms such as lip smacking or picking at clothes.	Involves an **impaired level of consciousness.**
Postictal	Todd's paralysis may be seen, presenting with weakness or paralysis that is often unilateral and resolves over 24 hours.	–

TABLE 5-23. Antiepileptic Therapy

Seizure Type	Anticonvulsant Therapy
Adult partial seizures	Phenytoin (Dilantin), carbamazepine (Tegretol), oxcarbazepine (Trileptal), phenobarbital, valproate (Depakote), lamotrigine (Lamictal), levetiracetam (Keppra), zonisamide (Zonegran), gabapentin (Neurontin), topiramate (Topamax), rufinamide (Banzel), lacosamide (Vimpat).
Pediatric partial seizures	Phenobarbital.
Absence seizures	Ethosuximide is first-line treatment; valproic acid or zonisamide may also be used.
Generalized tonic-clonic seizures	Phenytoin, phenobarbital, valproate, lamotrigine, levetiracetam, zonisamide, gabapentin, topiramate, rufinamide.

GENERALIZED SEIZURES

The 2 most common types of generalized seizures are absence (petit mal) and tonic-clonic (grand mal).

Absence (Petit Mal) Seizures

Absence seizures begin in childhood, are often familial, and typically subside before adulthood.

Signs and Symptoms

- Characterized by brief, often unnoticeable episodes of impaired consciousness lasting only seconds and occurring up to hundreds of times per day. Present as staring spells.
- There is no loss of muscle tone, and patients have no memory of these events.
- Eye fluttering or lip smacking is common during absence seizures.

Workup

The EEG shows a classic **3-per-second generalized spike-and-wave tracing.**

Treatment

See Table 5-23.

Tonic-Clonic (Grand Mal) Seizures

Signs and Symptoms

- Tonic-clonic seizures begin suddenly with **loss of consciousness** and tonic extension of the back and extremities, continuing with 1–2 minutes of repetitive, symmetric clonic movements.
- Seizures are sometimes marked by **incontinence** and **tongue biting** (check for bite marks on the lateral tongue).
- Patients may also appear cyanotic during the ictal period owing to poor respiratory function during the seizure.
- Consciousness is slowly regained in the postictal period.
- Postictally, the patient may complain of fatigue, muscle aches, and headaches.

DIFFERENTIAL

Syncope, cardiac dysrhythmias, brainstem ischemia, pseudoseizures.

TREATMENT

- Emergent treatment with benzodiazepines to abort the seizure.
- Protect the airway.
- Manage the underlying cause.
- Give antiepileptics for 2° prevention (see Table 5-23).

Weakness

The key to working up a patient with complaints of weakness is to think anatomically. There are several locations in the chain of executing a movement where pathology can occur, and you should consider them all: the cortex, corticospinal tract (including brainstem pathology), spinal cord, anterior horn cells, nerve roots, plexus, peripheral nerves, neuromuscular junction, and muscle. True weakness involves a loss of motor power or strength and is exclusively a disorder of the motor system, localizing somewhere between the motor cortex and the muscles themselves.

You should first seek to differentiate UMN from LMN disease (see Table 5-24). Then try to pinpoint the location using your examination, thinking about what the affected muscles have in common (eg, all are proximal; all are innervated by 1 nerve). As is always the case, the history, the physical examination, and the remainder of the neurologic examination are crucial in this process.

DIFFERENTIAL

- The etiology of weakness is generally classified by anatomic localization. Although in most cases the physical examination and history will indicate a certain anatomic level, don't get pigeonholed into a small differential; remember to consider all possible etiologies of weakness each time.
- Table 5-25 lists the location of lesions, the pattern of weakness expected, and associated etiologies. The principal causes of weakness, including demyelinating/degenerative disorders, disorders of the neuromuscular junction, and peripheral nerve disorders, are discussed in the sections that follow.

TABLE 5-24. Anatomic Localization: UMN vs. LMN Disease

Clinical Features	UMN	LMN
Pattern of weakness	Pyramidal (arm extensors, leg flexors).	Variable.
Tone	Spastic (↑; initially flaccid).	Flaccid (↓).
DTRs	↑ (initially ↓).	Normal, ↓, absent.
Miscellaneous signs	Babinski, other CNS signs.	Atrophy, fasciculations.

TABLE 5-25. Lesions in the Motor Pathways

Location of Lesion	Disease Term	Weakness Pattern	Etiologies
Intracranial	—	UMN, as described below.	Stroke, neoplasm, MS, hemorrhage, trauma, infection.
Spinal cord	Myelopathy	UMN at spinal level.	Compression, trauma, MS.
Anterior horn cell	Motor neuron disease	UMN/LMN; variable.	ALS, spinal muscular atrophy, poliomyelitis.
Nerve root	Radiculopathy	LMN at root level.	Compression, infection, meningeal mets, trauma.
Peripheral nerve	Neuropathy	LMN, by nerve.	Metabolic, toxic, inflammatory, neoplastic.
Neuromuscular junction	—	Diffuse weakness.	Myasthenia gravis, Lambert-Eaton syndrome.
Muscle	Myopathy	Proximal weakness.	Muscular dystrophy, polymyositis, EtOH, steroid myopathy.

Workup

The physical examination and history will largely shape the differential diagnosis and indicate which labs and tests to order. The patterns of laboratory and test results observed for the different etiologies of weakness are outlined in Table 5-26.

- If a central lesion or UMN syndrome is suspected, CT or MRI of the brain (including the brainstem) and MRI of the spinal cord are often ordered.
- If a peripheral neuropathy or a muscle-related weakness is suspected, tests should include CK, EMG, nerve conduction studies, and lab studies for treatable causes of peripheral neuropathy and myopathy. If there is a high index of suspicion for a demyelinating peripheral neuropathy, an LP may also be ordered.
- In cases of high suspicion of myopathy, a muscle biopsy may be indicated.

DEMYELINATING/DEGENERATIVE DISORDERS

Multiple Sclerosis (MS)

An autoimmune demyelinating disorder of the CNS that is most likely T-cell mediated. Patients present with neurologic complaints that are separated in time and space and cannot be explained by a single lesion. MS has a female-to-male ratio of 2:1, shows a peak incidence at 20–40 years of age, and is thought to have a genetic component. MS grows more common with increasing distance from the equator, and these geographic differences have led to the hypothesis that it may be the result of a genetic predisposition coupled with a heretofore uncharacterized viral infection. The clinical course varies with type—which, in order of decreasing frequency, are relapsing-remitting, 2° progressive, 1° progressive, and progressive relapsing (see also Figure 5-8):

- **Relapsing-remitting:** Characterized by periods of symptom exacerbation following by a periods of remission when symptoms partially or completely resolve.
- **2° progressive:** Occurs when patients with previously relapsing-remitting symptoms begin to have a progressive decline without episodes of remission.

TABLE 5-26. Investigation of Patients with Weakness

Test	Spinal Cord	Anterior Horn Cell Disorders	Peripheral Nerve Plexus	Neuromuscular Junction	Myopathy
Serum enzymes	Normal.	Normal.	Normal.	Normal.	Normal or ↑.
Electromyography	With lesions causing axonal degeneration, there may be abnormal spontaneous activity (eg, fasciculations, fibrillations) if sufficient time has elapsed after onset; with reinnervation, motor units may be large, long, and polyphasic.			Often normal, but individual motor units may show abnormal variability in size.	Small, short, abundant polyphasic motor unit potentials. Myositis—abnormal spontaneous activity.
Nerve conduction velocity	Normal.	Normal.	Slowed, especially in demyelinating neuropathies.	Normal.	Normal.
Muscle response to repetitive motor nerve stimulation	Normal.	Normal except in the active stage of disease.	Normal.	Abnormal decrement or increment depending on stimulus frequency and disease.	Normal.
Muscle biopsy	May be normal in the acute stage but subsequently suggestive of denervation.			Normal.	Changes suggestive of myopathy (eg, atrophy, fiber-type grouping).
Myelography or spinal MRI	May be helpful.	Helpful in excluding other disorders.	Not helpful.	Not helpful.	Not helpful.

- **1° progressive:** Rare, but characterized by a slow, steady decline from disease onset.
- **Progressive relapsing:** Characterized by a steady worsening of symptoms with acute periods of relapse.

> **KEY FACT**
>
> Factors exacerbating MS include infection, heat (referred to as **Uhthoff's phenomenon**), trauma, the postpartum period, and vigorous activity.

Signs and Symptoms

Signs of MS are abundant, as the disease can affect any white-matter region of the CNS. They include the following:

- **Ocular symptoms/signs:**
  - Optic pallor or atrophy.
  - Medial longitudinal fasciculus lesions leading to internuclear ophthalmoplegia and diplopia.
  - Optic neuritis involving painful visual loss.
- **Bulbar symptoms:** Dysarthria, vertigo.
- **Spinal cord symptoms:**
  - Hyperreflexia, spasticity.
  - Limb weakness.
  - Paresthesias and pain. Patients will often present with a sensory level (eg, numbness and tingling below a given dermatome) depending on where the lesion is located.

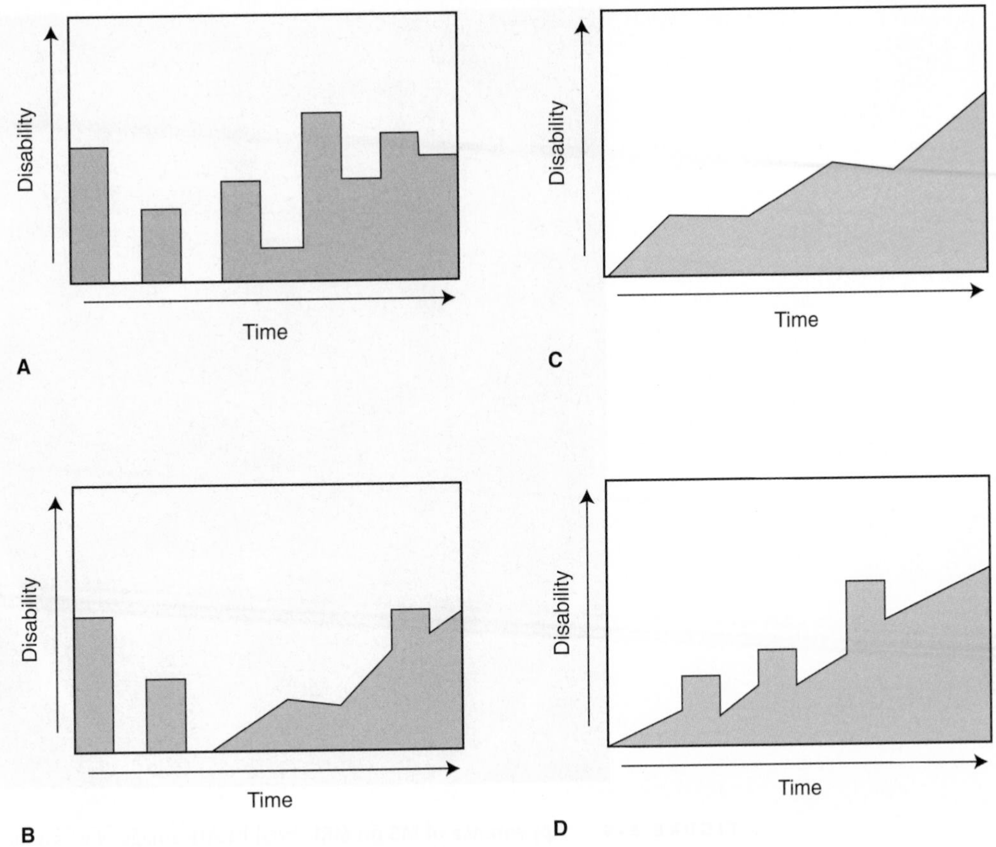

FIGURE 5-8. Clinical course of MS. (A) Relapsing-remitting. (B) Secondary progressive. (C) Primary progressive. (D) Progressive relapsing. (Reproduced with permission from Longo DL et al. *Harrison's Principles of Internal Medicine,* 18th ed. New York: McGraw-Hill, 2012, Fig. 380-2.)

- Urinary incontinence or retention (leading to an ↑ risk of UTI).
- **Lhermitte's sign** appears in some MS patients and presents as an electrical sensation running down the spine and into the lower extremities with neck flexion.

KEY FACT

Pregnancy is often associated with a ↓ frequency of MS exacerbations.

Differential

CNS tumors or trauma, multiple CVAs, vasculitis, vitamin B_{12} deficiency, CNS infections (Lyme disease, neurosyphilis), sarcoidosis, atypical presentations of other autoimmune diseases (eg, SLE, neurosarcoid, Sjögren's syndrome).

Workup

- Diagnosed clinically by a history of multiple, separate neurologic attacks consisting of the following:
  - Two attacks and clinical evidence of 2 separate lesions, **or**
  - Two attacks with clinical evidence of 1 lesion and laboratory evidence of another lesion.
- MRI shows multiple, asymmetric, often periventricular lesions in white matter, called plaques (see Figure 5-9). Plaques extending as long spindles perpendicular to the ventricles are referred to as Dawson's fingers. Corpus callosum lesions are usually pathognomonic. Active lesions enhance with gadolinium on MRI.
- CSF analysis may show mononuclear pleocytosis (> 5 cells/μL) in 25% of cases, elevated free kappa light chains in 60% of cases, ↑ CSF IgG in 80% of cases, and oligoclonal bands in 90% of cases (nonspecific). Typi-

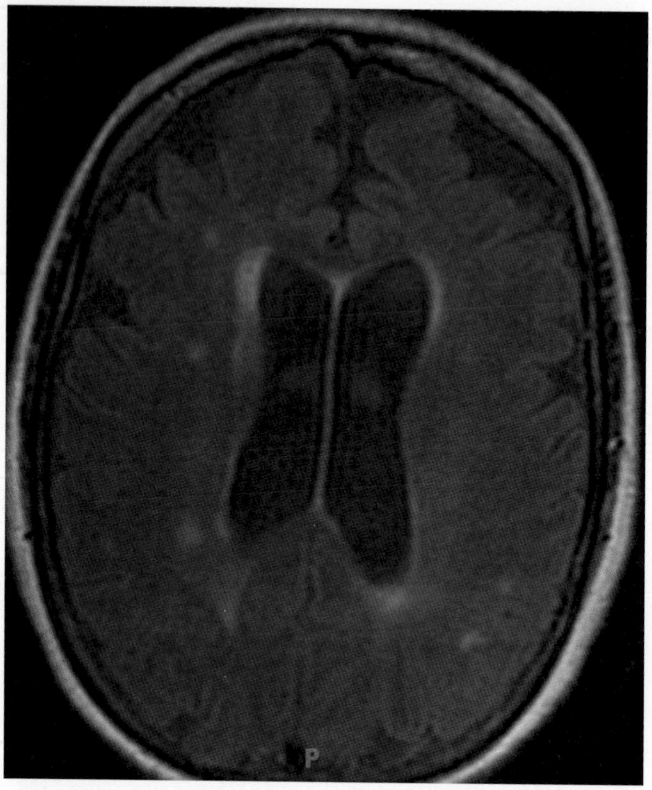

FIGURE 5-9. Appearance of MS on MRI. Axial FLAIR image of a 35-year-old woman with intermittent muscle weakness showing several bright lesions in the periventricular and subcortical white matter. This is a typical appearance for MS. (Reproduced with permission from USMLERx.com.)

cally, there are no more than 50 WBCs in CSF (in contrast to patients with meningitis).

- Other laboratory tests include visual, somatosensory, or brainstem evoked potentials.

Treatment

- There is no cure for MS.
- Immunomodulatory and immunosuppressive treatments can ↓ the number of relapses (by 30% or more) and can also reduce the severity of relapses in relapsing-remitting disease. First-line immunomodulators include **A**vonex (interferon-β1a), **B**etaseron (interferon-β1b), and **C**opaxone (copolymer 1). Newer agents with somewhat more restricted use and a higher side-effect profile include natalizumab (Tysabri) and fingolimod (Gilenya).
- IV steroids should be given during acute exacerbations to speed recovery.
- Patients may also benefit greatly from physical therapy and symptomatic treatment of spasticity, pain, fatigue, and depression.

Complications

- The **Kurtzke 5-year rule** states that the absence of significant motor or cerebellar dysfunction 5 years after diagnosis correlates with limited disability at 15 years. Fifteen years after diagnosis, approximately 20% of MS patients have no functional limitation; 70% are limited or are unable to perform major activities of daily living; and 75% are not employed.
- Morbidity and mortality are related to the accumulation of physical disabilities due to incomplete recovery from sequential attacks.

KEY FACT

Think MS with multiple neurologic lesions separated in time and space.

MNEMONIC

MS treatment is as easy as–

ABC

Avonex
Betaseron
Copaxone

KEY FACT

MS patients with the best prognosis have a relapsing-remitting course with discrete exacerbations, full recovery of function after each episode, and an early age of onset of the initial attack.

KEY POINT: KEY DISTINCTIONS BETWEEN MS AND GBS

- GBS produces no sensory level, whereas spinal cord demyelination does produce a sensory level.
- GBS produces hypo- or areflexia, whereas chronic MS often leads to hyperreflexia. Be careful, however, as an acute MS exacerbation can lead to areflexia for several days.

Guillain-Barré Syndrome (GBS)

An acute, rapidly progressive peripheral demyelinating disease, GBS is believed to be autoimmune in nature and is often associated with a viral URI prodrome or *Campylobacter jejuni* infection. Approximately 3500 cases are diagnosed each year in the United States, and some 85% of patients make a complete or near-complete recovery. The mortality rate is roughly 5%.

Signs and Symptoms

- Presents with rapidly progressive ascending paralysis. Classically, weakness and sensory symptoms begin distally (as with all peripheral nerve diseases) and ascend rapidly to involve the trunk, diaphragm, and cranial nerves.
- Reflexes are absent (this is a peripheral nerve disorder).
- Sensory symptoms such as numbness, tingling, and muscle aches are common, especially in the lower back.
- Autonomic deficits may be present.

Differential

- Key conditions in the differential include botulism, diphtheria, polio, myasthenia gravis, and poisoning or toxin-mediated conditions.
- Chronic inflammatory demyelinating polyneuropathy (CIDP) is similar to GBS except that symptoms have progressed to 8 weeks or longer.

Workup

- EMG and nerve conduction studies will eventually show diffuse demyelination but may not be present in the early course of the disease.
- LP reveals a CSF protein level > 55 mg/dL with little or no pleocytosis **(albuminocytologic dissociation).**
- MRI of the spinal cord to exclude cord compression.

Treatment

- Admit to the ICU for close monitoring. Be prepared to intubate patients if they develop impending respiratory failure (from paralysis of the diaphragm and accessory respiratory muscles).
- Watch for autonomic instability, including cardiac arrhythmias and gastroparesis. Autonomic instability is a **major cause of mortality.**
- Follow FVCs, not ABGs.
- Plasmapheresis and IVIG are first-line treatments. Steroids are **not** indicated in GBS but may be used in CIDP.
- Aggressive rehabilitation is imperative. Most patients will regain premorbid function, but in severe cases this may take up to a year.

KEY FACT

Not all neurologic disorders are responsive to steroids. While IV steroids are useful in MS relapses, they are not indicated in GBS.

> **KEY FACT**
>
> - UMN lesions—everything is **up** (tone, DTR, toe).
> - LMN lesions—everything is **lowered.**
> - UMN cell bodies are in the motor cortex and go to the spinal cord. LMN cell bodies are in the spinal cord and go to muscles.

Amyotrophic Lateral Sclerosis (ALS)

A chronic, progressive degenerative disease of unknown etiology characterized by loss of UMNs and LMNs. There are no associated sensory symptoms.

Signs and Symptoms

- Presents with asymmetric, slowly progressive weakness affecting the arms, legs, and cranial nerves. Some patients may present first with fasciculations.
- Also presents with UMN and/or LMN signs:
  - **UMN signs:** Spasticity, ↑ reflexes, upgoing toes.
  - **LMN signs:** Flaccidity, ↓ or absent reflexes, fasciculations, atrophy.
- Eye movements and sphincter tone are usually spared.

Workup

- The clinical presentation is often diagnostic. Rule out systemic causes.
- EMG/nerve conduction studies show widespread denervation and fibrillation potentials.
- CT/MRI of the spine to exclude structural lesions that might account for UMN signs.

Treatment

- Supportive measures and patient education.
- Riluzole, a glutamate inhibitor, may prolong survival time.

DISORDERS OF THE NEUROMUSCULAR JUNCTION

Myasthenia Gravis

An autoimmune disease caused by circulating antibodies to postsynaptic acetylcholine receptors. It occurs at all ages, most often affecting young adult women. The disease can be associated with thymoma, thyrotoxicosis, and autoimmune disorders such as rheumatoid arthritis (RA) and SLE.

Signs and Symptoms

- Patients most often present with fluctuating ptosis or double vision due to weakness of the levator palpebrae and EOM.
- Weakness worsens with activity and throughout the day.
- Difficulty swallowing and proximal muscle weakness (eg, difficulty climbing stairs, rising from a chair, or brushing hair) can also be present.
- Respiratory compromise and aspiration are rare but potentially lethal complications and are termed **myasthenic crises.**

Workup

- Often diagnosed on the basis of clinical findings. On examination, you can have the patient look up at your finger for a prolonged period of time (look for development of ptosis or disconjugate gaze/diplopia during this test). You can also assess for fatigability of muscles by having the patient do forced repetitions of the deltoid.
- Carefully monitored testing with **edrophonium** (Tensilon, a short-acting cholinesterase inhibitor) is diagnostic; in a symptomatic patient, IV injection of edrophonium leads to rapid (and temporary) improvement of clinical symptoms.
- An abnormal EMG and a decremental response to repetitive nerve stimulation can yield additional confirmation.

- AChR antibodies are ⊕ in 85–90% of patients. Twenty percent of patients who are ⊖ for anti-AChR antibodies will have anti–muscle-specific kinase (anti-MuSK) antibodies.
- Antistriatal (striated muscle) antibodies are present in 85% of patients with thymoma. CT of the chest is used to evaluate for thymoma.

Treatment

- Long-acting anticholinesterase inhibitors prolong the action of acetylcholine in the synapse and overcome the antibodies by competition. These medications include neostigmine and pyridostigmine (Mestinon), which provide symptomatic relief.
- Prednisone and other immunosuppressive agents are the mainstays of treatment. Because symptoms can worsen with prednisone, however, patients must be closely monitored.
- In severe cases, known as myasthenic crises, plasmapheresis or IVIG may provide temporary relief (days to weeks).
- Thymectomy (regardless of the presence of thymoma) is associated with an ↑ rate of clinical remission and a better clinical outcome (especially in younger patients).

Lambert-Eaton Myasthenic Syndrome

A paraneoplastic disorder characterized by muscle weakness that often improves with repetitive contraction of the muscle (vs. myasthenia gravis, in which repetitive muscle contraction causes ↑ weakness).

Signs and Symptoms

- Often associated with small cell lung carcinoma (90% of cases).
- Weakness of the proximal muscles is seen, with the extraocular or bulbar muscles typically spared.
- DTRs are depressed or absent.
- Table 5-27 contrasts myasthenia gravis with Lambert-Eaton myasthenic syndrome.

Workup

- Autoantibodies to presynaptic calcium channels.
- Chest CT for lung neoplasm.

Treatment

Guanidine hydrochloride is the mainstay of treatment. Anticholinesterases may also mitigate symptoms. Tumor resection can cure symptoms.

TABLE 5-27. Myasthenia Gravis vs. Lambert-Eaton Syndrome

	Cause	Site of Defect	Symptoms
Myasthenia gravis	Autoantibodies to the postsynaptic acetylcholine receptor prevent neurotransmitter binding.	Postsynaptic.	Fatigable weakness, ie, weakness worsens with increasing activity.
Lambert-Eaton syndrome	Autoantibodies to presynaptic calcium channels cause inadequate release of acetylcholine.	Presynaptic.	Strength improves with repeated contraction as the amount of neurotransmitter builds up in the neuromuscular junction.

PERIPHERAL NERVE DISORDERS

Carpal Tunnel Syndrome

Results from compression of the median nerve at the wrist where it passes through the carpal tunnel. Most commonly seen in women 30–55 years of age. Risk factors include repetitive use injury, pregnancy, diabetes, hypothyroidism, acromegaly, RA, and obesity.

> **KEY FACT**
>
> The carpal tunnel is located between the carpal bones and the flexor retinaculum.

SIGNS AND SYMPTOMS

- Wrist pain; numbness and tingling of the thumb, index finger, middle finger, and medial half of the ring finger on the palmar aspects; weak grip; ↓ thumb opposition.
- Pain and symptoms are exacerbated by activities that require wrist flexion, such as typing, holding a cup of coffee, or opening a jar.
- Symptoms may awaken patients at night and are relieved by shaking out the wrists. Patients often complain of nocturnal pain and paresthesias.
- Thenar atrophy may occur in severe cases.

WORKUP

- Two clinical examinations should be performed on suspected carpal tunnel patients:
  - **Tinel's sign** (approximately 60% sensitivity and 65% specificity): Tapping on the palmaris longus tendon at the wrist over the median nerve to elicit a tingling sensation in the thumb and affected fingers.
  - **Phalen's sign** (roughly 75% sensitivity and 35% specificity): Requires that the patient appose the dorsal aspects of the hands with the wrists flexed at 90 degrees for at least 30 seconds. The onset of paresthesias confirms the diagnosis.
- EMG and nerve conduction studies can be used to make a diagnosis, evaluate the degree of neural and motor compromise, and assess the severity of compression, especially in patients who exhibit persistent symptoms despite conservative management.
- Patients should also be evaluated for risk factors, including diabetes and hypothyroidism (myxedema). Pregnant patients may also develop carpal tunnel syndrome due to soft tissue edema.

TREATMENT

- Neutral wrist splints to wear both during the day and at night.
- Modification of repetitive activities and creation of a more ergonomic work environment.
- NSAIDs to control inflammation of the tendons.
- Direct injection of corticosteroid into the carpal space may also provide temporary relief.
- Surgical division of the transverse carpal ligament if symptoms persist.

Spinal Cord Compression

> **KEY FACT**
>
> Cauda equina syndrome presents with saddle anesthesia (↓ perianal sensation), bowel/bladder dysfunction, low back pain, and lower extremity weakness.

A condition that develops when the spinal cord is compressed by any swelling or lesion, such as a tumor, an abscess, a ruptured or slipped intervertebral disk, hematoma, or bone fragments from a vertebral fracture. Regardless of its cause, spinal cord compression is a medical emergency that requires swift diagnosis and treatment in order to prevent long-term disability from irreversible nerve damage. Other key spinal cord lesions that you should be familiar with for your clerkship include cord hemisection, Brown-Séquard syndrome, and central cord syndrome.

SIGNS AND SYMPTOMS

- Presents with back pain and with ↓ sensation below the level of compression and/or with paralysis of the limbs below the level of compression.
- Urinary and fecal incontinence and/or urinary retention may also be seen.
- Hyperreflexia and Lhermitte's sign (an intermittent shooting electrical sensation with neck flexion) may be present.

WORKUP

- Conduct a thorough neurologic examination, and emergently obtain radiographs and an MRI of the spine or CT myelography if the patient has a pacemaker (see Figure 5-10).
- Investigate common causes, including tumors (especially metastatic non–small cell lung cancer, breast cancer, prostate cancer, renal cell carcinoma, lymphoma, and multiple myeloma) and infection leading to abscess. Look for track marks in patients with a history of IV drug use.

TREATMENT

- IV dexamethasone (a glucocorticoid) should be given to reduce edema around the lesion.
- Urgent surgery is warranted if a localized lesion is identified and some hope of regaining function is predicted.
- In the setting of cancer-related compression, emergent radiation therapy may ↓ tumor bulk and help reduce compression.
- If complete paralysis is present for > 24 hours, the chances of recovery are significantly reduced.

KEY FACT

"Cauda equina" refers to the spinal nerve roots located below the sacral spinal cord (around L1).

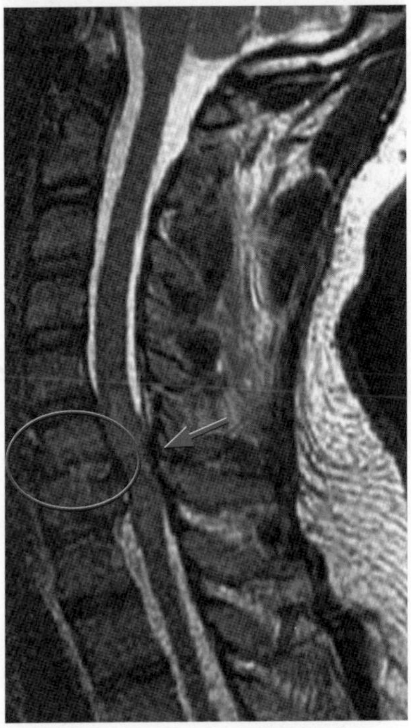

FIGURE 5-10. Spinal cord compression. Sagittal T2-weighted MRI of the cervical spine in a trauma patient with neurologic symptoms shows a C6–C7 fracture (circle) with displaced fragments compressing the spinal cord. Note the increased signal intensity in the cord at this level (arrow). (Reproduced with permission from Doherty GM. *Current Diagnosis & Treatment: Surgery,* 13th ed. New York: McGraw-Hill, 2010, Fig. 36-12.)

Ophthalmology

Although you may not encounter many ophthalmologic cases during your neuro rotation, it can be beneficial to have a grasp of at least some of the more common visual conditions seen in practice. A few of these are described briefly below.

CLOSED-ANGLE GLAUCOMA

SIGNS AND SYMPTOMS

- Characterized by extreme, sudden pain and blurred vision that may be accompanied by nausea and vomiting.
- Presents as a hard, red eye (from acute closure of the narrow anterior chamber angle) and is unilateral.
- The pupil is dilated and nonreactive to light.

WORKUP/TREATMENT

- **This is a medical emergency!** Perform a slit-lamp examination and measure intraocular pressure by tonometry. It is important to emergently ↓ intraocular pressure with acetazolamide, mannitol, pilocarpine, and timolol to prevent damage that can lead to blindness.
- Peripheral laser iridotomy can be curative.

KEY FACT

Closed-angle glaucoma, but **open** pupil.

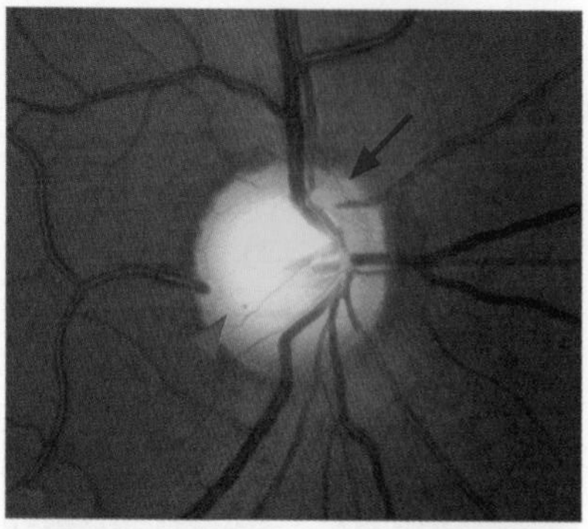

FIGURE 5-11. Open-angle glaucoma. Funduscopic image of a 68-year-old woman with decreased peripheral vision shows abnormal increased cupping (bright circle, arrowhead) of the optic disk (arrow). (Reproduced with permission from USMLERx.com.)

OPEN-ANGLE GLAUCOMA

Signs and Symptoms

- Can be asymptomatic, especially in the early stages.
- Suspect in patients > 40 years of age with frequent eyewear prescription changes, visual disturbances, and headaches.
- Visual defects start in the peripheral nasal fields.

Workup

Perform visual field testing, funduscopy, slit-lamp examination, and tonometry; look for cupping of the optic disk on slit lamp or funduscopy (see Figure 5-11).

Treatment

- Treat with topical β-blockers (eg, timolol) to ↓ aqueous humor production or with pilocarpine to ↑ aqueous humor outflow.
- Laser trabeculoplasty if medications fail.
- Patients > 40 years of age should have a yearly eye examination; those with a family history or diabetes should have more frequent examinations.

MACULAR DEGENERATION

The leading cause of bilateral visual loss among the elderly in the United States.

Signs and Symptoms

Presents with painless loss of central vision.

Workup/Treatment

- On funduscopy or slit-lamp examination, look for pigment or hemorrhagic changes in the macular region.
- Laser photocoagulation may delay the loss of central vision, but the disease will often continue to progress.

DIABETIC RETINOPATHY

Patients with DM should get regular eye examinations for early detection of retinopathy. Good glucose control is key to minimizing the risk of developing retinopathy.

Workup

- **Nonproliferative retinopathy:** On slit-lamp examination, look for dot-blot hemorrhages, microaneurysms, exudates, and edema.
- **Proliferative retinopathy:** On slit-lamp examination, look for retinal neovascularization. The more advanced the disease, the more likely it is to progress to blindness.

Treatment

- **Nonproliferative retinopathy:** Focal laser photocoagulation to affected areas, especially when the process starts to affect the macula.
- **Proliferative retinopathy:** Treat with panretinal photocoagulation, in which laser burns are applied to the entire periphery of the retina to destroy ischemic areas (which release the vessel-growth signals).

Common Clerkship Topics

The following is a list of topics that you should review during this rotation:

- **The complete neurologic examination:** Mental status, cranial nerves, motor, sensory.
- **Imaging basics:** CT, MRI.
- **Lumbar puncture:** Procedure and results.
- **Management of intracranial pressure.**
- **Aphasias:** Broca's, Wernicke's, transcortical, conduction, and global aphasias.
- **Coma:** Etiologies, assessing a comatose patient (Glasgow Coma Scale), primitive brainstem reflexes, workup and treatment, coma vs. persistent vegetative state vs. "locked-in" syndrome.
- **Cord compression/cord syndromes.**
- **Delirium and dementia,** Wernicke's encephalopathy, DTs, Alzheimer's disease.
- **Demyelinating/degenerative diseases:** MS, Guillain-Barré syndrome, ALS.
- **Disequilibrium:** Central vs. peripheral, nystagmus.
- **Headache:** Migraine, cluster, tension, temporal arteritis.
- **Infections:** Meningitis, bacterial and viral (see Pediatrics), HIV infection (1° and opportunistic), TB and HSV infection, encephalitis, cerebral abscess, polio and post-polio syndrome.
- **Intracranial hemorrhages:** Subarachnoid, epidural, subdural, intraparenchymal (see the Emergency Medicine chapter for all).
- **Intracranial neoplasms:** 1°, metastatic, presentation, children vs. adults.
- **Low back pain, spinal cord injuries:** Cord lesions, cord compression, myelopathies, cervical spine injury.
- **Movement disorders:** Parkinson's, Huntington's, and Wilson's disease.
- **Seizures:** Partial, generalized, absence (petit mal), tonic-clonic (grand mal), status epilepticus (see Emergency Medicine).
- **Stroke:** Clinical features, risk factors, prevention, treatment/management.
- **Weakness:** UMN vs. LMN, differential based on anatomy, carpal tunnel syndrome.

CHAPTER 6

OBSTETRICS AND GYNECOLOGY

Ward Tips

Welcome to obstetrics and gynecology! This rotation is dedicated to acquainting future physicians with the basic principles of labor and delivery (L&D) and managing gynecologic issues, including medical, surgical, and social issues. You will be involved in prenatal care, annual well-woman examinations, contraceptive counseling, and numerous surgical procedures ranging from cesarean sections (C-sections) to a variety of gynecologic operations. Obstetrician/gynecologists are surgeons by nature who keep extremely demanding schedules and spend minimal time rounding and discussing differentials. For the next few weeks, you will thus be exposed to a whirlwind of activities covering a wide range of issues. Regardless of the field you ultimately enter, more than half of your patients will be women with potential gynecologic problems. So take advantage of this learning opportunity and have a good time!

WHAT IS THE ROTATION LIKE?

OB/GYN rotations last approximately 6–8 weeks and differ vastly from school to school as well as from site to site. The basic setup consists of inpatient obstetrics, inpatient gynecology, and the outpatient clinic, where both obstetric and gynecologic patients are seen. Obstetrics can be one of the most rewarding and pleasant experiences in medical school, but it is not an easygoing discipline. The following outline summarizes the nature and duties of the rotation.

Obstetrics. When you are in the obstetrics portion of your rotation, you will spend much of your time in the L&D suite.

- **Responsibilities:**
  - Prerounding on antepartum **and** postpartum patients, and presenting those patients on ward rounds.
  - Evaluating patients in the triage area.
  - Writing the admission history and physical (H&P).
  - Monitoring the progress of laboring patients with residents and nurses. Patients in the L&D suite generally need an examination every 2–3 hours, so you can become a great resource by helping write progress notes.
  - Delivering babies, writing delivery notes, and checking labs.
- **You should:**
  - Get to know the nursing staff well, as much of L&D is often handled by nurses or midwives.
  - Read about the basics of L&D (eg, steps of labor, signs and symptoms of true labor, steps of delivery, and fetal heart tracing [FHT]), and learn about common complications that can arise (eg, failure to progress, hypertension, fetal distress) and their appropriate management.
  - Always keep in mind that competence is only half the story. Knowing your patient well by periodically checking in on her to see if she needs anything—or just to comfort her—will impress not only your patient but your residents and attendings as well.

Inpatient gynecology. As a surgically oriented specialty, inpatient gynecology is similar to general surgery. Rounding is early and fast; all the notes, rounding, and daily management planning for patients must be done prior to the surgeries that are planned for the day, which can start as early as 7:30 A.M.

- **Responsibilities:**
  - Prerounding on postoperative patients.
  - Presenting patients on ward rounds.
  - Writing notes (preoperative, operative, postoperative) on patients whose surgeries you are involved with.
- **You should:**
  - **Try to plan out** which surgery you want to participate in the next day; read up on the surgery and on relevant anatomy; and learn something about the patient's history. Practice some basic suturing and knot-tying skills in the event that you are presented with a rare opportunity to help close an incision.
  - Learn some of the medical jargon common to surgeries, and be willing to **ask questions** pertaining to technique or to the prognosis of the surgery being performed.
  - Be ready to **answer questions** about the basic anatomy, surgical procedure, and prognosis of the surgery being performed.

Outpatient clinics. The outpatient clinic is a great place to see both common and uncommon gynecologic and obstetric cases. The clinic experience is extremely helpful in that the skills and knowledge you will acquire there are likely to be applicable to most fields you may ultimately pursue, such as internal medicine, family practice, or surgery.

- **Gynecology clinic:**
  - **Responsibilities:** Common gynecologic clinic issues are requests for birth control, routine health maintenance (breast examinations, pelvic examinations, Pap smears), abnormal vaginal bleeding, vaginal discharge, and lower abdominal pain.
  - **You should:** Perform a **focused H&P.** Like other clinics at the hospital, this is a fast-paced place, and your efficiency in taking a history and figuring out what the patient needs (eg, prescriptions, results of diagnostic tests/labs, pelvic examination) will be greatly appreciated by residents and attendings alike.
- **Obstetric clinic:**
  - **Responsibilities:** Patients are seen in the obstetric clinic to assess the adequacy of pregnancy progression, to screen for potential maternal-fetal complications, to help mothers adjust to their pregnancies, and to prepare mothers for childbirth. In addition, postpartum patients are seen for their regular 6-week checkup or for any postpartum complications that may arise.
  - **You should:** Familiarize yourself with the **time course of prenatal labs** so that you are aware of which labs your clinic patients need at their visits. You can also impress your outpatient attendings, residents, and nurse practitioners if you familiarize yourself with the details and timing of various screening techniques, such as the first-trimester screen, the quad screen, chorionic villus sampling (CVS), amniocentesis, the gestational diabetes screen, and important pregnancy-related infectious disease panels.

> **KEY FACT**
>
> You should try to follow your patients from admission to delivery and postpartum care.

WHO ARE THE PLAYERS?

Team OB/GYN consists of a senior resident (R3 or R4), at least 1 junior resident (R2), and an intern (from OB/GYN, family practice, psychiatry, emergency medicine, or medicine). There may also be a fourth-year medical student doing his or her senior elective as well as 1 or 2 third-year medical students. Generally there is 1 ward attending, although there may also be sev-

KEY FACT

Midwives can be your strongest allies in the L&D suite.

eral private attendings, subspecialty attendings (maternal-fetal, gynecologic oncology), and fellows. Other important players on the team include the nursing staff and midwives (especially in L&D), who can teach you invaluable obstetric skills, and the anesthesiologists, who are needed for pain control both during labor and postoperatively.

HOW IS THE DAY SET UP?

A typical day on an OB/GYN service may look like this:

	OB Service	GYN	Clinic
5:30–6:30 A.M.	Prerounds	Prerounds	
6:30–7:30 A.M.[a]	Work rounds	Work rounds	
7:30 A.M.–4:00 P.M.	L&D	Operating room	Outpatient clinic (8:00 A.M.–5:00 P.M.)
4:00–6:00 P.M.	Wrap up work; do P.M. rounds if on GYN		

[a]Once or twice a week, there will usually be a morning report, lecture, or grand rounds that residents and medical students will be attending. On these days, be prepared to be finished half an hour earlier with a brief work round completed either before or just after the morning report.

Call days are usually busy and are always in house. After you are done with your regular workday, you start call in L&D (usually at 5:00 P.M.) and see patients in triage while also following any laboring patients you might have. You and your resident will also see and potentially admit patients from the ED for acute obstetric or gynecologic care. You will usually be up all night—or, if you are lucky, will get 1 or 2 hours of sleep. This is because there will often be someone delivering in the early hours of the morning or an emergency to keep you busy. Other medical schools will have you do 1 week of night float within the 6- or 8-week rotation block instead of taking overnight call. Night float can be difficult to adjust to for just 1 week, but most students enjoy this experience because of the opportunity it affords to get involved. Just make sure you are equipped to sleep during the day (eg, get good curtains/blinds and eye covers)!

WHAT DO I DO DURING PREROUNDS?

Depending on the size of your inpatient gynecologic service, prerounds should begin 30 minutes to 1 hour before work rounds. You should anticipate spending roughly 20–30 minutes on each patient you are following, depending on your stage in the year. As in surgery, most of your patients will be postoperative. The following outline lists prerounds activities by service.

- **Inpatient gynecologic service:**
  - Check vital signs overnight. Watch out for fever, hypotension, and ↓ O_2 saturation, which could indicate infection, loss of fluids, and pulmonary embolism (PE)/pulmonary edema/atelectasis, respectively.
  - Assess overnight fluid balance ("ins and outs"), including urine output. Since many gynecologic surgeries involve procedures that could poten-

tially damage the ureters, it is imperative that you check for adequate urine output in order to rule out urinary obstruction.
- Check labs, especially hematocrit if the patient lost a significant amount of blood during the operation.
- Go in to see the patient and ask her how she is doing. Be mindful of the fact that it is likely very early in the morning, and most people will not be as alert and chirpy as you are. A good way to start is by quietly entering the room after knocking, apologizing for waking the patient up, and asking if you can turn the light on for a few minutes. Ask about standard postoperative concerns such as fever, pain control, incision care (if there is one), ambulation, diet, and bowel movements. Then ask specific questions regarding the procedure the patient had (eg, vaginal bleeding if she had a transvaginal procedure).
- Do a quick physical examination, and check the surgical wound to assess for drainage and possible infection. As you leave, turn the light back off and rearrange anything you might have moved for your examination, such as food or water trays.
- Write up your findings, assessment, and plan into a brief progress note, usually in SOAP format, before work rounds. If possible, discuss your note with the intern on the team before presenting to your chief or attending.

- **Obstetric service:**
  - For **postpartum patients,** you should seek to accomplish the following:
    - Examine your patients' breasts.
    - Check the fundus for size, firmness, and tenderness, the extent of vaginal bleeding, and any wounds, such as sewn lacerations or cesarean incisions. A common complication of C-section is endometritis, and it is always good to let your residents know that you have considered that possibility during your examination.
    - Make sure your notes are always cosigned by your residents; not only is this good medical practice, but you'll also get helpful feedback.
  - For **antepartum patients,** you should ask the following questions during prerounds:
    - Do you feel the baby moving as much as usual?
    - Are you having any vaginal bleeding?
    - Are you having any abnormal vaginal discharge or gush of fluid?
    - Are you feeling contractions or pain?
    - Do you have any pain or discomfort with urination?

HOW DO I EXCEL IN OB/GYN?

- **Be assertive.** Assertiveness is key to furthering your education and to scoring points with the people who evaluate you. So ask good questions (you should know something about the subject matter before doing so); get to know other patients on the service (for your own learning and in case you are asked to fill in); take the initiative to ask for demonstrations of procedures; volunteer for drawing blood (you need to practice anyway); do pelvic examinations; participate in as many deliveries as you can; and try to dig up interesting and informative articles for your team.
- **Be visible.** The L&D suite is a busy, crowded place, so unless you take the initiative, you may easily be forgotten. With this in mind, don't wait for your residents to call you for deliveries or interesting physical examination findings; instead, know ahead of time which patients are likely to deliver during your shift, and anticipate that. Also bear in mind that most of the patients in the L&D suite need a progress note written every 2–3

KEY FACT

Don't get shut out of learning the pelvic examination.

> **KEY FACT**
>
> The key to success on the wards is to be a step ahead of your interns and residents. Write notes on triage patients **before** they ask you to do so!

hours, especially if they are on magnesium for tocolysis, so volunteer to write those notes before you are asked to do so.

- **Be the intern for your patients.** You will have patients assigned to you by your residents. Among other things, you will be responsible for obtaining each patient's H&P, writing progress notes, following up on diagnostic studies and pathology results, and presenting your patients to the team. In order to fulfill your responsibilities diligently, you will need to know and do everything you can for your patient. This means reading up on each case, carefully reviewing your patient's history, staying updated, and talking to your patient. These measures will allow you to actively participate in patient care and hence to act as your patient's strongest advocate.
- **Be knowledgeable in a general sense.** It is important to recognize that once residents become involved in a specialty, they tend to spend less time keeping up to date on everything else they learned in medical school. You can thus serve as a great asset to your team by providing new information about your patients' medical problems (eg, diabetes, hepatitis, hypertension) and by recognizing psychiatric or social issues (eg, postpartum depression, drug dependence, domestic violence).
- **Work quickly, independently, and efficiently.** Residents appreciate students who can effectively contribute to the team—so order lab tests, make necessary phone calls, and write notes for patients. In addition, be focused, organized, and brief when presenting the patient. Remember, again, that in many ways this rotation is similar to surgery.
- **Use the medical staff.** Midwives and nurses are your friends! Remember that they have been in the field much longer than you have and will be extremely knowledgeable regarding all aspects of patient care. So if you have questions, don't be afraid to ask them! In some institutions, midwives and nurses have a say in your clinical evaluation as well. Therefore, it is always important to introduce yourself and get to know them.
- **Don't be afraid to mess up.** In many circumstances, you may have an opportunity to try something, ask something, or say something that could end up changing your entire experience. It only takes one well-thrown suture, one astute question, or one correct response to potentially define someone's opinion of you. So don't be afraid that you might do, ask, or say the wrong thing! (Well, as long as you make sure that what you say is not inappropriate.) You can never predict in what moment you will shine, but if you don't go for it, you will never give yourself that chance.
- **Learn the language.** The vocabulary you will come across during your OB/GYN rotation, as in all rotations, will be like learning a new language. But instead of shying away from this challenge, embrace it. If you learn to speak and write like a knowledgeable professional in the field, you will be viewed and treated as such. This means using abbreviations for common signs, symptoms, diagnoses, and treatments in your notes and presentations (as long as you have seen or heard a resident/attending use them; it would probably be ill advised to make them up). The highest compliment you can receive from an attending (other than outright being told something wonderful) is to be treated the same way residents are treated. In a funny way, by learning how to "blend in," you will help yourself stand out.
- **Know the expectations.** At the beginning of the rotation, be straightforward and ask the residents on your team exactly what they expect of you. You should also find out your attending's preferred format for patient presentations. Midway through the rotation, it is equally important to **get feedback** both from residents and from attendings with whom you have worked. As part of this process, try to be assertive and ask for constructive feedback on what you should continue to do and areas in which you can improve. Be tactful, and communicate with the goal of maximizing your

performance, education, and contribution to the team while on the clerkship.

While you are on this rotation, you may fall in love with OB/GYN and want to pursue it as a career. If this is the case, you should take additional steps. If you make your team aware of your sincere interest in the field, they will be more than happy to lead you down the right track. Ask the interns and residents for advice on the politics of residency (eg, which programs are good, which key people to get to know better, whom to ask for letters of recommendation, which senior electives to take). If possible, try to work with one of the key faculty members, who can write an influential letter of recommendation or serve as your adviser in your quest to match into the residency of your choice.

KEY FACT

Ask about expectations at the beginning of the rotation and for feedback midway through the rotation.

SURVIVAL TIPS

In the course of your rotation, you may encounter a patient who does not want a medical student to deliver her baby or even to be involved in her care. Many mothers want as little intrusion as possible into this sacred, personal moment in their lives, while others may be concerned about the prospect of having an inexperienced student touch their newborn infant. Occasionally, male students may encounter some gynecologic patients who are uncomfortable with the notion of having a male in the examining room, much less a male student.

On a rotation such as OB/GYN, in which you will be working hard over long shifts, it can be easy to become frustrated when issues like these arise. It is nonetheless important to respect a patient's wishes and to bear in mind that there may be specific reasons these requests are made, such as a previous history of sexual abuse. So do not take it personally if a patient does not want you in the examination room. If this continues to happen frequently, you should discuss it with your resident. If you are a male medical student, being with an affable yet assertive female resident who cares about your educational experience may also help you get your foot in the door.

KEY FACT

Don't be discouraged if the patient does not initially want you in the examination room or delivering her baby.

Here are a few additional tips for this rotation:

- Talk to OB patients early in labor and throughout the delivery. Establishing a rapport early on will increase the likelihood that you will be able to help with the delivery.
- Learn how to "count" and coach a patient through labor. A calm yet clear and assertive voice is usually appreciated.

KEY NOTES

Obstetrics admission note. The obstetric H&P is similar to a standard H&P but should include the following additional information:

- **Gravida:** The total number of times a patient has been pregnant, including the current pregnancy.
- **Para:** Four numbers that represent term deliveries, preterm deliveries, abortions (including elective, therapeutic, and spontaneous), and number of living children. This is often referred to as TPAL (term, preterm, abortion, living).
- **Gestational age (GA):** Information on GA should be included along with information on the patient's last menstrual period (LMP) and estimated

KEY FACT

How would you designate a currently pregnant patient with 1 prior miscarriage and 1 prior term delivery? G3P1011.

> **KEY FACT**
>
> When presenting a patient on L&D, always include the GA both by dates and by ultrasound.

date of delivery, or EDD (which is the same as the due date and is often referred to as EDC, or estimated date of confinement).

- **Uterine contractions (UCs):** Information on the time of onset, frequency, and intensity of contractions should be noted.
- **Rupture of membranes (ROM):** The time of rupture and the color of the fluid should be described.
- **Vaginal bleeding (VB):** This should include the duration of bleeding, its consistency (bright red bleeding vs. old dark blood), and the number of pads.
- **Fetal movement (FM):** Notation should be made as to whether fetal movement is normal, decreased, or absent.
- **Ultrasound history:** This should include GA at the time of the first ultrasound, whether anatomy was evaluated, and whether the size on ultrasound is equivalent to that expected based on the LMP, or "size equal to dates" (S = D).
- **Lab studies:** Include current lab results such as UA, CBC, and cultures.
- **Physical examination:** This should include a thorough physical, including a pelvic examination, which is commonly referred to as a sterile vaginal examination.
- **FHT:** Record baseline heart rate, variability, accelerations, and decelerations.
- **Tocometer:** Note the frequency of UCs and whether a regular or an irregular pattern is seen.
- **Ultrasound:** Describe findings such as vertex, breech, amniotic fluid index (AFI), and the location of the placenta.
- **Estimated fetal weight (EFW):** Specify whether the EFW was determined by Leopold's maneuver (feeling with hands) or measured by ultrasound.

Prenatal care. Key notes associated with prenatal care should include the following elements on the first visit:

- **Obstetric history:** Dates of pregnancies with GA at time of delivery, route (vaginal, C-section), and complications (including preeclampsia, abruption, previa, preterm labor, and unusually long labor).
- **Gynecologic history:** Menstrual history, STIs, OCP use.
- **Family history (FH):** Congenital abnormalities, twins, bleeding disorders, hypertension, diabetes.
- **Social history (SH):** Note any tobacco, alcohol, or drug use during pregnancy; occupational exposures (eg, a nurse preparing chemotherapy agents); and the patient's involvement and/or relationship with the father of the baby. Also assess the patient's living situation.
- **Medical history:** Note any history of diabetes, hypertension, asthma, SLE, and the like.
- **Allergies.**
- **Medications:** List current medications and their dosages as well as medications used during pregnancy.
- **Prenatal labs:** Include blood type, Rh type, antibody screen, CBC, VDRL/RPR, rubella, HBsAg, UA and culture, Pap smear, gonorrhea culture (GC), chlamydia culture, PPD placement, VZV titer if there is no history of exposure, HIV if performed, maternal serum α-fetoprotein (MSAFP) if performed, Down syndrome screening results if performed, and 1-hour plasma glucose (PG) screening.
- **Diagnostic tests:** Ultrasound, amniocentesis if performed, CVS if performed.
- **Physical examination:** A thorough examination is critical, particularly the thyroid, heart, and lung evaluation and pelvic examination. It is important

to evaluate the size of the uterus on pelvic examination in order to determine if it is consistent with gestational weeks. It is also vital to document the initial cervical examination so as to have a reference point in the event that there are future issues with preterm contractions or preterm labor.

Key notes for all subsequent visits should record the following:

- Fetal heart tones
- BP
- Urine dip
- Fundal height
- Weight gain
- Fetal movement
- Vaginal bleeding
- Contractions or cramping
- ROM
- Unusual vaginal discharge
- Dysuria
- Pelvic pressure

Delivery note. Some hospitals have preprinted delivery forms that allow you to simply fill in the blanks and check off appropriate boxes. If this is not the case, the following is a summary of the information that should be included in a delivery note:

- Age, gravida, para, therapeutic abortion (TAB), spontaneous abortion (SAB), GA.
- Onset of labor, ROM (with or without meconium).
- Indications for induction (if applicable).
- Obstetric, maternal, or fetal complications.
- Anesthesia/pain control (IV, epidural, general).
- Time of birth.
- Type of birth (NSVD, forceps assist, vacuum suction, C-section).
- Bulb suction, sex, weight, Apgar scores, presence of nuchal cord (tight or loose), number of cord vessels.
- Time of placental delivery, placenta expressed or delivered spontaneously, whether or not the placenta is intact.
- Episiotomy (how done, degree, how repaired) and/or lacerations (locations, degree, how repaired).
- Estimated blood loss (EBL).
- Disposition—eg, mother to recovery room in stable condition; infant to newborn nursery in stable condition; future contraceptive plan (pills or condoms); breastfeeding vs. formula feeding.

Postpartum note. The postpartum note is similar to the routine progress note that is written on most inpatients (subjective, objective—vitals, routine physical examination). Additional items that should be included in the postpartum note are as follows:

- Breast examination (soft, tender, engorged, signs of mastitis [erythema, warmth]).
- Fundus check (firmness, tenderness, location described relative to the umbilicus).
- Lochia (scant, minimal, heavy).
- Perineum (intact or separating).
- Breastfeeding status (problems with feeding; breastfeeding exclusively or supplementing with formula).
- Contraception desired, if any (Depo-Provera injection, OCPs, condoms).

GYN operative note. The gynecology operative note contains the same information as the operative note for any other surgical service. This includes the following:

- Preoperative diagnosis (eg, symptomatic uterine fibroids, cervical cancer, ovarian cyst).
- Postoperative diagnosis (usually "same").
- Procedure (eg, total abdominal hysterectomy, ovarian cystectomy).
- Surgeons.
- Anesthesia (eg, general endotracheal tube).
- EBL.
- IV fluids.
- Urinary output.
- Findings.
- Complications (eg, enterotomy).
- Pathology specimens (eg, uterus, cervix, ovary).

SAMPLE ADMISSION H&P

26 yo G3P1011 at 39 1/7 weeks by LMP 5/11/11 c/w 10-week ultrasound presents c/o UCs 3–4 min, ⊕ FM, ⊖ ROM, ⊖ VB, ⊖ unusual vaginal discharge, ⊖ dysuria. Her due date is 2/15/12.

Prenatal care with Dr. Smith since 7 weeks for 11 visits.

Pregnancy complicated by:

UTI—treated with Keflex. TOC ⊖.

Pap smear c/w ASCUS—needs follow-up Pap smear 6 weeks postpartum.

PPD ⊕, CXR ⊖.

PNL: A+/–, RPR ⊖, rubella immune, HBsAg ⊖, HIV ⊖, Pap smear ASCUS, GC ⊖, chlamydia ⊖, 1-hour PG 121 (at 26 wks), PPD ⊕, CXR ⊖, declined screening for Down syndrome.

PMH: None.

PSH: Appendectomy age 9.

Meds: PNV, $FeSO_4$.

All: NKDA.

OB/GYN Hx:

Menarche age 13/menses q 28 days/lasts 3–5 days.

2008 NSVD, full term, uncomplicated 8-lb, 3-oz boy. No epidural.

2006 SAB in first trimester. No D&C needed.

H/o abnormal Pap smears—never had colposcopy or biopsy.

No h/o STIs.

SH:

Single, father of baby involved and supportive.

Denies T/E/D.

Key:

ASCUS = atypical squamous cells of undetermined significance
b = bilateral
BP = blood pressure
c/o = complaining of
CTAB = clear to auscultation bilaterally
CV = cardiovascular
c/w = consistent with
CXR = chest x-ray
D&C = dilation and curettage
DTRs = deep tendon reflexes
$FeSO_4$ = ferrous sulfate
h/o = history of
Hx = history
IUP = intrauterine pregnancy
NKDA = no known drug allergies
NSVD = normal spontaneous vaginal delivery
P = pulse rate
PMH = past medical history
PNL = prenatal labs
PNV = prenatal vitamins
PPD = purified protein derivative
PSH = past surgical history
RPR = rapid plasma reagin

FH: Maternal grandmother with hypertension. No h/o birth defects or mental retardation.

Physical exam:

VS: T 37.2 BP 120/70 P 82 RR 18.

Gen: Uncomfortable with UCs.

Lungs: CTAB.

CV: RRR, II/VI SEM.

Abd: Soft, gravid, nontender.

Ext: 1+ edema, DTRs 2+ b.

SSE: No pooling. Nitrazine ⊖. Ferning ⊖.

FHT: 130 bpm, accelerations, reactive. No decelerations.

Toco: 4–5 min UCs.

Ultrasound: Vertex, AFI 11.4, placenta fundal.

EFW: 3650 g by Leopold's.

Assessment/Plan: 26 yo G3P1011 at 39 1/7 weeks with uncomplicated IUP in active labor.

1. Admit to L&D.
2. Obtain routine labs (type and screen, RPR, CBC).
3. Expectant management. Will start pitocin augmentation if UCs ↓ in frequency and there is insufficient cervical change.
4. FHT reassuring. No signs of fetal distress.
5. Anticipate normal spontaneous vaginal delivery.

RR = respiratory rate

RRR = regular rate and rhythm

SEM = systolic ejection murmur

SSE = sterile speculum exam

T/E/D = tobacco/alcohol (EtOH)/drugs

TOC = test of cure

Toco = tocometer

UTI = urinary tract infection

VS = vital signs

SAMPLE POSTPARTUM PROGRESS NOTE

S—Eating solid foods. Breastfeeding without difficulty. No urinary complaints. Desires OCPs for contraception.

O—T_{max} 37.2, $T_{current}$ 37.6, BP 120–127/70–76, P 82–85, RR 18–20, I/O 1200/1370.

Gen: NAD, awake and alert.

Lungs: CTAB.

CV: RRR, no murmurs.

Abd: Soft, nontender, minimally distended, BS.

Fundus: Firm, at umbilicus, not tender.

Perineum: 2nd-degree laceration repair intact.

Lochia: Minimal.

Extremities: No edema; no tenderness or evidence of DVT.

Key:

A/P = assessment and plan

BS = bowel sounds

d/c = discharge

DVT = deep venous thrombosis

I/O = intake/output

NAD = no acute distress

O = objective data

OCPs = oral contraceptive pills

PPD = postpartum day

S = subjective data

s/p = status post

A/P—26 yo G3P2012 PPD#1 s/p NSVD at 39 1/7 weeks with uncomplicated labor course and delivery.

1. Ice packs to perineum.
2. Continue to encourage breastfeeding.
3. OCPs for contraception.
4. Anticipate d/c home tomorrow.

KEY PROCEDURES

Delivering babies, cervical checks, Pap smears, cervical/vaginal cultures, external fetal monitoring, IV lines, basic suturing and knot tying, and retracting for visualization during procedures are the principal procedures on this rotation. Descriptions of most of these procedures can be found in major textbooks. However, the best way to learn is by observing and practicing, so let your residents know you are interested in these procedures.

WHAT DO I CARRY IN MY POCKETS?

- ❑ Pregnancy wheel to calculate and double-check EDC (now available as an app on most smartphones)
- ❑ OB/GYN handbook of your choice
- ❑ Penlight
- ❑ Stethoscope
- ❑ Index cards to keep track of your patients. Create cards with high-yield information, including the following:
  - ❑ Steps of a vaginal delivery.
  - ❑ Normal and abnormal labor patterns (eg, duration, cervical dilation).
  - ❑ Indications for C-section.
  - ❑ Outlines of frequently written notes (pre-op, op, post-op, delivery notes).
  - ❑ The diagnosis and management of preeclampsia/eclampsia and other common maternal or obstetrical complications (eg, abruptio placentae, placenta previa, preterm labor).

High-Yield Clinical Topic Checklist

Read about these topics before you start the rotation. A full list of common clerkship topics can be found at the end of this chapter.

- ❑ Normal physiology of pregnancy
- ❑ Gestational diabetes
- ❑ Hypertension during pregnancy; gestational hypertension; preeclampsia/eclampsia
- ❑ First-trimester bleeding
- ❑ Third-trimester bleeding
- ❑ Normal labor and preterm labor

- ❑ Premature rupture of membranes
- ❑ Postpartum hemorrhage
- ❑ Common vaginal infections
- ❑ Pelvic inflammatory disease
- ❑ Contraception
- ❑ Infertility

Obstetrics

NORMAL PHYSIOLOGY OF PREGNANCY

In pregnancy, multiple adaptations occur in each of the mother's organ systems to support the maternal-fetal unit (see Table 6-1).

TABLE 6-1. Maternal Changes During Pregnancy

System	Changes	Effects
Metabolic	↑ proteins, lipids. ↑ need for iron and folate. ↑ insulin sensitivity **early** in pregnancy; ↓ glucose tolerance later in pregnancy.	↑ maternal fat deposition. Maternal anemia. Narrow euglycemic range (normal 84 +/– 10).
Blood	↑ plasma volume by 50%; ↑ RBC mass by 20–40%. ↑ WBCs, fibrinogen, and coagulation factors 7, 8, 9, and 10.	Physiologic anemia of pregnancy. Hypercoagulable state of pregnancy.
Endocrine	↑ estrogen, progesterone, and aldosterone. ↑ prolactin.	Water retention and mood changes. Breast engorgement; preparation for milk production.
Skin, hair	↑ estrogen and progesterone. ↑ testosterone. ↑ α-melanocyte-stimulating hormone.	Spider angiomata, palmar erythema. Mild hirsutism, acne. ↑ skin pigmentation (areolae, axillae, vulva).
Respiratory	↑ tidal volume; ↑ vital capacity. Slight ↑ in respiratory rate; upward displacement of the diaphragm late in pregnancy.	Dyspnea; mild respiratory alkalosis.
Cardiovascular	↑ cardiac output by 45% (primarily due to ↑ stroke volume). ↓ peripheral vascular resistance.	Physiologic flow murmur; dependent edema. ↓ BP; supine hypotensive syndrome.
Renal	Dilation of the collecting system; ↑ GFR up to 60%. ↑ renal blood flow by 30–50%. ↑ aldosterone, renin, and ADH.	↑ UTI frequency, hydroureter, pyelonephritis. ↑ urinary frequency, nocturia, glycosuria. Salt and water retention.
GI	↓ muscle tone leading to hypomotility. ↓ LES tone; prolonged gastric emptying time. Bile stasis.	Constipation, hemorrhoids. Gastric reflux, hiatal hernia. Gallstones.

PRENATAL CARE

KEY FACT

Nägele's rule for determining EDC: EDC = LMP − 3 months + 7 days. Exact dating uses EDC = LMP + 280 days.

KEY FACT

Women planning a pregnancy should take supplemental folate (400 μg/day) beginning 4 weeks prior to conception to ↓ the risk of neural tube defects.

KEY FACT

The typical quadruple-screen finding in Down syndrome is ↓ MSAFP, ↓ estradiol, ↑ hCG, and ↑ inhibin.

MNEMONIC

On quad screen, Down syndrome patients wave–

HI UP in the air

Hcg **elevated**
Inhibin **elevated**

Prenatal care is critical to the uneventful delivery of a healthy baby. Patients with little or no prenatal care can have complications arising from undiagnosed gestational diabetes, gestational hypertension, and intrauterine growth retardation (IUGR) as well as an inability to accurately estimate GA. The following are key aspects of prenatal care:

- **Frequency of visits:**
  - **0–28 weeks' gestation:** Every month.
  - **28–36 weeks' gestation:** Every 2–3 weeks.
  - **36 weeks' gestation until delivery:** Every week until delivery.
- **Estimated date of confinement:**
  - **Nägele's rule:** LMP − 3 months + 7 days + 1 year.
  - **Example:** If LMP is April 14, 2011, then EDC will be January 21, 2012.
- **Key definitions:**
  - **Embryo:** Fertilization to 8 weeks.
  - **Fetus:** Eight weeks to birth.
  - **Previable:** < 24 weeks.
  - **Preterm:** 24–37 weeks.
  - **Term:** 37–42 weeks.
- **Prenatal visits:** At each prenatal visit, the following subjective and objective findings should be addressed and documented:
  - **Subjective findings:**
    - Fetal movement.
    - Vaginal discharge and/or bleeding.
    - Abdominal cramps or UCs.
    - Leakage of fluid or signs of ROM.
    - Dysuria.
    - Blurred vision, headache, rapid weight gain, edema (after 24 weeks).
  - **Objective findings:**
    - Weight, fundal height, BP, edema.
    - Dipstick urine protein and glucose.
    - Fetal heart tones (heard after 10–12 weeks).
- **Fundal height:** Measured with a tape measure from the top of the pubic symphysis to the top of the fundus. Fundal height should correspond to GA as follows (see also Figure 6-1):
  - **At 12 weeks:** At the pubic symphysis.
  - **At 16 weeks:** Midway between the pubis and umbilicus.
  - **At 20 weeks:** At the umbilicus.
  - **At 20–32 weeks:** Height above the pubic symphysis should equal GA in weeks.
- **Nutrition:** During pregnancy, the caloric requirement is ↑ by 300 kcal/day. Iron and folate supplementation is recommended. Guidelines are as follows:
  - **Normal weight gain:** 25–35 lbs for the entire pregnancy.
  - **First trimester:** 3–5 lbs total.
  - **Second trimester:** 0.5 lb/week.
  - **Third trimester:** 1 lb/week.
- **Prenatal labs:** Table 6-2 outlines common prenatal laboratory studies.

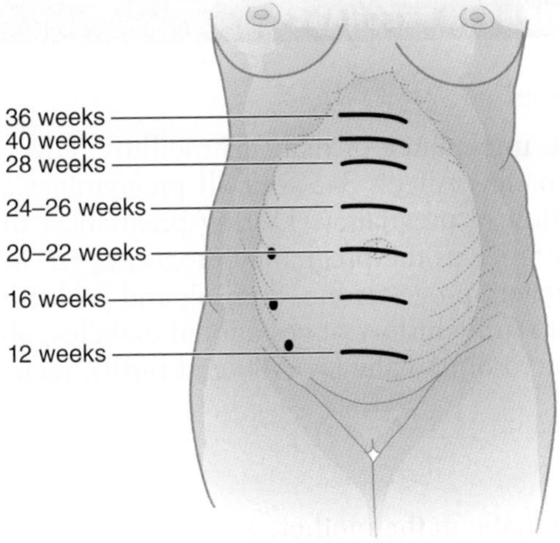

FIGURE 6-1. Height of the fundus during pregnancy. (Reproduced with permission from DeCherney AH et al. *Current Obstetric & Gynecologic Diagnosis & Treatment,* 8th ed. Stamford, CT: Appleton & Lange, 1994: 187.)

TABLE 6-2. Standard Prenatal Labs and Studies

Gestation	Labs to Be Obtained
Initial visit	Hematocrit/hemoglobin, type, Rh, and antibody screen. Infectious screen: rubella antibody titer, VDRL for syphilis, HBsAg, VZV titer (in patients with no history of exposure), PPD, HIV. Cervical gonorrhea and chlamydia cultures. Cystic fibrosis screening if desired. Pap smear; UA and urine culture; sickle prep in high-risk groups. Glucose test if the patient has risk factors for diabetes. First-trimester screening (nuchal thickness, PAPP-A, hCG) for Down syndrome or other trisomies if desired. A ⊕ screen will show ↑ nuchal thickness, ↓ PAPP-A, and significantly ↑ hCG.[a] Ultrasound for dating purposes if the LMP is unknown or is discrepant with the examination. CVS if indicated (eg, for advanced maternal age, a fetus at risk for genetic abnormality, or abnormal first-trimester screening as stated above).
16–20 weeks	Quad screen (hCG, inhibin, AFP, estradiol) to test for Down syndrome, Edwards' syndrome, and neural tube defects if desired. ▪ A ⊕ screen for Down syndrome will result in ↑ hCG and inhibin levels and ↓ AFP and estradiol. ▪ A ⊕ screen for Edwards' syndrome will yield low levels of hCG and estriol with variable AFP. ▪ A fetus with a neural tube defect will show high levels of AFP in the maternal serum. Offer MSAFP if the patient previously had a normal first-trimester screening or CVS. Amniocentesis if indicated. Ultrasound for anatomy evaluation at 18–20 weeks. This is the best time during fetal development to assess the anatomy of the fetus.
26–28 weeks	Diabetes screening test for everyone (risk factors or not). Administer RhoGAM to patients initially determined to be Rh antibody ⊖. CXR if PPD ⊕.
34–38 weeks	CBC, VDRL, cervical chlamydia and gonorrhea (repeated if the patient is at high risk). Group B streptococcus (GBS) culture at 35–37 weeks.

[a] If a patient has a ⊕ screen, either CVS at 10–12 weeks' GA or amniocentesis at 15–18 weeks is required to confirm the diagnosis. However, both tests are associated with a risk of miscarriage, and CVS is associated with a particularly high risk for birth defects such as limb deformities.

MEDICAL CONDITIONS IN PREGNANCY

Gestational Diabetes

> **KEY FACT**
>
> Gestational diabetes is the most common medical complication of pregnancy.

Defined as glucose intolerance or diabetes mellitus (DM) that is first recognized during pregnancy. Affects 3–5% of all pregnancies and is the leading medical complication of pregnancy. During pregnancy, there is a tendency toward insulin resistance as the pregnancy progresses (2° to the effects of human placental lactogen, progesterone, cortisol, and prolactin). Risk factors include a previous or family history of gestational diabetes; obesity; and a previous history of a macrosomic baby (> 4500 g at birth), recurrent miscarriages, and stillbirths.

Signs and Symptoms

- Largely asymptomatic in the mother.
- Presents with glycosuria, hyperglycemia, and/or an abnormal glucose tolerance test on routine prenatal screening at 26–28 weeks' gestation.
- Findings may include a fetus that is large for GA.

Differential

Pregestational DM type 1 or 2, volume overload, simple sugar overload, urinary tract abnormalities.

Workup

- **Glucose challenge test at 26–28 weeks:**
  - Give a 50-g glucose load (a special sweet orange liquid).
  - Check blood glucose level 1 hour later.
  - If > 140 mg/dL, follow up with a 3-hour glucose tolerance test.
  - If > 200 mg/dL, diagnose with gestational diabetes.
- **Three-hour glucose tolerance test if glucose challenge test is > 140 but < 200 mg/dL:**
  - Check blood glucose level at fasting (normal < 95 mg/dL).
  - Give a 100-g glucose load.
  - Check blood glucose level at 1-, 2-, and 3-hour intervals.
  - Findings are abnormal if levels are > 180 mg/dL at 1 hour, > 155 mg/dL at 2 hours, and > 140 mg/dL at 3 hours. The patient has gestational diabetes if at least 2 levels are abnormal.
  - Repeat glucose tolerance test 2–4 months postpartum to diagnose those few women who will remain diabetic.

Treatment

- Start with the American Diabetes Association (ADA) diet and monitor fasting blood glucose and 1- or 2-hour postprandial glucose levels.
- Facilitate patient education and diabetic clinic/dietitian consults.
- If studies reveal a persistent (1- to 2-week) fasting blood glucose level > 95 mg/dL or a 2-hour postprandial glucose level > 120 mg/dL, start glyburide or insulin.
- Although oral hypoglycemic agents were initially thought to be contraindicated in pregnancy, glyburide has recently been used in the third trimester with success.

> **KEY FACT**
>
> Some 25–35% of women with gestational diabetes will develop diabetes in 5 years.

Complications

Complications from gestational diabetes can be divided into maternal and fetal (see Table 6-3).

TABLE 6-3. Complications of Pregestational/Gestational Diabetes

MATERNAL	FETAL
Preterm labor	Macrosomia
Polyhydramnios	Shoulder dystocia
C-section for macrosomia	Perinatal mortality (2–5%)
Preeclampsia/eclampsia (fourfold)	Congenital defects (threefold)
Risk of future glucose intolerance or type 2 DM	Delayed organ maturity

Hypertension in Pregnancy

Risk factors for hypertension in pregnancy include nulliparity or multiple gestations, extremes of age at pregnancy (< 15, > 35), vascular disease (eg, hypertension 2° to lupus or diabetes), diabetes, and chronic hypertension. Subtypes are defined as follows:

- **Chronic hypertension:** Hypertension (BP > 140/90 mm Hg measured 2 times at least 6 hours apart) prior to 20 weeks' gestation. However, new-onset hypertension prior to 20 weeks' gestation is a molar pregnancy until proven otherwise.
- **Gestational hypertension (formerly known as pregnancy-induced hypertension):** Hypertension after 20 weeks in a patient without a previous history of hypertension and without proteinuria.
- **Preeclampsia:** Gestational hypertension plus proteinuria (> 300 mg/24 hrs) with or without edema. The etiology remains unclear but likely results from a systemic release of vasoconstrictors induced by the placenta. Therefore, the only cure is delivery (ie, removal of the placenta).
  - **Mild preeclampsia:** BP > 140/90 mm Hg on 2 occasions at least 6 hours apart and proteinuria 300 mg to 5 g/24 hrs.
  - **Severe preeclampsia:** Any of the following factors bumps up the diagnosis from mild to severe preeclampsia: BP > 160/110 mm Hg on 2 occasions at least 6 hours apart; proteinuria > 5 g/24 hrs; platelets < 100; AST/ALT more than twice normal; oliguria; severe IUGR; pulmonary edema/cyanosis; CVA; severe headache; scotomata; RUQ pain; epigastric pain; nausea/vomiting.
- **HELLP syndrome:** A variant of preeclampsia with a poor prognosis (see mnemonic). A patient with HELLP has severe preeclampsia even without other signs or symptoms of preeclampsia.
- **Eclampsia:** Preeclampsia plus seizures (not due to neurologic disease). Its exact etiology remains to be elucidated, but it may be due to vasospasm-induced neuronal irritability.

Signs and Symptoms

Table 6-4 lists the clinical presentation of hypertension in pregnancy.

Differential

- **Preeclampsia:** Renal disease, renovascular hypertension, 1° aldosteronism, Cushing's disease, pheochromocytoma, SLE.
- **Eclampsia:** 1° seizure disorder, TTP.

KEY FACT

The 3 most common symptoms preceding an eclamptic attack are headache, visual changes, and RUQ/epigastric pain.

MNEMONIC

HELLP syndrome:

Hemolysis
Elevated **L**FTs
Low **P**latelets (thrombocytopenia)

MNEMONIC

Signs and symptoms of severe preeclampsia—

BBLLKK

Blood—thrombocytopenia
Brain—vision changes, headache
Liver—elevated LFTs, RUQ pain
Lung—pulmonary edema
Kidney—oliguria
Kid—IUGR

Q

A gravid 27-year-old female at 32 weeks' gestation complains of a headache. She has had no other complications with her pregnancy. Her BP is 180/110 mm Hg, and her legs are swollen with 2+ pitting pedal edema. What labs should you order, and how should she be treated?

TABLE 6-4. Signs and Symptoms of Preeclampsia and Eclampsia

Mild Preeclampsia	Severe Preeclampsia	Eclampsia
Rapid weight gain, edema, JVD Hyperactive reflexes, clonus	Cerebral/visual changes (severe headaches, blurred vision, scotomata) RUQ/epigastric pain Pulmonary edema/cyanosis ↑ LFTs, ↓ platelet count ↓ urine output IUGR	Seizures

KEY FACT

If gestational hypertension occurs in the first trimester, suspect a molar pregnancy!

KEY FACT

Preeclamptic and eclamptic patients are at highest risk for seizure in the first 24 hours postpartum, but seizures have been reported up to 6 weeks after delivery.

KEY FACT

The presence of fetal cardiac activity on ultrasound is reassuring.

A

She needs a CBC to check for hemolysis and thrombocytopenia, LFTs, and, most importantly, a 24-hour urine test for proteinuria. Treatment for preeclampsia depends on severity and GA and may include antihypertensives, steroid injections to enhance fetal lung maturity, magnesium for seizure prophylaxis, and, ultimately, delivery.

Workup

- **Blood tests:** CBC, platelet count, BUN/creatinine, LFTs.
- **Coagulation tests:** Fibrinogen, fibrin split products (where indicated), PT/aPTT.
- **Urine studies:** UA, serial urine protein, urine toxicology screen (an ↑ BP may be 2° to drugs).
- **Fetal tests:** Ultrasound (to rule out oligohydramnios and IUGR), nonstress test (NST), biophysical profile (BPP).

Treatment

- **Preeclampsia:** The only cure for preeclampsia is delivery of the fetus and placenta (see Figure 6-2).
- **Eclampsia:** Treatment is as follows:
  - Monitor ABCs; give supplemental O_2.
  - Seizure control with $MgSO_4$.
  - Limit fluids; insert Foley catheter to check I/Os; monitor magnesium levels and fetal status.
  - Deliver when stable.
  - Continue $MgSO_4$ for the first 24 hours postpartum, or at least for 24 hours after the last seizure. Follow BP and heme, liver, and renal labs.

COMPLICATIONS OF PREGNANCY

First-Trimester Bleeding

Affects 20–30% of all pregnancies. Etiologies are as follows:

- SAB (complete, incomplete, missed, threatened, and septic abortion; intrauterine fetal death), ectopic pregnancy (see the Emergency Medicine chapter for more details), cervical carcinoma, hydatidiform mole, genital tract trauma, or infections (eg, cervicitis, genital tract trauma or infection). Can also be a normal part of pregnancy.
- It is best to place SAB and ectopic pregnancy at the top of your list and rapidly rule out both of these common causes of first-trimester bleeding.

Workup

- Qualitative/quantitative β-hCG.
- Transvaginal ultrasound.
- Pelvic examination to assess cervical dilation and possible ectopic pregnancy (adnexal mass).
- Type and screen (for RhoGAM administration if Rh ⊖).

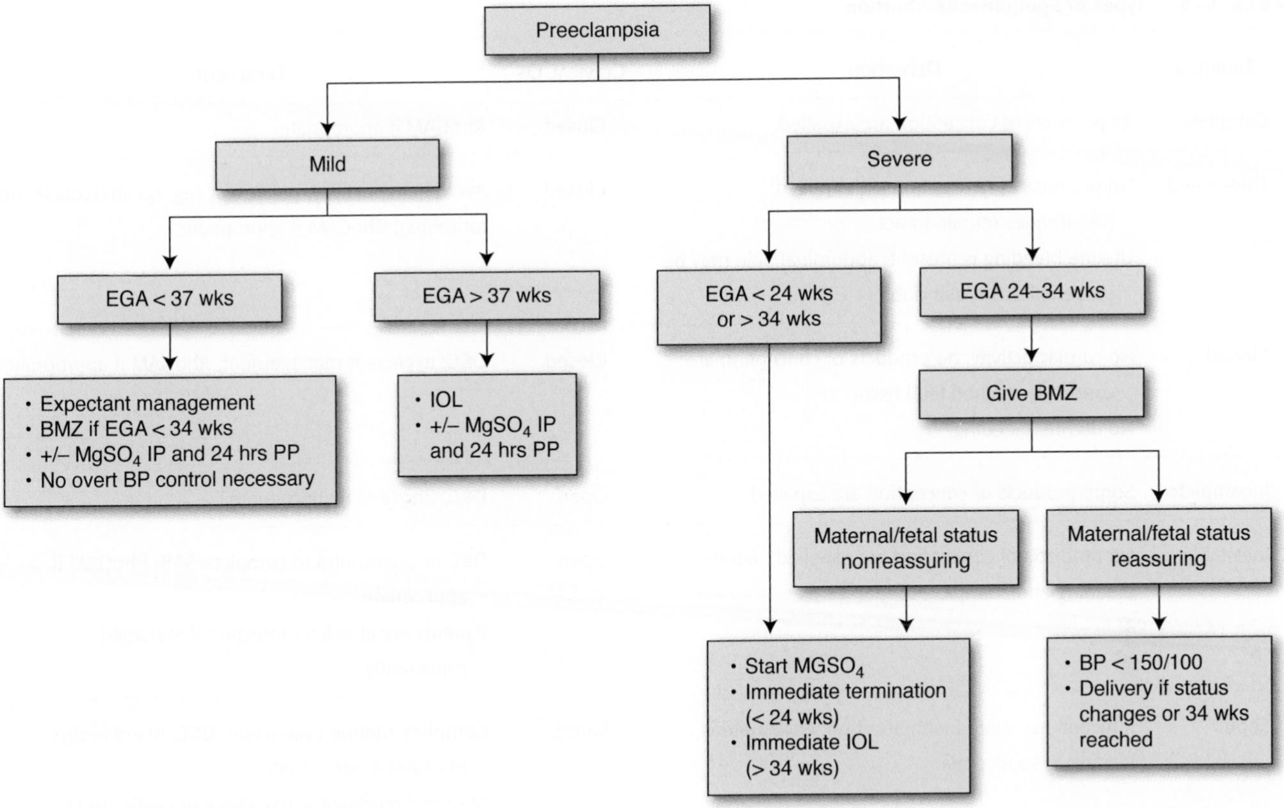

FIGURE 6-2. Algorithm for the treatment of preeclampsia. (BMZ = betamethasone; EGA = estimated gestational age; IOL = induction of labor; IP = intrapartum; PP = postpartum.)

TREATMENT

Etiology specific.

Spontaneous Abortion (SAB)

Abortion is the termination of pregnancy at < 20 weeks' GA or with an EFW < 500 g. It occurs in 13–26% of all pregnancies. The various types of abortion are outlined and compared in Table 6-5. Etiologies are as follows:

- **Chromosomal abnormalities:** The most common etiology (roughly 60%).
- **Infections.**
- **Anatomic defects:** Septate/bicornuate uterus, cervical incompetence, adhesions.

KEY FACT

In a patient who presents with first-trimester bleeding, ask about past pregnancies, a history of abnormal Pap smears, and a history of PID.

KEY POINT

NORMAL (INTRAUTERINE) VS. ABNORMAL PREGNANCIES

- In normal pregnancy, an intrauterine pregnancy (IUP) can be visualized by transvaginal ultrasound when β-hCG is > 1800–2000 mIU/mL and by transabdominal ultrasound when β-hCG is > 3500–5000 mIU/mL. The level at which an IUP should be able to be visualized is known as the "discriminatory zone."
- If hCG levels are above this cutoff and an IUP is not visualized, there is a strong likelihood of an ectopic or other abnormal pregnancy.

TABLE 6-5. Types of Spontaneous Abortion

Abortion	Definition	Cervical Os	Treatment
Complete	All products of conception are expelled.	Closed.	RhoGAM if appropriate.
Threatened	No products of conception are expelled; membranes remain intact. Uterine bleeding is present; abdominal pain may be present; fetus is still viable.	Closed.	Avoid heavy activity; pelvic rest (eg, no intercourse, no tampons); RhoGAM if appropriate.
Missed	No cardiac activity; no products of conception are expelled; retained fetal tissue. No uterine bleeding.	Closed.	D&C; expectant management; RhoGAM if appropriate.
Incomplete	Some products of conception are expelled.	Open.	D&C; RhoGAM if appropriate.
Inevitable	No products of conception are expelled; uterine bleeding and cramps.	Open.	D&C or uterotonics to complete SAB; RhoGAM if appropriate. Patients are at risk for infection if managed expectantly.
Septic	Infection associated with abortion; endometritis leading to septicemia.	Varies.	Complete uterine evacuation, D&C, IV antibiotics, RhoGAM if appropriate. Maternal mortality is 10–50% if in septic shock.

KEY FACT

Women with 3 or more consecutive SABs should be worked up for recurrent abortion (> 3 successive abortions).

- **Endocrine factors:** Progesterone deficiency, polycystic ovarian syndrome (PCOS).
- **Immunologic factors:** Lupus anticoagulant, antiphospholipid syndrome.

Signs and Symptoms

- Vaginal bleeding; passage of tissues.
- Abdominal pain.
- Hemodynamic instability in the presence of retained placental tissue or severe hemorrhage.

Treatment

- Establish hemodynamic stability.
- Administer RhoGAM to all Rh-⊖ patients (see Figure 6-3).

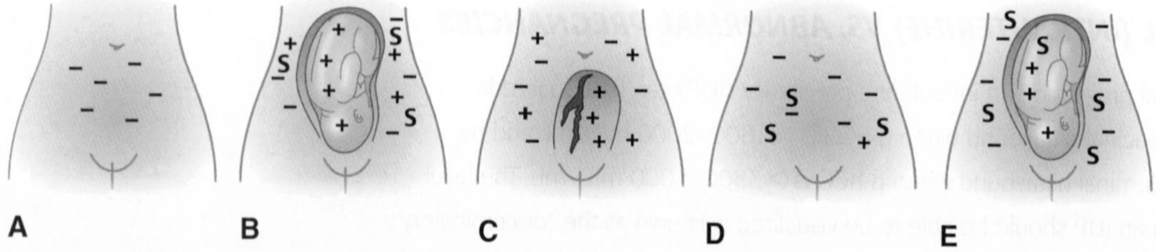

FIGURE 6-3. The significance of identifying Rh-⊖ mothers and giving them RhoGAM. (**A**) Rh-⊖ woman before pregnancy. (**B**) Pregnancy occurs; the fetus is Rh ⊕. (**C**) Separation of the placenta. (**D**) Following delivery, Rh isoimmunization occurs in the mother, and she develops antibodies (S = antibodies). (**E**) The next pregnancy with an Rh-⊕ fetus. Maternal antibodies cross the placenta, enter the bloodstream, and attach to Rh-⊕ RBCs, leading to hemolysis. RhoGAM (Rh IgG) is given to the Rh-⊖ mother to prevent sensitization. (Reproduced with permission from DeCherney AH et al. *Current Obstetric & Gynecologic Diagnosis & Treatment,* 8th ed. Stamford, CT: Appleton & Lange, 1994: 339.)

- Expectant management vs. uterine evacuation. If D&C is performed, chorionic villi should be identified.
- Antibiotics if infection is present.

KEY FACT

Antiphospholipid antibody syndrome is present in 5–15% of women with recurrent abortions.

Third-Trimester Bleeding

Defined as any bleeding that occurs after 28 weeks' gestation. Complicates approximately 5% of all pregnancies.

Signs and Symptoms

- Bleeding ranges from small amounts of spotting to passage of large clots.
- Abdominal pain and/or uterine tenderness suggests abruptio placentae.
- Profuse, painless bleeding is suggestive of placenta previa.

Differential

- **Obstetric causes** (see Table 6-6): Abruptio placentae (30%; see Figure 6-4), placenta previa (20%; see Figure 6-5), bloody show (loss of mucous plug with cervical dilation during the first stage of labor), uterine rupture.
- **Nonobstetric causes:** Genital tract lesions, infections, intercourse, friable cervix, cervical carcinoma.

KEY FACT

The 2 most common causes of third-trimester bleeding are abruptio placentae and placenta previa.

TABLE 6-6. Abruptio Placentae vs. Placenta Previa

Variable	Abruptio Placentae	Placenta Previa
Pathophysiology	Separation of normally implanted placenta from attachment to the uterus.	Abnormal implantation of the placenta near or at the cervical os. Classified as follows: ■ **Total:** The placenta covers the cervical os. ■ **Partial:** The placenta partially covers the os. ■ **Marginal:** The edge of the placenta extends to the margin of the os. ■ **Low lying:** The placenta is within reach of the examining finger, reached through the cervix.
Incidence	Incidence is 1 in 120, but accounts for 15% of perinatal deaths.	Incidence is 1 in 200.
Risk factors	Hypertension, abdominal or pelvic trauma, tobacco or cocaine use, previous abruption.	Prior C-sections, grand multiparity (> 5 previous deliveries).
Symptoms	**Painful** vaginal bleeding (although 10% of bleeding cases are concealed and there will be no overt bleeding). Bleeding usually does not spontaneously cease. Abdominal pain, uterine hypertonicity, tenderness. **Fetal distress** is often present.	**Painless** bright red bleeding. The bleeding source is usually the mother's (with the exception of vasa previa, which occurs when fetal rather than placental vessels are obstructing the cervical os). Bleeding occurs at 29–30 weeks and often ceases within 1–2 hours with or without UCs. Usually **no fetal distress.**

(continues)

TABLE 6-6. Abruptio Placentae vs. Placenta Previa *(continued)*

VARIABLE	ABRUPTIO PLACENTAE	PLACENTA PREVIA
Workup	On transabdominal/transvaginal ultrasound, look for a retroplacental clot. One can rule in the diagnosis but cannot rule it out! Not highly sensitive. Abdominal examination may reveal tenderness. Clinical examination reveals signs of fetal distress, frequent UCs, and hypertonicity.	On transabdominal ultrasound, look for an abnormally positioned placenta; this test is very sensitive for ruling out this diagnosis.
Treatment	Stable patient with premature fetus—expectant management with continuous monitoring. Moderate to severe abruption—immediate delivery (vaginal delivery if fetal heart rate is stable; C-section if the mother or the fetus is in distress). Close fetal monitoring at all times. Amniocentesis to check fetal lung maturity if indicated.	No vaginal examination! Premature fetus (stable patient)—bed rest, tocolytics, serial ultrasound to check fetal growth; resolution of partial previa. If at or near term, amniocentesis to check fetal lung maturity; betamethasone to augment fetal lung maturity if indicated. Delivery by C-section (vaginal route if it resolves). Delivery in the presence of persistent labor, unstable bleeding requiring multiple transfusions, coagulation defects, or documented fetal lung maturity.
Complications	Hemorrhagic shock. Coagulopathy (DIC complicates 10% of all abruptions). Ischemic necrosis of distal organs. Recurrence rate is 5–16%; this risk ↑ to 25% after 2 previous abruptions. Fetal anemia.	Placenta accreta (up to 25% with 1 previous C-section and anterior placenta). Vasa previa. ↑ risk of congenital abnormalities. ↑ risk of postpartum hemorrhage. Fetal anemia.

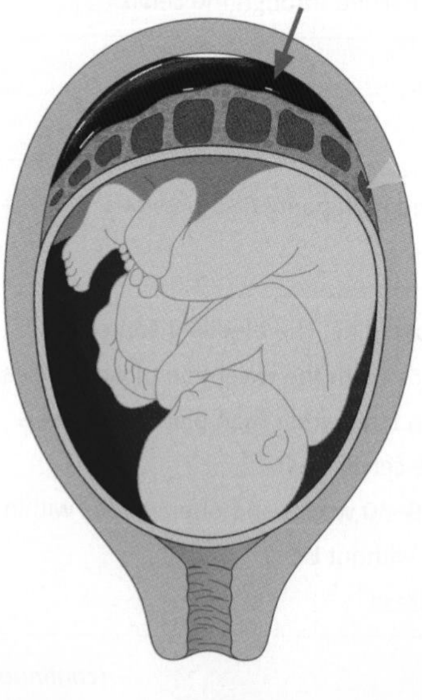

FIGURE 6-4. Placental abruption. The placenta (arrowhead) is separated from the uterus, causing bleeding (arrow). (Reproduced with permission from Tintinalli JE et al. *Tintinalli's Emergency Medicine: A Comprehensive Study Guide*, 7th ed. New York: McGraw-Hill, 2011, Fig. 104-1.)

WORKUP

- CBC and PT/aPTT to rule out DIC; type and cross; UA and cervical cultures to rule out infection.
- If the location of the placenta is unknown, perform an ultrasound to rule out placenta previa before performing a vaginal examination.
- If no previa is found, perform a sterile speculum examination to evaluate the source of bleeding or ruptured membranes.
- Perform a vaginal examination to rule out labor.
- Fetal well-being tests:
  - Check for fetal heart tones and conduct an NST.
  - Consider amniocentesis for fetal lung maturity for the assessment of delivery options.
  - Administer RhoGAM if Rh ⊖ and send a Kleihauer-Betke test to assess for the extent of fetomaternal bleed.

TREATMENT

- Delivery for term patients.
- Bed rest and cautious tocolysis for stable preterm patients.
- In a mature fetus or in the presence of severe placental abruption, close fetal monitoring, amniotomy, and delivery are indicated (see Table 6-6).

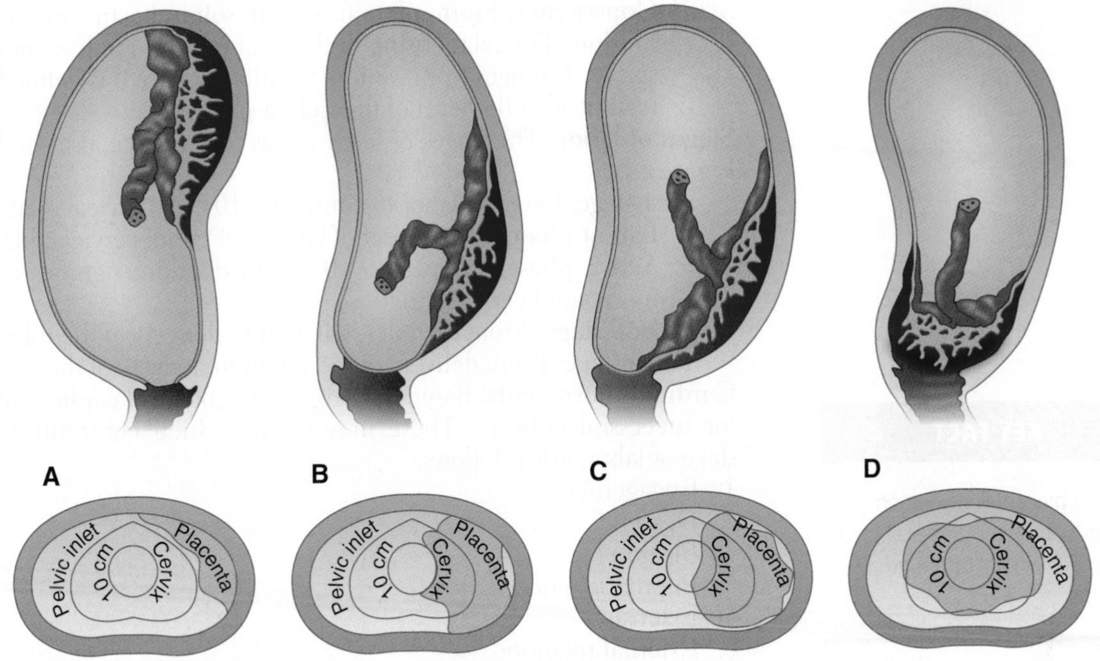

FIGURE 6-5. Implantation of the placenta. (**A**) Normal placenta. (**B**) Low implantation. (**C**) Partial placenta previa. (**D**) Complete placenta previa. (Reproduced with permission from DeCherney AH et al. *Current Obstetric & Gynecologic Diagnosis & Treatment,* 8th ed. Stamford, CT: Appleton & Lange, 1994: 404.)

LABOR AND DELIVERY

Normal Labor

Labor has 2 components: (1) UCs of sufficient frequency, duration, and intensity; and (2) cervical changes, including effacement (thinning) and dilation. Cervical dilation that occurs without UCs is not considered true labor. Similarly, UCs without cervical effacement and dilation are referred to as Braxton Hicks contractions, or false labor. The following are additional characteristics of normal labor:

- **Onset of labor:**
  - **Lightening:** A change in the shape of the abdomen with the sensation that the baby is less heavy. This event results from the descent of the fetal head into the pelvis.
  - **Bloody show:** Passage of blood-tinged mucus that is produced when the cervix begins to thin out (effacement). Cervical effacement commonly occurs before the onset of true labor, particularly in nulliparous patients.
- **Assessment of labor:**
  - Instruct the patient to report to the hospital for evaluation when:
    - Contractions occur every 5 minutes for at least 1 hour.
    - There is ROM (a large gush of fluid or continuous leakage).
    - There is significant bleeding.
    - There is a significant ↓ in fetal movement.
  - Cervical examination should evaluate the following:
    - **Effacement:** The length of the cervix as the cervix thins out and softens (%).
    - **Dilation:** The size of the cervical opening at the external os (cm).
    - **Position:** The location of the cervix with respect to the fetal presenting part.

- **Consistency:** From soft to firm, with soft indicating onset of labor.
- **Station:** The relationship of the fetal head to the level of the ischial spines. It ranges from −5 to +5 station (where 0 is defined to be the fetal head at the level of the ischial spines).

- **Stages of labor:** The stages of labor are as follows (see also Table 6-7 and Figure 6-6):
  - **First stage:** Onset of labor to complete (10-cm) cervical dilation.
    - **Latent phase:** From onset of labor to 4 cm of cervical dilation.
    - **Active phase:** From 4 to 10 cm of dilation; signifies a period of more rapid cervical dilation.
  - **Second stage:** From complete dilation to delivery of the infant.
  - **Third stage:** From delivery of the infant to delivery of the placenta.
- **Cardinal movements:** Babies undergo 7 stereotypical cardinal movements for successful delivery. These movements, which constitute the second stage of labor, are as follows:
  1. Engagement
  2. Descent
  3. Flexion
  4. Internal rotation
  5. Extension
  6. External rotation
  7. Expulsion
- **Fetal lie, presentation, and position:** The orientation of the baby is described in relation to the maternal pelvis in the following manner:
  - **Fetal lie:** The long axis of the baby in relation to the long axis of the mother (longitudinal, transverse, oblique).
  - **Fetal presentation:** That part of the fetus that enters the pelvis first—eg, vertex (head first), breech (buttocks or leg first), face, brow.
  - **Fetal position:** The reference point of the fetal presenting part (for ver-

KEY FACT

The 3 signs of placental separation: gush of blood; apparent umbilical cord lengthening; the fundus of the uterus rises and firms.

KEY FACT

Leopold's maneuver is used to determine fetal lie and presentation.

TABLE 6-7. The 3 Stages of Labor

Phase	Starts/End	Events	Average Duration (hrs) Nulli[a]	Multi[b]
First Stage				
Latent	Regular UCs/cervix dilated up to 4 cm.	Highly variable duration; cervix effaces and slowly dilates.	6–20	4–14
Active	4-cm cervical dilation/complete cervical dilation (10 cm).	Regular and intense UCs; cervix effaces and dilates more quickly; fetal head progressively descends into the pelvis.	4–12	2–5
Second Stage				
None	Complete cervical dilation/delivery of the baby.	Baby undergoes all stages of cardinal movements.	1–3	0.5–1.0
Third Stage				
None	Delivery of the baby/delivery of the placenta.	Placenta separates and uterus contracts to establish hemostasis.	0–0.5	0–0.5

[a] Nulli = nulliparous (first-time mother).

[b] Multi = multiparous (delivered vaginally before).

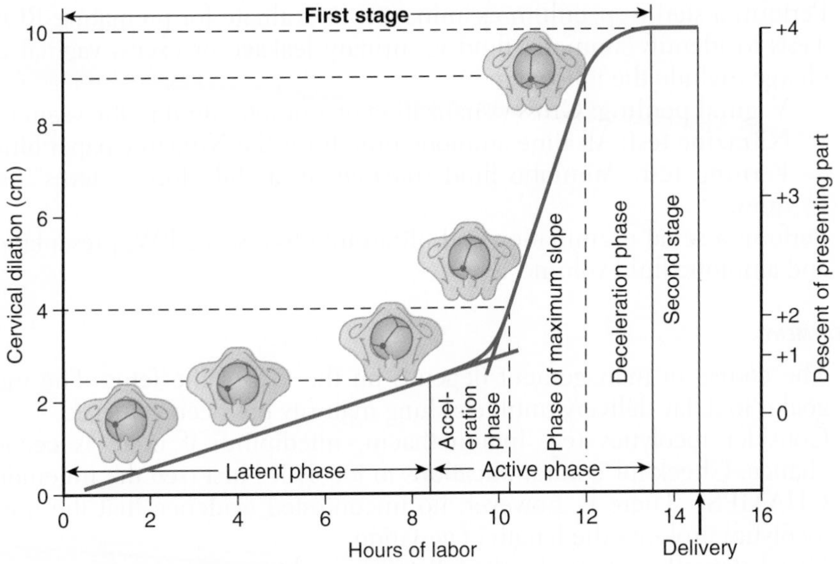

FIGURE 6-6. Stages of labor. Cervical dilation, level of descent, and orientation of occipitoanterior presentation are shown during various stages of labor. (Reproduced with permission from DeCherney AH et al. *Current Obstetric & Gynecologic Diagnosis & Treatment,* 8th ed. Stamford, CT: Appleton & Lange, 1994: 211.)

tex presentation, the presenting part is the occiput; for breech presentation, the presenting part is the sacrum) to the maternal pelvis (right, left, anterior, posterior).

Preterm Labor

- Preterm labor complicates 5–10% of all pregnancies. Risk factors can be described by the mnemonic **MAPPS.** However, half of all cases occur in patients with no risk factors. Diagnostic criteria are as follows:
  - **Preterm:** < 37 weeks' gestation.
  - **True labor:** UCs of sufficient duration and intensity to result in cervical dilation of > 2 cm or effacement of > 80%.

Signs and Symptoms

- Abdominal, pelvic, or back pain.
- Vaginal discharge; bloody show.
- UCs; cervical dilation and/or effacement.
- ROM.

Differential

- **False labor:** Contractions without cervical dilation or change.
- **Appendicitis.**
- **Local causes:** Cervicitis, genital tract infections, trauma, physiologic discharge.

Workup

- **Perform a cervical examination.**
- **Rule out infectious causes of preterm labor** with cervical cultures and a wet mount. Labs to send include CBC, a urine tox screen, a UA and urine culture, and vaginal and cervical cultures for GBS, chlamydia, and gonorrhea.

MNEMONIC

Risk factors for preterm labor–

MAPPS

Multiple gestations
Abdominal surgery during pregnancy
Previous **P**reterm labor or delivery
Surgery of the cervix

KEY FACT

- **Premature ROM:** Rupture of membranes that occurs before the onset of labor regardless of GA.
- **Preterm ROM:** Rupture of membranes that occurs before 37 weeks' gestation.

KEY FACT

When premature and preterm ROM occur together, it is termed premature preterm rupture of membranes (PPROM).

KEY FACT

A false-⊕ Nitrazine test can be caused by contamination from blood, semen, or vaginitis.

KEY FACT

Tocolytics are ineffective if the patient is in active labor (cervical dilation ≥ 4 cm).

MNEMONIC

Contraindications to tocolytics–

CHAMPS

Chorioamnionitis
Hemorrhage
Abruption of placenta
Maturity of fetus
Preeclampsia/eclampsia
Severe IUGR

- Perform a sterile speculum examination to evaluate for premature ROM. Tests to identify amniotic fluid vs. urinary leakage or excess vaginal discharge include the following:
  - **Vaginal pooling:** Gross visualization of amniotic fluid in the vagina.
  - **Nitrazine test:** Alkaline amniotic fluid turns the Nitrazine paper blue.
  - **Ferning test:** Amniotic fluid smeared on a slide forms "ferns" as it dries.
- Perform a serial examination and ultrasound to assess EFW, presentation, and amniotic fluid volume.

TREATMENT

- The course of management depends on the GA of the fetus. The main goal is to delay delivery until fetal lung maturity has been achieved.
- Consider tocolytics (eg, indomethacin, nifedipine) if there is cervical change. Check for contraindications to tocolytics first (see the mnemonic **CHAMPS**). There is, however, no uncontested evidence that the use of tocolytics prolongs the length of gestation.
- Give betamethasone under the following conditions:
  - Estimated GA of 24–34 weeks with preterm labor; estimated GA of 24–32 weeks with PPROM.
  - Absence of uncontrolled maternal diabetes.
  - No need for immediate delivery (eg, placental abruption with nonreassuring heart tracing).
- Amniocentesis may be considered, especially at 35–36 weeks' GA, to check for fetal lung maturity. Amniotic fluid may also be collected from vaginal pooling and sent for testing in the setting of PPROM.
- Notify pediatrics on admission, not only for counseling of the patient as to the expected neonatal outcome but also to ensure that the pediatricians are aware of a potential preterm infant delivery.

Abnormal Labor Patterns

A diagnosis of abnormal labor is considered in any case in which there is a variation in the normal pattern of cervical dilation or descent of the fetal presenting part. It occurs in 8–11% of all cephalic deliveries.

SIGNS AND SYMPTOMS

Table 6-8 describes patterns of abnormal labor. Also beware of false labor, which may be confused with arrest of dilation and has the following distinguishing characteristics:

- Irregular intervals and duration of UCs with no cervical dilation.
- Unchanged contraction intensity.
- Lower back and abdominal discomfort.
- Relief with sedation.

DIFFERENTIAL

Normal or false labor; ineffective UCs; fetal malposition/fetopelvic disproportion.

WORKUP

- Obtain a graphic demonstration of cervical dilation and effacement.
- Document on each vaginal examination the dilation of the cervix, the presence of the caput or molding of the fetal head, and the station and position of the fetal presenting part.
- The results of each examination should be assessed dynamically.

TABLE 6-8. Abnormal Labor Patterns

Abnormal Pattern	Threshold Duration of Labor: Nulliparous	Threshold Duration of Labor: Multiparous	Possible Causes
Precipitous	Completion of stages 1 and 2 in < 3 hours		Unknown.
Protracted latent phase	> 20 hours	> 14 hours	Ineffective UCs; unripe cervix; abnormal fetal position; false labor.
Protracted active phase	> 12 hours or rate of cervical dilation < 1.2 cm/hr	> 6 hours < 1.5 cm/hr	Abnormal fetal position; fetopelvic disproportion; excess sedation; ineffective UCs.
Arrest of dilation in active contraction phase	Cervical dilation stops for > 2 hours		Ineffective UCs; fetopelvic disproportion; abnormal fetal lie, presentation, or position.
Arrest of fetal descent in second stage	> 2 hours without epidural > 3 hours with epidural	> 1 hour without epidural > 2 hours with epidural	Ineffective UCs; fetopelvic disproportion.

- Workup should then proceed with the systematic assessment of the "3 P's" of labor (see mnemonic):
  - **Powers (uterine forces):** Frequency and duration can be evaluated through manual palpation of the gravid abdomen during a contraction, by a tocodynamometer, and by an internal pressure catheter (this is the only way to measure the pressure generated by each UC).
  - **Passenger:** Estimation of fetal weight and clinical evaluation of fetal lie, presentation, and position.
  - **Passage:** Measurement of the bony pelvis is often a poor predictor of abnormal labor unless the pelvis is extremely contracted. Also assess for other physical obstacles (eg, distended bladder or colon, uterine myoma, cervical mass).

TREATMENT

- **Precipitous labor:**
  - Stop any oxytocin use. Tocolytics have not been shown to be of benefit.
  - Complications include uterine atony leading to postpartum hemorrhage and genital tract trauma.
- **Prolonged latent phase:**
  - Rest or augmentation of labor with oxytocin if "power" is the problem.
  - Amniotomy (ie, artificial ROM [AROM]).
- **Protracted/arrested active phase:**
  - Intrauterine pressure catheter to measure the force of UCs.
  - AROM.
  - Augmentation with oxytocin if "power" is the problem.
  - C-section in the presence of fetopelvic disproportion or maternal/fetal distress.
- **Arrest in second stage:**
  - Attempt vaginal delivery if the mother and baby are doing well.
  - Augmentation with oxytocin.
  - Operative vaginal delivery (forceps, vacuum) if the vertex is low in the pelvis.
  - C-section in the presence of maternal/fetal distress, breech, or fetopelvic disproportion.

MNEMONIC

Causes of abnormal labor—

The 3 P's

Powers (uterine contractions)
Passenger (fetus)
Passage (pelvic)

KEY FACT

Shoulder dystocia is due to impaction of the fetal shoulder behind the pubic symphysis after delivery of the head.

MNEMONIC

Risk factors for shoulder dystocia—

MOMS on L&D

Maternal
Obesity
Macrosomia
Second stage prolonged
Late (postdate pregnancy)
Diabetes

FETAL HEART RATE (FHR) MONITORING

The FHR is usually monitored continuously throughout labor to evaluate its effects on fetal intrapartum events. **External monitoring** is conducted with an ultrasound transducer affixed to the maternal abdomen and is the current standard of care. **Internal monitoring** is done through an electrode attached to the fetal scalp and requires that the membranes have been ruptured. Internal monitoring with scalp electrodes is safe, but since it is more invasive than external monitoring, it is generally reserved for circumstances in which more stringent fetal monitoring is desired—eg, protracted labors, abnormal labors, or signs of fetal distress. Relevant variables are as follows:

- **Baseline FHR:** The normal range of the human FHR is 110–160 bpm. Abnormal patterns include the following:
  - **Baseline tachycardia:** A baseline heart rate > 160 bpm for > 10 minutes. Etiologies include fetal hypoxia, maternal fever, fetal infection, maternal thyrotoxicosis, fetal anemia, fetal arrhythmias, and the use of β-sympathomimetic drugs such as terbutaline (see the mnemonic **FFAAST Heart**).
  - **Baseline bradycardia:** A baseline heart rate < 110 bpm for > 10 minutes. Etiologies include fetal hypoxia, damage to the conduction system of the fetal heart, maternal autoimmune disease, and treatment with drugs such as β-blockers.
- **Heart rate variability:** Represents the interplay between cardioinhibitory and cardioacceleratory centers in the fetal brainstem.
  - **Beat-to-beat variability is the most reliable indicator of fetal well-being** and is one of the best indicators of intact integration between the CNS and heart of the fetus.
  - **Short-term variability:** Variation on a "beat-to-beat basis" usually ranges from 3 to 5 bpm.
  - **Long-term variability:** Fluctuations with amplitudes of 5–20 bpm occurring at 3–5 cycles per minute.
- **Periodic changes:** Table 6-9 and Figure 6-7 outline patterns in FHR. Relevant definitions are as follows:
  - **Accelerations:** Transient increases in FHR above the determined baseline. Accelerations are reassuring and usually indicate fetal well-being.
  - **Early decelerations:** Decreases in FHR that begin with a contraction, reach a nadir at the peak of the contraction, and end with the comple-

MNEMONIC

Causes of fetal baseline tachycardia–

FFAAST Heart

Fetal infection
Fever
Arrhythmia of fetus
Anemia of fetus
Sympathomimetics
Thyrotoxicosis of mother
Hypoxia

TABLE 6-9. Fetal Heart Rate Patterns

Variable	Early Deceleration	Late Deceleration	Variable Deceleration
Significance	Benign	Abnormal	Benign/abnormal
Onset	Gradual	Gradual	Abrupt
When	End with UC	End after UC	Variable
Etiology	Head compression	Uteroplacental insufficiency	Umbilical cord compression/head compression
Initial treatment	None required	O_2, lateral decubitus position, oxytocin off	Amnioinfusion

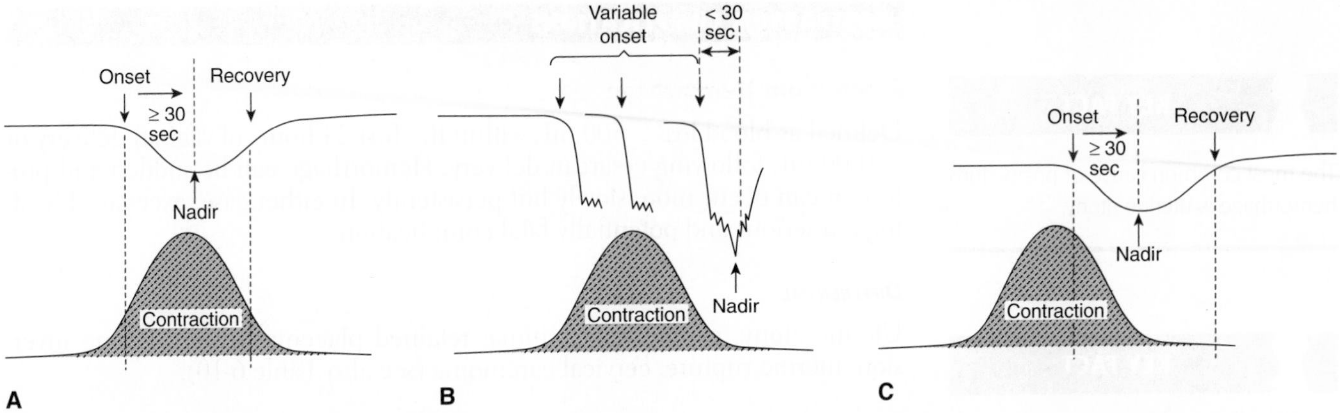

FIGURE 6-7. Fetal heart rate tracings. (**A**) Early deceleration. (**B**) Late deceleration. (**C**) Variable deceleration. (Reproduced with permission from Cunningham FG et al. *Williams Obstetrics,* 23rd ed. New York: McGraw-Hill, 2010, Figs. 18-14, 18-18, and 18-15.)

tion of the contraction. Early decelerations result from pressure on the fetal head through a reflex response mediated by the vagus nerve with release of acetylcholine at the sinoatrial node. Early decelerations are innocuous and can be observed throughout labor without alteration in fetal condition or acid-base status.

- **Variable decelerations:** Slowing of the heart rate that may start before, during, or after the UC and is characterized by a rapid fall in FHR, often below 100 bpm, with a rapid return to baseline.
  - Decelerations are associated with umbilical cord compression and are mediated through the vagus nerve with sudden and often erratic release of acetylcholine at the fetal sinoatrial node.
  - This pattern is often seen with oligohydramnios or after ROM 2° to "decreased cushioning" of the umbilical cord. If the variable decelerations are severe and repetitive, hypoxia and metabolic acidosis may result.
- **Late decelerations:** Begin after the UC starts, reach their nadir after the peak of the contraction, and end after the contraction ceases.
  - Late decelerations are a sign of uteroplacental insufficiency resulting from ↓ uterine perfusion or ↓ placental function.
  - Associated with progressive fetal hypoxia and acidemia. May occur with any process that would predispose to insufficient blood flow and oxygenation of the fetus, such as placental abruption, excessive uterine activity, maternal hypotension, anemia, and IUGR.
  - Although repetitive late decelerations are considered nonreassuring, they have very poor positive predictive value. Ninety percent of the time, a fetus with repetitive late decelerations actually has a normal acid-base status.

KEY FACT

Early decelerations mirror the contraction as it happens and are innocuous. Repetitive late decelerations are a delayed mirror image and may be a sign of uteroplacental insufficiency.

KEY FACT

A reactive tracing is a sign of fetal well-being. It is characterized by at least 2 accelerations in which the heart rate peaks 15 beats above baseline for at least 15 seconds during a 20-minute period.

KEY FACT

A fetus < 28 weeks' GA is neurologically immature and thus is not expected to have a "reactive" FHR.

KEY POINT

WHAT DO THE 3 TYPES OF DECELERATIONS REPRESENT?

- **Variable** = cord compression.
- **Early** = head compression.
- **Late** = uteroplacental insufficiency.

Only late decelerations are considered worrisome.

POSTPARTUM COMPLICATIONS

> **KEY FACT**
>
> The most common cause of postpartum hemorrhage is uterine atony.

> **KEY FACT**
>
> Remember serial hematocrits in postpartum hemorrhage.

Postpartum Hemorrhage

Defined as blood loss > 500 mL within the first 24 hours of vaginal delivery or > 1000 mL following cesarean delivery. Hemorrhage can be sudden and profuse or can occur more slowly but persistently. In either case, excessive bleeding is a serious and potentially fatal complication.

DIFFERENTIAL

Uterine atony, genital tract trauma, retained placental tissue, uterine inversion, uterine rupture, cervical carcinoma (see also Table 6-10).

WORKUP/TREATMENT

The diagnosis and treatment of the 3 major causes of postpartum hemorrhage are discussed in Table 6-10.

"Postpartum Blues"/Postpartum Depression

"Postpartum blues" is a common disorder affecting new mothers, many of whom experience mild, short-lived crying, irritability, anxiety, and emotional lability. However, when symptoms are of at least 2 weeks' duration and in-

TABLE 6-10. Common Causes of Postpartum Hemorrhage

VARIABLE	UTERINE ATONY	GENITAL TRACT TRAUMA	RETAINED PLACENTAL TISSUE
Risk factors	Overdistention of the uterus (multiple gestations, macrosomia). Abnormal labor (prolonged labor, precipitous labor). Conditions interfering with UCs (uterine myomas, $MgSO_4$, general anesthesia). Uterine infection.	Precipitous labor. Operative vaginal delivery (forceps, vacuum extraction). Large infant. Inadequate laceration repair. Unrecognized cervical laceration.	Placenta accreta/increta/percreta. Preterm delivery. Placenta previa. Previous C-section/curettage. Uterine leiomyomas.
Workup	Palpation of a softer, flaccid, "boggy" uterus without a firm fundus.	Careful visualization of the lower genital tract to look for any laceration > 2 cm in length or bleeding.	Careful inspection of the placenta for missing cotyledons. Ultrasound may also be used to examine the uterus.
Treatment	The most common cause of postpartum hemorrhage (90%). Bimanual uterine massage. Oxytocin infusion. Empty bladder (an overdistended bladder can prevent UCs). Methylergonovine maleate (Methergine) if the patient is not hypertensive and/or prostaglandin F2-α (Hemabate) if the patient is not asthmatic. Rectal misoprostol may also be used.	Surgical repair of the physical defect.	Manual removal of the remaining placental tissue. Curettage with suctioning may also be used, with care taken to avoid perforating the uterine fundus. In cases of true placenta accreta/increta/percreta where the placental villi invade into the uterine tissue, hysterectomy may be required as a life-preserving therapy.

clude anhedonia, insomnia, changes in appetite, feelings of guilt, suicidality, or feelings of wanting to hurt the baby, the diagnosis is likely to be postpartum depression. Treatment includes support groups, psychotherapy, and pharmacologic agents such as antidepressants.

Gynecology

ABNORMAL UTERINE BLEEDING

Subtypes of abnormal uterine bleeding are distinguished as follows:

- **Polymenorrhea:** Menses with intervals that are too short (< 21 days).
- **Menorrhagia:** Menses that are too long (> 7 days) and/or are associated with excessive blood loss (> 80 mL) at **normal** intervals.
- **Hypermenorrhea:** Menses that are too long (> 7 days) and/or are associated with excessive blood loss (> 80 mL) at **regular but not necessarily normal intervals.**
- **Oligomenorrhea:** Menses with intervals that are too long (> 35 days).
- **Metrorrhagia:** Menses occurring at irregular intervals with intermenstrual bleeding.
- **Menometrorrhagia:** A combination of menorrhagia and metrorrhagia.

DIFFERENTIAL

- Premenopause:
  - **Pregnancy:** The most common cause. Keep in mind that abnormal pregnancies such as ectopic pregnancy, threatened abortion, and incomplete abortion are included.
  - **Organic causes:** Blood dyscrasias, hypersplenism, hypothyroidism, sepsis, ITP, leukemia.
  - **Anatomic causes:** Malignancies, infections, endometriosis, ruptured corpus luteum cyst, fibroids, endometrial polyp, trauma.
  - **Dysfunctional uterine bleeding (DUB):** Bleeding that is not due to pregnancy or to an organic or anatomic etiology. Anovulatory cycles are the most common cause of DUB, especially around the time of menarche (onset of menstrual cycles) and menopause (cessation of menstrual cycles), and constitute the second most common cause of abnormal uterine bleeding overall.
- Postmenopause:
  - **Atrophic vaginitis:** Most common. Due to the loss of estrogen after menopause and subsequent drying and atrophy of vaginal dermal tissue.
  - **Endometrial cancer:** Must be ruled out in any postmenopausal woman with vaginal bleeding by performing an endometrial biopsy.
  - **Other:** Cervical cancer, vulvar cancer, hormone replacement therapy (HRT).

WORKUP

- Obtain an H&P, including a thorough menstrual and reproductive history.
- Assess the rate of bleeding, hemodynamic status, and orthostatic vitals; obtain a CBC.
- Conduct a pregnancy test.
- Determine whether the patient is having ovulatory or anovulatory cycles. The patient is ovulating if she has menstrual cycles at regular intervals.

KEY FACT

The most common cause of abnormal uterine bleeding is pregnancy.

KEY FACT

Vaginal bleeding in a postmenopausal woman is cancer until proven otherwise!

Q

A 65-year-old obese female with a history of infertility and hirsutism presents with vaginal bleeding. She has 2 adopted children and currently lives alone. Ultrasound shows endometrial thickening. What is the next step in management?

- If the patient **is not ovulating,** suspect DUB, most likely 2° to hormonal irregularities.
- If the patient **is ovulating,** conduct further workup to rule out pathology:
  - Order a PT/aPTT to rule out coagulopathy, particularly if the patient is an adolescent and has just begun menstruating.
  - Evaluate for skin and hair changes, thyroid enlargement, galactorrhea, obesity, hirsutism, cervical motion tenderness (CMT), uterine size, cervical lesions, and adnexal tenderness.
  - Obtain an endometrial biopsy for women > 35 years of age.
  - Consider transvaginal ultrasound to check for uterine and ovarian masses/endometrial thickening (normally < 5 mm in postmenopausal women).

TREATMENT

- **Anovulatory bleeding:** After ruling out pathologies (uterine polyps, endometrial cancer), place patients on medroxyprogesterone acetate (Provera) or OCPs. Also consider HRT if the patient is perimenopausal (see Table 6-11).
- **DUB:**
  - For mild cases (hemoglobin > 11), treat with iron supplements, NSAIDs, and OCPs. Alternatively, high-dose progestins (norethindrone) can be used to normalize menses.
  - For severe cases (hemoglobin < 7), stabilize the patient first (blood transfusion, saline) and then start on IV estrogen or OCPs.
  - For recurrent, severe cases, start on OCPs, Provera, or Depo-Provera with or without an estrogen supplement. The levonorgestrel-releasing IUD is also indicated for treating heavy bleeding.
  - If medical therapy fails, consider surgical options for DUB, which include hysteroscopy with D&C, endometrial ablation with laser or electrocautery, and hysterectomy.

ENDOMETRIOSIS

Defined as the presence of endometrial glands and stroma outside the uterine cavity. Affects 5–15% of premenopausal women, accounting for 40–50% of all surgeries for infertility. Sites affected include the ovaries, the broad ligament, and the cul-de-sac (see Figure 6-8). Etiologies include direct implantation of endometrial cells by retrograde menstruation, vascular and lymphatic dissemination of endometrial cells, and coelomic metaplasia of multipotential cells in the peritoneal cavity.

KEY FACT

Fibroids are benign uterine tumors that may cause excessive menstrual bleeding, pelvic pain, and frequent urination. That doesn't seem so benign!

TABLE 6-11. General Management of Abnormal Uterine Bleeding

Acute Uterine Bleeding	Recurrent Uterine Bleeding
High-dose estrogen (oral or IV)	GnRH agonists (Lupron)
High-dose OCPs	Danazol (multiple side effects)
D&C	D&C/endometrial biopsy to aid in diagnosis
	Endometrial ablation

A

Biopsy the endometrial lining by D&C. A postmenopausal woman with vaginal bleeding has endometrial carcinoma until proven otherwise. This patient has multiple risk factors, including obesity, nulliparity, and PCOS, all of which involve chronic, isolated increases in estrogen levels.

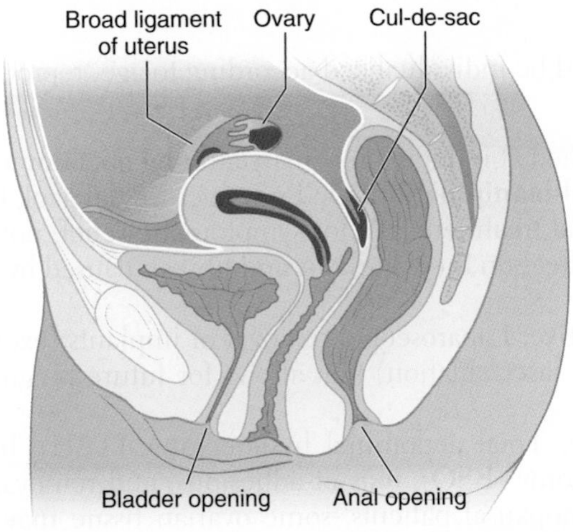

FIGURE 6-8. Common sites of endometriosis. Red-shaded regions outside the uterus are abnormal locations of endometrial tissue. (Adapted with permission from Doherty GM, Way LW. *Current Surgical Diagnosis & Treatment,* 12th ed. New York: McGraw-Hill, 2006: 1075.)

Signs and Symptoms

- Presents with pelvic pain (dysmenorrhea, dyspareunia, dyschezia), abnormal bleeding, and infertility.
- The disease is hormone dependent and usually improves after menopause.
- Physical examination reveals nodular thickening along the uterosacral ligament; a fixed, retroverted uterus; and tender, fixed adnexal masses (endometriomas).

Differential

Most women with endometriosis are asymptomatic. However, patients can present with a wide range of symptoms, and the differential depends on the patient's specific complaints.

- **Chronic abdominal pain:** Chronic PID and pelvic adhesions.
- **Amenorrhea:** Causes of 1° and/or 2° amenorrhea.
- **Sudden-onset lower abdominal pain:** Ectopic pregnancy, appendicitis, PID, adnexal torsion, rupture of the corpus luteum, endometrioma.

Workup

- **Laparoscopy:** Offers a definitive diagnosis.
- **Biopsy:** Biopsy of "endometriosis-appearing lesions" reveals functional endometrial glands and stroma together with hemosiderin-laden macrophages.
- **Labs/imaging:** Pregnancy test, UA, ultrasound, MRI.

KEY POINT

ENDOMETRIOSIS VS. ADENOMYOSIS

What is the difference between endometriosis and adenomyosis?

- **Endometriosis** is endometrial tissue found outside the uterus.
- **Adenomyosis** is endometrial tissue found in the myometrium.

KEY FACT

Endometriosis lesions are described as "powder burns" or "chocolate cysts" because old blood on the uterine wall or in the ovarian cysts looks dark brown or black.

KEY FACT

For endometriosis, disease severity does not necessarily correlate with symptoms.

Q

A 20-year-old female is concerned because she has never had a menstrual period. She also notes a lack of pubic and axillary hair growth. She is found to be 4'11", is Tanner stage 1, and has a systolic murmur. What is the pathognomonic finding, and how is it detected?

TREATMENT

Treatment should be individualized according to age, reproductive plans, and extent of disease.

- **Medical:** Aimed at inducing inactivity/atrophy of endometrial tissue.
  - **Hormonal manipulation:** OCPs, progestin, danazol, GnRH agonists.
  - All medical treatments are for symptomatic relief, not for cure, as they have no effect on the adhesions and fibrosis caused by endometriosis.
- **Surgical:**
  - **Conservative:** Laparoscopic removal of implants (excision, electrocauterization, laser ablation) that allows for future pregnancy (see Figure 6-9).
  - **Definitive:** Total abdominal hysterectomy (TAH), bilateral salpingo-oophorectomy (BSO), lysis of adhesions, and removal of all implants. In premenopausal patients, some ovarian tissue may be left intact to prevent early menopause, although there may be a recurrence of endometriosis. In patients without endogenous estrogen production (eg, patients who have no ovaries), HRT should be initiated. Some experts advocate waiting before starting HRT.

KEY FACT

Medical treatment of endometriosis is symptomatic and will not improve a patient's ability to conceive.

AMENORRHEA

KEY FACT

The workup for a patient with 1° amenorrhea is the same as that for 2° amenorrhea if the patient has both a uterus and breasts. If not, do a karyotype.

1° **amenorrhea** is defined as the absence of menses by age 16. 2° **amenorrhea** is defined as the absence of menses for 3 cycles or for 6 months with normal prior menses. Etiologies are as follows:

- **1° amenorrhea:** Constitutional delay (physiologic), pituitary failure, gonadal failure/agenesis, androgen insensitivity syndrome, müllerian abnormality, genital tract outflow obstruction, pregnancy.

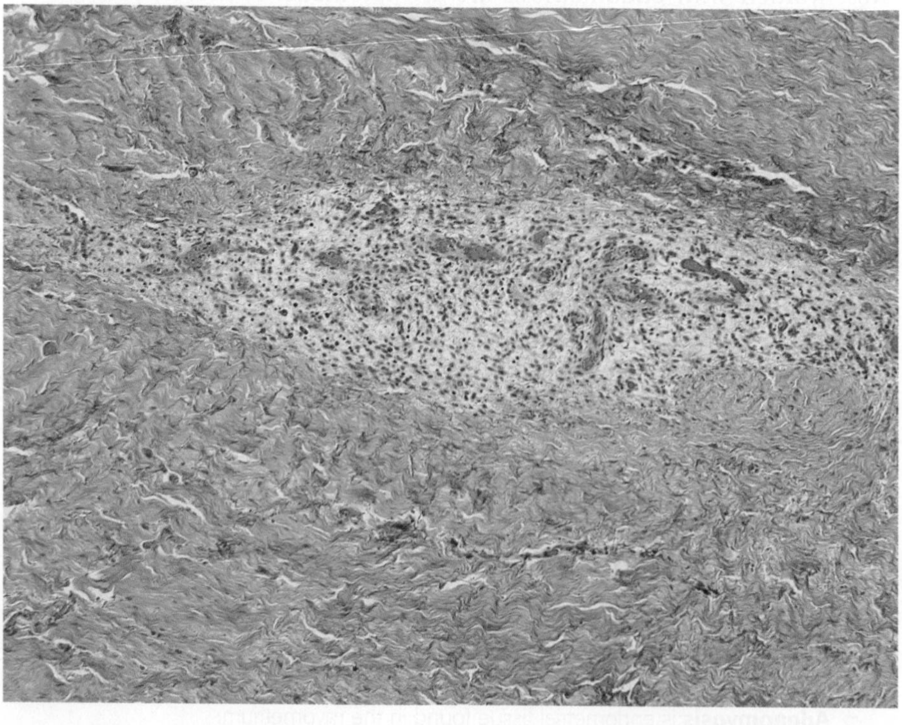

FIGURE 6-9. Endometriosis. Pathologic evaluation of an abdominal wall implant from a patient with endometriosis shows endometrial glands and stroma within dense abdominal wall connective tissue. (Reproduced with permission from USMLERx.com.)

A

Streaked ovaries are detected by pelvic ultrasound. This patient has Turner's syndrome. She presents with short stature, 1° amenorrhea, and lack of 2° sexual characteristics due to defective ovaries. Turner's is also associated with coarctation of the aorta and renal anomalies such as horseshoe kidney.

- 2° amenorrhea:
  - **Pregnancy:** The most common cause of amenorrhea.
  - **Hypothalamic causes:** Hypothyroidism, hyperprolactinemia, anorexia.
  - **Pituitary causes:** Tumor, hemosiderosis.
  - **Ovarian causes:** PCOS, premature menopause (premature ovarian failure).

WORKUP/TREATMENT

Begin by determining if the amenorrhea is 1° or 2°. If it is 1°, refer to the workup described in Figure 6-10. 2° amenorrhea is divided into 2 groups: without galactorrhea and with galactorrhea. Workup should thus proceed as follows:

- **First rule out pregnancy.**
- **With galactorrhea** (see Figure 6-11):
  - Check TSH. If abnormal, evaluate for thyroid disease.
  - If TSH is normal, check prolactin. If high, evaluate for pituitary tumor and drugs affecting pituitary function.
- **Without galactorrhea** (see Figure 6-12):
  - Do a progestin challenge. If ⊕ (withdrawal bleeding), there is adequate estrogen production, indicating anovulation. If ⊖, check LH and FSH levels.
  - Low LH/FSH indicates that the main problem lies in the hypothalamic-pituitary axis (eg, stress, nutritional imbalance, tumors) or is attributable to constitutional delay in a patient with 1° amenorrhea.
  - High LH/FSH levels indicate that the problem lies in the ovaries.
  - Consider hysteroscopy to rule out Asherman's syndrome.

KEY FACT

What should you always check in a patient with amenorrhea? That's right, a pregnancy test! Pregnancy can cause bleeding when you wouldn't expect it, and not cause bleeding when you would expect it.

KEY FACT

Do not start a patient on OCPs for amenorrhea until you are satisfied that you have determined an etiology. It may interfere with your workup.

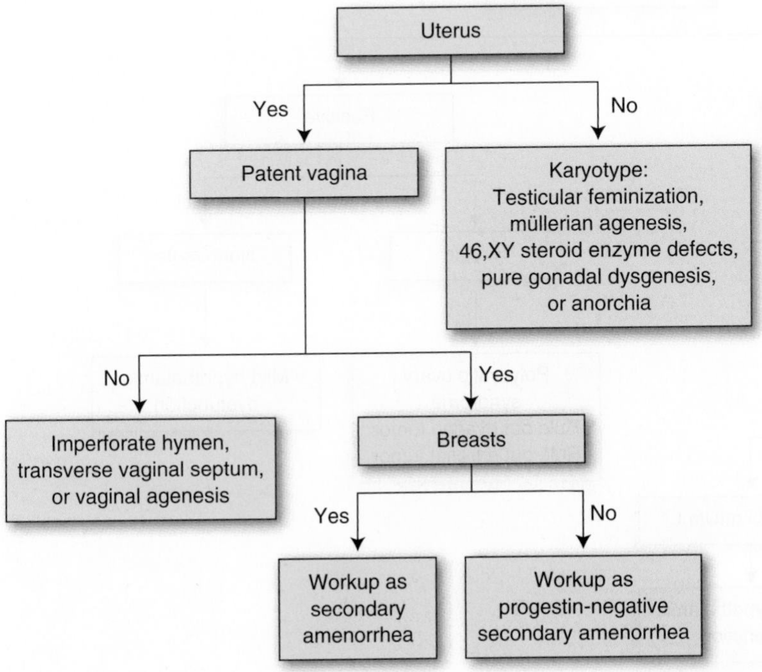

FIGURE 6-10. Workup for 1° amenorrhea. (Reproduced with permission from DeCherney AH et al. *Current Obstetric & Gynecologic Diagnosis & Treatment,* 8th ed. Stamford, CT: Appleton & Lange, 1994: 1010.)

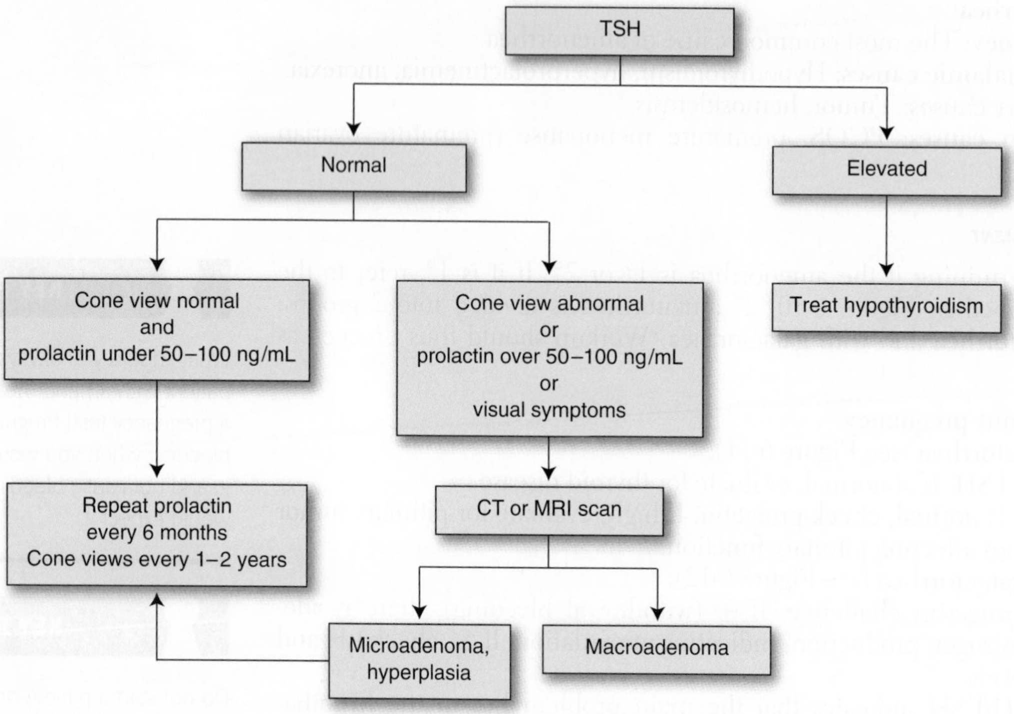

FIGURE 6-11. Workup for 2° amenorrhea with galactorrhea and hyperprolactinemia. (Reproduced with permission from DeCherney AH et al. *Current Obstetric & Gynecologic Diagnosis & Treatment,* 8th ed. Stamford, CT: Appleton & Lange, 1994: 1011.)

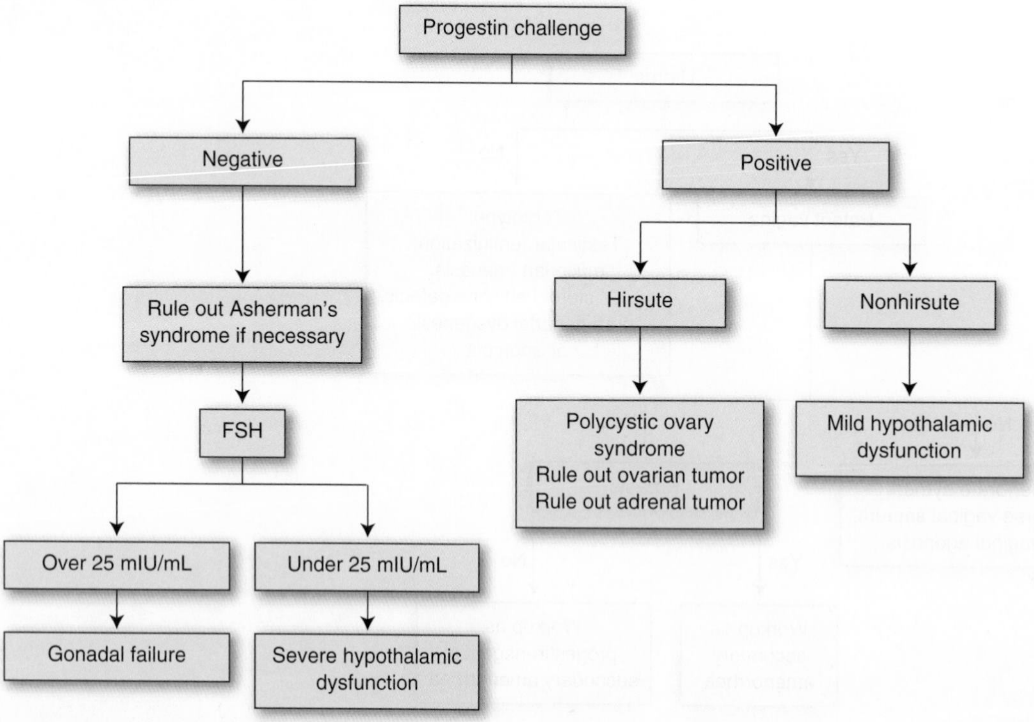

FIGURE 6-12. Workup for 2° amenorrhea without galactorrhea or hyperprolactinemia. (Reproduced with permission from DeCherney AH et al. *Current Obstetric & Gynecologic Diagnosis & Treatment,* 8th ed. Stamford, CT: Appleton & Lange, 1994: 1010.)

CONTRACEPTION

Table 6-12 summarizes the various forms of contraception available and their failure rates during the first year of use (both "lowest expected" and "typical,"

TABLE 6-12. Forms of Contraception and Their Failure Rates

Method	How Used	Percentage of Women with Pregnancy (%)[a] Lowest Expected	Typical
No Method			
None	No form of contraception	85.0	85.0
Hormonal Agents			
Combination pill	Once-daily pill	0.3	8.0
Progestin-only pill	Once-daily pill	0.3	8.0
Depo-Provera	IM injection every 12 weeks	0.3	3.0
Barrier Methods			
Male condom	With each intercourse	2.0	15.0
Female condom	With each intercourse	5.0	21.0
Diaphragm/spermicide	With each intercourse	6.0	16.0
Spermicide	With each intercourse	18.0	29.0
Cervical cap—parous	With each intercourse	26.0	32.0
Cervical cap—nulliparous	With each intercourse	9.0	16.0
IUD—Copper T	Inserted every 10 years	0.6	0.8
IUD—levonorgestrel	Inserted every 5 years	0.1	0.1
Sterilization			
Female	One-time operation	0.5	0.5
Male	One-time operation	0.10	0.15
Behavioral Methods			
Periodic abstinence	Calendar method	9.0	25.0
	Ovulation method	3.0	25.0
	Symptothermal	2.0	25.0
	Postovulation	1.0	25.0
Withdrawal	With each intercourse	4.0	27.0

[a] Data apply to the first year of use.

KEY FACT

What form of contraceptive is recommended in nursing mothers? Progestin-only pills. What is the only contraceptive effective against STIs? Condoms.

KEY FACT

Overall, the risk of any pregnancy, including ectopic pregnancy, ↓ with IUD use. In the event that a woman with an IUD does become pregnant, a greater proportion of the pregnancies will be ectopic.

KEY FACT

↑ serum FSH levels in postmenopausal women are due to feedback from fewer oocytes (and thus ↓ estrogen production) and a perceived ↑ in FSH requirement.

meaning the rate actually seen in the population). Common contraindications for combination estrogen/progesterone OCPs include the following:

- Women > 35 years of age who smoke.
- Those with a history of the following conditions:
  - **Vascular:** Thromboembolic disorders, DVT/PE, CVA, CAD, diabetes with vascular involvement, uncontrolled hypertension.
  - **Gynecologic:** Known/suspected pregnancy or undiagnosed abnormal genital bleeding.
  - **Oncologic:** Estrogen-dependent carcinoma or known/suspected breast cancer.
  - **Liver:** Active liver disease or jaundice with pill use.
  - **Other:** Migraines with aura.

MENOPAUSE

Defined as the permanent cessation of natural menses that marks the end of a woman's reproductive life. The average age of onset ranges from 45 to 55 years, with the median age 51 years. The climacteric period is the extended period of ↓ ovarian function beginning several years before and lasting years after menopause itself.

Signs and Symptoms

- **Perimenopausal symptoms:**
  - Irregular and infrequent menses.
  - Hot flashes, sleep disturbances, vaginal dryness, volatility of affect, sexual dysfunction, hair and nail brittleness.
- **Postmenopausal symptoms:** Genital tract atrophy (eg, urinary incontinence), osteoporosis, cardiovascular diseases.

Differential

Premature ovarian failure (menopause occurring prior to 42 years of age), which may be due to alkylating chemotherapy, smoking, autoimmune diseases, hysterectomy, or genetic predisposition.

Workup

- FSH, LFTs, cholesterol panel, CBC, UA.
- Obtain a mammogram, a Pap smear, and a bone density study (to screen for osteoporosis).
- Definitive diagnosis is made when serum FSH is > 25 mIU/mL at 2 separate times or when the FSH/LH ratio is > 2.

Treatment

- **HRT:** Estrogen plus progestin.
  - In light of the landmark 2002 Women's Health Initiative study correlating ↑ cardiovascular morbidity and breast cancer with prolonged HRT use, it is generally advised that HRT be used only in symptomatic patients for short durations, and only after patients have been thoroughly informed about relevant risks and benefits.
  - However, there has been substantial debate about the NIH trial that prompted these recommendations, since the majority of patients studied had been postmenopausal years before starting HRT. Therefore, it remains unclear how well the results apply to perimenopausal women.

- **Side effects** of HRT include irregular bleeding (especially in the first 6 months), weight gain, fluid retention, and endometrial hyperplasia (rare if the patient is also taking progesterone).
- **Contraindications** include a history of breast cancer, endometrial cancer, liver disease, thromboembolic disease, or MI.

- Patients should be advised to take calcium supplements, stop smoking, and exercise to prevent or minimize osteoporotic changes. A pelvic examination should be performed and a Pap smear and mammogram obtained based on the patient's own risk factor profile.
  - Women > 30 years of age who have had 3 consecutive ⊖ Pap smears, have no history of CIN 2/3 or immune compromise (including HIV infection), and were not exposed to DES in utero can have Pap smears every 3 years until age 65 or 70.
  - If the patient has these risk factors, more frequent screening may be required.

KEY FACT

If a woman still has her uterus, a combined estrogen-progestin regimen should be used for HRT to prevent endometrial hyperplasia.

INFERTILITY

Defined as the inability to get pregnant after trying for 1 year. The most important determinant of infertility in a couple is the woman's age, as conception rates are more than halved by age 35 and over. However, infertility is just as often attributed to the male as to the female. Specific etiologies are as follows:

- **Males:** Often due to a ↓ sperm count, dysfunctional sperm, or impaired sperm delivery.
- **Females:** Often due to structural damage (eg, damage to the fallopian tubes resulting from STIs or from endometriosis or fibroids), hormonal imbalances that can affect ovulation (including PCOS), or ovarian failure.
- **Both males and females:** Obesity, EtOH, smoking, improper nutrition, and age may all affect fertility.

Workup

- **Females:**
  - Workup should include measurement of body mass index (BMI); FSH and LH levels to assess ovarian function; evaluation of midluteal progesterone levels to confirm ovulation; cervical cytology and testing for STIs; ultrasound to image the ovaries and uterus; and/or hysterosalpingography to assess tubal patency.
  - If the woman has a history of irregular menses, prolactin and thyroid levels may be tested, and androgen levels may be evaluated if hyperandrogenism is suspected.
- **Males:** Workup involves semen analysis, possible hormone testing, and ultrasound imaging to visualize structural abnormalities.

Treatment

- Often begins with lifestyle modification (eg, smoking cessation and weight loss) and, if possible, treating underlying issues such as repair of a varicocele in the male.
- The next step often involves stimulation of ovulation with drugs such as clomiphene citrate or metformin in women with PCOS.
- Assisted reproductive technology includes in vitro fertilization and intracytoplasmic sperm injection. Some couples choose donor insemination.

Q

A 30-year-old female presents with infertility. She also notes pain during intercourse and rectal pain during menses. Bimanual examination reveals palpable, tender ovarian masses bilaterally. What is the gold standard for making the diagnosis?

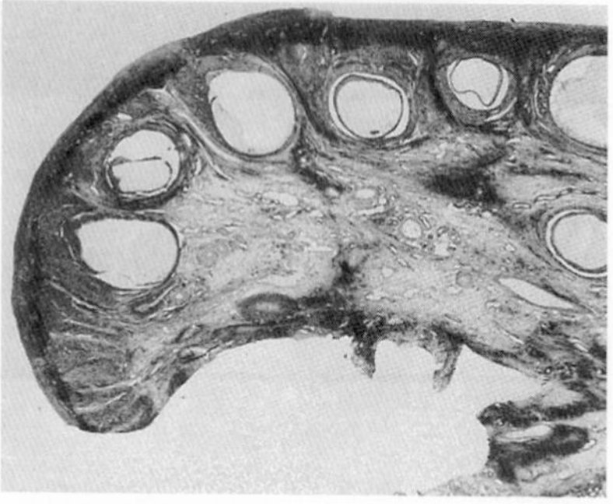

FIGURE 6-13. Polycystic ovarian syndrome. Gross specimen from a PCOS patient shows multiple enlarged peripheral ovarian follicles. (Reproduced with permission from DeCherney AH, Nathan L. *Current Diagnosis & Treatment Obstetrics & Gynecology,* 10th ed. New York: McGraw-Hill, 2007, Fig. 40-3.)

KEY FACT

In PCOS, the ovaries have a characteristic "string of pearls" appearance due to multiple follicles lined up in the ovary. There is usually no dominant follicle, and ovulation does not occur.

KEY FACT

The "whiff test," which consists of adding KOH to a vaginal prep and noting the presence of a fishlike amine odor, is pathognomonic for bacterial vaginosis.

A

This patient likely has endometriosis, best diagnosed by laparoscopy. Dyspareunia and rectal pain during menses are signs of endometrial gland hyperplasia around the cervix and pouch of Douglas. The tender ovarian masses are likely "chocolate cysts." Endometriosis can cause infertility from scarring, adhesions, and cystic infiltration of the ovaries.

POLYCYSTIC OVARIAN SYNDROME (PCOS)

Affects 5–7% of females of reproductive age. Characterized by oligo- or amenorrhea, evidence of hyperandrogenism (eg, hirsutism, acne, male-pattern hair loss), and multiple cysts in the ovaries (see Figure 6-13), which can be seen on ultrasound. Lab abnormalities include elevated LH and testosterone levels. May also be associated with insulin resistance, fertility problems due to anovulation, and metabolic syndrome.

Differential

Includes other hormonal imbalances, such as Cushing's syndrome, hyperprolactinemia, and thyroid abnormalities.

Workup

- Obtain prolactin and TSH levels to rule out other causes of the characteristic signs and symptoms.
- Measure testosterone and DHEAS levels, both of which may be elevated (if excessively elevated, consider an androgen-secreting tumor).
- Transvaginal/pelvic ultrasound to visualize the ovaries.
- A fasting blood glucose or glucose tolerance test is often performed to screen for insulin resistance.

Treatment

- Weight loss in obese patients; treatment of insulin resistance; OCPs to normalize menstrual cycles and inhibit androgens.
- Women with PCOS who experience infertility may respond to weight loss, metformin, clomiphene citrate, and/or gonadotropin therapy.

COMMON VAGINAL INFECTIONS (VAGINITIS)

The normal vaginal flora consists of approximately 25 bacterial species. The vaginal environment is normally acidic (pH 3.3–4.2) 2° to lactic acid production by colonizing lactobacillus. This acidic environment inhibits the growth of pathologic organisms. A less acidic environment can lead to bacterial proliferation and result in possible clinical infection. Table 6-13 outlines common etiologies of vaginitis.

Signs and Symptoms

- Vulvovaginal itch with or without a burning sensation.
- An abnormal odor.
- ↑ vaginal discharge.
- In examining the patient, always check the quantity, odor, and color of vaginal discharge.

Differential

The differential diagnosis for ↑ vaginal discharge includes STIs and UTIs.

Workup

- **Wet prep:** Slide smears with saline and KOH.
- **Labs:**
  - Obtain a Gram stain of the vaginal discharge and a gonorrhea and chlamydia antigen test to rule out STIs.
  - UA of a clean-catch urine specimen to rule out UTIs.

TABLE 6-13. Causes of Vaginitis

VARIABLE	BACTERIAL VAGINOSIS (USUALLY *GARDNERELLA*)	*TRICHOMONAS*	YEAST (USUALLY *CANDIDA*)
Relative frequency (%)	50	25	25
Discharge	Homogenous, grayish-white, watery; **fishy and stale odor.**	Profuse, malodorous, grayish, frothy; **"strawberry spots"** on the cervix and vaginal wall.	Thick, white, **cottage-cheese** texture.
Vaginal pH	> 4.5	> 4.5	Normal.
Saline smear[a]	**Clue cells** (epithelial cells coated with bacteria; see Figure 6-14).	**Motile** trichomonads.	Pseudohyphae; budding yeast.
KOH smear	Fishy odor.	Nothing.	Pseudohyphae; budding yeast.
Treatment	Metronidazole 500 mg PO BID × 7 days or 2 g PO single dose.[b] Alternatives include clindamycin or tinidazole. Metronidazole or clindamycin vaginal cream may also be considered.	Metronidazole 2 g PO single dose. Treat the partner, as this is considered an STI.	Miconazole (Monistat) or nystatin.

[a] If you see many WBCs and no organism on saline smear, suspect chlamydia.

[b] Patients taking metronidazole should not drink alcohol, as this can result in an Antabuse-like effect.

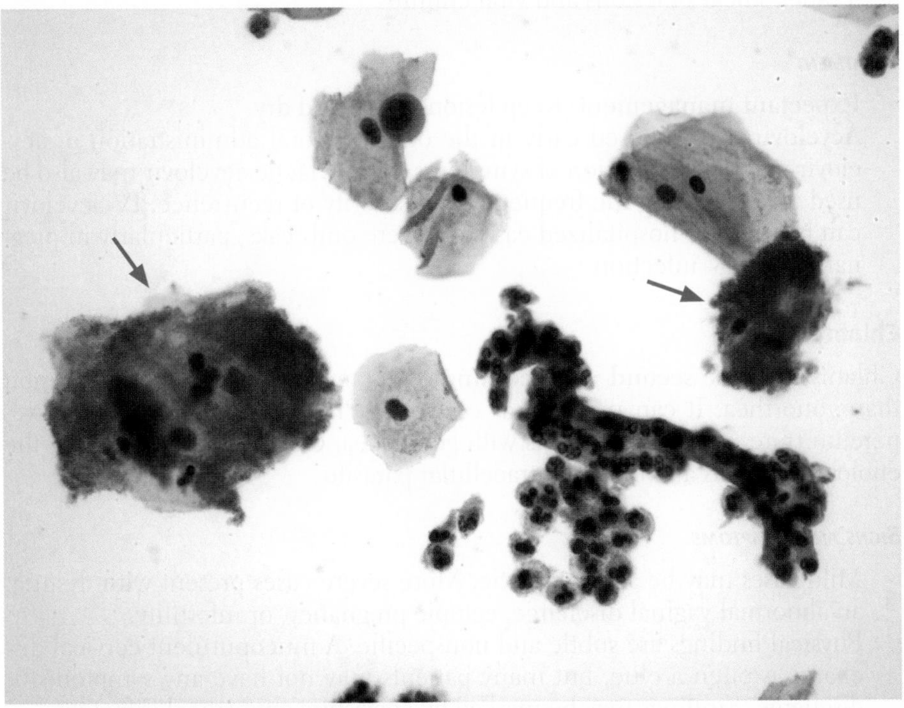

FIGURE 6-14. Bacterial vaginosis. Pap smear shows several "clue cells" (arrows) that are epithelial squamous cells coated by *Gardnerella vaginalis*, giving them a purple coat. (Reproduced with permission from USMLERx.com.)

KEY FACT

Some 20–50% of patients with an STI have coexisting infections, creating a low threshold for detecting other infectious diseases. All contacts of the patient must be treated.

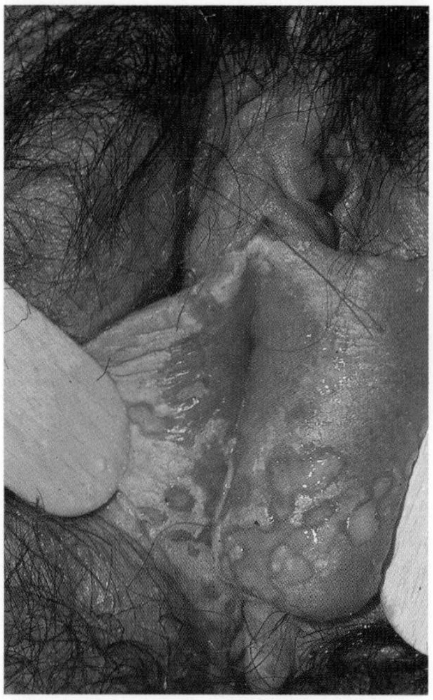

FIGURE 6-15. Genital herpes. Large, painful erosions on the labia minora are seen in a patient with recurrent genital herpes. (Reproduced with permission from Wolff K, Johnson RA. *Fitzpatrick's Color Atlas & Synopsis of Clinical Dermatology*, 6th ed. New York: McGraw-Hill, 2009, Fig. 30-16.)

KEY FACT

Look for multinucleated giant cells on Tzanck smear in patients with genital herpes.

KEY FACT

Gonorrhea and chlamydia travel together. When gram-⊖ diplococci are seen, add azithromycin or doxycycline to cover for chlamydia.

TREATMENT

Treatments for specific types of vaginitis are discussed in Table 6-13.

SEXUALLY TRANSMITTED INFECTIONS (STIs)

Taken together, STIs are one of the most common gynecologic problems encountered in the outpatient setting. All sexually active patients must therefore be examined with an awareness of a possible STI. Patients often have a past history of STIs, which can be elicited through careful and tactful history taking.

Genital Herpes

Herpes simplex is the **most common** STI and is highly infectious (75% transmission rate). Etiologies are HSV type 2 (90%) and type 1 (10%).

SIGNS AND SYMPTOMS

- **1° infection:** Characterized by malaise, low-grade fever, and adenopathy.
  - The **prodromal phase** presents with mild paresthesia and burning.
  - Painful vesicular lesions arise 3–7 days after exposure.
- **Physical findings:** Physical examination reveals multiple clear vesicles that may have lysed, progressing to painful ulcers with red borders that coalesce and become secondarily infected. Lesions can be found on the vulva, vagina, cervix, perineum, and perianal area (see Figure 6-15).

WORKUP

- Obtain a thorough sexual history and look for the physical findings outlined above.
- Tzanck smear of lesions and viral cultures.

TREATMENT

- **Expectant management:** Keep lesions clean and dry.
- **Acyclovir:** If diagnosed early in the outbreak, oral administration of acyclovir may ↓ the duration of symptoms. Prophylactic acyclovir may also be used for decreasing the frequency and severity of recurrence; IV acyclovir can be used for hospitalized cases or severe outbreaks, particularly in pregnancy or HIV infection.

Chlamydia

Chlamydia is the **second most common** STI and is 10 times more common than gonorrhea. It can manifest as cervicitis, PID, or lymphogranuloma venereum (rare) and often coexists with gonorrhea. *Chlamydia trachomatis*, the etiologic agent, is an obligate intracellular parasite.

SIGNS AND SYMPTOMS

- Mild cases may be asymptomatic. More severe cases present with dysuria, an abnormal vaginal discharge, ectopic pregnancy, or infertility.
- Physical findings are subtle and nonspecific. A mucopurulent cervical discharge is often a clue, but many patients may not have any symptoms or discharge. Findings may be masked by coexisting gonorrheal infection.

WORKUP

- Monoclonal antibody test (faster).
- Enzyme immunoassay of the cervical secretion (has 95% specificity).
- Always check for **concomitant gonorrheal infection** (cultures, smear).

TREATMENT

Azithromycin, tetracycline, or doxycycline (erythromycin may be substituted in allergic or pregnant patients). Treatment is associated with a 95% cure rate.

COMPLICATIONS

Insidious tubal damage leading to infertility.

> **KEY FACT**
>
> Lymphogranuloma venereum is an STI caused by *Chlamydia* that is usually seen outside the United States. It is characterized by painless ulcers and large draining lymph nodes.

Gonorrhea

Gonorrhea remains a very common infection. An ↑ frequency has also been observed with penicillin-resistant strains in asymptomatic infections. *Neisseria gonorrhoeae*, the etiologic agent, is a gram-⊖ intracellular diplococcus.

SIGNS AND SYMPTOMS

- Presents with a malodorous, purulent, yellow-green discharge from the cervix, vagina, Skene's ducts, urethra, or anus.
- Some 10–20% of affected heterosexual women also have gonorrhea infection in the pharynx.

WORKUP

- Gram stain of discharge.
- Cultures from the discharge on Thayer-Martin medium (80–95% sensitivity).
- Obtain an enzyme immunoassay for gonorrhea and chlamydia antigen, as there is a high rate of coinfection.

> **KEY FACT**
>
> A 1-time dose of azithromycin will cover both chlamydia and gonorrhea but may cause GI upset.

TREATMENT

Maintain a low threshold for treating patients for gonorrhea; it is valid to treat on clinical grounds alone. The choice of antibiotics depends on the site of infection and has recently been updated on the basis of the CDC's 2010 treatment guidelines:

- **Urethral, cervical, or rectal infection:** Ceftriaxone 250 mg IM single dose or cefixime 400 mg orally single dose. Include an azithromycin or doxycycline regimen for chlamydia coverage.
- **Pharyngeal infection:** Ceftriaxone 250 mg IM single dose. Include an azithromycin or doxycycline regimen for chlamydia coverage.

> **KEY FACT**
>
> Roughly 15% of women infected with gonorrhea will progress to PID if untreated.

Condylomata Acuminata (Venereal Warts)

Condylomata acuminata are almost as common as gonorrhea infection. Unlike other STIs, however, the sequelae may take years to manifest. The etiologic agent is HPV. Condylomata acuminata are commonly associated with serotypes 6 and 11; cervical neoplasia is associated with serotypes 16, 18, and 31.

> **KEY FACT**
>
> Venereal warts and cervical dysplasia are associated with different serotypes of HPV.

> **KEY FACT**
>
> HPV serotypes 16, 18, and 31 are highly associated with cervical cancer.

SIGNS AND SYMPTOMS

- Presents with painless bumps, discharge, and pruritus.
- Physical findings include soft, fleshy, exophytic, papular, verrucous, flat, or macular growths on the cervix, vagina, vulva, urethral meatus, perineum, or perianal area. Lesions are often symmetrical.
- Coinfection with *Trichomonas* or *Gardnerella* is common.

WORKUP

The presumptive diagnosis is made with physical findings. The diagnosis can be confirmed with a biopsy of warts following 5% acetic acid staining.

> **Q**
>
> A 30-year-old female with a history of multiple sexual partners and recent unprotected intercourse presents with 3 days of fever and a mucus-like vaginal discharge. On bimanual examination, the cervix is extremely tender to palpation. What is the danger if this patient goes untreated?

KEY FACT

Pap smear of the cervix diagnoses only about 5% of patients infected with HPV.

KEY FACT

Argyll Robertson pupil, which refers to pupils that accommodate but do not react, is a pathognomonic finding for 3° syphilis.

KEY FACT

Argyll Robertson pupil = "prostitute's pupil": It will accommodate but will not react.

KEY FACT

A false RPR can be caused by pregnancy, lupus, antiphospholipid antibodies, and certain viral infections, including HIV, Lyme disease, and yaws.

A

This patient has acute PID, which is most often caused by *N gonorrhoeae* and/or *C trachomatis.* Without prompt antibiotic treatment, the infection can lead to abscess formation and septic shock or to eventual scarring of the uterus, fallopian tubes, and/or ovaries.

TREATMENT

- **External and vaginal lesions:** Condylox, cryotherapy, CO_2 laser, or trichloroacetic acid.
- **Cervical lesions:** Colposcopy and potential biopsy of the cervix; cryotherapy, laser, or loop electrosurgical excision procedure (LEEP).
- Lesions are often more resistant to therapy in pregnant, diabetic, and immunosuppressed patients.

Syphilis

The incidence of syphilis has been rising over the past few years owing to the increasing prevalence of drug-resistant strains. *Treponema pallidum*, a motile spirochete, is the etiologic agent.

SIGNS AND SYMPTOMS

Presentation depends on disease stage:

- **1° (10–60 days after infection):** Presents with a **painless ulcer** (chancre) of the vulva, vagina, cervix, anus, rectum, pharynx, lips, or fingers. The chancre heals spontaneously in 3–9 weeks.
- **2° (4–8 weeks after the appearance of the chancre):**
  - Low-grade fever, headache, malaise, generalized lymphadenopathy.
  - A diffuse, symmetric, asymptomatic maculopapular rash on the soles and palms.
  - Condyloma latum, which heals spontaneously in 2–6 weeks.
- **3° (1–20 years after the initial infection):** Destructive, granulomatous **gummas** can be seen that cause systemic damage to the CNS, heart, or great vessels. Complicated by aortitis, meningovascular disease, and tabes dorsalis.

WORKUP

- **Screening test:** VDRL or RPR (rapid but nonspecific).
- **FTA-ABS/MHA-TP:** Very specific; perform if RPR is ⊕.
- Dark-field microscopy (motile spirochetes) of 1° or 2° lesions.

TREATMENT

- **Penicillin** is the treatment of choice for 1°, 2°, and 3° syphilis.
- Tetracycline or penicillin desensitization for allergic patients. In light of the risk of congenital syphilis, patients must be treated with penicillin during pregnancy.
- Transplacental spread can occur at any stage of syphilis and can lead to congenital syphilis.

PELVIC INFLAMMATORY DISEASE (PID)

An upper genital tract infection that usually results from an ascending infection from the cervix. The lifetime risk is 1–3%. Causative organisms include *N gonorrhoeae* (one-third of cases), *C trachomatis*, and anaerobes/aerobes (eg, *E coli, Bacteroides*). Risk factors include multiple sexual partners, unprotected intercourse, new partners within 30 days of becoming symptomatic, cigarette smoking, and recent placement of an IUD or surgical instrumentation.

SIGNS AND SYMPTOMS

- Presents with a 1- to 3-day history of lower abdominal pain with or without fever; a vaginal discharge, recent menses, a history of sexual exposure, and a past history of PID may also be seen.

- Other findings include the following:
  - Lower abdominal tenderness.
  - CMT.
  - An adnexal mass and/or tenderness.

DIFFERENTIAL

Ectopic pregnancy, endometriosis, ovarian torsion, hemorrhagic ovarian cyst, appendicitis, diverticulitis, UTI.

WORKUP

- **Diagnostic criteria** are as follows:
  - A history of abdominal pain and findings of abdominal tenderness with or without rebound (90%).
  - CMT.
  - Adnexal tenderness (should be bilateral).
- **Additional criteria,** 1 of which is required to establish the diagnosis, are as follows:
  - A temperature > 38°C (> 100.4°F).
  - A WBC count > 10,000 cells/mm^3.
  - An inflammatory mass (tubo-ovarian abscess) on examination/sonography.
  - Culdocentesis that yields peritoneal fluid with bacteria and WBCs.
  - The presence of *N gonorrhoeae* and/or *C trachomatis* on the endocervix.
- **Labs:**
  - CBC (WBC > 10,000 cells/mm^3), ESR (> 15 mm/hr), β-hCG (to assess for possible ectopic pregnancy).
  - Gram stain of cervical discharge.
  - RPR/VDRL (to rule out syphilis); HIV and hepatitis screen.
- **Imaging:**
  - Ultrasound to detect an inflammatory mass.
  - Laparoscopy for the definitive diagnosis of edema and erythema of the fallopian tubes and purulent exudate. Note that laparoscopy has been shown to confirm the clinical diagnosis in approximately 60% of cases.

TREATMENT

- **Inpatient vs. outpatient management:** Most patients can be treated with outpatient therapy. However, inpatient management should be considered for patients with severe nausea/vomiting that precludes the use of oral antibiotics, as well as for those who are pregnant, are immune deficient, or have a suspected tubo-ovarian abscess from untreated PID. Otherwise, inpatient management can be reserved for those who do not clinically improve after 72 hours of outpatient therapy.
  - **Outpatient treatment:** Oral cefoxitin or ceftriaxone and doxycycline.
  - **Inpatient treatment:** IV cefotetan and doxycycline (orally or IV).
- Admit patients for IV antibiotics in the presence of the following:
  - A temperature > 38°C (> 100.4°F).
  - Suspected pelvic or tubo-ovarian abscess.
  - Nausea and vomiting that would prevent compliance with the administration of oral medications.
  - Signs of peritonitis.
  - Pregnancy.
  - A possible surgical emergency such as appendicitis.
  - Lack of clinical response to an oral regimen.
- **Surgery:** Warranted if the diagnosis is uncertain or if the patient has a tubo-ovarian abscess that is unresponsive to parenteral antibiotics.

KEY FACT

The insertion of IUDs carries an ↑ risk of PID. IUDs are indicated in monogamous women at low risk for STIs.

KEY FACT

The chandelier sign is severe CMT on examination that makes the patient "jump for the chandelier."

KEY FACT

Fitz-Hugh–Curtis syndrome is perihepatitis from ascending infection, generally from gonorrhea or chlamydia infection. It presents with RUQ pain, ↑ LFTs, and perihepatic adhesions that can lead to infertility.

KEY FACT

Ask your patients about urinary incontinence. Much of the time, they will not volunteer this information.

KEY FACT

All patients with urinary incontinence should have a UA and urine culture.

COMPLICATIONS

- ↑ (tenfold) risk of an ectopic pregnancy.
- ↑ (fourfold) risk of chronic pelvic pain.
- Infertility (15% after a single episode and 75% after 3 episodes).
- Recurrent PID.
- Fitz-Hugh–Curtis syndrome (found in 15–30% of PID cases).

URINARY INCONTINENCE

At some point in their lives, almost half of all women will be affected by urinary incontinence. Many women will not volunteer that this is an issue unless the subject is broached by their care provider. As women age, they experience greater degrees of pelvic relaxation and a greater incidence of urinary incontinence, especially daily incontinence. Table 6-14 summarizes the main types of urinary incontinence as well as their risk factors, diagnosis, and treatment.

TABLE 6-14. Types of Urinary Incontinence

	STRESS	URGE	OVERFLOW	TOTAL
Symptoms	Urine loss with coughing, laughing, or straining.	Dribbling/leaking regardless of whether the bladder is full. Sense of not being able to reach the bathroom in time.	Urinary retention, poor stream, straining to void.	Continuous urine leakage.
Risk factors	Menopause, pelvic relaxation, chronically ↑ intra-abdominal pressure (eg, cough, ascites).	Most cases are idiopathic. Recurrent UTIs. Neurologic disease (eg, Alzheimer's, diabetes, Parkinson's). Bladder foreign bodies or irritants.	Epidural anesthesia (95% of cases). Neurologic disease (eg, MS, spinal cord injury).	Pelvic surgery, pelvic radiation, PID.
Diagnostic tests	Standing stress test, cotton swab test, urethroscopy. Cystometrogram (distinguishes stress from urge incontinence). Normal residual volume.	Cystometrogram; normal/↓ residual volume.	Uroflowmetry; ↑ residual volume.	Localize the fistula with indigo carmine, methylene blue, or cystourethroscopy.
Treatment	Kegel exercises, estrogen replacement, α-agonists, pessaries, surgery to restore hypermobile bladder neck to anatomic position.	Anticholinergics, β-agonists, smooth muscle relaxants, TCAs, Kegel exercises, behavior modification.	α-agonists, striated muscle relaxants, cholinergic agents, self-catheterization, surgical removal of obstruction if present.	Surgery to repair fistula.

GYNECOLOGIC ONCOLOGY

Table 6-15 summarizes the essentials of the 3 important gynecologic cancers.

TABLE 6-15. Common Gynecologic Cancers

Variable	Cervical Cancer	Endometrial Cancer	Ovarian Cancer
Symptoms	Postcoital bleeding; foul discharge. May be asymptomatic.	Postmenopausal uterine bleeding; palpable abdominal and pelvic masses.	↑ abdominal girth (ascites). Often asymptomatic until late stages. GI and GU complaints; thrombophlebitis; lower abdominal pain/pressure.
Risk factors	Anything that ↑ the risk of or indication of HPV infection, including venereal warts, early sexual activity, multiple sexual partners, and smoking.	Chronic, unopposed estrogen stimulation (eg, PCOS, estrogen-only contraceptives, DES exposure). Obesity, nulliparity, endometrial hyperplasia, DM, hypertension, early menarche, late menopause, anovulation, family history.	Nulliparity, breast cancer, family history. OCPs may have a protective role in ↓ the risk of ovarian cancer.
Screening	Pap smears should be obtained once every 2 years starting at age 21 regardless of the age at which sexual activity commenced. Women > 30 years of age with 3 consecutive ⊖ results can be screened once every 3 years until age 65. Patients with risk factors such as HIV, immunosuppression, in utero DES exposure, or prior CIN 2, CIN 3, or cervical cancer treatment should be screened more frequently. If HPV infection is detected, colposcopy should follow for diagnostic testing.	None (Pap smear is only 50% effective in detecting uterine cancer).	None (routine ultrasound and CA-125 are not cost-efficient).
Diagnosis	Punch and/or cone biopsy.	Ultrasound (see Figure 6-16), endometrial biopsy, D&C.	Ultrasound, pelvic MRI, abdominal CT, CA-125 for epithelial cancers; AFP and β-hCG for germ cell cancers.
Treatment	**Early stage:** Cervical conization, hysterectomy (see Figure 6-17), radiotherapy, radical lymphadenectomy. **Advanced stage:** Irradiation/chemotherapy only (surgery would harm the bladder and rectum without being effective).	TAH-BSO, and peritoneal washing for cytology +/– pelvic and aortic node sampling. Radiotherapy, chemotherapy, progesterone.	TAH-BSO, omentectomy, and peritoneal washing for cytology +/– pelvic and aortic node sampling. Tumor debulking, chemotherapy.

(continues)

TABLE 6-15. Common Gynecologic Cancers *(continued)*

VARIABLE	CERVICAL CANCER	ENDOMETRIAL CANCER	OVARIAN CANCER
Prevention	Safe sex (condoms) to ↓ the risk of HPV infection. Smoking cessation; routine Pap smears.	Progesterone to oppose estrogen; low-fat diet, weight control.	OCPs. Oophorectomy in patients with a strong family history of ovarian cancer.
Notes	Some 85% are squamous cell carcinoma and 15% adenocarcinoma. Unless nephrostomy tubes are placed, renal failure is the most common cause of death in patients with end-stage cervical cancer.	The **most common gynecologic cancer.** The fourth most common cancer in women (after breast, colorectal, lung). Most are adenocarcinoma. Endometrial hyperplasia is the precursor lesion and is treated with progesterone.	The **most lethal** gynecologic cancer. Complications include ovarian rupture, torsion, hemorrhage, infection, and infarction. The most common cause of death in end-stage ovarian cancer is bowel obstruction.

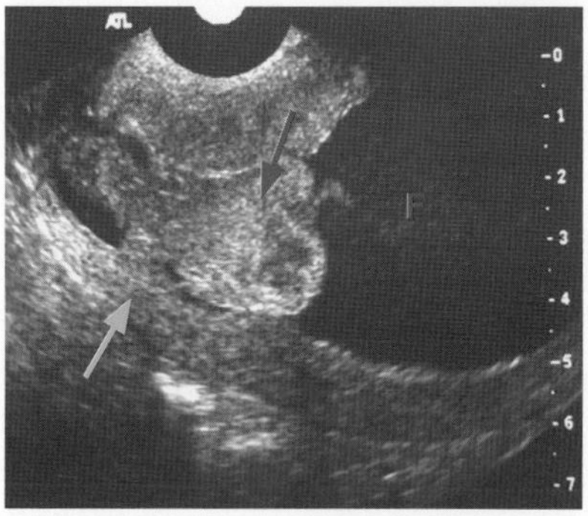

FIGURE 6-16. Endometrial cancer. Endovaginal ultrasound of a 53-year-old postmenopausal woman with vaginal bleeding shows a lobulated mass (red arrow) within the endometrial canal originating from the lower uterine segment (yellow arrow). Note the abnormal fluid (F) distending the endometrial cavity beyond the mass. Biopsy showed endometrial carcinoma. (Reproduced with permission from USMLERx.com.)

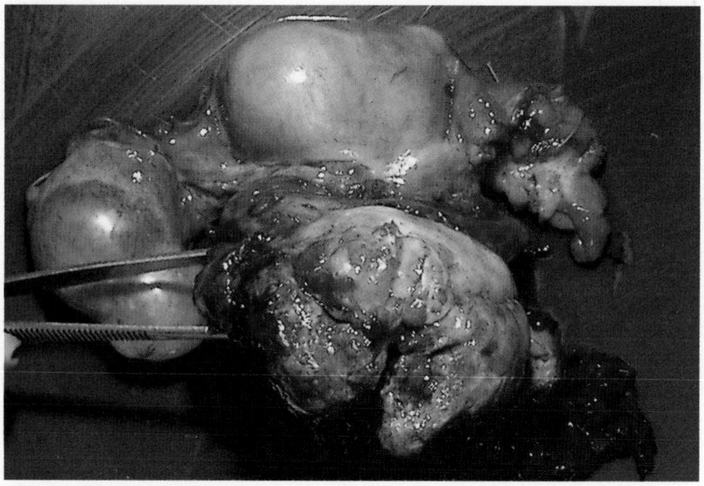

FIGURE 6-17. Cervical cancer. Gross specimen from a hysterectomy and bilateral salpingo-oophorectomy shows a large irregular fungating cervical mass that was proven on biopsy to be cervical cancer. (Reproduced with permission from USMLERx.com.)

Common Clerkship Topics

In OB/GYN, you should be able to generate a differential diagnosis for common problems; perfect a systematic way of working up a patient; gain experience in performing a thorough pelvic examination with a Pap smear; and, it is hoped, find an appreciation of the process of birth. You can also learn about commonly used modalities such as ultrasonography, cervical biopsies, and fetal monitoring. The following list outlines common disease entities, conditions, and topics that you are likely to encounter during your OB/GYN rotation and on a shelf examination.

- **Obstetrics:**
  - Normal physiology of pregnancy
  - Prenatal care
  - Medical conditions in pregnancy
    - Gestational diabetes
    - Hypertension in pregnancy
  - Complications of pregnancy
    - PROM/PPROM
    - First-trimester bleeding
    - Spontaneous abortion
    - Ectopic pregnancy (see Emergency Medicine)
    - Hydatidiform mole
    - Third-trimester bleeding
- **Labor and delivery:**
  - Normal labor
  - Preterm labor
  - Abnormal labor patterns
  - Fetal heart rate monitoring
  - Postpartum hemorrhage
- **Gynecology:**
  - Abnormal uterine bleeding
  - Amenorrhea
  - Common vaginal infections (vaginitis)
  - Contraception
  - Endometriosis
  - Gynecologic oncology
  - Infertility
  - Menopause
  - Pelvic inflammatory disease
  - Premenstrual syndrome
  - Preventive care (primarily HPV, breast cancer, and STI screening guidelines)
  - Sexually transmitted infections
    - Genital herpes
    - Chlamydia
    - Gonorrhea
    - Condylomata acuminata
    - Syphilis
  - Urinary incontinence

CHAPTER 7

PEDIATRICS

Ward Tips

Welcome to pediatrics! The pediatric rotation is a 6- to 8-week block at most medical schools, with time split between inpatient and outpatient settings. In the past, more time has traditionally been devoted to the inpatient service, but this may change given the current emphasis on outpatient primary care. The outpatient portion of the pediatrics rotation may be completed in a community pediatrician's office, the hospital's outpatient clinic, or the emergency department (ED). In addition, a week or less is generally devoted to the newborn nursery.

WHO ARE THE PLAYERS?

The ward team typically consists of an attending, 1–2 upper-level residents, 2–4 interns, and 1–4 medical students.

Attendings. The attending may be a member of the general pediatric faculty or one of the pediatric subspecialties. The attending is responsible for the majority of patients on the service, and depending on your institution, you may or may not present to him or her on a daily basis. You will have an opportunity to formally present patients during attending rounds and will also interact with your attending during didactic teaching sessions. It is therefore advisable that you become familiar with your attending's area of interest, as he or she is likely to focus on those topics during rounds. It would also be helpful to clarify expectations and set clear goals for the rotation with your attending at the start of the rotation.

Residents. Residents are responsible for running the service and supervising the interns and medical students. They perform most of the daily teaching and are a great source of knowledge. They report directly to the attending and play a critical role in your clinical evaluations.

Interns. Interns are responsible for monitoring patients' daily progress and doing the "grunt work." They are extremely busy and are often thankful if you can help them by comanaging patients and writing the daily progress note. Discuss each patient's assessment and plan (A&P) with your intern so that you understand the rationale behind all orders, tests, and consults you have requested. By doing so, you will be more informed when you present to the residents and attending.

Nurses, social workers, nutritionists, child life specialist. As on other services, these specialists are invaluable sources of information about your patients. In particular, make sure you always speak to nurses before morning rounds and shift change, as nurses spend the most time with patients and can usually summarize overnight events. Always inform nurses of the daily plan regarding your patients, and include them on decisions made by the team. Social workers, child life specialists, and nutritionists are also commonly consulted in pediatrics, so it is imperative that you build a good relationship with these providers and make use of their knowledge whenever you can.

HOW IS THE DAY SET UP?

The schedule of a typical day on the ward is as follows:

6:30–8:00 A.M.	Prerounds
8:00–9:00 A.M.	Team rounds
9:00–10:00 A.M.	Attending rounds
10:00 A.M.–12:00 noon	Complete progress notes; order labs, imaging, medications, and other tests; obtain consults, speak with primary care providers, and obtain outside hospital records
Noon–1:00 P.M.	Lunch or noon conference
1:00–5:00 P.M.	Check afternoon labs; check in on patient and family; follow up on consult notes and daily goals; sign out to the intern and senior resident; admit new patients

WHAT DO I DO DURING PREROUNDS?

In general, prerounding should begin by getting sign-out from the overnight intern or medical student and checking in with the nurses who are caring for your patients. Children should be examined during prerounds even if they are still sleeping. However, you should ask your resident if there are any patients who should not be examined prior to morning rounds. You may also wake a patient's parents to ask how their child is doing. Be sure to check the chart for any important labs, imaging, diagnostic testing results, and vitals. Allow yourself some extra time, as calculations often need to be done prior to rounds. Also note that most numbers are reported on a per-kilogram basis. For example, input (fluids and formula) is reported as cc/kg/day or kcal/kg/day, and urine output is reported as cc/kg/hr. Medication dosages are also reported on a per-kilogram basis.

KEY FACT

In pediatrics, most numbers (I's and O's, medication dosages) are reported on a per-kilogram basis.

HOW DO I EXCEL IN PEDIATRICS?

The following are some useful tips on how to maximize your performance on the pediatrics rotation.

- **Know your patient.** Remember that you have the time to investigate patients thoroughly so that your busy interns, residents, and attendings can turn to you for the detailed information they may not have obtained during their workups. Important but often not thoroughly investigated aspects of the admission history and physical (H&P) are diet, immunization history, developmental milestones, birth history, and social history.
- **Communicate with your patient and parents.** This rotation is unique in that you will need to interact with concerned (and, unfortunately, sometimes unconcerned) parents in addition to your patients. You will likely have the most time to speak with a child's family and may enjoy a closer relationship with them than anyone else on the team. For this reason, you

should attempt to earn the trust of your pediatric patient and parents by maintaining open lines of communication with regard to the child's condition, prognosis, and planned procedures. No one knows the patient better than the primary caregiver, so listen carefully. At times, parents may ask you questions that lie beyond your medical knowledge. An incorrect answer could undermine their trust in you, so you should never give them an answer if you are unsure of its validity. You will not lose face for not having all the answers; to the contrary, parents will respect you for being honest and keeping them informed.

- **Read about the patients you admitted as soon as you get the chance.** The sooner you read about a patient's problem, the more likely it will be that you will remember the topic—and the more knowledgeable you will be when you present to your team. Review articles are a great learning tool and will help you discover questions you should have asked and new labs, diagnostic tests, and imaging you could have ordered. If you want to be a superstar, do a quick PubMed search and learn about a hot topic of ongoing research to discuss with your team on rounds the following morning.
- **Practice your presentation.** Typically, the only time your attending has the chance to see you at work is during rounds, so use this time to your advantage. Make sure your presentations are organized, precise, accurate, and, whenever possible, done from memory. Also make sure that the A&P sections are well thought out and have been discussed with the intern or resident beforehand. Pointing to a review article or pertinent evidence-based guidelines about your topic will show your commitment and enthusiasm.
- **Ask for feedback.** The attendings and residents will usually schedule a time for feedback halfway through the rotation. If they don't schedule such time, ask for it, but always be mindful of their time commitments and daily responsibilities. Request that they give you a detailed evaluation of your performance, emphasizing areas in which you can improve. Try not to accept the answer that you are "doing fine," and always get some constructive feedback. However, avoid repeatedly asking for feedback, as you may come across as being overbearing.
- **Act professionally and respect your colleagues.** Nothing looks worse than a situation in which team members are overtly criticizing one another, especially in front of a patient. This undermines a patient's trust and can also compromise care. So if you need to say something to a colleague, save it until you have left the patient's room, and express your thoughts tactfully. It is crucial to maintain morale so that your team can continue to work together as a cohesive unit.
- **Read about bread-and-butter pediatric topics on a daily basis.** These topics are listed later in this chapter and are critical to success both in the clerkship and on the shelf examination. A great resource to use is the journal *Pediatrics in Review*, which contains excellent review articles about important pediatrics topics.

KEY NOTES

The H&P and daily progress notes for pediatrics are similar to those of medicine, but there are a few variations:

- **Source:** You may obtain the history from the parent, the patient, other caregivers, or any combination of the above.

- **History of present illness (HPI):** Key questions include recent diet history (changes in appetite, feeding history), number of wet diapers, bowel movements, changes in energy or irritability, sick contacts, recent travel, and other environmental changes.
- **Past medical history (PMH):** This should include maternal history (mother's age, gravida, para, abortions, pregnancy course); details of the pregnancy (onset of prenatal care, weight gain, complications such as diabetes or hypertension, blood type, Coombs' test, rubella immunity status, RPR/VDRL); group B strep, chlamydia, HIV, PPD, and HBV status; drug/alcohol/tobacco use; labor and delivery details (spontaneous or induced, duration, complications, presentation, method of delivery, presence of meconium); neonatal history (birth weight, gestational age [GA], nursery complications, length of stay); and a history of other hospitalizations, surgeries, or injuries. Note that the pregnancy and neonatal history may not be relevant to all admissions.
- **Nutrition:** For infants, include information on breast milk or formula type, frequency, and amount. For toddlers, include the introduction of cereal and baby foods as well as the amount of milk intake per day. For older children, discuss appetite and types of food eaten.
- **Growth:** For infants, plot length, weight, weight-for-length, and head circumference on the growth chart and assess for trends. For children > 2 years of age, plot height, weight, and body mass index (BMI) on the growth chart. Remember to use the correct CDC and WHO growth charts, as these charts differ based on age.
- **Immunization:** This is a very important section. Ask to see the patient's immunization record, and obtain records from the family's pediatrician if necessary. Always ask about influenza status.
- **Developmental history:** Ask the parents when the child first began to sit, walk, and talk and when he or she completed toilet training. For children < 6 years of age, the Denver Developmental Assessment is a useful tool with which to gauge a child's language acquisition, motor development, and social interactions. For older children, be sure to ask about school performance.
- **Family history (FH):** Simply asking if there are medical problems that run in the family will often prove unproductive, so it is important to specifically ask about childhood illnesses or diseases. Focus on inherited diseases, consanguinity, sudden infant death syndrome (SIDS), miscarriages, early deaths, congenital anomalies, developmental delay, mental retardation, sickle cell disease, asthma, seizure disorders, atopy, and cardiovascular diseases. It is also helpful to include a pedigree chart.
- **Social history (SH):** This is an important section in pediatrics and should include information about the home environment such as who lives at home, tobacco/alcohol/drug use in the home, and childproofing. Asking and carefully counseling caregivers about smoking cannot be emphasized enough. Other components include the child's interaction with the family, the primary caregiver in the household, and parental contact information. For younger children, ask about day care (↑ exposure to communicable diseases) and pets in the house (eg, cats or dogs provoking asthma exacerbations; pet baby turtles causing *Salmonella*). Also include information about school history, activities, and hobbies. A psychosocial assessment should be tailored to the age of the child; the basic components for adolescent patients are outlined in the mnemonic **HEADDSSS.**

KEY FACT

Don't forget to plot **all** children on growth charts and assess trends! This may require obtaining information from the child's pediatrician.

MNEMONIC

Components of a pediatric social history—

HEADDSSS

Home life
Education, **E**mployment
Activities (sports, school, friends)
Drugs (alcohol, tobacco, illicit drugs)
Depression
Suicide
Safety
Sexual activity

TIPS FOR EXAMINING CHILDREN

Starting at around 8 months, infants often have anxiety toward strangers, and it is thus very common for children to cry during the examination. Here are some useful tips:

- While taking the history, sit near the child so that he or she will become accustomed to your presence. Children will often become interested in you and your examination tools. You can start to examine the child while you are taking the history.
- Take off your white coat before entering the room (unless your attending prefers otherwise). Consider wearing a tie with cartoon characters on it, or perhaps wearing a sticker on your shirt. Take time to play with the young patient before attempting a physical examination.
- For infants and toddlers, perform as much of the examination as possible with the child in the parent's lap. If the patient is in respiratory distress (which may worsen with agitation), the child should be left in the parent's arms.
- Distraction with a toy, name badge, mirror, or penlight works well for young children (those < 2 years of age) and can help you assess how well a child visually tracks objects. Giving older children a "task" to perform during your examination will help ensure their cooperation.
- Let the child touch and play with the instruments. Demonstrate what you are about to do on yourself, a parent, or a stuffed animal to let the child know that the procedure is not painful. Save the invasive and painful parts of the examination for the end.
- Perform the cardiac and pulmonary portion of the examination first, while the child is still quiet. Leave the ear, eye, and throat examination to the very end, as this examination tends to cause the most agitation.
- With newborns, infants, and toddlers, observe, auscultate, and then palpate.
- Use age-appropriate terms. Smile and speak in a soft tone. Tell the child how well he or she is doing. Be funny whenever possible.
- To boost the likelihood of obtaining an accurate sexual and social history, always speak with teenage patients for a few minutes with their parents outside the room.

Variations in the physical examination are as follows:

- **Vital signs:** Include the method by which temperature was obtained: axillary, rectal, oral (only in children > 3 years of age), or tympanic. Rectal temperatures are the gold standard, whereas axillary and tympanic temperatures are often inaccurate and unreliable; temporal temperatures are currently seeing increasing use. Oral temperatures are generally 1°F below rectal. Include weight, height, and head circumference (in units and percentile range). Head circumference is routinely measured in children up to 2 years of age. Finally, do not say "vital signs are stable"; instead, it is more accurate to state that "vital signs are age appropriate" and to report the relevant ranges. Resting heart rate is also important and must be obtained when the child is calm, familiar with you, or asleep.
- **General appearance:** This is an often forgotten but important component of the physical examination. Be descriptive and comment on alertness, playfulness, consolability, hydration status (tearing, drooling), respiratory status, social interactions, responsiveness (smiling, laughing), and nutritional status (well nourished, malnourished, obese).

KEY FACT

Report vital signs as ranges with maximum and current values.

- **Skin:** Check for jaundice, cyanosis, acrocyanosis, mottling, birthmarks, cradle cap, rashes, and capillary refill (note the location where you check capillary refill, as it can vary).
- **Head:** Note circumference, sutures, shape, and fontanelles.
- **Eyes:** Note red reflex in newborns/infants, strabismus (cover test in preschoolers and corneal light reflex in infants), scleral icterus, and conjunctival injection/pallor.
- **Ears:** Use the largest speculum you can. One option to facilitate the ear examination is to have the parent hold the child so that he or she is facing you. Ask the parent to cross his or her leg over both of the child's legs. Also ask the parent to wrap 1 arm around the child's arm and body and to use the other arm to hold the child's head. In an infant, pull the auricle backward and downward. In an older child, pull the external ear backward and upward to straighten the ear canal. Brace your hand with the child's head and use an insufflator bulb to assess tympanic membrane (TM) mobility.
- **Nose:** Look for patent nares, boggy turbinates, a deviated nasal septum, nasal polyps, and nasal flaring (a sign of respiratory distress).
- **Mouth:** Note dentition, palate (cleft), tonsils, oropharynx, midline uvula, and thrush. Use a gloved finger to evaluate the infant's palate and suck reflex.
- **Heart:** The average heart rate in a newborn is 140–160 bpm; in an older child it is 85–120 bpm (keeping a reference list of vital signs according to age will come in handy). Always check for femoral pulses in infants to evaluate for coarctation. Innocent murmurs are found in most children and are characterized by low intensity (I–II/VI), occurrence in systole, variation with position and respiration, and a musical quality.
- **Chest:** The average respiratory rate in a newborn is 40–60; in an older child it is 15–25. Expiration is more prolonged in infants than in adults; in young infants, respiratory movements are produced by abdominal movements. Look for any skin retraction between the rib or above the clavicles (a sign of respiratory distress).
- **Abdomen:** Deep palpation should be performed on every infant. Check the umbilicus (or stump), check for hepatosplenomegaly and masses, and check for hydronephrosis (enlarged kidneys). This portion of the examination often requires the most patience, so distraction is essential. Examining from the head of the patient and cupping your fingers under the ribs can help you palpate the liver, an olive, or other masses. Flexing the patient's hips and knees can relax the abdominal musculature.
- **Back:** Check for scoliosis, tufts of hair, and deep sacral dimples.
- **Genitalia:** Circumcision, testes (descended bilaterally), hernias, labia (adhesions), hymenal opening, and Tanner stage should be noted.
- **Musculoskeletal:** Check for developmental hip dysplasia. With the infant supine, stabilize the pelvis with 1 hand, and then flex and adduct 1 hip and apply gentle posterior pressure on the thigh. Feel for hip dislocation, which will usually relocate spontaneously upon release of pressure (Barlow maneuver). To reduce a dislocated hip, place 1 finger on the greater trochanter and 1 on the inner thigh, flex and abduct the hip, and lift the femoral head anteriorly, feeling for a clunk as it relocates into the acetabulum (Ortolani maneuver). Check range of motion, leg length, and symmetry of skin creases.
- **Neurologic:** Check tone, strength, symmetry of movement, neonatal reflexes (eg, root, suck, grasp, Moro, stepping), Babinski, DTRs, and development.

Key:

AFOSF = anterior fontanelle open, soft, and flat

A/P = assessment and plan

AXR = abdominal x-ray (also known as a KUB, or kidney, ureter, bladder)

BMP = basic metabolic panel

BP = blood pressure

BS ⊕ = bowel sounds present

CBC = complete blood count

CC = chief complaint

C/C/E = clubbing/cyanosis/edema

CN = cranial nerve

CTAB = clear to auscultation bilaterally

c/w = consistent with

d/c = discharge

DOA = day of admission

DTRs = deep tendon reflexes

EOMI = extraocular movements intact

F/C = fever/chills

G1P1 = gravida 1, para 1

GU = genitourinary

HBV = hepatitis B vaccine

HC = head circumference

HEENT = head, eyes, ears, nose, and throat

h/o = history of

HR = heart rate

HSM = hepatosplenomegaly

ID = identification

LAD = lymphadenopathy

MAE = moves all extremities

MMM = mucous membranes moist

M/R/G = murmurs/rubs/gallops

MS = mental status

NAD = no acute distress

NBNB = nonbilious, nonbloody

NC/AT = normocephalic, atraumatic

SAMPLE PEDIATRIC ADMIT NOTE

Source: Parents, reliable.

CC: "Throwing up."

ID: 7-week-old previously healthy Caucasian male presents with progressive emesis × 1 week.

Referring physician: Dr. Paul Smith, pediatrician, (310) 555-8798.

HPI: Adam is a 7-week-old, previously healthy Caucasian male who was in his USOH until 1 week PTA, when parents describe onset of emesis after feedings. Emesis occurred 1–2 times/day, looked like formula, and was NBNB. In the 3 days PTA, emesis ↑ in frequency, occurring within 10 minutes of every feeding, and became projectile in nature. On the DOA, the mother noted projectile emesis to 2–3 feet of a dark brown color and decided to bring him to the ED. Patient has no prior history of similar symptoms. He feeds avidly and appears hungry after vomiting. He had 4 wet diapers in the past 24 hours. Parents deny F/C, diarrhea or constipation, weight loss, irritability, rashes, cough, rhinorrhea, or other URI symptoms. No h/o recent travel or ill contacts. In the ED, patient was given a 20-cc NS bolus × 1 and was admitted to pediatrics for further evaluation.

Medications: None.

Allergies: NKDA.

Immunizations: UTD. Received HBV at birth. Well-child visit next week for 2-month vaccines.

Diet: Initial breastfeeding × 4 weeks. Now Enfamil with iron q 4 h at 2–4 oz per feed.

Birth history: 3000-g 38-week-GA term male born via C-section for failure to progress to a 25 y/o G1P1 Caucasian female at Mercy Hospital. Apgar scores of 7 at 1 min and 9 at 5 min. Home in 2 days without complications. Pregnancy had been uneventful. Mother denies infections, exposures, tobacco, medication, or drug use.

PMH/PSH:

1. **Past illnesses:** None.
2. **Surgical history:** None.

FH: Father with pyloric stenosis at age 8 weeks. No other family history of congenital illness, developmental delay, or GI disease. Firstborn son.

SH: Patient lives with his mother and father in an apartment. There are no siblings (patient is firstborn). Parents are college educated. Father works

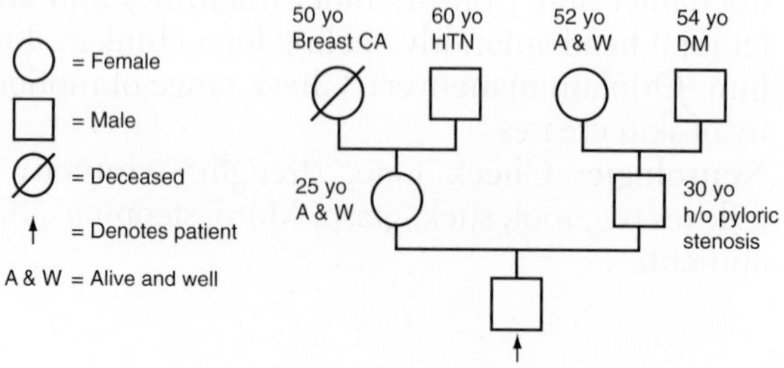

as an accountant, and mother works part time as a lawyer. Paternal grandmother babysits. No smoking, pets, or firearms in the home.

ROS: Unremarkable except as above.

PE: VS: T 98.4°F (rectal), HR 144, RR 48, BP 95/60 (right arm).

Growth: Wt 4.8 kg (50%), length 57 cm (50%), HC 38.7 cm (50–75%).

General: WD/WN 7-week-old male resting quietly in NAD.

Skin: Dry, warm, pink with good turgor. No jaundice, ecchymoses, or rashes.

HEENT:

Head: NC/AT, AFOSF 1 × 1 cm, head shape symmetric.

Eyes: PERRL, EOMI, RR intact bilaterally, anicteric, conjunctivae clear and moist.

Ears: TMs nonerythematous, mobile; normal landmarks bilaterally.

Nose: Patent nares, no nasal flaring or d/c, pink and moist turbinates.

Mouth: Palate intact, no thrush, MMM, O/P clear without erythema or exudates.

Neck: No LAD, no masses, no thyromegaly.

Chest: No respiratory distress, symmetric excursion, CTAB, no W/R/R.

Cardiac: RRR, nl S1/S2, no M/R/G, femoral and brachial pulses 2+ bilaterally.

Abdomen: Soft, NT/ND, occasional peristaltic waves visible, BS ⊕, no masses or palpable "olive," no HSM.

GU: Circumcised male, both testes descended without masses or tenderness, no hernias present, no discharge from penis.

Back: No dimples or tufts.

Extremities: Brisk cap refill < 2 seconds, no C/C/E. No Barlow's/Ortolani's sign or hip clicks; skin folds symmetric.

Neuro: MS: Alert and active. CNs: Pupillary light reflex/face/palate symmetric, tongue midline. Motor: MAE, normal tone and bulk, strong suck; no sensory abnormalities noted. Reflexes: Moro present and symmetric, DTRs 2+ bilaterally, palmar and plantar grasp intact, both toes upgoing.

Labs: CBC and BMP pending.

Studies: AXR: Nonspecific bowel gas pattern. No masses seen. Abdominal U/S: Hypoechoic mass > 1.5 cm, c/w pyloric stenosis.

A/P: 7-week-old previously healthy male with 1-week h/o progressive projectile emesis with confirmed pyloric stenosis on U/S.

1. **Emesis:** The clinical picture of progressive, projectile, nonbilious emesis in a firstborn term male is consistent with the diagnosis of pyloric stenosis, which was confirmed on U/S. Other etiologies, such as GERD or metabolic disease, are much less likely given the ultrasound report and classic history. Patient does not appear dehydrated. However, prior to surgical intervention, must r/o electrolyte

NKDA = no known drug allergies

nl = normal

NPO = nothing by mouth

NS = normal saline

NT/ND = nontender, nondistended

O/P = oropharynx

PERRL = pupils equal, round, and reactive to light

PSH = past social history

PTA = prior to admission

r/o = rule out

ROS = review of systems

RR = respiratory rate, red reflex

RRR = regular rate and rhythm

URI = upper respiratory infection

U/S = ultrasound

USOH = usual state of health

UTD = up to date

VS = vital signs

WD/WN = well developed and well nourished

W/R/R = wheezes/rhonchi/rales

abnormalities such as hypokalemic hypochloremic metabolic alkalosis 2° to persistent vomiting.

- Check BMP results for electrolyte abnormalities.
- Surgery consult to evaluate for pyloromyotomy.
- NPO until surgery.
- IV fluids at 1 × maintenance for hydration.

2. **Routine health maintenance:** Patient is UTD on his vaccinations.

THE NURSERY ROTATION

Most students will spend a week or less on the nursery service. As part of the nursery team, you will be paged to attend deliveries in which newborns may be at risk. The pediatric team is called for issues such as multiple gestations, preterm deliveries, cesarean sections, possible meconium aspiration, and known fetal anomalies. On arrival, the team obtains a brief history, sets up the infant warmer, and prepares resuscitation equipment such as O_2, suction, and intubation apparatus. The newborn is then shuttled from the obstetrician to the warmer, where the team goes to work. The baby is immediately dried off, the nose and mouth are suctioned, and the baby is rubbed and stimulated. The team provides ventilatory support, CPR, and/or advanced life-support measures if necessary. Apgar scores are assessed at 1 and 5 minutes, and the baby receives an initial head-to-toe examination. If the baby appears vigorous and healthy, a brief delivery note is written, and the team's role may end there. If there are potential problems, the baby may be taken to the nursery for observation or admitted to the neonatal ICU (NICU).

The team will also take care of newborns in the nursery, write daily progress notes, and talk with and provide important anticipatory guidance for new mothers. This portion of the pediatric rotation gives you a great opportunity to interact with neonatologists and newborns and to practice physical examinations (before the onset of stranger anxiety). The nursery can have a fair amount of downtime, so this is a great time to get lectures or bedside teaching from your residents.

KEY PROCEDURES

The key procedures in pediatrics are lumbar puncture (LP), urine catheterization, IV line placement, and blood drawing. Drawing blood in newborns < 1 month of age is often accomplished with a heel or arterial stick. Ask a nurse or a resident to demonstrate the technique for you. Always be proactive and ask to perform procedures.

PEDIATRIC PRESCRIPTIONS

Writing pediatric prescriptions is unique because dosing is done on a per-kilogram basis, and drugs must often be dispensed in a liquid form. You

KEY POINT

SAMPLE PRESCRIPTION

Amoxicillin 400 mg/5 mL

Sig: 800 mg (10 mL) by mouth every 12 hours for 10 days

Disp: 200 mL

Refills: zero

should refer to a pharmacology manual to help you with dosing. The following is a list of steps to help you write a pediatric prescription for the treatment of acute otitis media in a 20-kg child:

- **Find the dose range of amoxicillin:** 40–45 mg/kg/dose every 12 hours.
- **Calculate the amount of drug per dose:** 800–900 mg every 12 hours.
- **Determine the dosage form you need (liquid or tablet):** Liquid suspension.
- **Find the available compositions of your dosage forms:** 125 mg/5 mL or 400 mg/5 mL.
- **Choose an appropriate dosage composition to minimize volume:** 400 mg/5 mL.
- **Calculate the amount to dispense per dose:** 800 mg/(400 mg/5 mL) = 10 mL.
- **Find the duration of treatment:** 10 days for otitis media.
- **Calculate the total amount to dispense:** 10 mL × 10 days × 2 doses/day = 200 mL.
- **Write your prescription** (see boxed item).

WHAT DO I CARRY IN MY POCKETS?

The white coat is generally not used in pediatrics, so don't rely on those handy oversized pockets to store your peripheral brain and instruments of the trade.

- ❑ Toy for distraction
- ❑ Stethoscope
- ❑ Ophthalmoscope
- ❑ Otoscope with tips of different sizes and an insufflator bulb
- ❑ Penlight
- ❑ Reflex hammer
- ❑ Pocket immunization card from WHO or CDC Web site
- ❑ Extra prescription pads
- ❑ Alcohol wipes
- ❑ Tongue blades
- ❑ Calculator (to determine dosages for meds)
- ❑ Notebook
- ❑ Optional: stickers for a reward; cartoon Band-Aids

High-Yield Clinical Topic Checklist

Read about these topics before you start the rotation. Most are discussed in this chapter. A full list of common clerkship topics can be found at the end of this chapter.

- ❑ Acute otitis media
- ❑ Asthma
- ❑ Bronchiolitis
- ❑ Congenital heart disease
- ❑ Developmental milestones
- ❑ Fever management
- ❑ Immunizations
- ❑ Infant nutrition
- ❑ Lead poisoning
- ❑ Neonatal hyperbilirubinemia
- ❑ Sickle cell disease

Well-Child Care

DEVELOPMENTAL MILESTONES

Pediatricians use a sequence of milestones to monitor a child's developmental progress and to identify developmental delays. Assessments are typically divided into gross motor, fine motor, language, and social development. Table 7-1 summarizes key developmental milestones. Obtain a copy of the Denver Developmental Screening Test II for more extensive guidelines. Table 7-2 describes classical neonatal reflexes. Most neonatal reflexes disappear by the sixth month of life. Persistent primitive reflexes can be a clue to developmental or neurologic disorders.

> **KEY FACT**
>
> For children born before 38 weeks' gestation, age should be corrected for prematurity up to 2 years.

FAILURE TO THRIVE (FTT)

A condition of undernutrition that is generally identified in the first 3 years of life. Traditionally, FTT has been defined as either medical (**organic**) or psychosocial (**nonorganic**) in origin, but the current teaching is that there is considerable overlap between these categories. Table 7-3 summarizes the etiologies of FTT.

> **KEY FACT**
>
> In FTT, children fall off the weight curve first, then the height curve, and then the head circumference curve.

Signs and Symptoms

- Weight below the fifth percentile for age.
- Weight-for-length below the fifth percentile for age.
- A decline of > 2 major percentile lines on the growth chart over 3–6 months.
- Other signs and symptoms are usually specific to the etiology (see Table 7-3).

> **KEY FACT**
>
> It is crucial to ask caretakers for detailed information about formula (eg, powder, concentrate, or ready-to-feed formula and how formulas are being prepared).

Workup

- Obtain a detailed birth, feeding, developmental, and social history (most important).
- Conduct a thorough physical examination.
- Trend height, weight, and head circumference on the growth chart.

TABLE 7-1. Key Developmental Milestones

Age	Gross Motor	Fine Motor	Language	Social
Birth	–	Visually fixes.	–	–
1 month	Raises head from prone position.	Tracks to midline.	Alerts to sound.	Regards face.
2 months	Holds head midline.	Tracks past midline.	Smiles socially.	Recognizes parent.
3 months	Holds head up.	Tracks in circles.	Coos.	Anticipates feeding.
4 months	Rolls over.	Brings hands to midline.	Laughs; orients to voice.	Enjoys looking around.
6 months	Sits upright.	Transfers objects.	Babbles.	Exhibits stranger anxiety.
9 months	Crawls, pulls to stand, cruises.	Immature pincer grasp.	Says "mama, dada"–nonspecific.	Plays pat-a-cake.
12 months	Walks alone.	Uses mature pincer grasp.	Says "mama, dada"–specific.	Imitates actions; comes when called.
15 months	Creeps up stairs; walks backward.	Builds tower of 2 blocks.	Uses 4–6 words.	Uses spoon and cup.
18 months	Runs; throws objects from standing position.	Builds tower of 3 blocks.	Uses 7–10 words.	Plays in the company of other children.
24 months	Walks up and down steps without help.	Turns pages 1 at a time.	Knows 50 words; uses 2-word sentences.	Engages in parallel play.
3 years	Pedals a tricycle.	Copies a circle.	Knows 250 words; uses 3-word sentences.	Engages in group play.
4 years	Hops and skips.	Copies a square.	Knows colors.	Plays cooperatively.
5 years	Jumps over low obstacles.	Copies a triangle.	Prints first name.	Abides by rules.

- Order a CBC, electrolytes, BUN, creatinine, albumin, protein, TSH, and a UA and urine culture.
- With GI symptoms, order stool guaiac, culture, and O&P.
- Other tests include a sweat chloride test (for cystic fibrosis [CF]) and assessment of bone age. Tests for malabsorption (stool pH and reducing substances) may also be appropriate.

Treatment

- Varies according to etiology.
- Keeping a food diary that includes calorie count may be helpful.
- Encourage nutritional supplementation if breastfeeding is inadequate.
- Hospitalize for feeding, calorie counts, and observation if there is evidence of neglect or severe malnourishment or if no growth results from dietary modification.

Q

A child smiles spontaneously, babbles, sits without support, reaches, and feeds herself a cookie but has no pincer grasp. What is her approximate developmental age?

TABLE 7-2. Selected Neonatal Reflexes

Reflex	Timing	Description
Moro	Present at birth; disappears by 3–6 months.	Sudden neck extension while supine leads to extension, adduction, and then abduction of the upper extremities.
Palmar or plantar grasp	Present at birth; disappears by 9 months.	Infants grasp a finger placed in the palm or perform plantar flexion if the bottom of the foot is stimulated.
Rooting	Present at birth; disappears by 6–12 months.	Infants pursue an object placed around the mouth or next to the cheek.
Stepping	Present at birth; disappears by 2–3 months.	Infants move their legs in a walking movement when they are held upright and leaning forward.
Asymmetric tonic neck ("fencer")	Present at birth; disappears by 4–9 months.	Turning the head laterally 45–90 degrees while supine leads to ipsilateral extremity extension and contralateral flexion (fencer position).
Galant	Present at birth; disappears by 2–6 months.	Stroking the paravertebral region while the infant is in prone suspension causes the pelvis to move toward the stimulated side.
Babinski	Present at birth; disappears by 6 months.	Stroking the lateral plantar surface causes fanning and upgoing motion of the toes.

GROWTH PARAMETERS

At each pediatric visit, the weight, height, and head circumference of the patient are plotted on growth charts specific for gender and age. It is recommended that the WHO growth charts be used for children 0–2 years of age and that the CDC growth charts be used for children > 2 years of age. Over time, the clinician uses these growth charts to recognize potential growth abnormalities. Specialized growth charts exist for prematurity as well as for Down, Prader-Willi, Cornelia de Lange, Marfan's, Noonan's, Turner's, and Williams syndromes. Some helpful rules of thumb are summarized in Table 7-4.

KEY FACT

As a general rule, babies triple in weight and double in length from birth to 12 months.

IMMUNIZATIONS

Tables 7-5 and 7-6 summarize recommended childhood immunization schedules. Contraindications to vaccination include the following:

- Current moderate to severe acute illness.
- Severe allergy to a vaccine component or to a prior dose of vaccine.
- Anaphylactic reaction to eggs (influenza vaccine), gelatin (MMR), neomycin (MMR, IPV), polymyxin B (IPV), or streptomycin (IPV). Perform prior skin testing.
- Encephalopathy within 7 days of prior pertussis vaccination (use DT instead of DTaP).
- Pregnancy, immune compromise, or use of high-dose steroids (oral polio, MMR, varicella).
- Recent administration of antibody-containing blood products (live injected vaccines).

KEY FACT

Prematurity, malnutrition, current antibiotic therapy, and the presence of mild acute illness and/or low-grade fever are **not** contraindications to immunization.

A

Eight or 9 months. An immature pincer grasp is seen at 9 months, and a fine pincer grasp is observed at 10 months.

TABLE 7-3. Etiologies of Failure to Thrive

System	Causes
GI	**Feeding disorders:** Cleft palate, dentition disorders. **Vomiting:** Reflux, pyloric stenosis, Hirschsprung's disease. **Diarrhea:** Milk protein allergy/intolerance, infection. **Malabsorption:** CF, celiac disease, IBD.
Hepatic	Chronic hepatitis, glycogen storage disease.
Pulmonary	CF, bronchopulmonary dysplasia, asthma, obstructive sleep apnea.
Cardiac	Congenital heart malformations.
Renal	Chronic pyelonephritis, renal tubular acidosis, Fanconi's syndrome, UTI, diabetes insipidus, chronic renal insufficiency.
Endocrine	Hypothyroidism, rickets, vitamin D deficiency/resistance, growth hormone resistance/deficiency, adrenal insufficiency/excess, diabetes mellitus (DM), parathyroid disorders, hypophosphatemia.
CNS	Pituitary insufficiency, cerebral palsy.
Infectious	TB, HIV.
Congenital	Inborn errors of metabolism, trisomy 13/18/21, Prader-Willi syndrome, Cornelia de Lange syndrome, fetal alcohol syndrome, TORCH infections, skeletal dysplasias.
Nutritional	Kwashiorkor, marasmus, zinc/iron deficiency.
Other organic	Prematurity, oncologic disease/treatment, immunodeficiency, collagen vascular disease, lead poisoning.
Nonorganic	Child neglect/abuse, poverty, lack of true caregivers, maternal depression, marital discord, spousal abuse, inadequate food intake, low socioeconomic status.

TABLE 7-4. Growth Pearls

Variable	Guidelines
Weight	**Average birth weight (BW):** 3.5 kg (7.7 lbs). ▪ 5–10% of BW is usually lost over the first 5–7 days. ▪ Babies return to BW by the second week of life. ▪ BW should double by 5 months, triple by 1 year, and quadruple by 2 years. **Average weight gain:** 20–30 g/day or 1 kg/month for the first 3 months; 10–20 g/day for 4–12 months; 5 lbs/year from age 2 to puberty. **BMI growth curve:** Used for those 2–20 years of age; > 85% are overweight and > 95% are obese.
Height	**Average birth length:** 50 cm (20 inches). **Average height:** 30 inches at 1 year; 3 feet at 3 years; 40 inches at 4 years (2 times birth length); 3 times birth length at 13 years. **Average growth:** 2–3 inches per year from age 4 to puberty.
Head circumference	**Average birth head circumference:** 35 cm. **Average head circumference ↑:** 1 cm/month for 1 year. Some 90% of head growth occurs by age 2.

TABLE 7-5. 2012 CDC Immunization Schedule: 0–6 years

Vaccine	Birth	2 Mos	4 Mos	6 Mos	12–15 Mos	15–18 Mos	2 Years	4–6 Years
HBV[a]	x	x		x				
Rotavirus[b]		x	x	x				
DTaP		x	x	x		x		x
Hib		x	x	x	x			
IPV[c]		x	x	x				x
Influenza[d]				x	x	x	x	x
PCV[e]		x	x	x	x			
MMR					x			x
Varicella					x			x
HAV[f]					x		x	
MCV4[g]							x	

[a] The first dose of HBV should be given before discharge; the second dose at 1 or 2 months; and the third dose no earlier than 6 months but no later than 18 months. Infants who did not receive a birth dose should receive 3 doses on a schedule of 0, 1, and 6 months.

[b] The first dose of rotavirus vaccine should be given at 6–14 weeks. No vaccine should be initiated for infants ≥ 15 weeks of age. The maximum age for the final dose is 8 months.

[c] The third dose of IPV can be given between 6 and 15 months.

[d] The influenza vaccine is recommended yearly for all children 6–59 months of age. The minimum age is 6 months for trivalent inactivated influenza vaccine and 2 years for the live attenuated influenza vaccine. Children < 9 years of age who are receiving influenza vaccine for the first time should receive 2 doses separated by > 4 weeks.

[e] PCV13 is also given to high-risk children > 24 months of age. In addition, PCV13 is recommended for all children < 5 years of age, and 1 dose should be given between 24 and 59 months in healthy children who are not completely immunized for their age.

[f] HAV is recommended for all children 1 year of age. The 2 doses in the series should be administered at least 6 months apart.

[g] MCV4 is recommended for children 2–10 years of age with persistent complement component deficiency and anatomic or functional asplenia. Two doses are given at least 8 weeks apart followed by 1 dose every 5 years thereafter.

KEY FACT

High school seniors about to enter a college dormitory, as well as children with sickle cell disease or functional asplenia, may need a meningitis vaccine.

KEY FACT

"Breast is best": For the vast majority of infants, breastfeeding is preferred over commercially available infant formulas.

Also look for prior reactions to pertussis vaccine—eg, a fever > 40.5°C (> 105°F), a shock-like state, persistent crying for > 3 hours within 48 hours of vaccination, or seizure within 3 days of vaccination.

INFANT NUTRITION

Breast Milk

The American Academy of Pediatrics (AAP) recommends exclusive breastfeeding for the first 6 months of life and continuation of breastfeeding through 12 months of age for optimal infant nutrition. At 4 months of age, breastfed infants may require iron supplementation, as maternal stores of iron are often depleted by that time. Advantages to breastfeeding include the following:

- **Infant benefits:** Facilitates mother-infant bonding; ↓ the risk of eczema and cow's-milk protein allergy; ↓ the risk of serious infections due to the

TABLE 7-6. 2012 CDC Immunization Schedule: 7–18 Years

VACCINE	7–10 YEARS	11–12 YEARS	13–18 YEARS
Tdap[a]		x	
HPV[b]		x	
MCV4[c]		x	
PCV[d]	x	x	x
Influenza	x	x	x
HAV[e]	x	x	x

[a] Children 11–18 years of age who have not received Tdap should receive a dose followed by a Td booster every 10 years thereafter. Those 7–10 years of age who are not fully immunized against pertussis should receive a single dose of Tdap.

[b] A 3-dose series of HPV vaccine should be administered to females starting at 11–12 years of age. The series may also be administered to males 9–18 years of age to reduce their likelihood of genital warts. The second and third doses should be administered 1–2 months and 6 months after the first dose.

[c] The MCV4 vaccine should be given at 11–12 years of age with a booster dose at 16 years. One dose should be administered at 13–18 years of age to those who have not previously been vaccinated. Those who received their first dose at 13–15 years of age should receive a booster at 16–18 years. Administer 1 dose to previously unvaccinated college freshmen living in dormitories.

[d] PCV23 is recommended for certain high-risk groups.

[e] HAV is recommended for certain other groups of children, including those in areas where vaccination programs target older children.

presence of maternal IgA antibodies; ↓ the incidence of chronic disease; ↑ cognitive development.
- **Maternal benefits:** ↑ oxytocin levels; ↓ postpartum bleeding; allows for more rapid involution of the uterus; delays ovulation; improves bone mineralization; ↓ the risk of breast and ovarian cancer; promotes earlier return to prepregnancy weight.
- **Other benefits:** ↓ cost in comparison to formula; ↑ convenience (correct temperature, no preparation, no risk of mixing errors).

Breastfeeding is **not** recommended for:

- Mothers infected with HIV-1, HIV-2, HTLV-1, or HTLV-2.
- Mothers with active, untreated TB.
- Mothers with active herpetic breast lesions.
- Mothers who are using or are dependent on illicit drugs.
- Mothers who are taking chemotherapeutic drugs or are undergoing radiation therapy.

Formulas

Formulas may be based in cow's milk or soy. Table 7-7 outlines the major types of formula. Table 7-8 delineates recommended foods for the first year of life. Remember the following when guiding parents on infant nutrition:

- In the first 2 months of life, babies will eat 2–3 ounces (or approximately 10–20 minutes per breast) every 2–3 hours.

KEY FACT

Do not leave formula bottles in the crib overnight, as this may cause milk-bottle tooth caries.

TABLE 7-7. Comparison of Formulas

Formula	Indications
Cow's-milk based (Enfamil, Similac, Good Start)	Most infants.
Soy (ProSobee, Isomil, Good Start Soy)	Milk allergy; galactosemia.
Hydrolyzed protein (Alimentum, Nutramigen)	Milk and soy allergy.
Amino acid based (Neocate, EleCare)	Severe food allergy not responding to hydrolyzed formulas; malabsorption.
Preterm formulas (EnfaCare, NeoSure; both are 22 calories)	Prematurity.

KEY FACT

All breastfed infants should receive vitamin D (400 IU/day) to prevent rickets.

- New foods should be introduced after 6 months of age at a rate of 1 every 2–3 days to allow for the identification of potential allergies.
- Avoid honey in children < 1 year of age in light of the risk of infant botulism.
- Avoid foods that may lead to choking, including nuts, raisins, and hot dogs.
- The only supplementation breastfed babies need is vitamin D.
- Some 40–50% of patients who have milk protein allergy are also allergic to soy, so do not give soy formulas to infants suspected of having milk protein allergy.

TABLE 7-8. Infant Nutrition

Age	Recommended Foods
Birth	Breast milk or formula with iron.
4 months	Iron-fortified single-grain cereal.
6 months	Pureed fruits and vegetables; fluoride supplementation.
8 months	Well-chopped meats.
9–10 months	Cheese, egg yolk, protein-rich foods.
10–12 months	Soft finger foods: cookies, fruits, vegetables, meats.
12 months	Soft table foods; egg whites; can start whole cow's milk.
24 months	Can start nuts or shellfish.

TABLE 7-9. Tanner Stages

STAGE	MALE GENITALIA	FEMALE BREASTS	PUBIC HAIR
I	Preadolescent.	Preadolescent.	Preadolescent.
II	↑ scrotum and testis size; scrotum darkening (12 years).	Breast bud (11 years).	Sparse, long, slightly pigmented, downy hair (female 12, male 13.5).
III	↑ penis length (13 years).	↑ breast and areola size; single contour (12 years).	Darker, coarse, curled hair (female 12.5, male 14).
IV	↑ penis breadth, glans development (14 years).	2° mound; projection of areola and papilla (13 years).	Adult-type hair limited to the genital area (female 13, male 14.5).
V	Mature stage (15 years).	Mature stage (15 years).	Mature stage (female 14.5, male 15).

TANNER STAGING

Puberty follows a predictable sequence in all adolescents, but with variations in timing and rate of change. The Tanner staging system is outlined in Table 7-9. Normal progression is as follows:

- **Males:** Testicular enlargement → penile enlargement → growth spurt → pubic hair.
- **Females:** Thelarche → growth spurt → pubic hair → menarche.

KEY FACT

- **Menarche:** Onset of menses.
- **Pubarche:** Pubic hair development.
- **Thelarche:** Breast development.

Cardiology

CONGENITAL HEART DISEASE (CHD)

CHD is generally divided into acyanotic disease ("pink babies") and cyanotic disease ("blue babies"). Cardiac defects with right-to-left shunts are cyanotic, and those with left-to-right shunts are acyanotic. Workup includes CXR, ECG, and an echocardiogram.

Acyanotic CHD

Table 7-10 presents a detailed discussion of acyanotic congenital heart diseases. Lesions are often asymptomatic in early childhood, but as fetal circulation transitions into adult circulation over the first several weeks of life, left-to-right shunting ↑ and symptoms of CHF develop, usually between 1 and 3 months. Large ASD or VSD lesions may lead to Eisenmenger's syndrome, in which a left-to-right shunt causes pulmonary hypertension and shunt reversal.

MNEMONIC

The 5 major causes of cyanotic heart disease:

1 finger up – **T**runcus arteriosus (1 = 1 vessel)
2 fingers up–**T**ransposition of the great vessels (2 = 2 vessels transposed)
3 fingers up–**T**ricuspid atresia (3 = tri)
4 fingers up–**T**etralogy of Fallot (4 = tetra)
5 fingers up–**T**otal anomalous pulmonary venous return (5 = 5 words)

Q

A 3-month-old female born at full term was in her USOH until 3 weeks ago, when she became dyspneic and had difficulty feeding. On examination, a loud holosystolic murmur is heard at the LLSB, and an ECG shows LVH and RVH. What lesion does this child have, and how should it be treated?

TABLE 7-10. Acyanotic Congenital Heart Diseases

Lesion	Epidemiology	Presentation	ECG	CXR	Treatment
VSD	Accounts for 20–25% of cases of CHD; incidence is 2 in 1000 births.	**Small:** Asymptomatic. **Large:** CHF/pulmonary hypertension. Holosystolic murmur at the left lower sternal border (LLSB).	Normal LVH	Cardiomegaly ↑ pulmonary vascular markings (PVMs)	Spontaneous closure (30–50%). Diuretics, digitalis. Surgical closure.
ASD	Accounts for 10% of cases.	Asymptomatic. Widely fixed, split S2 at the left upper sternal border (LUSB).	Normal RVH Right atrial enlargement (RAE) RBBB	Cardiomegaly ↑ PVMs	Spontaneous closure (90%). Surgical closure if ASD is > 8 mm.
PDA	Accounts for 5–10% of cases; females > males.	Machine-like murmur at the LUSB. Wide pulse pressure. Common in prematurity.	Normal LVH Biventricular hypertrophy	Cardiomegaly ↑ PVMs	Indomethacin and NSAIDs. Surgical ligation.
Pulmonary stenosis	–	Ejection click at the LUSB. Systolic ejection murmur (SEM) at the LUSB.	Normal Right axis deviation (RAD)/RVH RAE	Normal size ↓ PVMs	Valvotomy/valve replacement.
Aortic stenosis	Some 85% of stenotic valves are bicuspid.	Crescendo-decrescendo systolic murmur. Systolic ejection click.	Normal LVH +/– strain	Normal	Valvotomy/valve replacement.
Coarctation of the aorta	Accounts for 8–10% of cases; males > females; associated with Turner's syndrome.	Infant in CHF; ↓ lower extremity pulses; acidosis; murmur over the left scapula. Child with upper extremity hypertension and leg weakness/pain.	RVH in infants LVH in children	Cardiomegaly Pulmonary venous congestion Rib notching	Resection of coarctation. Balloon dilatation.

Cyanotic CHD

Table 7-11 presents a detailed discussion of cyanotic congenital heart diseases, which typically present after the ductus arteriosus closes in the first week of life. Nonoxygenated blood bypasses the lungs into the systemic circulation, and infants may present with cyanosis, respiratory distress, or shock.

A

The infant likely has a large VSD causing left-to-right shunting and pulmonary hypertension. Left-sided volume overload and RVH are suggestive of a large VSD. She will need treatment for CHF (diuretics, digitalis) and surgical closure of the VSD.

TABLE 7-11. Cyanotic Congenital Heart Diseases

Lesion	Epidemiology	Presentation	ECG	CXR	Treatment
Tetralogy of Fallot	The most common type of cyanotic CHD.	FTT. Variable cyanosis ("tet" spells). Right ventricular impulse, single S2, SEM at the LUSB.	RAD RVH	Boot-shaped heart Normal size ↓ PVMs	Surgery.
Transposition of the great vessels	The most common cyanotic heart lesion of the newborn period; associated with DiGeorge syndrome.	To be compatible with life, either the PDA needs to remain open or there needs to be a septal defect such as a VSD.	RAD RVH	"Egg on a string" Cardiomegaly ↑ PVMs	**No VSD:** PGE1 and balloon atrial septostomy (BAS). **VSD:** Pulmonary artery band. Surgery.
Tricuspid atresia	ASD/VSD are usually present.	Cyanosis in the first week. Left ventricular impulse displaced laterally. Single S2.	Superior QRS axis RAE LVH	Normal or enlarged Might be boot shaped	PGE1/BAS/surgery.
Total anomalous pulmonary venous return	Males > females.	Right ventricular impulse. Fixed and widely split S2. SEM at the LUSB. Cyanosis.	RAD RVH	Cardiomegaly ↑ PVMs "Snowman" sign	BAS/surgery.
Truncus arteriosus	Associated with DiGeorge syndrome.	CHF, cyanosis in the first week. Single S2. Strong, bounding pulses.	RAD RVH	Cardiomegaly ↑ PVMs	Surgery.

Dermatology

NEONATAL DERMATOLOGIC CONDITIONS

While in the nursery, you will see a variety of neonatal rashes in newborn babies. It is sometimes hard to differentiate between benign and pathologic rashes. Table 7-12 and Figures 7-1 and 7-2 outline benign neonatal dermatologic disorders.

TABLE 7-12. Benign Neonatal Dermatologic Conditions

Condition	Etiology	Appearance	Timing
Sebaceous hyperplasia	Maternal hormones.	Shiny yellow papules (see Figure 7-1A).	A few weeks.
Acne neonatorum	Maternal hormones.	Similar to minor acne vulgaris (see Figure 7-1B).	Peaks at 2 months.
Milia	Dead skin/oil in hair follicles.	White papules on the face.	Within the first month.
Erythema toxicum	Uncertain (occurs in 50% of full-term infants).	Blotchy red spots with overlying white or yellow papules or pustules (see Figure 7-2A).	Presents shortly after birth and resolves in a few days.
Mongolian spots	Melanocytes.	Congenital blue-gray macules (non-Caucasian infants) (see Figure 7-2B).	Presents at birth and resolves in the first few years of life; some never disappear.

KEY FACT

Avoid ASA when treating fever in the setting of a viral infection, as it is associated with **Reye's syndrome,** a disorder that presents with acute, severe encephalopathy and degenerative liver disease.

EXANTHEMS

There are many causes of rash in children. The clinical history is often the key tool used to make the diagnosis. Common rashes caused by viruses are discussed in Table 7-13 and are depicted in Figures 7-3 and 7-4. Note that the treatment of viral exanthems consists mainly of supportive measures (eg, fluids, treatment of discomfort from fever with acetaminophen) along with isolation while patients are contagious.

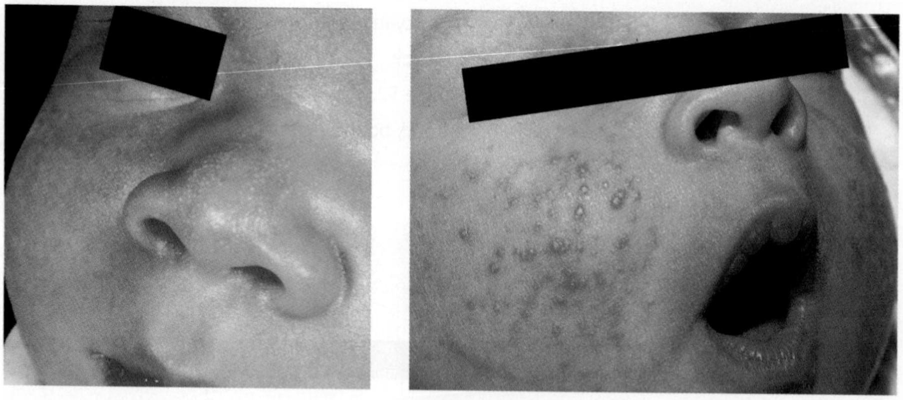

A B

FIGURE 7-1. Benign neonatal dermatologic conditions of the face. (A) Sebaceous hyperplasia. Note the papules on the nose. (B) **Neonatal acne.** Note the tiny papulopustules on the cheeks. (Reproduced with permission from Wolff K et al. *Fitzpatrick's Dermatology in General Medicine,* 7th ed. New York: McGraw-Hill, 2008, Figs. 106-2 and 106-5.)

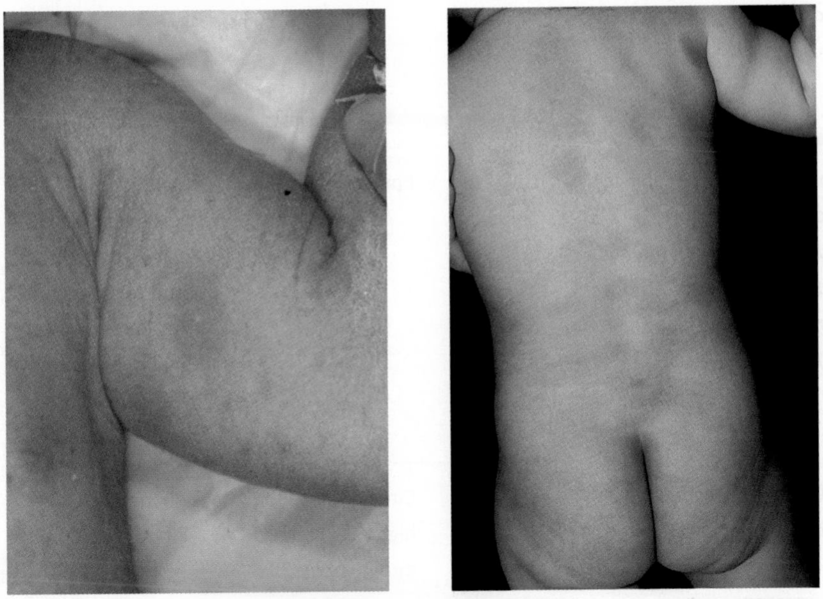

FIGURE 7-2. Benign neonatal dermatologic conditions of the trunk and extremities. (A) **Erythema toxicum.** Note the erythematous macules on the arm. (B) **Mongolian spots.** Note the multiple, ill-defined, bluish lesions scattered on the child's back. (Image A reproduced with permission from Wolff K, Johnson RA. *Fitzpatrick's Color Atlas & Synopsis of Clinical Dermatology,* 6th ed. New York: McGraw-Hill, 2009, Fig. 9-12. Image B reproduced with permission from Wolff K et al. *Fitzpatrick's Dermatology in General Medicine,* 7th ed. New York: McGraw-Hill, 2008, Fig. 106-3.)

TABLE 7-13. Common Exanthems

Infection/ Pathogen	Sequence	Rash	Fever	Hallmarks	Complications
Measles (rubeola)—paramyxovirus	Fever and the **"3 C's"—C**oryza, **C**ough, and **C**onjunctivitis × 3–4 days—**precede** the rash.	Erythematous descending maculopapular rash that spreads from the head to the body (see Figure 7-3A).	High.	**Koplik's spots**—whitish-gray spots on the buccal mucosa.	Otitis media (common), encephalitis, pneumonia, subacute sclerosing panencephalitis (rare).
Rubella (German or 3-day measles)—RNA/togavirus	Low-grade fever for 1–2 days precedes the rash.	Descending maculopapular rash that spreads from the face to the body (see Figure 7-3B); resolves in 3–5 days.	First day of rash only.	Enlargement of the suboccipital lymph nodes; palatal petechiae (Forschheimer spots).	Devastating if a fetus is infected during gestation. Rarely, encephalitis and thrombocytopenia.
Roseola (exanthema subitum)—HHV-6 and -7	**High** fever for 4–5 days; the rash occurs **after** the fever has resolved.	Discrete maculopapular rash on the trunk; lasts < 24 hours.	High fever for 4–5 days.	Enlargement of the suboccipital lymph nodes; red eardrums.	Febrile seizures.

(continues)

TABLE 7-13. Common Exanthems *(continued)*

Infection/ Pathogen	Sequence	Rash	Fever	Hallmarks	Complications
Erythema infectiosum (fifth disease)—parvovirus B-19	Flulike illness for 7–10 days followed by red **"slapped cheeks."**	"Slapped cheek" appearance and circumoral pallor followed by an erythematous, maculopapular, lacy rash on the trunk and legs (see Figure 7-3C). Lasts 2–3 weeks.	Low grade or none.	Epidemics in spring.	Rare arthritis of the knee, aplastic crisis (sickle cell disease and other anemias), fetal anemia/hydrops fetalis (in utero infection), encephalopathy.
Scarlet fever—group A streptococcus	Fever with sore throat; desquamation (peeling) in week 2.	**Sandpaper**-like, confluent rash (erythroderma); accentuated in folds, where darker Pastia's lines are seen.	Resolves in 2–7 days.	Circumoral pallor; high ASO titer; ⊕ throat culture.	Rheumatic fever, glomerulonephritis.
Varicella (chickenpox)—VZV	Fever and malaise for 1 day followed by a rash of different stages over 3–7 days.	Crops of "dew drops on a rose petal"; evolve from papule to vesicle to pustule to excoriation.	Preceding rash; fever for 1 day.	Rash in different stages of evolution; starts on the trunk; the palms and soles are spared.	Meningoencephalitis, hepatitis, pneumonitis.
Hand-foot-and-mouth disease—coxsackievirus	Fever, rash, URI/GI infection symptoms.	"Football-shaped" vesicles with surrounding erythema on the hands and feet (see Figure 7-4A); oral ulcerations (see Figure 7-4B). Resolves in 1 week.	Present.	Involvement of the palms and soles; erosions on the pharynx, tongue, and palate (enanthema).	—

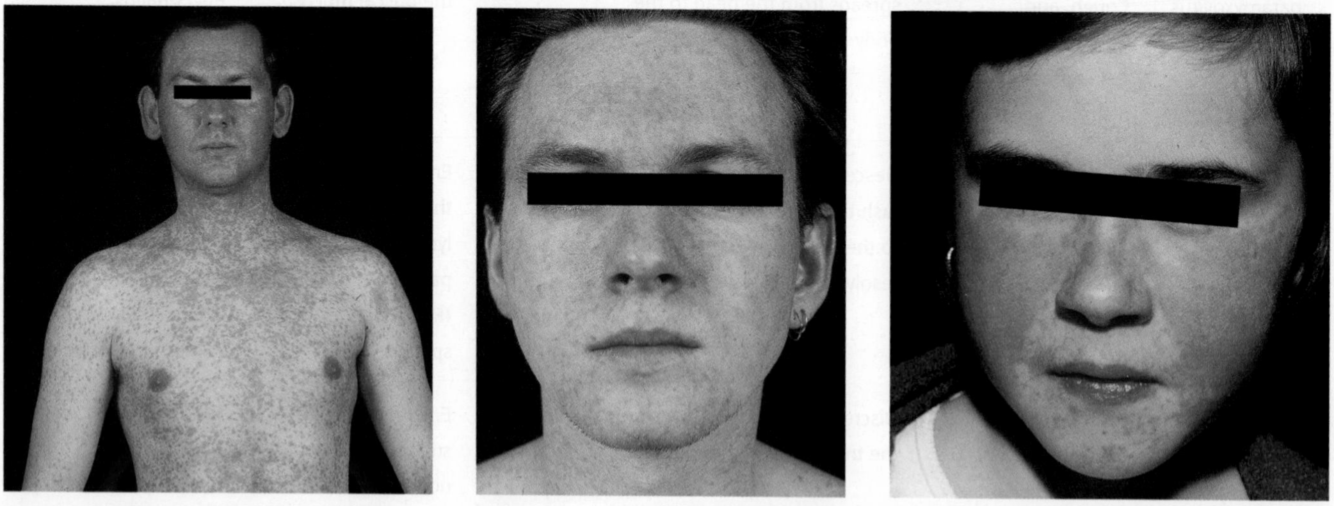

A B C

FIGURE 7-3. Viral exanthems of the face, trunk, and extremities. (A) **Rubeola (measles).** Erythematous papules appear on the face and neck, become confluent, and spread to the trunk and arms. (B) **Rubella.** Erythematous macules and papules initially appear on the face before spreading to the trunk and extremities. (C) **Erythema infectiosum (fifth disease).** Note the diffuse erythema and "slapped cheek" appearance. (Reproduced with permission from Wolff K, Johnson RA. *Fitzpatrick's Color Atlas & Synopsis of Clinical Dermatology,* 6th ed. New York: McGraw-Hill, 2009, Figs. 27-21, 27-22, and 27-24A.)

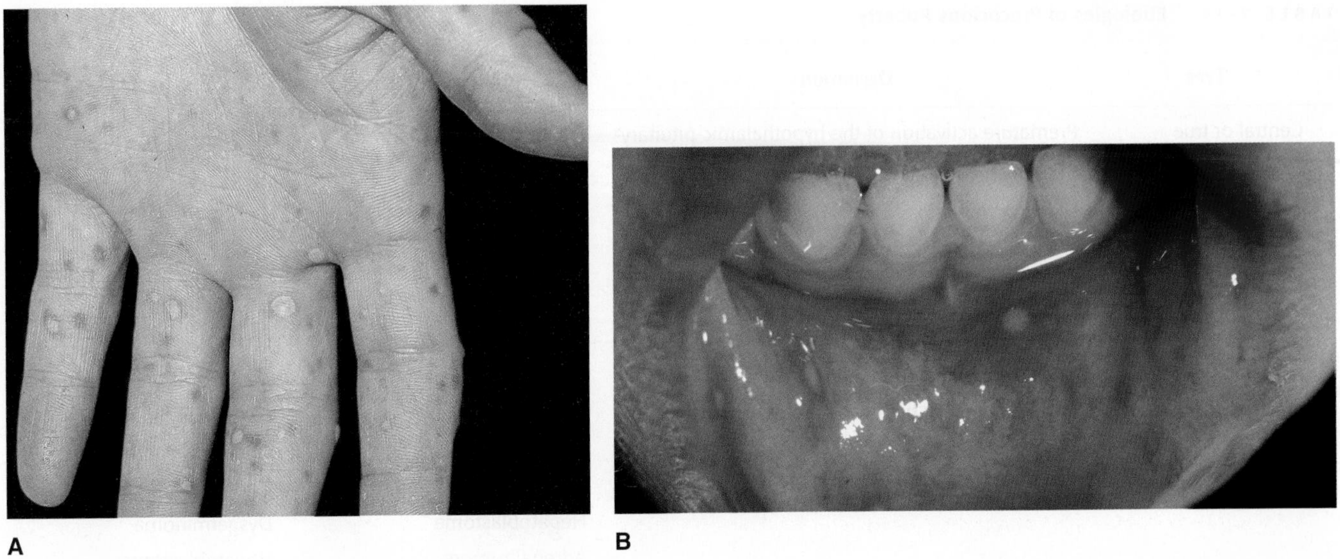

FIGURE 7-4. Hand-foot-and-mouth disease. (**A**) Multiple discrete vesicular lesions are seen on the fingers and palms. (**B**) Multiple superficial erosions and small vesicular lesions surrounded by an erythematous halo are seen on the lower labial mucosa. (Reproduced with permission from Wolff K, Johnson RA. *Fitzpatrick's Color Atlas & Synopsis of Clinical Dermatology,* 6th ed. New York: McGraw-Hill, 2009, Fig. 27-23A and B.)

Endocrinology

PRECOCIOUS PUBERTY

Defined as premature onset of 2° sexual characteristics. In girls, the criterion is < 8 years of age for Caucasians and < 7 years of age for African Americans and Hispanics. In boys, it is defined as < 9 years of age. Etiologies are outlined in Table 7-14.

Signs and Symptoms

- Growth acceleration; advanced bone age.
- Progressive sexual development.
- Premature thelarche (breast development); premature pubarche/adrenarche (pubic hair development).

Workup

- FSH, LH, estradiol, testosterone, DHEAS, 17-hydroxyprogesterone, and androstenedione can help distinguish central from peripheral causes.
- **α-fetoprotein (AFP), hCG:** Elevated levels can indicate the presence of germ cell tumors.
- **Gonadotropin-releasing hormone (GnRH) stimulation:** In peripheral precocious puberty, no ↑ in gonadotropins is seen following GnRH stimulation; in central precocious puberty, a pubertal LH-dominant response is seen.
- **Scrotal or pelvic ultrasound:** To look for peripheral etiologies (eg, Leydig cell tumor).
- **MRI of the brain:** To look for central etiologies (eg, hypothalamic hamartoma).
- **CT of the abdomen and pelvis:** To look for peripheral etiologies (eg, adrenal tumor).
- **Radiographs:** To determine bone age vs. true chronological age.

Q

A 6-year-old girl develops enlarged breasts and then develops pubic and axillary hair a few months later. Her menses began at age 9. What is the cause of her condition, and how should she be evaluated?

TABLE 7-14. Etiologies of Precocious Puberty

Type	Definition	Male Causes	Female Causes
Central or true	Premature activation of the hypothalamic-pituitary-gonadal axis. Gonadotropin dependent. High FSH, LH, sex steroids.	Hypothalamic hamartoma Head injury Hydrocephalus Radiation Surgical trauma Brain tumors	Same as male causes
Peripheral or pseudo-precocious puberty	Gonadotropin independent. Low FSH and LH; high sex steroids.	Testotoxicosis Leydig cell tumor Choriocarcinoma Dysgerminoma Hepatoblastoma Adrenal tumors Congenital adrenal hyperplasia McCune-Albright syndrome Exogenous steroid use	McCune-Albright syndrome Granulosa cell tumor Gonadoblastoma Choriocarcinoma Dysgerminoma Hepatoblastoma Adrenal tumors Exogenous steroid use

Treatment

- Treat the underlying cause in both central and peripheral etiologies.
- GnRH analogs are used for central precocious puberty.
- Androgen antagonists and aromatase inhibitors are given for peripheral precocious puberty.

DIABETIC KETOACIDOSIS (DKA)

An acute complication of DM that is usually precipitated by stress, infection, and trauma. Defined as hyperglycemia (a blood glucose level > 200 mg/dL), a pH < 7.30, a bicarbonate level < 15 mmol/L, ketonuria, and ketonemia (> 3 mmol/L). Other lab findings include an anion gap (> 12–16 mEq/L), hemoconcentration, leukocytosis, pseudohyponatremia, and hyperkalemia.

Signs and Symptoms

Polyuria, polydipsia, dehydration, fatigue, headache, nausea, vomiting, abdominal pain, tachycardia, and tachypnea.

Treatment

- **Fluids:** Give 10- to 20-mL/kg boluses of NS over 1 hour, followed by repletion of remaining fluid over 24–48 hours plus maintenance fluids. Beware of more rapid volume repletion, as it may precipitate cerebral edema, the most feared complication of DKA.
- **Electrolytes:** Fluids should contain one-half NS, since sodium will correct as glucose drops; potassium should be given as one-half KCl or potassium acetate plus one-half potassium phosphate. Bicarbonate is rarely given except in extreme acidosis.
- **Insulin:**
  - Begin with an insulin drip at 0.1 U/kg/hr after the first fluid bolus with a goal glucose drop of 80–100 mg/dL/hr. When glucose levels reach

A

Idiopathic precocious puberty. Evaluation should include serum FSH, LH, estradiol, and bone age. A brain MRI should be obtained to rule out intracranial lesions.

250–300 mg/dL/hr or there is a change in blood glucose > 100 mg/dL/hr, D5 should be added to fluids.
- Once pH is > 7.30, bicarbonate is > 16 mmol/L, anion gap is resolved, and the patient is eating food, start SQ insulin and discontinue the insulin drip after 1 hour.

Complications

- **Before therapy:** Severe dehydration, cardiac arrhythmias due to hyperkalemia, cerebral edema (treat with immediate reduction in IV fluid rate, hyperventilation, and mannitol).
- **After initiation of therapy:** Hypokalemia due to low total body potassium and insulin administration, hypoglycemia, cerebral edema.

Gastroenterology

INTUSSUSCEPTION

Occurs when 1 portion of the bowel telescopes into an adjacent portion, usually proximal to or involving the ileocecal valve. It is the most common cause of acute intestinal obstruction in the first 2 years of life and affects males more often than females. Risk factors include viral infections (enterovirus in summer, rotavirus in winter) and "lead points" caused by polyps, Meckel's diverticulum, Henoch-Schönlein purpura, intestinal lymphoma, celiac disease, and CF.

Signs and Symptoms

- The classic triad consists of colicky abdominal pain, bilious vomiting, and red "currant jelly" stool (a rare and late finding).
- Neurologic signs include lethargy (very important as a sole sign).
- An ill-defined, "sausage-shaped" mass is palpated in the RUQ.
- Dance's sign, or absence of bowel in the RLQ, is also seen.

Differential

Constipation, GI infection, Meckel's diverticulum, lymphoma (in children > 6 years of age), meconium ileus (neonates).

Workup

- AXR shows a paucity of bowel gas, loss of liver tip, and the "target" sign.
- Ultrasound is the test of choice and shows a "target" or "doughnut" sign or a "pseudokidney" sign (see Figure 7-5).
- Barium enema shows a cervix-like mass (not useful for ileoileal intussusceptions). Contraindications to this test include peritonitis, perforation, and profound shock.
- Air enema is preferred over barium enema.

Treatment

- Correct dehydration.
- NG tube for decompression.
- Barium/air enema for reduction.
- If enema reduction is unsuccessful or peritoneal signs are present, surgery is indicated.

KEY FACT

The classic triad of intussusception (intermittent colicky abdominal pain, bilious vomiting, and "currant jelly" stool) is found in only 20% of cases.

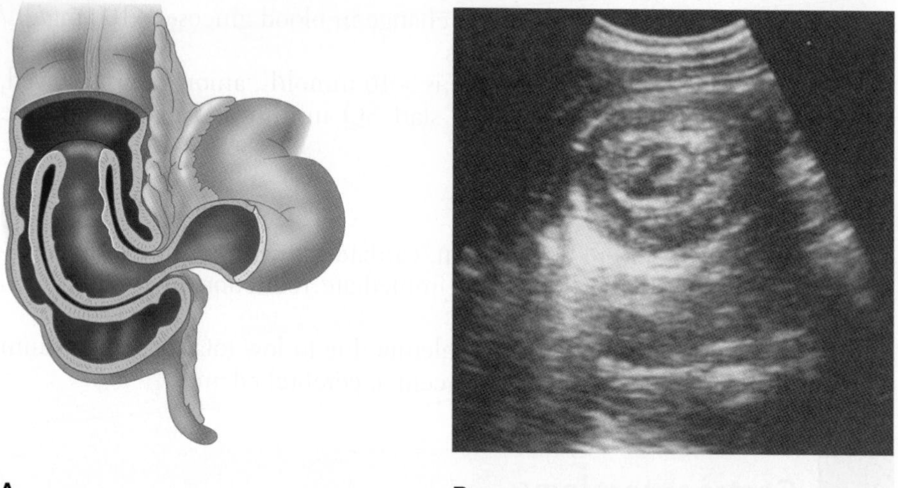

FIGURE 7-5. Intussusception. (A) Ileocolic intussusception, the most common location in children. (B) Transabdominal ultrasound shows the classic "target" sign or doughnut appearance of bowel-within-bowel. (Image A reproduced with permission from Doherty GM. *Current Diagnosis & Treatment: Surgery,* 13th ed. New York: McGraw-Hill, 2010, Fig. 43-12. Image B reproduced with permission from Ma OJ et al. *Emergency Ultrasound,* 2nd ed. New York: McGraw-Hill, 2008, Fig. 9-15A.)

> **KEY FACT**
>
> Pyloric stenosis is most often seen in firstborn males.

> **KEY FACT**
>
> Erythromycin use is associated with an ↑ risk of pyloric stenosis.

PYLORIC STENOSIS

A gastric outlet obstruction caused by hypertrophy of the pyloric sphincter in the first 2–8 weeks of life. It is more common in firstborn males, exhibiting a male-to-female ratio of 4:1. Incidence is approximately 1 in 500 births. Risk factors include administration of erythromycin.

Signs and Symptoms

- Presents with projectile nonbilious emesis after feedings that gradually ↑ in intensity and frequency.
- An olive-shaped mass may be palpable in the epigastric area.
- Gastric peristaltic waves may be visible after feeding.
- Hypochloremic hypokalemic metabolic alkalosis with dehydration is commonly seen.

Differential

Pylorospasm, overfeeding, gastroenteritis, hiatal hernia, duodenal atresia ("double bubble" sign on x-ray), esophageal stenosis, malrotation/volvulus, incarcerated hernias, meconium ileus, milk protein allergy, gastroesophageal reflux.

Workup

- BMP.
- Ultrasound, which can detect pyloric muscle diameter and thickness, has 90% sensitivity.
- AXR may show a dilated, air-filled stomach.

Treatment

- NG tube placement.
- Correction of dehydration and electrolyte abnormalities (crucial).
- Surgical pyloromyotomy after dehydration and electrolytes are corrected.

MECKEL'S DIVERTICULUM

Prolonged persistence of the omphalomesenteric (vitelline) duct, which should normally disappear by the seventh week of gestation. Usually occurs proximal to the ileocecal valve.

Signs and Symptoms

- Intermittent painless rectal bleeding is the most common presenting sign.
- Intestinal obstruction and diverticulitis are also seen.

Differential

Acute appendicitis, intussusception, volvulus, GI infection.

Workup

- Stool guaiac.
- Meckel's scan (scintigraphy); uptake is enhanced by cimetidine, glucagon, or gastrin.

Treatment

Surgical resection with transverse closure of the enterotomy.

> **MNEMONIC**
>
> ***Meckel's rules of 2:***
>
> **2**% of population
> **2** inches long
> **2** feet from the ileocecal valve
> < **2** years of age
> **2**% symptomatic

HIRSCHSPRUNG'S DISEASE

Defined as absence of ganglion cells in the bowel, leading to abnormal innervation. Males are affected more often than females, and incidence ↑ with a ⊕ family history. Associated with Down syndrome.

Signs and Symptoms

- Delayed passage of meconium at birth (after 48 hours of age).
- ↑ abdominal distention → ↓ intestinal blood flow → deterioration of the mucosal barrier → bacterial proliferation → enterocolitis.
- Chronic constipation and abdominal distention are seen in older children.

Workup

- Rectal manometry to measure the pressure of the anal sphincter.
- Barium enema shows a narrowed rectal segment with a sharp transition from the dilated proximal bowel.
- Definitive diagnosis can be made with rectal suction biopsy, but submucosa must be obtained to evaluate for rectal ganglion cells.

Treatment

Surgery is definitive.

> **Q**
>
> A full-term male infant develops progressive abdominal distention on the second day of life, with no stool since birth. AXR shows distended loops of bowel. Contrast enema reveals a narrowed distal segment of colon and a distended proximal loop. What is the diagnosis, and how should the infant be managed?

Genetic Disorders

AUTOSOMAL TRISOMIES (21, 18, 13)

There are many important chromosomal abnormalities in pediatrics. Table 7-15 outlines the 3 major autosomal trisomies with which you should be familiar.

TABLE 7-15. Autosomal Trisomies

Disorder	Clinical Features	Epidemiology/Prognosis
Trisomy 21 (Down syndrome)	Mental retardation, hypotonia. Brushfield spots (speckled irises), transverse palmar crease, flat nasal bridge and epicanthal folds, short stature, endocardial cushion/septal defects. ↑ incidence of ALL and AML. Duodenal atresia, Hirschsprung's disease, hypothyroidism. Alzheimer's disease is seen in adulthood (affects 25% of Down patients > 35 years of age).	Incidence is 1 in 600 live births and ↑ with advanced maternal age. Life expectancy is 30s–40s. Maternal serum AFP ↓; maternal β-hCG ↑.
Trisomy 18 (Edwards' syndrome)	Severe mental/growth retardation, seizures, hypertonia. Prominent occiput, low-set ears, small mouth, short sternum, rocker-bottom feet, camptodactyly (overlapping fourth and fifth digits/clenched hands). Horseshoe kidney, VSD.	Incidence is 1 in 6000 live births; has a male-to-female ratio of 1:3. Roughly 50% of patients die in the first week of life; 90% die in the first year of life.
Trisomy 13 (Patau's syndrome)	Severe mental/growth retardation. Holoprosencephaly, microphthalmia, polydactyly, agenesis of the corpus callosum. Scalp aplasia cutis, cystic kidneys, VSD.	Incidence is 1 in 10,000 live births; 60% of those affected are female. Some 80% of patients die in the first month of life; 5% survive past 6 months.

A

The infant has Hirschsprung's disease. Definitive diagnosis is made by rectal biopsy; surgery is indicated for bowel resection.

Hematology and Oncology

SICKLE CELL DISEASE (SCD)

An autosomal recessive disorder resulting from a mutation in the β-globin chain. Occurs in 1 in 500 African Americans. Median life expectancy is 42 years for men and 48 years for women. Patients endure a chronic hemolytic anemia with intermittent acute events or "crises." These crises generally require hospital admission and include the following:

- **Vaso-occlusive crisis or "pain crisis":** The most common cause of hospital admissions. Microvascular infarcts occurring in any tissue in the body lead to pain and organ dysfunction. Examples include hand-foot syndrome (dactylitis), priapism, and avascular necrosis of the femoral head. Pain crises typically occur in bones.
- **Acute chest syndrome:** The second leading cause of hospital admissions. Defined by the radiologic appearance of a new pulmonary opacity along with fever and respiratory symptoms (see Figure 7-6); hypoxia may be present but is not required for diagnosis. The etiology is often unknown, but infection and fat emboli (from bone marrow infarcts) are known causes.

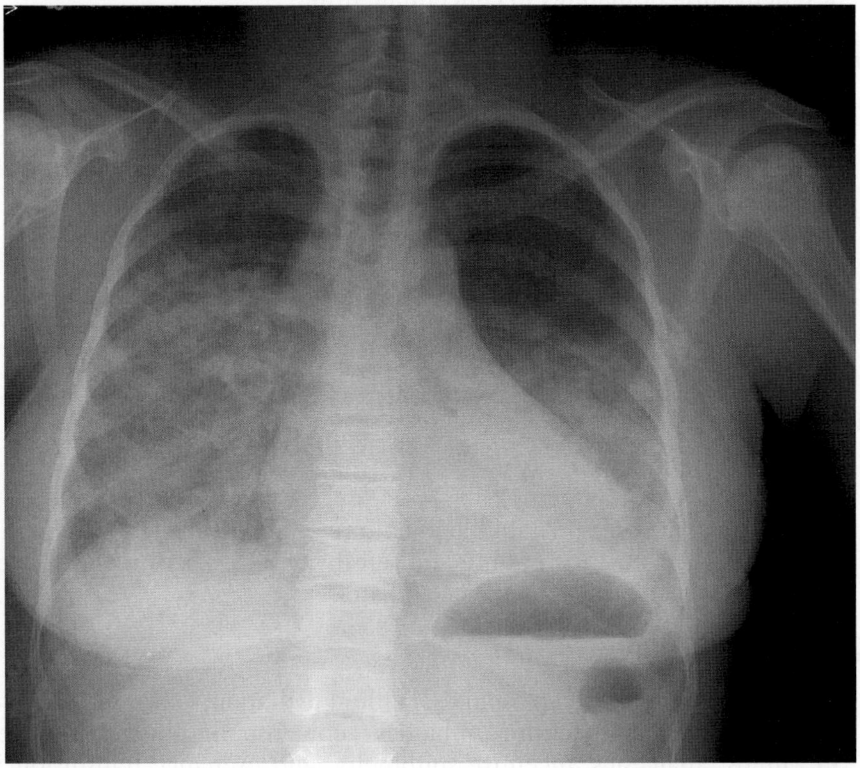

FIGURE 7-6. Acute chest syndrome. Frontal CXR of a 19-year-old female with sickle cell disease and acute chest pain. Note the bilateral lower and midlung opacities and mild cardiomegaly. (Reproduced with permission from USMLERx.com.)

- **Aplastic anemia:** Transient suppression of RBC precursors in bone marrow, often due to parvovirus B19 infection; leads to an acute and reversible reticulocytopenia. Most patients need transfusions for 1–2 weeks. Anemia in sickle cell disease results from the much shorter half-life of a sickled RBC relative to a normal RBC.
- **Hemolytic crisis:** An acute ↓ in hemoglobin resulting from exposure to oxidative stress, typically in patients with G6PD deficiency.
- **Acute splenic sequestration:** An acute ↓ in hemoglobin 2° to splenic pooling of RBCs with splenomegaly and hypovolemic shock. Typically occurs between 6 months and 2 years of age. Splenectomy should be considered if patients have had 2 or more events.
- **Serious infection:** By 2–4 years of age, sickle cell patients are also susceptible to life-threatening infections with encapsulated organisms (*Streptococcus pneumoniae, H influenzae, Salmonella, Neisseria meningitidis*) due to functional asplenia.
- **Cerebrovascular disease:** Overt occlusive stroke involving large cerebral arteries affects 11% of patients by age 20, and silent infarcts (involving sickling in microcirculation) are detected by neuroimaging studies in an additional 22%.
- **Other:** Pulmonary artery hypertension, renal papillary necrosis, hematuria, cholelithiasis (pigment stones), retinopathy. Heterozygotes with "sickle cell trait" generally have no manifestations of disease but may show painless hematuria or inability to concentrate urine.

KEY FACT

Sickle cell patients are at higher risk for *Salmonella* osteomyelitis than the general population.

Signs and Symptoms

- A progressive hemolytic anemia develops after 6 months of age as HbF ↓.
- Patients may exhibit pallor, splenomegaly, cardiomegaly, a systolic ejection murmur, short stature, and delayed puberty. Gallstones/jaundice are also seen.
- Dactylitis (swollen hands and feet) is most often seen in toddlers.
- Complications of vaso-occlusive crisis include leg ulcers, stroke, priapism, and pain crises.
- Patients with a fever > 38°C (> 100.4°F) must be evaluated for bacterial sepsis, septic joints, and osteomyelitis.

KEY FACT

All sickle cell patients with fever need a workup for sepsis.

Workup

- Newborn screening at birth.
- Hemoglobin electrophoresis.
- During an acute crisis, obtain blood cultures and sensitivities, CBC, reticulocyte count, UA/urine culture and sensitivity, CXR, serum electrolytes, a peripheral blood smear, and type and cross.

Treatment

- **Pain crisis:** NSAIDs and/or opioids, IV fluid hydration, O_2 for hypoxia.
- **Acute chest:** Broad-spectrum antibiotics (cephalosporin plus a macrolide), O_2, fluids, analgesics, incentive spirometry, and exchange transfusion in the setting of hypoxia or a hematocrit < 18%.
- **Stroke, priapism, and other complications:** Chronic exchange transfusions to keep HbS < 30%.
- **Aplastic anemia, sequestration, hemolytic crisis:** Simple transfusion.

Prevention

- To prevent bacteremia, start prophylactic oral penicillin VK BID and folate at diagnosis and continue until the child is at least 5 years of age.

- In light of the high incidence of splenic autoinfarction, patients must be vaccinated against encapsulated organisms such as *S pneumoniae* (PCV23 pneumococcal vaccine), *H influenzae*, and *N meningitidis*.
- **Retinal examinations** for sickle retinopathy (yearly starting at age 8).
- **Transcranial Dopplers** for assessing stroke risk (every 1–2 years at age 2).
- **Hip radiographs** for avascular necrosis (yearly starting at age 10).
- **Echocardiography** for pulmonary artery pressures (every other year starting at age 10).
- Chronic transfusion therapy in patients at high risk for stroke as identified by transcranial Dopplers.
- Hydroxyurea in children > 5 years of age with severe complications to ↑ the proportion of HbF.
- Bone marrow transplantation has significant risks but has been curative in some children.
- Deferoxamine and deferasirox can be given with transfusions to prevent hemochromatosis.

CHILDHOOD CANCERS

Although there are many important pediatric cancers, the key features of selected malignancies are discussed below.

Acute Lymphocytic Leukemia (ALL)

ALL is a malignant disorder of lymphoblasts and is the most common childhood cancer, exhibiting a peak onset at age 4.

Signs and Symptoms

- Patients often present with lethargy, fever, fatigue, and anorexia.
- Bone pain, limp, and refusal to bear weight may also be seen.
- CNS manifestations include headache.
- Signs include petechiae, purpura and bleeding (from thrombocytopenia), pallor (from anemia), lymphadenopathy, hepatosplenomegaly, and testicular swelling.

Differential

Aplastic anemia, immune thrombocytopenic purpura, rheumatic diseases (SLE, JIA), other malignancies, mononucleosis or other viral infections.

Workup

- CBC reveals anemia, an abnormal WBC count, and a low platelet count.
- Peripheral smear shows immature lymphoblasts.
- Baseline CMP along with calcium, magnesium, and phosphorus (acts as a baseline prior to chemotherapy to monitor for tumor lysis syndrome).
- LDH and uric acid levels (often ↑).
- Bone marrow biopsy reveals hypercellular marrow with ↑ lymphoblasts.
- Flow cytometry.
- CXR, LP, and CT to screen for metastases.

Treatment

- **Induction:** Cytoxan, vincristine, prednisone, L-asparaginase, and/or doxorubicin are commonly used.
- **Consolidation:** 6-MP, 6-TB, or cytosine arabinoside may be added.

KEY FACT

Although ALL is a lymphocyte-proliferative disorder, WBC counts can be low, normal, or high.

- **Maintenance:** 6-MP and methotrexate; vincristine and prednisone may be added.
- **CNS prophylaxis:** Intrathecal methotrexate; patients may have radiation to the head.

COMPLICATIONS

- One of the major complications of treatment is **tumor lysis syndrome,** which occurs during the induction phase of chemotherapy.
- Rapid killing of tumor cells releases high concentrations of potassium, phosphate, and uric acid (from DNA breakdown).
- Untreated tumor lysis syndrome can result in acute renal failure (from uric acid deposition in the renal tubules) and cardiac arrhythmias (from hyperkalemia).
- Tumor lysis is treated with fluids, diuretics, allopurinol, alkalinization of urine, and reduction of phosphate.

Wilms' Tumor (Nephroblastoma)

> **KEY FACT**
>
> Wilms' tumor accounts for > 6% of pediatric cancers, more than lymphoma.

> **KEY FACT**
>
> Wilms' tumor has an overall cure rate of > 85%.

A tumor of embryonal origin and the most common renal tumor in children. Seen between 1 and 4 years of age and associated with a family history of Wilms' tumor, Beckwith-Wiedemann syndrome (hemihypertrophy, macroglossia, omphalocele, and embryonal tumors), Denys-Drash syndrome (nephropathy and genital abnormalities), **WAGR** syndrome (**W**ilms' tumor, **A**niridia, **G**enitourinary abnormalities, and mental **R**etardation), and neurofibromatosis. A small number of tumors are bilateral. Wilms' tumor spreads by contiguous invasion of adjacent organs, extension into the renal vein and IVC, and hematogenous spread to the lung and liver.

SIGNS AND SYMPTOMS

- The most common presentation is a painless abdominal or flank mass (classically discovered while parents are giving the child a bath).
- Fever, nausea, emesis, bone pain, weight loss, hematuria, dysuria, and polyuria may also be seen.
- Common findings include hypertension (due to ↑ renin secretion by tumor or compression of renal vasculature) and varicocele in boys (due to spermatic vein compression).

DIFFERENTIAL

Neuroblastoma, polycystic kidneys, hydronephrosis, other abdominal neoplasms.

WORKUP

- Renal ultrasound.
- CT scan to stage and find metastases (present at diagnosis in 10–15% of patients). Stages are as follows:
  1: Tumor limited to the kidney; operable.
  2: Growth beyond the kidney; operable.
  3: Nonhematogenous extension into the abdomen.
  4: Hematogenous metastases.
  5: Bilateral renal metastasis.
- Biopsy.
- CBC, LFTs, BUN/creatinine, UA.

TREATMENT

- **Stages 1–3:** Nephrectomy and chemotherapy with vincristine and dactinomycin.
- **Stage 4:** Pulmonary irradiation; 3-drug combination chemotherapy.

Neuroblastoma

A tumor of neural crest cells that make up the adrenal medulla and sympathetic nervous system. Neuroblastoma is the most common malignant tumor of infants and presents in children < 5 years of age. It may arise at any site of sympathetic nervous tissue, with the adrenals, retroperitoneal ganglia, and abdomen the most common sites. Associated with neurofibromatosis, Hirschsprung's disease, and fetal hydantoin syndrome.

KEY FACT

Neuroblastoma is the most common malignant tumor of infancy.

SIGNS AND SYMPTOMS

- Patients may present with abdominal distention, anorexia, weight loss, malaise, and muscular symptoms.
- Examination reveals a firm, smooth, nontender abdominal or flank mass.
- Hypertension (from compression of renal vasculature) is common; fever, pallor, and periorbital bruising ("raccoon eyes") are also seen.
- Metastases to the liver, bone, and lymph nodes can lead to hepatosplenomegaly, bone pain, or lymphadenopathy.
- Watery diarrhea (from secretion of VIP), opsoclonus/myoclonus ("dancing eyes/dancing feet"), and Horner's syndrome may also be present.

DIFFERENTIAL

Wilms' tumor, Ewing's sarcoma, rhabdomyosarcoma, lymphoma, hepatoblastoma.

WORKUP

- CT/MRI of the abdomen, chest, and pelvis.
- Bone scan and bone marrow aspirate; LP to look for metastasis.
- MIBG scan for detecting small 1° tumors and metastases.
- A 24-hour urine collection for catecholamines (VMA and HVA are ↑ in 95% of patients).
- CBC, LFTs, coagulation panel, BUN/creatinine.

KEY FACT

Infants tend to have neuroblastomas localized to the cervical/thoracic region, whereas older children have disseminated disease in the abdomen.

TREATMENT

- At diagnosis, 50% of children have distant metastases.
- Treat via excision of localized tumors.
- For intermediate- to high-risk stages, combination chemotherapy and/or radiation.

Immunology

AUTOIMMUNE DISORDERS

Juvenile Idiopathic Arthritis (JIA)

Formerly known as juvenile rheumatoid arthritis, JIA is a collagen vascular disease that is defined by persistent inflammation in 1 or more joints for 6 or

Q

A 1-year-old boy has refractory oral thrush despite nystatin treatment. He has a history of recurrent otitis media and uncontrolled eczema. His uncle died in infancy of infection. Both TMs are dull, and purpura and eczema are present. CBC reveals thrombocytopenia. What is the diagnosis?

more weeks in a patient < 16 years of age. Onset most commonly occurs at 1–3 years of age, with girls affected more often than boys. JIA is divided into 3 subtypes on the basis of clinical symptomatology: pauciarticular (50%), polyarticular (35%), and systemic (20%).

Signs and Symptoms

- **Pauciarticular:**
  - Affects < 5 joints in an asymmetric distribution; large weight-bearing joints (knees, ankles) are most commonly affected.
  - Iridocyclitis is found in 50% of cases.
  - Chronic asymptomatic uveitis (more likely in ANA-⊕ patients) can lead to blindness in young children if not diagnosed by slit-lamp examination. Acute-onset uveitis is more common in older children.
  - Systemic features are uncommon.
  - Has a good prognosis (~ 70% of patients go into remission after several years).
- **Polyarticular:**
  - A long-term arthritis whose symptoms wax and wane.
  - Affects 5 or more joints in a symmetric distribution. Both large (knees, ankles) and small joints (hands, feet) are affected. The TMJ and cervical vertebrae may also be involved.
  - Systemic features are less prominent.
  - RF seropositivity is associated with older age of onset, ⊕ ANA, and more severe disease.
- **Systemic (Still's disease):**
  - Characterized by recurrent high, spiking fevers to > 39.4°C (> 102.9°F) that may begin weeks prior to the arthritis; a salmon-pink macular rash that comes and goes with fever; and unremitting, severe arthritis.
  - RF and ANA are ⊖.
  - Myalgias, pericarditis, pleuritis, lymphadenopathy, hepatosplenomegaly, and growth retardation are also seen.
  - Labs reveal anemia of chronic disease, leukocytosis, ↑ ESR, ↑ CRP, and ↑ platelets.
  - Has the worst prognosis (complete resolution is rare, and ~ 50% develop destructive arthritis).

KEY FACT

Children with systemic JIA are at risk for **macrophage activation syndrome,** a life-threatening condition marked by high fever, pancytopenia, hepatosplenomegaly, liver dysfunction, DIC, hypofibrinogenemia, hyperferritinemia, and hypertriglyceridemia.

Differential

Lyme disease, seronegative spondyloarthropathies (for the pauciarticular type), rheumatic fever, SLE, occult infection, sarcoidosis, juvenile dermatomyositis, malignancy.

KEY FACT

A normal ESR does not exclude the diagnosis of JIA.

Workup

- CBC and ESR.
- RF/ANA serologies.
- Radiographs show soft tissue swelling, osteopenia, joint space narrowing, or bony erosions.
- MRI is more sensitive for early joint changes.
- Synovial fluid analysis reveals leukocytosis (5000–30,000 WBCs/mm^3) and elevated protein.

A

Wiskott-Aldrich syndrome, an X-linked recessive syndrome characterized by the triad of eczema, thrombocytopenia, and immunodeficiency. Definitive treatment consists of bone marrow transplantation.

Treatment

- Most patients respond to NSAIDs. ASA is contraindicated because of the risk of Reye's syndrome.

- Intra-articular steroids are of benefit for joint pain and swelling; systemic steroids are appropriate for severe systemic disease or uveitis.
- Methotrexate can be given for severe disease.
- Anti-TNF therapy (etanercept or infliximab) is appropriate for refractory polyarticular disease.
- Stretching and morning baths are helpful for morning stiffness.
- Steroid eye drops and dilating agents for uveitis.
- Calcium supplements and weight-bearing exercises to prevent osteoporosis.

Kawasaki Disease

An acute autoimmune vasculitis of unknown etiology, Kawasaki disease is the most common cause of acquired heart disease in children. It is more common among Asians and males and most often occurs in the winter and spring.

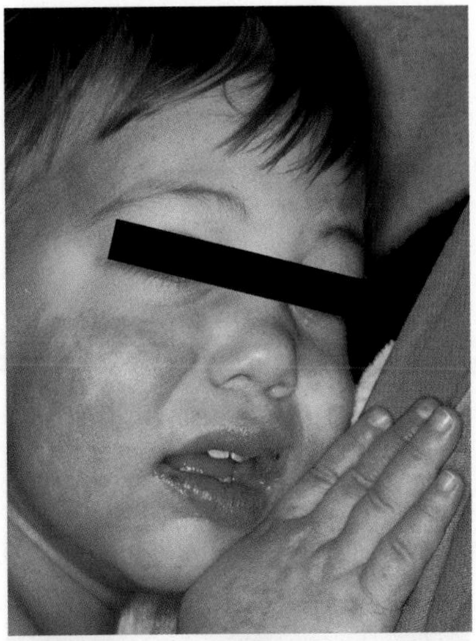

FIGURE 7-7. Kawasaki disease. Note the cherry-red lips with hemorrhagic fissures in this boy with prolonged high fever. The child also has a generalized morbilliform eruption, injected conjunctivae, erythema/edema of the fingertips, and "strawberry tongue." (Reproduced with permission from Wolff K, Johnson RA. *Fitzpatrick's Color Atlas & Synopsis of Clinical Dermatology,* 6th ed. New York: McGraw-Hill, 2009, Fig. 14-44.)

Signs and Symptoms

- Presents with a high fever, bilateral nonexudative conjunctivitis, mucocutaneous changes ("strawberry tongue," cracked or red lips), swelling and/or erythema of the hands and feet, cervical lymphadenopathy, a maculopapular or polymorphous rash (more common in infants), and a perineal rash with desquamation (see Figure 7-7).
- Extreme irritability, abdominal pain, diarrhea, and vomiting are commonly seen.
- Desquamation of the fingers and toes is seen in the subacute phase.
- Children who are suspected of having Kawasaki disease but do not meet the full diagnostic criteria are said to have incomplete Kawasaki disease. These children are still at risk for cardiac complications.

Workup

- CBC may show anemia, thrombocytosis, and leukocytosis with left shift.
- ESR and/or CRP may be elevated; LFTs are ↑.
- Blood cultures, LP (may reveal aseptic meningitis); UA and urine culture (may show sterile pyuria).
- ECG; baseline echocardiogram to evaluate for early coronary aneurysms.

Treatment

- Treatment is necessary to prevent cardiac sequelae.
- Give a 2-g/kg dose of IVIG over 10–12 hours.

KEY POINT

DIAGNOSTIC CRITERIA FOR KAWASAKI DISEASE

Fever for ≥ 5 days without other explanation plus 4 or more of the following:

- Bilateral conjunctivitis (without exudate)
- "Strawberry tongue"; dry, red, cracked lips; diffuse erythema of the oral cavity
- Erythema and/or edema of the hands and feet
- Polymorphic rash (usually truncal)
- Cervical lymphadenopathy (1 lymph node ≥ 1.5 cm)

Q

A 3-year-old Asian male presents with 7 days of high fever, nonexudative conjunctivitis bilaterally, erythema multiforme, anterior cervical lymphadenopathy, sterile pyuria, thrombocytosis, and erythematous lips, palms, and soles. What is the diagnosis and major complication, and how should the condition be treated?

- High-dose ASA (80–100 mg/kg/day in 4 doses) should be given until 48–72 hours after fever resolves, followed by low-dose ASA (3–5 mg/kg/day).
- Steroids should be given only if the disease is refractory to repeat doses of IVIG.

COMPLICATIONS

Coronary artery aneurysms (children < 1 year of age are less likely to meet all the criteria for Kawasaki but are more likely to develop aneurysms); pericardial effusion, CHF.

Henoch-Schönlein Purpura (HSP)

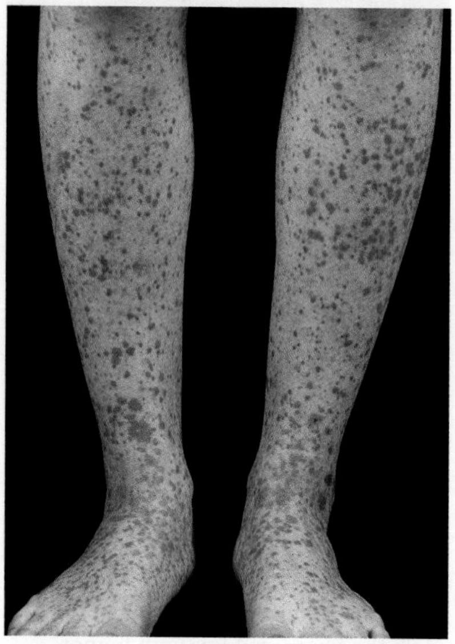

FIGURE 7-8. Henoch-Schönlein purpura. Classic palpable purpura on the lower legs is seen in a patient with colicky abdominal pain, arthritis, and microhematuria. (Reproduced with permission from Wolff K, Johnson RA. *Fitzpatrick's Color Atlas & Synopsis of Clinical Dermatology,* 6th ed. New York: McGraw-Hill, 2009, Fig. 14-35.)

The most common small vessel immune-mediated vasculitis in children; involves the GI tract, joints, and kidneys and produces a characteristic rash. Affects males more often than females, with a typical age of onset of 2–7 years. Most often occurs in the winter months following a group A streptococcal URI.

SIGNS AND SYMPTOMS

- **Palpable purpura:**
  - The most common presenting feature (see Figure 7-8).
  - Urticarial lesions → maculopapular rash → purpuric lesions.
  - Most commonly appears on the legs and buttocks.
  - New lesions can appear for 2–4 weeks.
- **Migratory polyarthritis and/or polyarthralgias:**
  - The presenting feature in 25% of cases.
  - Characterized by tender and painful periarticular joint swelling.
  - No joint effusion is present.
  - Involves the ankles and knees; usually transient with no permanent deformities.
- **Abdominal pain:**
  - Colicky in nature.
  - 2° to hemorrhage and edema of the small intestine.
  - Can result in ileoileal intussusception in 2% of cases.
  - Associated with vomiting and upper/lower GI bleeding.
- **Glomerulonephritis:**
  - Seen in 25–50% of cases; can develop months prior or after onset of rash.
  - IgA nephropathy is characteristic.
  - RBC casts and acute renal failure can develop.

WORKUP

- CBC, platelet function tests, bleeding time, coagulation studies.
- UA, stool guaiac.
- IgA levels may be elevated.

A

Kawasaki disease is associated with a significant risk of coronary aneurysms and must be treated with IVIG and high-dose ASA.

TREATMENT

- Provide adequate hydration.
- Monitor vital signs in light of GI bleeding and renal involvement.
- Analgesia for joint pain.
- Steroids may be given in the setting of GI and renal involvement.
- Prolonged immunosuppression is needed if renal disease develops.

- Typically self-limited, with full recovery seen in 4–6 weeks.
- Screening UAs will be necessary for at least 3–6 months following the acute disease.

Idiopathic Thrombocytopenic Purpura (ITP)

An acquired autoimmune hemorrhagic disorder that results from excessive destruction of platelets. ITP is the most common thrombocytopenia of childhood and is typically benign. It is often preceded by a viral illness (varicella, rubella, mumps, infectious mononucleosis).

Signs and Symptoms

- A diagnosis of exclusion.
- Presents with a petechial rash, easy bruising, and an antecedent viral illness (50–65% of cases).

Workup

- CBC and peripheral blood smear reveal thrombocytopenia.
- Platelet function tests, coagulation studies, bleeding time (prolonged).
- ESR/CRP.
- Bone marrow biopsy and aspirate (to differentiate from malignancy) reveal ↑ megakaryocytes (not always indicated).

Treatment

- Based on the severity of bleeding; > 80% of patients recover within several months without treatment.
- Admit if platelet count is < **20,000/mm³**.
- IVIG or anti-Rho antibodies.
- IV methylprednisolone.
- Splenectomy is appropriate for children > 4 years of age and those with severe or chronic ITP (> 1 year).
- Platelet transfusion is of no benefit.

IMMUNODEFICIENCIES

1° immunodeficiencies can be divided into T-cell specific, B-cell specific, T-cell/B-cell combined, and phagocytic disorders. Table 7-16 discusses select immunodeficiency disorders. Immunodeficiencies often present with recurrent infections, so when you are evaluating a child for an immunodeficiency, it is important to note the following:

- **Age of onset:** T-cell deficiencies present in the first 3–4 months of life; B-cell deficiencies present after 6 months of age, when maternal antibodies disappear.
- **Inheritance:** Wiskott-Aldrich syndrome, Bruton's agammaglobulinemia, and most cases of chronic granulomatous disease are X-linked recessive disorders, which means that the vast majority of patients affected by these disorders are male.
- **Sites and types of infection:** B-cell deficiencies result in sinopulmonary and GI infections; T-cell deficiencies are associated with disseminated intracellular diseases; phagocytic deficiencies result in sinopulmonary and soft tissue infections.

KEY FACT

Selective IgA deficiency can have fatal anaphylaxis with blood (IVIG) infusion.

TABLE 7-16. Immunodeficiency Disorders

Disorder	Defect	Clinical Features	Infections	Treatment
		B-Cell Disorders		
Bruton's congenital agammaglobulinemia	X-linked; tyrosine kinase deficiency blocks B-cell maturation.	No tonsils; no palpable lymph nodes. ↓ B cells; ↓ immunoglobulins of all classes. Recurrent bacterial infections are seen after 6 months of age.	Sinopulmonary (pneumococcal), GI (*Giardia,* rotavirus).	IVIG.
Selective IgA deficiency	Defect in isotype switching to IgA.	Milk allergies and diarrhea are common. Patients may have autoimmune disorders (IBD, arthritis). Fatal anaphylaxis occurs with administration of IVIG. IgA < 5 mg/dL.	Primarily respiratory (sinus and lung).	IVIG is contraindicated.
Common variable immunodeficiency (CVID)	Defect in B-cell maturation; has many causes.	A group of disorders with a bimodal age distribution at 1–5 and 16–20 years of age. Lymphadenopathy and splenomegaly are common. Patients may have autoimmune disorders (IBD, arthritis). Lymphoid interstitial pneumonitis; granulomas on various organs. Associated with an ↑ risk of lymphoma and gastric cancer.	Pneumococcal, *Giardia,* *Mycoplasma,* sinusitis.	IVIG if IgG is < 400.
		T-Cell Disorders		
DiGeorge syndrome	22q11 deletion.	Thymic aplasia → ↓ T cells and ↓ immunoglobulins. Absent thymic shadow on CXR. Hypoparathyroidism → hypocalcemia → tetany and seizures. CHD and great vessel defects are common. Hypertelorism and cleft palate are seen (see Figure 7-9). Diagnose with FISH.	Opportunistic infections: *Candida,* *Mycobacterium,* VZV, CMV, PCP.	Thymus transplant (ALC < 100); use irradiated blood products only.
Hyper-IgE syndrome (Job's syndrome)	T cells fail to produce IFN-γ, leading to a neutrophil chemotactic defect.	Characterized by the mnemonic **FATED:** coarse **F**acies, noninflamed **A**bscesses, retained primary **T**eeth, ↑ Ig**E**, and **D**ermatologic problems (eczema). Lax joints; eosinophilia.	Skin and lung, *Staphylococcus,* *Aspergillus.*	Penicillinase-resistant antibiotics; bone marrow transplantation (BMT).
Chronic mucocutaneous candidiasis	T-cell dysfunction; inability to recognize *Candida* antigens.	Refractory thrush; severe refractory diaper rash. Angular cheilitis; thickened nails; periungual edema and erythema. Hypo-/hyperthyroidism. Normal T and B cells.	*Candida albicans* infections of skin and mucous membranes.	Systemic antifungals, skin care.

TABLE 7-16. Immunodeficiency Disorders *(continued)*

Disorder	Defect	Clinical Features	Infections	Treatment
		Combined B- and T-Cell Disorders		
Severe combined immunodeficiency (SCID)	Various types: IL-2 receptor defect, adenosine deaminase (ADA) deficiency.	Onset is at 3 months of age. Diarrhea, pneumonia, otitis, sepsis. FTT, skin rashes, no palpable lymph nodes. Hypoplastic thymus. ALC < 500 with no T and B cells. ↓ serum immunoglobulins.	Opportunistic infections: *Candida, Mycobacterium,* VZV, CMV, PCP.	Antimicrobial treatment, recombinant ADA, BMT.
Ataxia-telangiectasia	Defect in DNA repair enzymes.	Presents with the triad of cerebellar defects (ataxia), spider angiomas (telangiectasia), and IgA deficiency. Red sclerae are the earliest sign. Associated with an ↑ incidence of lymphomas and leukemias. Onset is during the first 6 years of life; patients are confined to a wheelchair by 10–12 years of age. Absence of antibodies after vaccination. ↓ IgA, IgM, and T4 cells; ↑ AFP.	Opportunistic infections, sinopulmonary infections.	Supportive, antibiotics.
Wiskott-Aldrich syndrome	X-linked recessive cytoskeleton defect; progressive T and B cell deletion.	Characterized by the mnemonic **TIE: T**hrombocytopenic purpura, **I**nfection, and **E**czema. ↓ IgM; ↑ IgA and IgE. Absence of antibodies after vaccines. Normal T and B cells.	Opportunistic infections.	BMT.
		Phagocytic Disorders		
Chronic granulomatous disease (CGD)	X-linked; lack of NADPH oxidase → ↓ reactive oxygen species in neutrophils.	Gingivitis and seborrheic dermatitis are commonly seen. Associated with retinitis pigmentosa. Chemotaxis and phagocytosis are intact. Hepatosplenomegaly (granulomas). Can't kill **catalase-⊕** bugs. Diagnosed by the nitroblue tetrazolium test and by the presence of leukocytosis and hypergammaglobulinemia.	Deep soft tissue abscesses, lymphadenitis, *Staphylococcus, Aspergillus, Burkholderia cepacia.*	Antimicrobial treatment; surgical excision of abscesses.
Chédiak-Higashi syndrome	Defect in microtubular function → ↓ phagocytosis.	Partial oculocutaneous albinism is frequently found. Neurologic involvement in the form of progressive neuropathy. Hepatosplenomegaly. Giant gray granules are seen in the cytoplasm of nucleated cells. Leukopenia, neutropenia. Abnormal chemotaxis test.	*Staphylococcus* infections of the skin and lung.	Antibiotics, BMT.

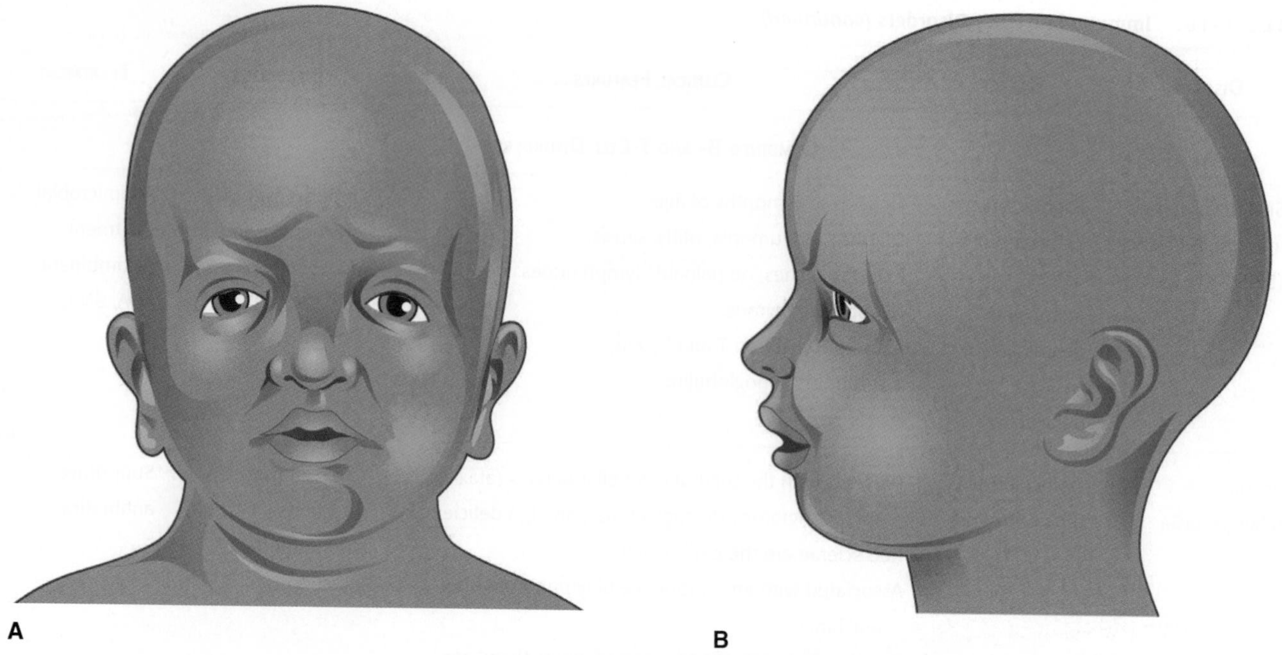

FIGURE 7-9. DiGeorge syndrome. Note the low-set ears, wide-set eyes (**A**), and small jaw (**B**). (Reproduced with permission from USMLERx.com.)

KEY FACT

All toxic-appearing children must be hospitalized for antibiotics and must receive a full workup for sepsis.

KEY FACT

Full sepsis workup:

- LP with CSF culture, Gram stain, cells, glucose, protein, and possibly HSV PCR
- Urine culture and UA
- CBC with differential, blood culture, and BMP (electrolytes, glucose, BUN/Cr)

KEY FACT

In neonates, group B streptococci (GBS), enteric gram-⊖ bacilli (*E coli*), and *Listeria* are the most common bugs.

Infectious Disease

FEVER WITHOUT A FOCUS

The management of a young child with fever depends on the age group of the child. Children are divided into 3 age groups for this purpose: < 28 days, 28–90 days, and 3–36 months. New management guidelines have diminished the number of hospitalizations for fever. To further clarify these new guidelines, a few definitions follow:

- **Fever:** A rectal temperature ≥ 38°C (≥ 100.4°F) in infants < 3 months of age, or ≥ 38.3°C (≥ 102°F) in those 3 months to 2 years of age.
- **"Toxic appearing":** Signifies lethargy, signs of poor perfusion, marked hypoventilation or hyperventilation, or cyanosis.
- **Lethargy:** An altered level of consciousness characterized by poor or absent eye contact or failure of the child to recognize the parents or interact with the environment.
- **Low-risk criteria (for infants 28–90 days):** Previously healthy, non–toxic appearing, no focal bacterial infection on examination (except otitis media), WBC count 5000–15,000/mm^3 (< 1500 bands), normal UA (< 5 WBCs/hpf) on Gram-stained smear; if diarrhea, < 5 WBCs/hpf in stool; if respiratory symptoms, normal CXR.

Febrile Infants < 28 Days

All febrile infants < 28 days old should be hospitalized for a full sepsis workup.

Workup

- Admit to the hospital.
- Blood culture, CBC with differential, BMP.
- UA and urine culture.
- LP for CSF culture, Gram stain, cell count, glucose, protein, HSV PCR.

Treatment

- Ampicillin + gentamicin or ampicillin + cefotaxime pending culture results (usually for a 48-hour rule-out).
- Antibiotics should be administered before the LP if any delay in the LP is anticipated.
- Acyclovir may be started empirically pending the results of CSF HSV PCR.

Febrile Infants 28–90 Days Without a Source

See Figure 7-10 for an algorithm on the management of infants in this age group.

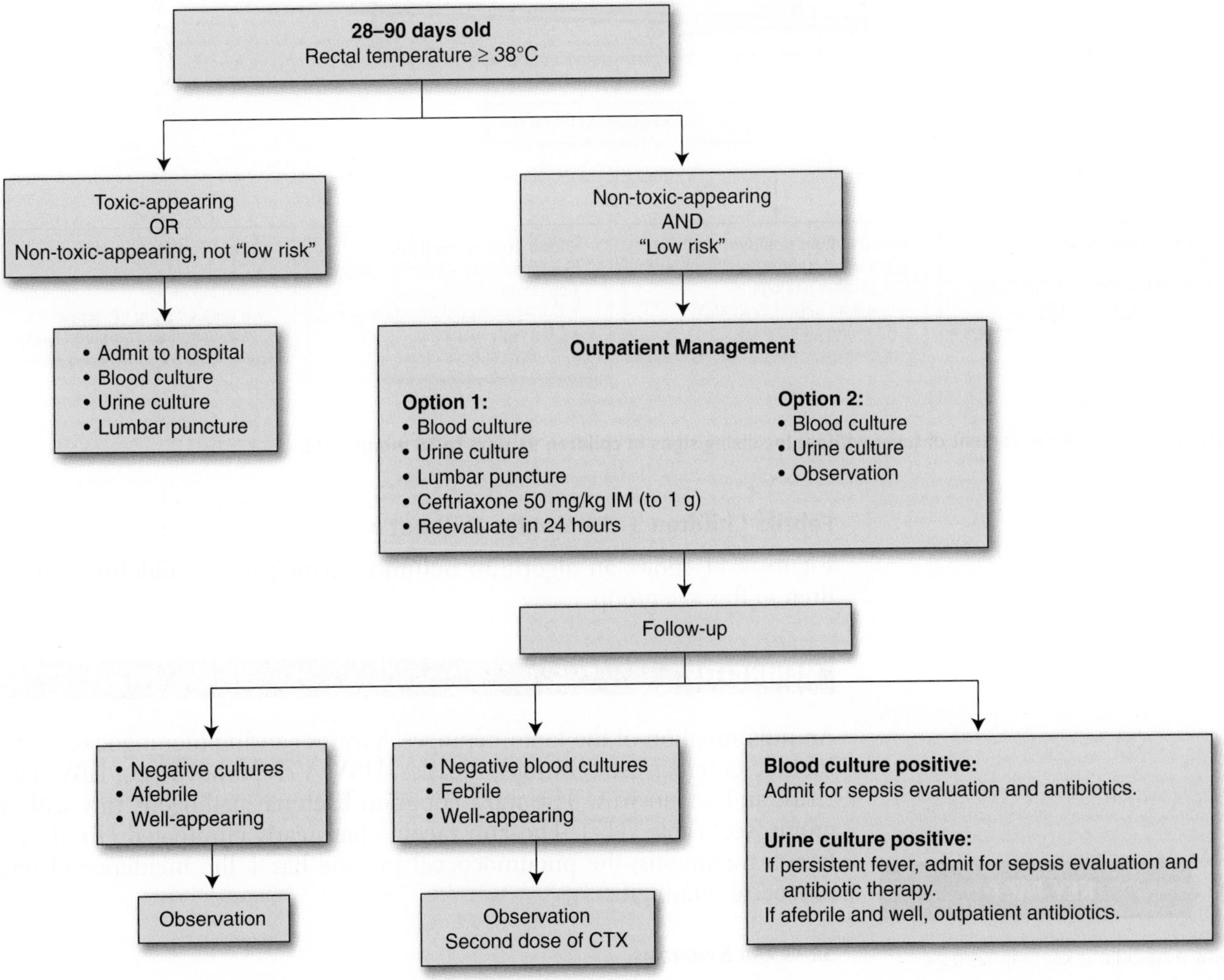

FIGURE 7-10. Management of fever without localizing signs in infants 28–90 days old.

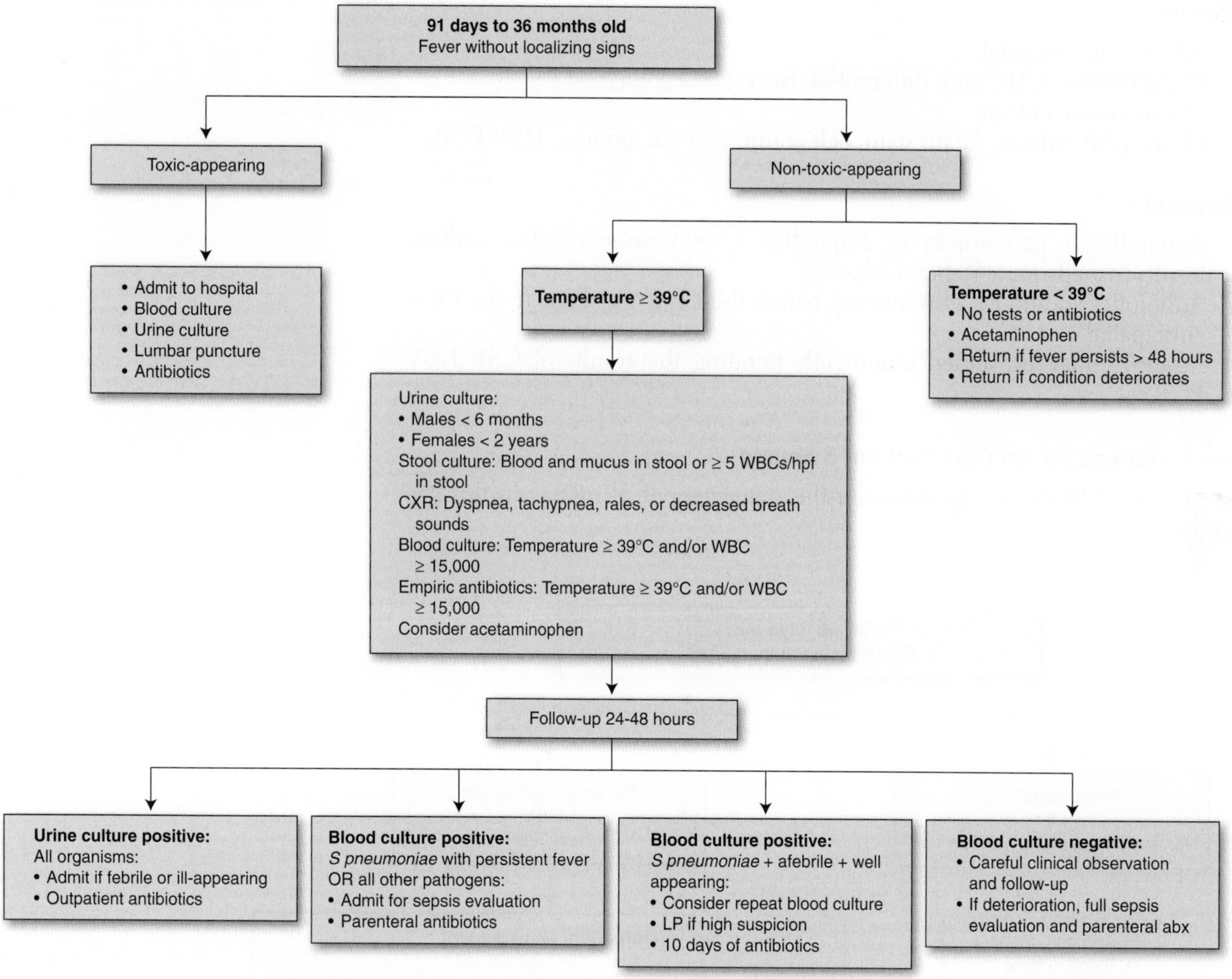

FIGURE 7-11. Management of fever without localizing signs in children 91 days to 36 months old.

Febrile Children 3–36 Months Without a Source

Figure 7-11 shows an algorithm outlining management guidelines for children in this age group.

MENINGITIS

An inflammation of the leptomeninges. Viruses causing meningoencephalitis include enteroviruses, mumps, measles, HSV, VZV, arboviruses, EBV, rabies virus, and adenovirus. The most common bacterial pathogens vary with age group (see Table 7-17). The Hib vaccine has nearly eliminated *H influenzae* type b meningitis; the pneumococcal vaccine has ↓ the incidence of pneumococcal meningitis.

KEY FACT

Having a hard time keeping Kernig's and Brudzinski's signs straight? Think "**K**nee" for **K**ernig's sign and "**B**rain" for **B**rudzinski's sign.

Signs and Symptoms

- **Kernig's sign:** Flexion of the hip to 90 degrees with pain on extension of the leg.
- **Brudzinski's sign:** Involuntary flexion of the knees/hips after neck flexion while supine.

TABLE 7-17. Common Bacterial Causes and Empiric Treatment of Meningitis

Age	Pathogens	Treatment
Neonates (< 1 month)	GBS *E coli* *Listeria monocytogenes*	Ampicillin + cefotaxime or ampicillin + gentamicin: ▪ × 14–21 days for GBS and *Listeria* ▪ × 21 days for *E coli*
Infants (1–3 months)	*S pneumoniae* *N meningitidis* GBS *H influenzae*	Ampicillin + cefotaxime: ▪ × 10–14 days for *S pneumoniae* ▪ × 7 days for *N meningitidis* ▪ × 7–10 days for *H influenzae*
Children (3 months–18 years)	*N meningitidis* *S pneumoniae* *H influenzae*	Cefotaxime or ceftriaxone. Vancomycin may be added for possible penicillin-resistant *S pneumoniae*. Duration is similar to that of infants.

- These signs are not always present in children and are not found in neonates.
- **Age-specific signs and symptoms:** See Table 7-18.

KEY FACT

In meningococcal meningitis (*N meningitidis*), a rapidly spreading petechial rash is typical and may precede other symptoms.

DIFFERENTIAL

Encephalitis, brain abscess, epidural or subdural empyema, mastoiditis, tumors, cysts, trauma, vasculitis, intracranial hemorrhage, bacterial endocarditis with septic embolism, demyelinating disorders, drug intoxication or side effects.

WORKUP

- **CT:** Obtain if there are signs of ↑ ICP such as focal neurologic findings or papilledema.
- **LP:** CSF culture with cell count, glucose, protein, and Gram stain (see Table 7-19).
- **Other studies:**
  - HSV PCR from LP may be appropriate in certain situations.
  - An opening pressure > 180 mm Hg may indicate bacterial meningitis.
  - CBC, electrolytes, glucose, blood culture.

TABLE 7-18. Age-Related Signs and Symptoms of Meningitis

Age	Symptoms	Signs
0–3 months	Fever, paradoxical irritation (irritable when held and less irritable when not held), altered sleep pattern, respiratory distress, vomiting, poor feeding, diarrhea, seizures.	**Early:** Lethargy, irritability, temperature instability. **Late:** Bulging fontanelle, shock, seizures.
4–24 months	Altered sleep pattern, lethargy, seizures.	**Early:** Fever, irritability. **Late:** Nuchal rigidity (after 18 months), coma, shock.
> 24 months	Headache, stiff neck, lethargy, photophobia, myalgia, seizures.	**Early:** Fever, nuchal rigidity, irritability, papilledema, Kernig's sign, Brudzinski's sign. **Late:** Seizures, coma, shock.

TABLE 7-19. CSF Findings in Meningitis

Component	Normal	Bacterial	HSV	Other Viral	TB
Glucose (mg/dL)	40–80	< 30	> 30	> 30	20–40
Protein (mg/dL)	20–50	> 100	> 75	50–100	100–500
WBCs/μL	0–6	> 1000	10–1000	100–500	10–500
Neutrophils (%)	0	> 50	< 50	< 20	< 20
RBCs/μL	0–2	0–10	10–500	0–2	0–2

KEY FACT

In aseptic meningitis, many patients feel better after the LP.

- WBC count is usually ↑ in bacterial meningitis but may be unremarkable in aseptic meningitis.
- EEG in patients who present with seizures generally shows nonspecific generalized slowing; focal slowing in the temporal area is characteristic of HSV infections.

Treatment

- The initial choice of antimicrobial is based on the most likely organisms involved given the patient's age group (see Table 7-17).
- Empiric antibiotics should be started immediately, even before the results of the LP and CSF analyses are known.
- Supportive care includes the following:
  - Strict fluid balance in light of the risk of SIADH.
  - Rehydration with isotonic solution until euvolemic followed by 2/3 maintenance fluids.
  - Frequent assessment of urine specific gravity.
  - Daily weights and daily measurement of head circumference in babies.
  - Neurologic assessment; seizure precautions.
  - Isolation may be necessary until the causative organism has been identified.

KEY FACT

Acute treatment with dexamethasone before or at the time of antibiotic administration may improve neurologic outcome in Hib meningitis but is not indicated in other types of meningitis.

Complications

- **Acute:** Shock, seizures, subdural effusions (common with Hib infection), SIADH, subdural empyema, cerebral edema, ventriculitis, abscess.
- **Long term:** Deafness, epilepsy, learning disabilities, blindness, paresis, ataxia, hydrocephalus.

PNEUMONIA

Inflammation of the lung parenchyma that may be infectious or noninfectious. Pneumonia can be classified according to etiologic agent, patient age, host reaction, and anatomic distribution (eg, lobar, interstitial, bronchopneumonia). Risk factors include anatomic malformations, immunodeficiencies, chronic lung disease 2° to prematurity, and exposure to cigarette smoke.

KEY FACT

Viruses are the leading cause of pneumonia in children.

- The most common cause of pediatric pneumonia is viral infection (RSV, influenza, parainfluenza virus [PIV], adenovirus); *S pneumoniae* is the most common bacterial agent.

TABLE 7-20. Presentation of Pneumonia by Etiology

Type	Symptoms	Lung Exam	CXR	WBC Count
Viral pneumonia	Cough, low-grade fever.	Diffuse crackles and wheezes.	Diffuse and streaky infiltrates.	Normal or ↑ with a lymphocyte predominance.
Bacterial pneumonia	High fever, cough, chills, dyspnea, chest pain.	Focal crackles, ↓ breath sounds, dullness to percussion, egophony.	Lobar consolidation.	Leukocytosis with left shift.

- In neonates, GBS and *Listeria* are potential agents.
- Infants 1–3 months of age may present with *Chlamydia trachomatis* pneumonia, while older children and teenagers are susceptible to *Mycoplasma pneumoniae* and *Chlamydia pneumoniae* infections.

SIGNS AND SYMPTOMS

Presents with tachypnea, tachycardia, cough, and shortness of breath; malaise, fever, chest pain, and retractions are also seen. Overall patterns of presentation may vary with the etiologic agent (see Table 7-20). Presenting symptoms also differ with age group:

- **Newborns:**
  - Tachypnea, cyanosis, nasal flaring, grunting, retractions.
  - Poor perfusion, hypotension, acidosis, leukopenia/leukocytosis.
  - Poor feeding, irritability, lethargy.
- **Young children:**
  - Abdominal pain, fever, malaise, GI symptoms, restlessness, apprehension, chills.
  - Tachypnea, cough, grunting, nasal flaring.
  - Children rarely expectorate even with a productive cough.
- **Older children:**
  - Mild upper respiratory tract symptoms such as cough and rhinitis.
  - Followed by abrupt fever, chills, tachypnea, chest pain, and productive cough.
  - Adolescents with *Mycoplasma* infections present with prolonged cough without fever.

KEY FACT

Infants with *C trachomatis* pneumonia are afebrile and may have conjunctivitis and a staccato cough.

DIFFERENTIAL

Gastric aspiration, foreign body aspiration, atelectasis, congenital malformation, bronchopulmonary dysplasia, CHF, neoplasm, chronic interstitial lung disease, collagen vascular disease, pulmonary infarct.

KEY FACT

On CXR, aspiration pneumonia shows right middle or upper lobe infiltrates.

WORKUP

- Viral nasal swab for respiratory pathogens such as RSV, influenza, and parainfluenza.
- Obtain a CXR in ill-appearing infants and children, those who need hospitalization, and those who worsen clinically on antibiotics.
- WBC count is often > 15,000/mm^3 in bacterial pneumonia.
- A WBC count < 5000/mm^3 in the newborn period may indicate sepsis.

Q

A previously healthy 7-year-old boy has a 1-week history of increasing cough, low-grade fever, and fatigue on exertion. CXR shows diffuse perihilar infiltrates. What is the diagnosis and treatment?

TABLE 7-21. Etiologies and Empiric Treatment of Pneumonia by Age Group

Organisms	Empiric Coverage
Neonates	
E coli (gram-⊖ enterics), GBS, *S aureus, Listeria monocytogenes, C trachomatis*	Ampicillin + gentamicin/cefotaxime × 10–21 days. Add vancomycin if MRSA is prevalent. Blood cultures should be obtained and effusions drained and Gram stained.
HSV	IV acyclovir.
3 Weeks to 4 Months	
C trachomatis, S pneumoniae	Ampicillin or amoxicillin or cefotaxime IV (if febrile) × 10 days.
HSV, RSV, CMV, enterovirus	IV acyclovir for suspected HSV; ribavirin for RSV; ganciclovir for CMV.
6 Weeks to 4 Years: Lobar Pneumonia	
S pneumoniae, S aureus, nontypable *H influenzae,* group A streptococcus	Amoxicillin or clindamycin PO OR ceftriaxone or cefotaxime IV × 7–10 days.
6 Weeks to 4 Years: Atypical Pneumonia	
Bordetella pertussis	Azithromycin × 5 days or clarithromycin × 7 days. Prophylaxis for close contacts. Avoid erythromycin in light of the link to pyloric stenosis.
Respiratory viruses (RSV/PIV)	No antibiotics indicated; supportive care.
Influenza A and B	Oseltamivir for influenza A and B (> 1 year); amantadine for influenza A (> 1 year). Antivirals can ↓ symptoms if given within 36 hours.
4 or More Years: Lobar Pneumonia	
S pneumoniae, S aureus	Amoxicillin or erythromycin PO × 7–10 days. Ceftriaxone or cefotaxime IV + PO/IV macrolide × 7–10 days. Vancomycin/clindamycin for *S aureus.*
4 or More Years: Atypical Pneumonia	
M pneumoniae, C pneumoniae	Clarithromycin or azithromycin OR doxycycline or erythromycin × 14–21 days (5 days if azithromycin).
Influenza	Supportive care. Zanamivir or oseltamivir can ↓ symptoms if given within 36 hours.

A

The child has *Mycoplasma pneumoniae* infection. Treat with clarithromycin or azithromycin.

TREATMENT

See Table 7-21 for empiric antibiotic therapy by age group. Criteria for hospitalization include the following:

- All children < 2 months of age.
- Children > 2 months of age with respiratory distress, hypoxia, inability to take oral medications, failure to respond to oral antibiotics, immunosup-

pression, underlying cardiopulmonary disease, or evidence of empyema on CXR.
- Hospitalized children should be treated with IV antibiotics until afebrile and then given oral antibiotics for 7–10 days of treatment.

ACUTE OTITIS MEDIA (AOM)

A suppurative infection of the middle ear cavity. Children are more susceptible to infection owing to the angle of entry, short length, and ↓ tone of the eustachian tube. Up to 75% of children will have at least 3 episodes of AOM by age 2.

- Bacteria such as *S pneumoniae*, nontypable *H influenzae*, and *Moraxella catarrhalis* are responsible for roughly 80% of cases.
- Viruses such as influenza A, RSV, and PIV account for approximately 20% of cases.
- Conditions that predispose to AOM include viral URIs, bottle feeding, pacifier use, passive exposure to tobacco smoke, day care, immunodeficiency, trisomy 21, hypothyroidism, and cleft palate.
- Breastfeeding ↓ the risk of AOM.

> **KEY FACT**
>
> The 3 most common bacterial pathogens that cause acute otitis media are *S pneumoniae,* nontypable *H influenzae,* and *M catarrhalis.*

Signs and Symptoms

- Presents with ear pain, fever, crying, irritability, and difficulty sleeping. Difficulty feeding, vomiting, and diarrhea are also seen.
- Young children may tug on their ears.
- Often preceded by URI symptoms (cough, congestion, rhinorrhea).
- Otoscopic examination reveals the following (see also Figure 7-12):
  - Abnormal color, opacification, and ↓ mobility.
  - Erythema and bulging of the affected TM. However, erythema alone is not sufficient for diagnosis, as it may also result from vigorous crying.

> **KEY FACT**
>
> A diagnosis of acute otitis media requires:
> 1. A history of acute onset of signs and symptoms.
> 2. The presence of a middle ear effusion.
> 3. Signs and symptoms of middle ear inflammation.

Differential

- Otitis media with effusion (OME)—fluid behind the TM without evidence of inflammation (see Table 7-22).

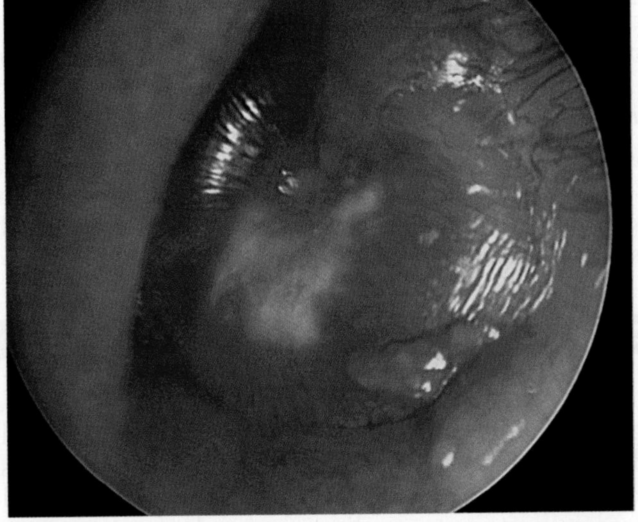

FIGURE 7-12. Acute otitis media. Otoscopic examination demonstrates purulent material behind a bulging tympanic membrane. (Reproduced with permission from Brunicardi FC et al. *Schwartz's Principles of Surgery,* 9th ed. New York: McGraw-Hill, 2010, Fig. 18-1.)

TABLE 7-22. Acute Otitis Media vs. Otitis Media with Effusion

FEATURE	AOM	OME
Signs/symptoms	Ear tugging, ear pain. Fever, malaise, irritability. Hearing loss.	No ear pain or tugging. No fever. Hearing loss.
Otoscopic examination	Erythema and bulging of TM. Loss of landmarks. Air-fluid levels. Opacification. **↓ mobility of TM.**	Retracted TM. Loss of landmarks. Air-fluid levels/bubbles. No opacification. No immobility of TM.
Treatment	Amoxicillin.	Usually supportive.

- Myringitis (inflammation of the eardrum with normal TM mobility).
- Otitis externa, mastoiditis, foreign body in the ear, ear trauma, a hard cerumen, mumps, teething, pharyngitis, nasal congestion, TMJ dysfunction.

TREATMENT

Treatment is controversial owing to widespread concern over the growing antibiotic resistance of respiratory pathogens.

- The AAP advocates an observational period of 48–72 hours with treatment after 72 hours for:
  - Children > 2 years of age with nonsevere illness.
  - Infants 6 months to 2 years of age with an uncertain diagnosis and mild symptoms.
- Antibiotic usage is as follows:
  - **First line:** High-dose amoxicillin 80–90 mg/kg/day × 5–10 days.
  - **Alternative for penicillin allergy:** Cefuroxime, cefdinir, cefprozil, azithromycin (5–7 days for patients > 2 years of age without a language or hearing deficit).
  - **Persistent otitis media (2–3 days):** High-dose amoxicillin/clavulanate (Augmentin), cefdinir, or IM/IV ceftriaxone.
- Children with > 3 infections in 6 months or 4 infections in 1 year should be considered for tympanostomy tube placement or myringotomy.

KEY FACT

Don't rush to antibiotics when evaluating AOM; instead, consider your patient and whether an observational period of 2–3 days might be appropriate.

COMPLICATIONS

Hearing loss with risk of language delay (for chronic otitis media with effusion), TM perforation, scarring (tympanosclerosis), cholesteatoma (growth of desquamated stratified squamous epithelium in the inner ear), chronic otitis media, mastoiditis, meningitis, labyrinthitis.

STREPTOCOCCAL PHARYNGITIS

Caused by group A β-hemolytic streptococcal infection (GABHS, or *Streptococcus pyogenes*); typically affects patients > 2 years of age. Complications are categorized as suppurative (peritonsillar and retropharyngeal abscesses) and nonsuppurative (acute rheumatic fever, postinfectious glomerulonephritis). Treatment can prevent most complications (scarlet fever, acute rheumatic fever, toxic shock syndrome), with the exception of postinfectious glomerulonephritis.

KEY FACT

Streptococcal pharyngitis is very rare in children < 2 years of age.

Signs and Symptoms

- High fever (> 40°C [>104°F]), sore throat, tender anterior cervical lymphadenopathy, enlarged hyperemic tonsils with exudates, and lack of upper respiratory symptoms (coryza, rhinorrhea) are more likely to be streptococcal pharyngitis than viral in nature.
- Other symptoms include abdominal pain, vomiting, headache, an erythematous oropharynx with a fetid odor, and uvular edema.
- If fever and pharyngitis are accompanied by a "sandpaper-like" rash, think **scarlet fever.**

KEY FACT

The sensitivity of rapid strep tests ranges from 80% to 90%, but their specificity is > 95%. This means that false-⊖ results occasionally occur, and you must base your treatment decisions on the entire clinical picture.

Workup

- A ⊕ throat culture or streptococcal antigen detection test ("rapid strep test") distinguishes streptococcal from viral pharyngitis.
- See Tables 7-23 and 7-24 for a description of the modified Centor criteria, which can help guide the diagnosis and management of streptococcal pharyngitis.

Treatment

- Penicillin VK or amoxicillin PO × 10 days.
- Benzathine penicillin G × 1 dose.
- Macrolides or clindamycin × 10 days for penicillin-allergic patients.
- Tetracycline and sulfonamides should not be used to treat GABHS.

Complications

- **Postinfectious glomerulonephritis:**
  - May follow streptococcal pharyngitis or streptococcal skin infections within 1–2 weeks.
  - **Not** prevented by timely antibiotic administration.
  - Presents with hematuria, proteinuria, ↓ urination, hypertension, pulmonary edema, and peripheral edema.
  - Complement levels (C3) may be low.
  - Typically self-limited and does not recur.

TABLE 7-23. Modified Centor Scoring

Criteria	Points
Temperature > 38°C	1
Absence of cough	1
Swollen, tender anterior cervical lymph nodes	1
Tonsillar swelling or exudate	1
Age:	
3–14	1
15–44	0
≥ 45	−1

TABLE 7-24. Treatment Guidelines for Streptococcal Pharyngitis

Centor Score	Risk of Infection (%)	Suggested Management
≤ 0	1–2.5	None.
1	5–10	None.
2	11–17	Culture.
3	28–35	Antibiotics only for ⊕ culture results.
≥ 4	51–53	Treat empirically with antibiotics and/or culture.

- **Acute rheumatic fever:**
  - An immune reaction that may arise 2–6 weeks after untreated streptococcal pharyngitis.
  - The diagnosis is made using the modified Jones criteria (see the mnemonic **JONES**) and requires 2 major or 1 major + 2 minor criteria + lab evidence of group A streptococcal infection:
    - **Major: J♥NES** (Joints = polyarthritis; ♥ = carditis; SQ Nodules; Erythema marginatum, Sydenham's chorea).
    - **Minor:** Arthralgia, fever, ↑ ESR or CRP, prolonged PR interval.
  - Treatment involves penicillin, anti-inflammatory medications, and supportive therapy.
  - Given the high rate of recurrence, indefinite daily prophylactic penicillin should be started.

MNEMONIC

Jones criteria (major criteria) for acute rheumatic fever–

JONES

Joints—migratory polyarthritis involving > 2 joints
♥ carditis—new murmur (mitral or aortic insufficiency or Carey Coombs murmur) or symptoms of CHF
Nodules—over the joints, scalp, or spine
Erythema marginatum—a circinate, erythematous maculopapular rash on the trunk and extremities
Sydenham's chorea—emotional instability, involuntary movements

URINARY TRACT INFECTION (UTI)

UTI is an abnormal number of bacterial colonies from the urine and can be classified as lower (cystitis, involving the bladder) or upper (pyelonephritis, involving the kidney). In infants, the source of bacteria is more often from hematogenous seeding of the kidneys, whereas in older children UTIs more frequently result from ascending infections of fecal flora. During the newborn period, the incidence of UTI is slightly higher in males; during childhood, it becomes 10 times more common in females.

- The predominant organisms responsible for UTI are *E coli*, *Proteus*, *Klebsiella*, *Staphylococcus saprophyticus* (especially in adolescent females), and the enteric streptococci.
- Risk factors include vesicoureteral reflux, obstructive uropathy, renal calculi, bladder dysfunction, and intermittent catheterization. Infection in a small child should prompt you to consider the possibility of abnormal anatomy.

MNEMONIC

UTI pathogens–

SEEKS PP

S *saprophyticus*
E *coli*
E*nterobacter*
K*lebsiella*
S*erratia*
P*roteus*
P*seudomonas*

Signs and Symptoms

- Varies by age (see Table 7-25).
- **Cystitis:** Presents with ↑ frequency, urgency, dysuria, incontinence, and suprapubic tenderness. Hematuria and a low-grade fever may also be seen.
- **Pyelonephritis:** Presents with high fevers, chills, flank pain, nausea, and vomiting. CVA tenderness (related to flank pain) and dehydration are also seen.

TABLE 7-25. Signs and Symptoms of UTI

Newborns	Infants	Preschool Age	School Age
Fever	Fever	Fever	Fever/chills
Hypothermia	Irritability	Enuresis	Enuresis
Poor feeding	Poor feeding	Dysuria	Dysuria
Vomiting	FTT	Urgency	Urgency
Jaundice	Diarrhea	Urinary frequency	Urinary frequency
FTT		Abdominal pain	CVA tenderness
Sepsis		Vomiting	Hematuria
Apnea			
Diarrhea			

Workup

- **UA:** Pyuria, hematuria, and bacteriuria suggests a UTI, but a urine culture is needed to confirm the diagnosis.
- **Urine culture:**
  - A culture is ⊕ if:
    - $> 10^5$ colonies/mL are obtained from a midstream clean-catch sample.
    - $> 10^4$ colonies/mL are obtained from an intermittent ("in and out") catheterization sample.
    - Any colonies are obtained from a suprapubic tap sample.
- If culture contains diphtheroid bacilli, *Staphylococcus*, or multiple organisms, suspect contamination and repeat the urine culture.
- Any toxic-appearing child should have a sepsis workup.

Treatment

- Initiate empiric antibiotic treatment while awaiting sensitivity results.
- **Uncomplicated cystitis:**
  - **PO:** TMP-SMX or cefixime × 7–14 days.
  - **IV:** Cefotaxime or ampicillin + gentamicin for neonates, toxic-appearing patients, or suspected pyelonephritis.
- **Abnormal host/urinary tract:**
  - Add *Pseudomonas* coverage.
  - Ampicillin + gentamicin, piperacillin/tazobactam, or ticarcillin/clavulanic acid × 14–21 days.
- All patients can switch to oral antibiotics once clinical improvement is seen.
- **Prophylactic antibiotic therapy** (TMP-SMX or nitrofurantoin) is indicated for the following:
  - Before a VCUG.
  - Reflux of any grade in infancy and early childhood.
  - Reflux of grades III–V in children > 5 years of age.
  - Patients with > 3 UTIs per year.

KEY FACT

Key tests to order for a child with flank pain and fever include CXR, UA, and urine culture. Flank pain can result from pyelonephritis or lower lobe pneumonia.

Neonatology

APGAR SCORE

An objective tool used for evaluating the need to resuscitate a newborn. Determined at 1 minute and 5 minutes after birth. The Apgar score alone should not be used to determine when to initiate resuscitation. Scores of 8–10 indicate no need for resuscitation; scores of 4–7 indicate a potential need for resuscitation. Scores of 0–3 indicate severe distress and the need for immediate resuscitation (see Table 7-26).

CONGENITAL INFECTIONS

> **KEY FACT**
>
> CMV and toxoplasmosis both lead to intracranial calcifications. CM**V** leads to peri**V**entricular calcifications, whereas to**X**oplasmosis results in diffuse calcifications in the corte**X**.

Infections acquired in utero or in the perinatal period are commonly referred to by the acronym **ToRCHeS.** These include **T**oxoplasmosis, **O**ther (parvovirus, *Borrelia*, VZV), **R**ubella, **C**ytomegalovirus, **H**SV/HIV/HBV, and **S**yphilis. Clinical findings common to many of these infections are intrauterine growth restriction, anemia and thrombocytopenia, hepatosplenomegaly, hydrops fetalis, jaundice, and chorioretinitis. Table 7-27 summarizes the distinctive clinical signs and symptoms of each.

NEONATAL HYPERBILIRUBINEMIA

Physiologic Jaundice

Generally benign jaundice that occurs in the first week of life with a peak bilirubin concentration up to 15 mg/dL (> 15 mg/dL is considered pathologic; see Table 7-28). Physiologic jaundice results from:

- ↑ RBC destruction as HbF is replaced with adult hemoglobin.
- ↓ clearance due to immature hepatocytes' inability to conjugate and excrete bilirubin.

Pathologic Jaundice

May be direct or indirect. Etiologies are as follows (see also Table 7-28):

- **Indirect (unconjugated) hyperbilirubinemia:**
  - Hemolysis of any cause (G6PD deficiency is common).
  - Blood group incompatibility.
  - Internal bleeding.

TABLE 7-26. Interpretation of the Apgar Score

Category	0	1	2
Appearance	Blue, pale	Body pink, extremities blue	Body and extremities pink
Pulse	Absent	< 100/min	> 100/min
Grimace	No response	Grimace	Cough or sneeze
Activity	Limp	Some extremity flexion	Full extremity flexion
Respiratory effort	Absent	Weak cry	Strong cry

TABLE 7-27. TORCHeS Infections

INFECTION	EPIDEMIOLOGY	CLINICAL FEATURES	TREATMENT
Toxoplasma gondii	Maternal exposure to cat feces or poorly cooked meat. Fetal disease with 1° infection only. The highest risk of exposure occurs at 10–24 weeks' gestation.	The classic triad consists of chorioretinitis, hydrocephalus, and intracranial calcifications. Microcephaly, severe mental retardation, and epilepsy are also seen. Infants may be asymptomatic at birth.	Pyrimethamine + sulfadiazine.
Other (VZV)	First-trimester maternal chickenpox infection. Infections that develop within 1 week before or after delivery are associated with severe disseminated disease.	Microphthalmia, cataracts, cutaneous and bony abnormalities, risk of zoster as an older child.	Acyclovir; prevent with VZIG after exposure to VZV.
Rubella	Non-rubella-immune mother. Fever, rash, lymphadenopathy, and arthritis in the mother. The highest transmission risk is in the first trimester (80%). The virus may persist in the infant's oropharynx for 1 year.	Presents with the classic triad of PDA or pulmonary artery hypoplasia, cataracts, and deafness. Microcephaly, glaucoma, microphthalmia, and "salt-and-pepper" chorioretinitis are also seen. A "blueberry muffin" rash is characteristic. B- and T-cell deficiencies. Infants may be asymptomatic at birth.	No treatment; vaccine preventable.
CMV	The most common congenital infection. 1° infection has the worst outcome; reinfection can also cause disease. Infants may shed virus in urine for 1–6 years.	Hearing loss, seizures, sepsis, and pneumonia are common. Periventricular calcifications, microcephaly, severe mental retardation, and hepatosplenomegaly are also seen. Infants may be asymptomatic at birth with late neurologic sequelae.	Ganciclovir; prevent with CMV-⊖ blood products.
HIV	Most mothers are asymptomatic with a high-risk history (prostitution, drug abuse, hemophilia).	Recurrent infections, chronic diarrhea, hepatosplenomegaly, neurologic abnormalities, FTT.	AZT, TMP-SMX (PCP prophylaxis); avoid breastfeeding.

TABLE 7-28. Physiologic vs. Pathologic Jaundice

PHYSIOLOGIC JAUNDICE	PATHOLOGIC JAUNDICE
Not present until 36 hours after birth.	Present in the first 24 hours.
Total bilirubin ↑ < 5 mg/dL/day.	Total bilirubin ↑ > 0.5 mg/dL/hr.
Total bilirubin peaks at < 15 mg/dL.	Total bilirubin rises to > 15 mg/dL in formula-fed term and preterm infants. Total bilirubin can rise to > 17 mg/dL in breastfed or full-term infants.
Jaundice resolves by 1 week in term infants and 2 weeks in preterm infants.	Jaundice persists beyond 1 week in term infants and 2 weeks in preterm infants.

  - Polycythemia.
  - Infants of diabetic mothers.
  - Congenital defects in bilirubin metabolism (Gilbert's syndrome, Crigler-Najjar syndrome).
  - Cephalohematoma.
  - Breast milk jaundice.
- **Direct (conjugated) hyperbilirubinemia:**
  - TORCHeS infections.
  - Metabolic disorders (galactosemia, α_1-antitrypsin deficiency, CF).
  - Bacterial sepsis.
  - Obstructive jaundice (biliary atresia).
  - Prolonged administration of TPN.
  - Neonatal hepatitis.

KEY FACT

Conjugated hyperbilirubinemia is always pathologic.

Signs and Symptoms

Jaundice starts in the head and progresses to the feet as bilirubin levels rise.

Workup

- **Indirect hyperbilirubinemia:** Blood typing, Coombs' test, CBC, blood smear, reticulocyte count.
- **Direct hyperbilirubinemia:**
  - LFTs, bacterial and viral cultures, metabolic screening tests.
  - Hepatic ultrasound; sweat chloride test.

Treatment

- Phototherapy for term infants with bilirubin levels 15–20 mg/dL, depending on the infant's age and the cause of the hyperbilirubinemia.
- Infants with risk factors for hyperbilirubinemia (prematurity, maternal blood type antibodies to infant blood type) are monitored and treated more aggressively.
- Skin bronzing may be seen after phototherapy in infants with direct hyperbilirubinemia.
- Exchange transfusions for bilirubin levels > 20 mg/dL if phototherapy fails.

Complications

Kernicterus (bilirubin encephalopathy) is the main complication.

- Unconjugated bilirubin is lipid soluble, crosses the blood-brain barrier, and precipitates in the basal ganglia (meningitis and prematurity cause

KEY POINT

BREAST MILK JAUNDICE VS. BREASTFEEDING JAUNDICE

- **Breast milk jaundice:** A syndrome of prolonged unconjugated hyperbilirubinemia that is thought to be due to inhibition of bilirubin conjugation in the breast milk of some mothers. It is an extension of physiologic jaundice, peaks at 10–15 days of age, and declines slowly by 3–12 weeks of age.
- **Breastfeeding jaundice:** Attributable to poor feeding or inadequate breast milk supply and ↑ enterohepatic circulation of bilirubin. It usually occurs during the first week of life and resolves when enteral intake improves. Treatment involves evaluating the breastfeeding pair and encouraging more feeding.

the blood-brain barrier to be more porous; therefore, these processes cause kernicterus at lower bilirubin levels).

- Kernicterus typically occurs at levels > 25 mg/dL without risk factors.
- Infants who survive often develop a neurologic syndrome characterized by hypotonia, seizures, choreoathetoid movements, deafness (manifested by delayed language acquisition), impairment of eye movements (especially upward gaze), and dental enamel hypoplasia.
- Cognitive function is relatively spared.

KEY FACT

Premature infants are more susceptible to kernicterus.

RESPIRATORY DISTRESS SYNDROME (RDS)

The most common form of respiratory failure in preterm infants, RDS (also known as hyaline membrane disease) results from a deficiency of surfactant that leads to poor lung compliance, atelectasis, and hyaline membrane formation in the alveoli. Risk factors include maternal diabetes, hypothermia, asphyxia, and prematurity. RDS is seen in 65% of infants born at 29–30 weeks' gestation.

Signs and Symptoms

- Tachypnea (respiratory rate > 60); progressive hypoxemia.
- Cyanosis, nasal flaring, intercostal retractions, and grunting.
- Symptoms occur in the first 72 hours of life.

Differential

Transient tachypnea of the newborn, meconium aspiration syndrome, congenital pneumonia, spontaneous pneumothorax, diaphragmatic hernia, cyanotic heart disease.

Workup

CXR shows bilateral atelectasis with a "ground-glass" appearance and air bronchograms (see Figure 7-13).

Treatment

- Intubation and ventilation may be required to maintain oxygenation.
- Mechanical ventilation is associated with barotrauma and oxygen toxicity.
- It is recommended that infants be extubated as quickly as possible and stabilized on CPAP.
- Surfactant replacement therapy ↓ mortality.
- Supportive care in a NICU is required.

KEY FACT

Treatment with surfactant ↓ mortality from neonatal RDS.

Prevention

- Measures to prevent premature birth.
- Pretreatment of at-risk mothers with corticosteroids (betamethasone).
- Fetal lung maturity can be monitored in utero with the amniotic fluid lecithin-to-sphingomyelin (L/S) ratio and the presence of phosphatidylglycerol.
- An L/S ratio < 2 indicates a possible surfactant deficiency and the need for steroids.

KEY FACT

Pretreatment of at-risk mothers with betamethasone ↓ the incidence of RDS by increasing the production of surfactant by type II pneumocytes.

Complications

Bronchopulmonary dysplasia; pneumothorax/interstitial emphysema.

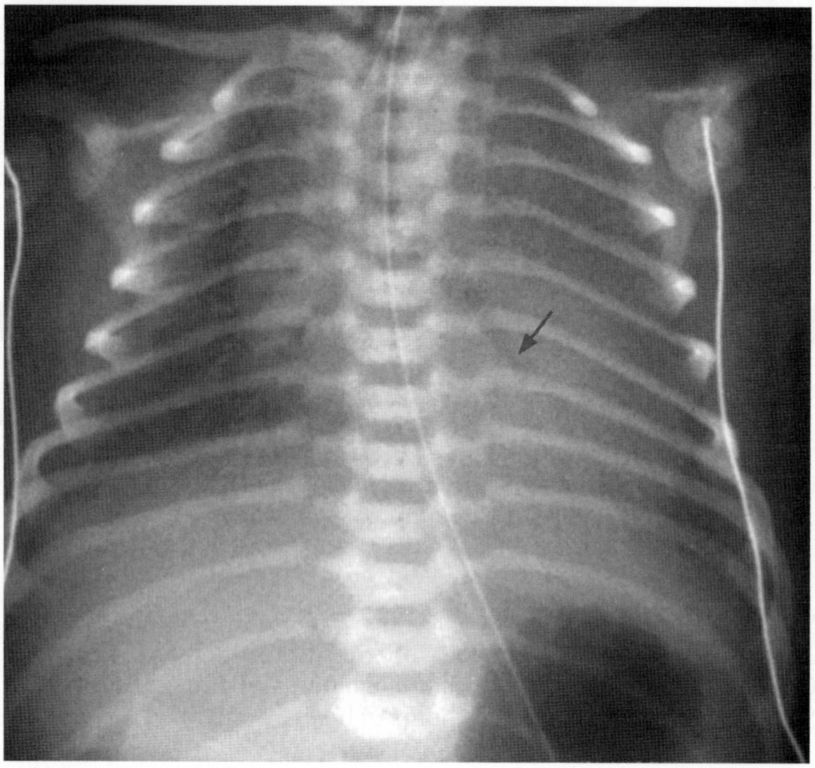

FIGURE 7-13. Respiratory distress syndrome. CXR in a premature neonate with RDS shows the typical findings of poor lung inflation and diffuse, granular "ground-glass" opacities with central air bronchograms (arrow). (Reproduced with permission from Tintinalli JE et al. *Tintinalli's Emergency Medicine: A Comprehensive Study Guide,* 7th ed. New York: McGraw-Hill, 2007, Fig. 4.0-1.)

Neurology

FEBRILE SEIZURES

Defined as seizures that arise in association with fever. They generally occur in children between 6 months and 6 years of age with an incidence of 3–4%. The risk of febrile seizures is slightly higher following the administration of some vaccines (eg, MMR), but there are no associated long-term consequences.

> **KEY FACT**
>
> Simple febrile seizures carry a better prognosis.

Signs and Symptoms

- Associated with a maximum temperature ≥ 39°C (≥ 102.2°F); may be due to a rapid ↑ in temperature.
- Classified as simple or complex (see Table 7-29).

Workup

- **History:** Determine the following:
  - Nature of the seizure (focal vs. generalized).
  - Duration (keep in mind that parents often overestimate duration).

TABLE 7-29. Simple vs. Complex Febrile Seizures

Simple Febrile Seizure	Complex Febrile Seizure
Short duration (< 15 minutes).	Long duration (> 15 minutes).
Generalized.	Focal features; postictal paralysis.
One seizure in a 24-hour period.	More than 1 seizure in a 24-hour period ("cluster").

- Number of seizures.
- Postictal state and events preceding the seizure.
- History of previous seizures; family history of febrile seizures.
- History of trauma or ingestions.

- **Examination:**
  - Check rectal temperature, vital signs, and mental status.
  - Look for nuchal rigidity (valid only for children > 18 months of age).
  - Check for fullness of the fontanelle.
  - Assess muscle strength and tone.
- **Labs:**
  - None in simple febrile seizures.
  - Sepsis workup for children < 12 months of age.
  - LP if CNS infection is suspected or in children > 6 months of age.
  - Serum glucose and/or D-stick in all seizure patients.
  - Head CT is indicated only if CNS disease is suspected (eg, macrocephaly, signs or symptoms of ↑ ICP).
  - EEG should be considered for complex febrile seizures.

Treatment

- Antipyretics may be helpful in overall management but do not ↓ the recurrence rate.
- Appropriate treatment of any underlying illness.
- Diazepam per rectum may be used to stop prolonged seizures (> 5 minutes).
- Phenobarbital or valproic acid prophylaxis may be given for complex febrile seizures.

Complications

- Seventy percent of children will never have another febrile seizure.
- The majority of recurrent seizures take place within 1 year of the initial episode.
- Simple febrile seizures carry no ↑ risk of developmental, intellectual, or growth problems.
- Febrile seizures ↑ the risk of epilepsy from a 0.5–1.0% baseline risk to 2–4% for patients with simple febrile seizures and by 6% for patients with complex febrile seizures.

KEY FACT

Risk factors for epilepsy include complex febrile seizures, abnormal neurologic examinations, neurologic or developmental abnormalities, and a ⊕ family history.

Orthopedics

DEVELOPMENTAL DYSPLASIA OF THE HIP (DDH)

Poor growth and development of the hip resulting in an abnormal relationship between the femoral head and acetabulum. DDH is progressive with growth and is reversible if corrected in the first few weeks. It occurs in 1 in 1000 live births, and there is a tenfold ↑ risk in siblings of children with DDH. Breech females are at highest risk for DDH. It is associated with anomalies such as torticollis, clubfeet, and metatarsus adductus.

Signs and Symptoms

- Newborn:
  - ⊕ **Ortolani or Barlow tests** (see Figure 7-14).
  - Asymmetric skin folds on the front and back of the legs and buttocks.
- **3–6 months:**
  - Limited abduction.
  - **Allis's or Galeazzi's sign:** The knee is lower on the affected side when the hips are flexed.
- **12 months (unilateral dislocation): Trendelenburg** sign—a painless limp and lurch to the affected side with ambulation.
- **12 months (bilateral dislocation):**
  - Waddling gait.
  - Lumbar lordosis due to flexion contractures.

KEY FACT

- **Ortolani test:** Slowly abduct the flexed hip; the femoral head will shift into the acetabulum, producing a clunk.
- **Barlow test:** Dislocate the hip by flexing and adducting the hip with axial pressure.

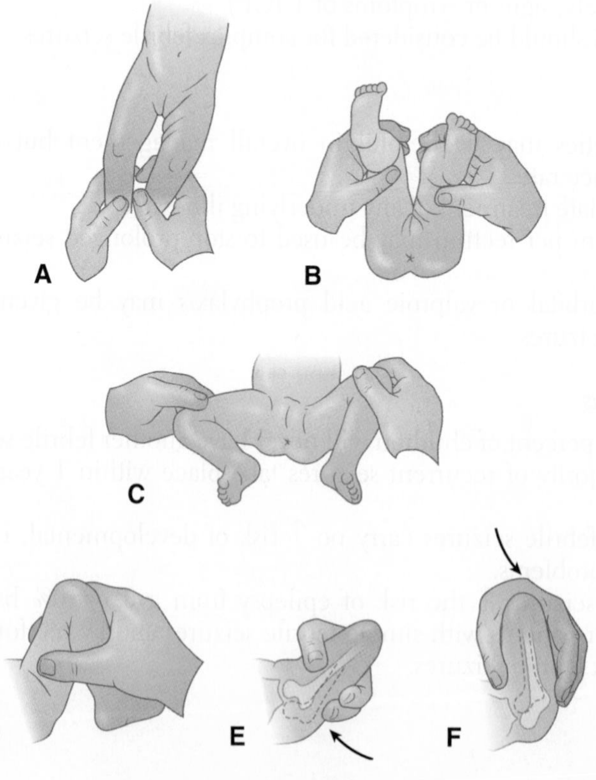

FIGURE 7-14. Clinical examination of developmental dysplasia of the hip. In all of these images, the child's left hip is the abnormal side. (A) Asymmetric skin folds. (B) Galeazzi test. (C) Limitation of abduction. (D–F) Ortolani and Barlow tests. (Reproduced with permission from Skinner HB. *Current Diagnosis & Treatment in Orthopedics,* 4th ed. New York: McGraw-Hill, 2006, Fig. 11-4.)

WORKUP

- Signs of instability are more reliable than x-ray in DDH.
- **< 6 months:** Ultrasound is most helpful due to cartilaginous acetabulum/proximal femur.
- **> 6 months:** X-rays are helpful because the proximal femoral epiphysis ossifies.

TREATMENT

- **< 6 months:** Pavlik harness (flexion and abduction of the hip).
- **6 months to 3 years:** Skin traction for 3 weeks to relax soft tissues around the hip prior to closed or open reduction. After 6 months of age, the failure rate for the Pavlik harness is > 50%.
- **> 3 years:** Operations to correct acetabular and femoral deformities.

PEDIATRIC FRACTURES

A number of fracture types are specific to pediatrics. These include the following:

- **Torus:** Involve "buckling" of the cortex with compression of the bone.
- **Greenstick:** Incomplete fractures that break 1 side of a bone and bend the other.
- **Epiphyseal:** Involve the growth plate (the weakest portion of a child's skeletal system) and are classified into 5 groups by the Salter-Harris system, which predicts the prognosis for a given fracture (see Figure 7-15).

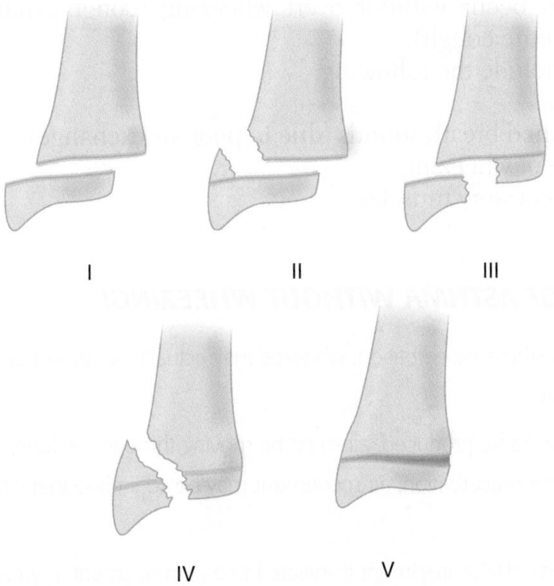

FIGURE 7-15. Salter-Harris classification of epiphyseal fractures. **I**—fracture line through physis only. **II**—fracture line through physis and metaphysis. **III**—fracture line through physis and epiphysis. **IV**—fracture through metaphysis, physis, and epiphysis. **V**—crush injury of the physis. (Reproduced with permission from Tintinalli JE. *Tintinalli's Emergency Medicine: A Comprehensive Study Guide,* 7th ed. McGraw-Hill, 2007, Fig. 264-7.)

MNEMONIC

Salter-Harris classification for epiphyseal fractures–

SALTer

I: **S**traight across (through physis)
II: **A**bove (through metaphysis and physis)
III: **L**ow (through epiphysis and physis)
IV: **T**hrough (through both epiphysis and metaphysis)
V: Crush injury on the physis

Q

At a 4-month-old girl's well-child checkup, the pediatrician notices that the child's left knee is lower when her hips are flexed. Her birth history is significant for a vaginal breech delivery. What maneuver should be performed, and how should the child be treated?

Pulmonology

ASTHMA (REACTIVE AIRWAY DISEASE)

A bronchial disorder characterized by the triad of inflammation, reversible smooth muscle constriction, and mucus production. The most common chronic condition of childhood, affecting 6% of all children and 40% of children in urban settings.

- 1° triggers include irritants such as cigarette smoke, air pollution, ozone, pollen, dust mites, pets, and cockroaches.
- Other triggers include exercise, cold weather, respiratory infections, drugs (ASA, β-blockers), stress, foods, and food additives.
- Be sure to elicit a history of past severity, frequency of attacks, ER visits, hospitalizations, ICU admissions, intubations, courses of steroids per year, number of school days missed, and a family history of asthma, allergies, and atopic disease.

KEY FACT

Ask about the allergic triad: asthma, atopic dermatitis, and allergic rhinitis.

Signs and Symptoms

- Parents may report congestion, persistent or nighttime cough, exercise intolerance, dyspnea, or pneumonia.
- Irritability or feeding difficulties may be found in younger children.
- Examination may reveal wheezing, coughing, tachypnea, tachycardia, and prolonged expiration.
- Hyperresonance, intercostal and subcostal retraction, and nasal flaring may also be present on examination.
- Asthma can occur without overt wheezing (cough-variant asthma produces a chronic cough).
- **Red flags** include the following:
  - Cyanosis.
  - Diminished breath sounds (due to poor air exchange).
  - Absence of wheezing.
  - Use of accessory muscles.

KEY POINT

BEWARE OF ASTHMA WITHOUT WHEEZING!

- During an asthma exacerbation, wheezes may actually be absent on lung examination.
- For wheezes to be produced, air must be moving through the lungs. In patients with a severe exacerbation, air movement may be so limited that wheezes are not heard.
- Once bronchodilator treatment is initiated and air movement ↑, wheezes may appear, indicating clinical improvement.
- Conversely, the disappearance of wheezes is important to note. While this may signal resolution of an exacerbation, it can also be an ominous sign that the patient's ability to move air through the lungs is decreasing. This finding indicates the need for more aggressive treatment.

A

Development dysplasia of the hip is diagnosed by the Galeazzi sign, which is an apparent shortening of the femur on the side of the dislocated hip. At this age the diagnosis should be confirmed by ultrasound, and the girl should be placed in a Pavlik harness.

- Increasingly labored breathing.
- Mental status changes (indicative of hypercarbia and/or significant hypoxemia).
- **Status asthmaticus:** Severe asthma attacks that may not be responsive to standard treatments.
  - A life-threatening condition that may lead to respiratory acidosis and respiratory arrest.
  - Patients are usually hospitalized, often in an intensive care setting.

KEY FACT

Key indicators of asthma severity:

- Frequent ED visits
- A history of intubation
- Past hospitalizations
- Past steroid use

DIFFERENTIAL

- Aspiration, foreign body.
- Bronchiolitis, pneumonia, bronchopulmonary dysplasia, CF, allergic bronchopulmonary aspergillosis.
- GERD.
- Vascular slings, tracheoesophageal fistula.

WORKUP

Diagnosis is based on clinical findings. However, the following may be helpful:

- **PFTs:** Look for ↓ vital capacity, ↑ functional residual capacity, ↑ residual volume, ↓ FEV_1, ↓ peak expiratory flow (PEF), and reversal of pulmonary abnormalities by inhalation of aerosolized albuterol.
- **Peak flow (PF) monitoring:** Measures how fast a patient can forcibly expire air after a maximal inhalation; reductions of 50–80% of predicted values indicate mild to moderate obstruction, and readings < 30% of predicted indicate severe obstruction. PFs are also helpful in monitoring treatment efficacy.
- **CXR:** Nonspecific findings include hyperinflation, depressed diaphragm, peribronchial thickening, and atelectasis.
- **ABGs:** Look for hypoxia and respiratory acidosis during acute exacerbations. It is important to recognize increasing $Paco_2$ as a sign of impending respiratory failure; with tachypnea, values should usually be well below 40.

TREATMENT

- **Acute therapy:**
  - Bronchodilators (nebulized albuterol 0.15 mg/kg in 2–3 cc NS or MDI 2 puffs q 1–6 h PRN) are immediately effective and are the mainstay of acute treatment.
  - A 5-day "pulse" of PO prednisone or IV methylprednisolone (Solu-Medrol) is highly effective but takes 4–6 hours to have an effect.
  - O_2 if hypoxemic.
  - For more severe exacerbations or for patients who do not respond to the therapies above, IV magnesium (for smooth muscle relaxation), epinephrine (for rapid bronchodilation), or heliox (↑ laminar flow of air) can be used.
- **Chronic therapy:**
  - Avoid triggers such as tobacco smoke, exercise, or allergens.
  - Give inhaled corticosteroids +/– long-acting β-agonists for prevention.
  - Leukotriene receptor antagonists can be used as an alternative to inhaled corticosteroids for mild persistent asthma or in combination with inhaled corticosteroids for moderate to severe persistent asthma.

- **Classification determining therapy:**
  - Asthma is classified by severity for the purpose of determining treatment (see Table 7-30).
  - It is recommended that treatment begin with more aggressive therapy in a "step-down" fashion.
  - In addition to the maintenance medications listed in Table 7-30, all patients should have short-acting bronchodilators (albuterol) as needed during an acute attack.

KEY FACT

The best way to prevent the spread of RSV in the hospital is to wash your hands before and after **every** patient encounter!

KEY FACT

All that wheezes is not asthma!

BRONCHIOLITIS

An acute inflammatory illness of the small airways occurring in children < 3 years of age, and the most common lower respiratory infection in children < 2 years of age. RSV is the 1° agent, although parainfluenza virus (especially type 3), adenovirus, influenza, and rhinovirus have also been implicated. Most cases occur in late fall to early spring. Risk factors for severe disease include prematurity (< 35 weeks' gestation), low birth weight, age < 12 weeks, chronic pulmonary disease, CHD, and immunodeficiency states.

Signs and Symptoms

- Presents with rhinorrhea, sneezing, cough, and low-grade fever followed by tachypnea and wheezing.
- Nasal flaring, retractions, and intermittent cyanosis may also be seen.
- Apnea may be the presenting sign in premature or young infants.

Differential

Asthma, pneumonia, heart failure, laryngomalacia, foreign body aspiration, GERD, CF.

TABLE 7-30. Classification of Asthma Severity

Step	Symptoms	Night Symptoms	PEF/ FEV_1	Maintenance Medications
Step 1: mild intermittent	Symptoms occur < 2 times per week. Patients are asymptomatic between exacerbations.	< 2/month.	> 80%	No daily medication is needed.
Step 2: mild persistent	Symptoms occur > 2 times per week but < 1 time per day. Exacerbations may affect activity.	> 2/month.	> 80%	Low-dose inhaled steroid.
Step 3: moderate persistent	Daily symptoms; ≥ 2 exacerbations per week. Exacerbations limit activity.	> 1/week.	60–80%	Medium-dose inhaled corticosteroids **or** low- to medium-dose inhaled steroid **and** long-acting bronchodilator. If needed, medium- to high-dose inhaled steroid **and** long-acting bronchodilator.
Step 4: severe persistent	Continual symptoms. Limited activity; frequent exacerbations.	Frequent.	< 60%	Daily inhaled high-dose corticosteroids **and** long-acting bronchodilator **and** PO steroids 2 mg/kg/day.

Workup

- Diagnosis is based primarily on clinical signs and symptoms.
- CXR may show hyperinflation but should be obtained only for ill or hypoxic patients or for recurrent episodes of wheezing.
- Nasopharyngeal swab and direct fluorescent antibody (DFA) testing or culture.
  - Although commonly used, nasopharyngeal swabs rarely change the nature of management.
  - Helpful for surveillance/grouping of RSV-⊕ patients in hospital wards to ↓ transmission.

Treatment

- Supportive care (oral hydration, antipyretics).
- Hospitalize patients with a respiratory rate > 50–60, hypoxemia, apnea, inability to tolerate feeding, chronic cardiopulmonary disease, or an unreliable home environment.
- Supplemental O_2 and contact isolation are appropriate for hospitalized patients.
- Bronchodilators may transiently improve symptoms.
- Inhaled steroids are not recommended, as no benefit has been shown.
- The use of ribavirin aerosol should be reserved for severely affected or high-risk children.
- High-risk infants < 2 years of age can be treated prophylactically with RSV IVIG or palivizumab.

KEY FACT

Breastfeeding has been shown to ↓ an infant's chance of developing bronchiolitis.

KEY FACT

Epiglottitis is life-threatening emergency. Patients are toxic appearing, with difficulty swallowing, drooling, and severe respiratory distress. **Urgent intubation** for airway protection is indicated.

CROUP

Viral croup (laryngotracheobronchitis) is an acute inflammatory disease of the upper respiratory tract that especially affects the subglottic space (see Figure 7-16). PIV types 1 and 3 are the most common cause; other organisms include RSV, influenza virus, rubeola virus, adenovirus, and *M pneumoniae*.

KEY FACT

Listen for a seal-like bark in croup.

Signs and Symptoms

- Presents with inspiratory stridor that worsens with agitation.
- Patients have a hoarse voice and a seal-like, barking cough.
- May be preceded by a prodrome of mild fever and coryza.
- Diminished breath sounds, restlessness, altered mental status, or cyanosis may be seen if the patient is hypoxic.

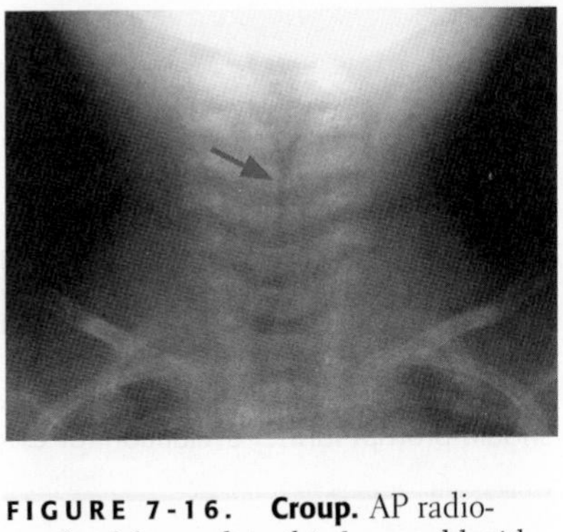

FIGURE 7-16. Croup. AP radiograph of the neck in this 1-year-old with inspiratory stridor and cough shows the classic "steeple sign" (arrow) consistent with the subglottic narrowing of laryngotracheobronchitis. (Reproduced with permission from Stone CK, Humphries RL. *Current Diagnosis & Treatment: Emergency Medicine*, 6th ed. New York: McGraw-Hill, 2008, Fig. 30-10A.)

Differential

- **Infectious:** Epiglottitis, bacterial tracheitis, retropharyngeal abscess (see Table 7-31). Consider tracheitis if the patient does not respond to aerosolized racemic epinephrine.
- **Other:** Foreign body aspiration, angioneurotic edema.

Workup

- CXR and neck x-ray if the diagnosis is in doubt.
- A PA x-ray of the neck shows subglottic narrowing or "steeple sign" (see Figure 7-16).

KEY FACT

On a neck x-ray, look for the "steeple sign," which indicates subglottic narrowing in croup.

Treatment

- **Mild cases** (no stridor at rest): Supportive measures, fluids, cool-mist therapy, humidity.

TABLE 7-31. Characteristics of Croup, Epiglottitis, and Tracheitis

Feature	Croup	Epiglottitis	Tracheitis
Age	Three months to 5 years.	Two to 7 years.	Older children.
Etiology	Viral, commonly parainfluenza.	Group A strep, *S aureus*, viral.	Often *S aureus*.
Onset	Develops over 2–3 days.	Rapid onset over several hours.	Acute decompensation after a 2- to 3-day gradual onset.
Fever	Low grade.	High grade.	High grade.
Respiratory distress	Usually mild to moderate.	Commonly severe.	Commonly severe.
Position preference	Prefers sitting up, leaning against the parent's chest.	"Tripod" position with neck extended.	May have position preference.
Response to aerosolized racemic epinephrine	Stridor improves.	No response.	No response.
Imaging	"Steeple sign" on PA neck films.	"Thumb sign" on lateral neck films.	Subglottic narrowing; hazy tracheal border.

- **Moderate cases** (with stridor at rest): Corticosteroids.
- **Severe cases** (respiratory distress, hypoxia): IV hydration, systemic steroids, nebulized racemic epinephrine, supplemental O_2 and intubation if necessary (rare; only for < 1% of hospitalized patients).

CYSTIC FIBROSIS (CF)

KEY FACT

Nasal polyps in any pediatric patient should prompt further evaluation for CF.

A multisystem autosomal recessive disorder characterized by a mutation in the CFTR gene, which is located on chromosome 7 and is involved in chloride conductance. CF is the most common lethal genetic disease affecting Caucasians (1 in 3000 live births); 93% of patients are diagnosed in childhood.

Signs and Symptoms

- Respiratory, GI, reproductive, endocrine, and musculoskeletal symptoms may be seen (see Table 7-32).
- The most common presentations are meconium ileus, recurrent respiratory infections, and FTT.

Workup

KEY FACT

About 1% of CF patients have a ⊖ sweat chloride test.

- Sweat test shows a chloride concentration > 70 mEq/L.
- PFTs reveal obstructive and restrictive disease.
- Sputum/throat cultures.
- CXR may show hyperinflation, airway thickening, and atelectasis in young children; later findings include bronchiectasis and scarring.
- Newborn screening programs (for ↓ amounts of trypsin) identify ~ 10% of cases.
- Genetic testing for common mutations (> 70% of CF cases result from the ΔF508 mutation).

TABLE 7-32. Signs and Symptoms of CF

SYSTEM	PRESENTATION
Respiratory	Asthma with clubbing of the digits. Nasal polyps; chronic pansinusitis. Recurrent pneumonia (especially staphylococcal). Chronic atelectasis, chronic pulmonary disease, pneumothorax, bronchiectasis, hemoptysis, or chronic cough. Colonization with mucoid *Pseudomonas aeruginosa*. X-rays showing persistent hyperaeration or atelectasis.
GI	Meconium ileus (pathognomonic). Intestinal obstruction (meconium plug or recurrent intussusception). FTT (protein-calorie malnutrition). Steatorrhea or chronic diarrhea. Rectal prolapse. Prolonged jaundice; hepatic cirrhosis and portal hypertension. Recurrent pancreatitis.
Musculoskeletal	Bone pain and joint effusion due to hypertrophic osteoarthropathy.
Reproductive	Infertility in men (due to obliteration of the vas deferens); infertility in women (due to thick, spermicidal cervical mucus).
Miscellaneous	Hypoproteinemia and edema. Fat-soluble vitamin deficiencies (vitamins A, D, E, and K). Hypoprothrombinemia. "Salty" taste or salt crystals on skin. Unexplained hyponatremic hypochloremic metabolic alkalosis. Impaired glucose tolerance or type 1 DM.

TREATMENT

- Aerosolized deoxyribonuclease (DNase) to ↑ mucus clearance.
- Chest physiotherapy with postural drainage.
- Bronchodilators and antibiotics if acute declines in lung function or pneumonia is suspected.
- Intermittent aerosolized tobramycin (BID × 4 weeks) for *Pseudomonas*.
- H_2 blockers, antacids.
- Pancreatic enzyme supplements; vitamin A, D, E, and K supplements.
- A high-calorie, high-protein diet with supplemental NG or gastrostomy tube feedings.
- Pulmonary exacerbations require hospitalization for IV antibiotics.
- Patients will require double-lung transplantation between the second and third decade of life.

KEY FACT

The average life expectancy of a CF patient is roughly 37 years, although improvements in treatment mean that a baby born today may expect to live longer.

Toxicology

LEAD POISONING

Most lead exposure comes from lead-containing paint remaining in buildings constructed before 1978. Other sources of exposure include industrial plants, lead solder in pipes, lead-containing pottery, paint on some imported toys and household items, and some traditional herbal remedies. Lead poisoning requiring medical evaluation refers to levels > 20 μg/dL, but levels of 10–19 μg/dL can also be toxic, and recent data have shown some neurocognitive effects at levels < 10 μg/dL. Lead levels > 70 μg/dL are considered severe.

Signs and Symptoms

- Presents with irritability, hyperactivity, listlessness, and a decline in school performance.
- Behavioral difficulties, attention disorders, and developmental delay may be seen.
- Anorexia, abdominal discomfort, vomiting, and constipation are common.
- Lead encephalopathy is associated with ↑ ICP, headache, vomiting, ataxia, seizures, coma, or death.
- Other findings include the following:
  - Peripheral neuropathy (wrist and foot drops).
  - Burton's lines (blue lines on the gums).
  - Reddish-brown discoloration of the urine.
  - Proximal tubule dysfunction (aminoaciduria, glycosuria, and hyperphosphaturia).
  - Pica.

KEY FACT

Check lead levels at 12 and 24 months in all children.

Workup

- Obtain lead levels for all children at 12 months and 2 years of age, and in others on the basis of risk.
- Peripheral smear shows basophilic stippling and hypochromic microcytic anemia.
- X-rays reveal lead lines.

Treatment

- Remove the source of lead in the child's environment.
- Succimer/DMSA or calcium disodium EDTA for levels > 45 μg/dL.
- EDTA and dimercaprol/BAL for levels > 70 μg/dL or symptoms of encephalopathy.
- Correct iron deficiency if present.

Trauma

CHILD ABUSE AND NEGLECT

KEY FACT

Suspect child abuse if the story and the injuries don't match.

Most clinicians will encounter at least 1 case of child abuse at some point in their careers. Almost half of reported cases occur in children < 1 year of age. Children at ↑ risk for abuse include those with special needs or behavioral problems, premature infants, and children of single, teenage, or substance-abusing parents. The presence of spousal abuse ↑ the risk of child abuse in the same household. Even after intervention, the abuse often continues, and the mortality rate for abused children is 5%.

Signs and Symptoms

- Injury is inconsistent with the description of events, or the history changes over time.
- There is unexplained delay in obtaining care.

- **Fractures:**
  - Mandibular fractures.
  - Rib fractures (often multiple and posterior in location).
  - Scapular fractures.
  - Long bone spiral fractures.
  - Often in different stages of healing.
- **Head injuries:**
  - Apnea, seizures, coma.
  - Subdural hematomas, retinal hemorrhages.
- **Burn marks:** Straight lines, symmetry, unusual geometry.
- **Sexual abuse:**
  - Genital trauma, STIs, recurrent UTIs, encopresis, enuresis.
  - Rectal or genital pain, discharge, bleeding.
  - Sleeping/eating disorders.
  - Behavioral and school difficulties.
  - Sexualized behavior with peers or objects.
- **Neglect:**
  - FTT; ↓ SQ fat in the cheeks, extremities, and buttocks.
  - Diaper rash and impetigo. Look for unwashed skin and clothing.
- **Development:**
  - Delayed social and speech development.
  - Avoidance of eye contact, depressed affect, and absence of a cuddling response.

WORKUP

- Skeletal survey, bone scan, ophthalmologic examination.
- Include a head CT in infants if head trauma or neurologic involvement is suspected.
- Osteogenesis imperfecta, bleeding disorders, and bullous skin disorders must be ruled out.
- Obtain a UA, a urine culture, and a stool culture if sexual abuse is suspected.
- Lab and clinical studies may be conducted without parental permission.
- Photograph and document injuries.

> **KEY FACT**
>
> Tests can be ordered without parental permission if abuse is suspected.

TREATMENT

- Immediately report suspected abuse to state protection agencies.
- Stabilize injuries as needed.

Common Clerkship Topics

The following is a list of core topics that you are likely to encounter in the course of your pediatrics rotation and on a shelf examination.

- **Well-child care:**
  - Anticipatory guidance and safety
  - Developmental milestones
  - Failure to thrive
  - Growth parameters
  - Immunizations
  - Infant nutrition
  - Tanner staging

- **Cardiology:**
  - Arrhythmias (supraventricular tachycardia, long QT syndrome, Wolff-Parkinson-White syndrome) (see Internal Medicine)
  - Congenital heart disease
  - Congestive heart failure
  - Pericardial disease
- **Dermatology:**
  - Atopic dermatitis
  - Diaper rash
  - Impetigo
  - Neonatal rashes (acne neonatorum, erythema toxicum, milia)
  - Psoriasis
  - Scabies and lice
  - Seborrheic dermatitis
  - Viral exanthems
- **Endocrinology:**
  - Adrenal dysfunction (congenital adrenal hyperplasia)
  - Diabetes
  - Thyroid dysfunction
- **Gastroenterology:**
  - Appendicitis (see Surgery)
  - Constipation
  - Gastroesophageal reflux
  - Hirschsprung's disease
  - Intussusception
  - Malrotation and volvulus
  - Meckel's diverticulum
  - Pyloric stenosis
- **Genetic disorders:**
  - Autosomal trisomies (21, 18, 13)
    - Common associations (CHARGE, VATER)
    - Common syndromes (DiGeorge, Marfan's, Noonan's, Prader-Willi, Williams)
  - Sex chromosome disorders (Turner's, Klinefelter's, fragile X)
- **Hematology and oncology:**
  - Anemia
  - Sickle cell disease
  - Thalassemia
  - Childhood cancers (acute lymphocytic leukemia, Wilms' tumor, neuroblastoma)
- **Immunology:**
  - Autoimmune disorders (Henoch-Schönlein purpura, idiopathic thrombocytopenic purpura, juvenile idiopathic arthritis, Kawasaki disease)
  - Immunodeficiencies (T cell, B cell, combined, complement, phagocytic, HIV)
- **Infectious disease:**
  - Acute otitis media
  - Cellulitis
  - Fever management
  - Gastroenteritis
  - Meningitis
  - Orbital and periorbital cellulitis
  - Osteomyelitis
  - Pneumonia
  - Sexually transmitted infections (see Obstetrics and Gynecology)

  - Sinusitis
  - Streptococcal pharyngitis
  - Urinary tract infection
- **Neonatology:**
  - Apgar score
  - Congenital infections
  - Neonatal hyperbilirubinemia
  - Prematurity
  - Respiratory distress syndrome
- **Nephrology/urology:**
  - Cryptorchidism
  - Fluid and electrolyte management (see Practical Information for All Clerkships)
  - Hematuria and proteinuria
  - Hemolytic-uremic syndrome
- **Neurology:**
  - Cerebral palsy
  - Febrile seizures
  - Hydrocephalus
  - Neural tube defects
  - Seizure disorders
- **Orthopedics:**
  - Developmental hip dysplasia
  - Limp
  - Nursemaid's elbow (subluxation of the radial head)
  - Pediatric fractures
- **Psychiatry:**
  - Attention-deficit hyperactivity disorder (see Psychiatry)
  - Learning disorders (see Psychiatry)
  - Mental retardation (see Psychiatry)
- **Pulmonology:**
  - Apnea/apparent life-threatening event/sudden infant death syndrome
  - Asthma (reactive airway disease)
  - Bronchiolitis
  - Croup
  - Cystic fibrosis
  - Epiglottitis
- **Toxicology:**
  - Acetaminophen and salicylate toxicity
  - Ingestions
  - Lead poisoning
- **Trauma:**
  - Child abuse
  - Head injury

CHAPTER 8

PSYCHIATRY

Ward Tips

Psychiatry is the study and management of behavioral disorders. Given ongoing advances in the neurobiologic understanding of major psychiatric disorders, together with continuing additions to the psychiatrist's pharmacologic arsenal, many find psychiatry to be an increasingly exciting field in which to practice and conduct research. Many psychiatric disorders interact with other medical illnesses to affect both prognosis and treatment. Ideally, the rotation should offer you valuable exposure to common psychiatric disorders (eg, depression, schizophrenia, bipolar disorder, anxiety disorders, dementia, delirium) that you will see for the rest of your career, regardless of the specialty you choose.

WHAT IS THE ROTATION LIKE?

In general, the psychiatry core rotation can feel more relaxed than other clerkships. Thus, if you have the option of choosing the order in which to take your third-year core rotations, psychiatry would be a good rotation to take after surgery or OB/GYN as a means of helping you "catch your breath."

On the other hand, the expectations and mechanics of this rotation are much different from those of the more conventional clerkships. Determining accurate diagnoses and treatment measures among complex differentials can be challenging and requires experience in addition to medical/neurologic knowledge. A medical student's exposure to the outpatient setting is often limited owing to the private nature of the activity. Consultation and liaison, as well as emergency crisis services, also play an important role in most psychiatric departments. Medical schools that are associated with a VA or children's hospital will allow students to focus on a unique psychiatric population, and students may rotate through any or a combination of these services.

Outpatient psychiatry encompasses a spectrum of activities ranging from one-time consultations and brief crisis intervention to medication management and long-term psychotherapy. Patients who require psychiatric hospitalization are admitted to an inpatient psychiatric service. Patients on other hospital services as well as those in the ED may develop or have a psychiatric illness, and these services may consult psychiatry for advice.

HOW DO I EXCEL IN PSYCHIATRY?

KEY FACT

Good listening and observational skills are a must on the psych rotation, as is an ability to organize observations into criteria for various diagnoses.

Emphasizing the biopsychosocial model, modern psychiatry combines biologic, experiential, and sociocultural factors into a single paradigm. Doing well in psychiatry therefore requires the development of interviewing skills, the study of psychopathology, and the acquisition of knowledge about psychopharmacology. Generally, psychiatry emphasizes the doctor-patient relationship in the healing process. Thus, the development of empathic skills and an ability to listen are critical to excelling in this rotation. The use of open-ended questions to acquire information about a patient's psychopathology is also a must.

In addition to developing interviewing skills, it is important that you acquire a solid fund of psychiatric knowledge. You will also need to hone your observational skills in order to monitor abnormalities in a patient's appearance, behavior, and affect. Specifically, this rotation will provide you with an opportunity to learn about disorders of feeling, thinking, and behavior that interfere with the way a person functions and relates to others. At the same time, you must also learn how to present a psychiatric history. As a medical student, you will often have more recent experience on medicine wards than any other member of the team. You can therefore prove to be a real asset in helping the team manage medical problems in psychiatric patients.

Many students initially find themselves disoriented by the unique organization and expectations of the psychiatry clerkship. Here are some tips from students and residents:

- Keep an open and inquiring mind. Psychiatric training benefits physicians in all fields, particularly given the high rates of comorbidity between psychiatric illness and other medical diagnoses.
- Be organized. For each patient, keep a card that includes a short history, a thorough medication list, and a checklist of things to do.
- Make a card with the generic and trade names, common dosages, and side effects of the most frequently used psychiatric drugs, as well as a card with an outline of the mental status exam (MSE).
- When interviewing a patient, obtain a thorough medication history, including dates of use, effectiveness, and side effects.
- Be friendly with the support staff, especially the nurses!
- Remember—safety first. If you feel threatened by a patient, leave the room immediately and get help. While on this rotation, you may witness a "take-down" in which the staff physically pins down a violent, labile patient. This may look frightening and unpleasant at first, but bear in mind that it is often the safest and kindest option available.
- When interviewing a patient, try to meet in a location that respects the patient's confidentiality while also allowing for an unobstructed departure from the room should this become necessary. If the patient is potentially dangerous, leave the door to the interview room open. In such instances, a third person might be asked to stand inside or outside the room to be available if trouble arises.
- Take the initiative. When discussing your patient, think ahead and consider issues such as housing, finances, social support, time of discharge, cultural issues, and community services.
- Try to pick up on how your patient makes you feel (eg, depressed, anxious). You'll often find that your patient has similar feelings.
- You may not need your white lab coat or any kind of uniform on this rotation. Some institutions even ban ties and necklaces, as patients can use them to strangle the caretaker. However, bring your white coat on the first day of your rotation, and wear it until you are told that you can leave it at home.
- Don't touch your patients. Touch is a powerful and volatile tool that should be used only after you have gained more experience. With appropriate discussion and information, however, consent can be acquired from patients in situations where contact may be clinically indicated (eg, in patients suffering from emotional trauma or paranoia).
- Don't share details of your life with your patients.
- Before you interview a patient, discuss the goals of your encounter with your resident or attending. Is the goal to gather information or to treat? Are there any sensitive topics that you should avoid?

You will often experience a mix of feelings when dealing with psychiatric patients. Be open to exploring these feelings with your team. Having such feelings will not be seen as a sign of weakness, but failing to deal with them can be detrimental.

KEY FACT

Never let a labile patient get between you and the door.

WHAT IS THE DSM-IV?

The DSM-IV, or the *Diagnostic and Statistical Manual of Mental Disorders*, 4th edition, is published by the American Psychiatric Association. The DSM is the standard diagnostic classification system used by all U.S. mental health workers (both clinicians and researchers) as well as by insurance companies and the federal government. The DSM, which is revised roughly once a decade to incorporate new research findings, consists of long lists of criteria that are required to assign specific psychiatric diagnoses to patients. At first glance, the DSM-IV may appear lengthy, complex, and confusing. However, you do not need to know the details of all the criteria it describes. The more important criteria will be found here under the appropriate headings.

It is important to note that despite its precise and detailed diagnostic criteria, the DSM-IV is not meant to be used by nonpsychiatrists in a "check the appropriate boxes" or "cookbook" fashion. To the contrary, the DSM-IV merely offers guidelines for trained psychiatrists to apply with a view toward ensuring better diagnostic agreement among clinicians and researchers. Practically speaking, the DSM-IV also provides useful criteria for billing for psychiatric care, and in some institutions this is its primary use. Regardless of the attention paid to the DSM-IV criteria, including an assessment of the 5 axes will impress your attendings and residents on rounds.

Although psychiatrists currently make wide use of the DSM-IV, the DSM-V is on the horizon and may ultimately affect the way in which some psychiatric diagnoses are defined. It may be useful to ask experienced psychiatrists' opinions on this milestone in the field.

KEY POINT

DSM-IV CLASSIFICATION

The DSM-IV uses a "multiaxial classification," which is just an elaborate way of saying that information is broken down into 5 categories (which should be used for presenting patients in rounds, write-ups, and the like):

Axis I: Psychiatric disorders, including substance dependence/abuse.

Axis II: Personality disorders and mental retardation.

Axis III: Physical and medical problems.

Axis IV: Social and environmental problems/stressors.

Axis V: The Global Assessment of Functioning (GAF), which rates a patient's overall level of social, occupational, and psychological functioning (current and best in the past year) on a scale of 1 (completely nonfunctional) to 100 (extremely high level of functioning in a wide number of areas). Note that in some instances, patients require a GAF of < 40 to warrant admission to the hospital.

KEY NOTES

The psychiatric admit note is similar to its medicine counterpart except for the emphasis it places on past psychiatric history, patients' personal history, and the development of a biopsychosocial formulation. Large portions of a psychiatric history often need to be obtained from other sources or collaterals. At a minimum, you must talk to a family member and to the patient's regular physician and review any old charts that may exist. Other pertinent information is outlined below.

- **Chief complaint (CC)/reason for admission:** Some psychiatric patients may not have a primary complaint, while others may voice a complaint that is incoherent, obscene, or irrelevant—so it is often necessary to briefly state how and why the patient ended up in the hospital or ED in addition to noting the patient's perception of what happened.
- **History of present illness (HPI):** This includes symptoms, precipitants, time course, any medication changes or medication noncompliance, effects on function at home and work, and current treatment.
- **Review of systems (ROS):** This includes a brief review of depressive symptoms, manic symptoms, anxiety symptoms, any symptoms of psychosis, and substance abuse with intoxication/withdrawal symptoms of note. Read the individual sections for these disorders and work with your residents/attendings to develop a concise set of questions to ask for each.
- **Past psychiatric history:** This includes age at onset of symptoms, first psychiatric contact, first psychiatric hospitalization, number of hospitalizations, the date and duration of the most recent hospitalization, suicide attempts (when, how, seriousness), and medications (what, how much, how long, what helped, side effects, why the patient stopped taking them). Also include any history of verbal, physical, or sexual abuse or neglect, as well as any traumatic life events.
- **Substance use:** Ask about substances used, including what, how much, how often, how long, what route, any withdrawal, shared needles, any history of inpatient or outpatient detox, and longest period of sobriety.
- **Past medical history (PMH):** The PMH should be obtained with the same thoroughness as in other specialties. However, a history of seizures, CNS infections, endocrine difficulties (eg, thyroid dysfunction), head trauma, or allergies, as well as the presence of acute or chronic pain, are particularly important to obtain.
- **Social history (SH):** In psychiatry, heavy emphasis is placed on the social/personal history, as a patient's health, lifestyle, and social interactions may heavily influence his or her current psychiatric illness. It is therefore important to flesh out the details of a patient's birth, childhood, school performance, marriage, education, religious and cultural beliefs, occupational history, family and social relations, sexual history, hobbies and special interests, community supports, and current living arrangements. The patient's legal history, any history of violence, and a history of physical or sexual abuse should be documented as well. Attention should also be paid to family structure and significant interpersonal dynamics (eg, whether the patient is divorced or adopted).
- **Family history (FH):** Ask about any psychiatric illnesses that run in the family. Get details on diagnoses, severity, outcomes, and which medications helped. Also ask about nonpsychiatric illnesses that run in the family, including a history of seizures or neurologic disorders or a family history of suicide.

Key:

A&O × 4 = alert and oriented to person, place, time, and situation
BAD = bipolar affective disorder
BID = twice daily
BP = blood pressure
CAD = coronary artery disease
CC = chief complaint
C/C/E = clubbing/cyanosis/edema
CM = Caucasian male
CN = cranial nerve
CTAB = clear to auscultation bilaterally
CV = cardiovascular
d/o = disorder
DTRs = deep tendon reflexes
EOMI = extraocular movements intact
EPS = extrapyramidal symptoms
EtOH = alcohol
FT = fine touch
FTN = finger to nose
HEENT = head, eyes, ears, nose, and throat
HIV = human immunodeficiency virus
h/o = history of
HSM = hepatosplenomegaly
HTN = hypertension
HTS = heel to shin
IVDU = intravenous drug use
LAD = lymphadenopathy
LOC = loss of consciousness
MDD = major depressive disorder
MI = myocardial infarction
MMSE = Mini-Mental Status Exam
M/R/G = murmurs/rubs/gallops
MS = mental status
NABS = normoactive bowel sounds
NAD = no acute distress
NC/AT = normocephalic/atraumatic

SAMPLE PSYCHIATRY ADMIT NOTE

ID/CC: TM is a 20-year-old CM college student brought into the ED by his parents because he has been bedridden and increasingly isolative for 2 weeks.

Source of information: Parents, who are reliable.

HPI: TM is a 20-year-old college student with a previous diagnosis of paranoid schizophrenia who presents with worsening isolation and odd behavior in the setting of noncompliance with antipsychotic medications. He was in his usual state of health until 2 weeks ago. Over the past 2 weeks, his parents report that he has isolated himself in his room and does not leave except to use the restroom. He continually lies in bed with the sheets over his head and the blinds drawn. He has stopped attending school and recently stopped leaving the house altogether. According to his parents, the patient appears "mute and tearful," answering questions with single words and acting differently from his "usual social self." They also report that at times he has occasionally appeared to be responding to voices or other sounds that no one else could hear. They grew concerned until they finally brought him to the ED today.

On initial interview at the time of admission, TM endorses a running debate in his head from a single, unrecognized voice. The conversation revolves around daily activities and decisions such as choosing a seat. He claims that the voice does not command him to do anything. He admits often feeling afraid that someone will harm him. He reports that he currently has no appetite (eats only a small sandwich a day), sleeps 4 hours per night, and is not participating in any of his usual activities. He has been noncompliant with his Zyprexa for the past 3–4 months and does not provide a rationale for his noncompliance.

On psychiatric ROS, the patent endorses poor mood but denies suicidal ideation at any time and has never made any suicide attempts. He denies homicidal ideation. He denies that the hallucinations are persecutory or command him in any way. He denies visual hallucinations. He denies any h/o anxiety, including panic attacks. He denies any episodes of abnormally elevated mood, reduced need for sleep, or increased impulsivity that might suggest mania. He endorses a h/o alcohol and cocaine use but denies using for the last 3 months. This history is corroborated by his parents at bedside.

At the time of interview, the patient did not feel that he was ill or that he needed medications to help him.

Past psychiatric history:

This is the patient's first inpatient admission for symptoms. Patient was in his usual state of health until 3 years ago, when he became depressed after failing a college class. Also at that time, he thought he was being "followed" and that "whispers were talking behind his back." A first diagnosis of schizophrenia of the paranoid type was made at that time by Dr. Jones, who started patient on Zyprexa (titrated up to 20 mg/day), which was effective. He has since seen 4 additional psychiatrists and has tried Prozac for depressive symptoms with no success. Patient has been able to continue school part time and to function fairly well.

Substance use: Tobacco: 1/2 ppd × 4 years; EtOH: drinks approx. 12 beers/week × 6 years, last used 3 weeks ago; cocaine: intranasal cocaine 2 times/week × 5 years, last used 3 weeks ago; denies h/o IVDU.

Trauma: The patient denies any h/o verbal, physical, or sexual abuse. He denies any h/o traumatic events.

PMH:

Childhood illnesses: None.

Medical illnesses: None.

Surgeries: None.

Hospitalizations: None.

Trauma: Head injury due to bicycle accident with brief LOC in 1995. No retrograde or anterograde amnesia. No hospitalization or treatment at that time.

Allergies: None.

Medications: Zyprexa 20 mg QD.

No herbal medications, supplements, or vitamins.

FH: H/o depression in all paternal male relatives, including father. One paternal uncle committed suicide at age 40. Mother with heavy EtOH use. No h/o schizophrenia or other psychiatric illnesses. No h/o CAD, HTN, MI, or cancer. No h/o seizures or other neurologic illness.

SH: Patient was raised by his mother and father. Parents state that childhood development was normal, and he was a good student with A's and B's until his diagnosis 3 years ago. He currently lives at home with his parents in Los Angeles and attends a local junior college. He has been unemployed × 1 month and worked most recently at a grocery store. He has held multiple odd jobs over the past 3 years; his longest job was 6 months. No h/o arrests or legal problems. No current romantic relationship, and patient is not sexually active. He has enjoyed playing the guitar since age 13.

Medical ROS: Poor sleep, appetite, and energy. No recent weight change. Otherwise unremarkable except as above.

PE:

Gen: Disheveled 20-year-old male sitting in a chair in NAD.

VS: T 36.8, RR 18, orthostatic BP: sitting 150/82 P 104; standing 156/87 P 107.

Skin: Tattoo on left shoulder; no rashes, scars, or lesions noted.

HEENT: NC/AT, PERRL, EOMI, no nystagmus, conjunctiva clear, O/P clear with good dentition.

Neck: Supple, no LAD.

Lungs: CTAB, no W/R/R.

CV: Tachycardic, regular rhythm, no M/R/G, normal S1/S2.

NR = normal range

NT/ND = nontender, nondistended

O/P = oropharynx

P = pulse rate

PE = physical examination

PERRL = pupils equal, round, and reactive to light

PO = by mouth

PP = pin prick

ppd = pack per day

PRN = as needed

QAM = every morning

QD = every day

QHS = every night

r/o = rule out

RPR = rapid plasma reagin

RR = respiratory rate

RUA = routine urinalysis

SAD = schizoaffective disorder

T = temperature

TSH = thyroid-stimulating hormone

VS = vital signs

W/R/R = wheezes/rhonchi/rales

Abd: Soft, NT/ND, NABS, no masses or HSM.

Ext: Warm and well perfused with cap refill < 2 sec. No C/C/E. Distal pulses 2+ bilaterally.

Neuro: MS: A&O × 4; CN: II–XII intact; motor: normal tone, bulk, and power throughout; sensory: FT/PP/temp intact and symmetric; cerebellar: FTN and HTS intact, Romberg ⊖; DTRs 2+ and symmetric; gait: normal, able to tandem gait.

MSE:

- Appearance: Alert young male who appears stated age. Clean shaven, but hair and clothing are disheveled; in no apparent acute distress.
- Speech: Slow rate, low volume, somewhat monotonous with prolonged speech latency. Coherent but with paucity of content.
- Mood: "Anxious."
- Affect: Blunted—patient tells stories with limited emotional expression. Mood congruent.
- Thought process: Linear and goal directed without circumstantiality or tangentiality.
- Thought content: No suicidal or homicidal ideation; no evident paranoia or delusions.
- Perception: Endorses auditory hallucinations; has "voices inside that are debating about where to sit," making it difficult for him to make decisions. Denies visual or tactile hallucinations.
- Cognition: MMSE 28/30. Missed 2 points on serial 7's. (Note: If the patient has greater than a high school education, he/she should be asked to do "serial 7's"—ask the patient to start at 100 and repeatedly subtract 7, eg, 100, 93, 86, 79, 72.)
- Judgment: Poor—patient wants to leave the hospital without treatment.
- Insight: Poor—patient does not feel that he is ill or that taking medication will help him.
- Impulsivity: Fair—patient does not feel he might take impulsive actions toward himself or others and has no history of doing so.

Labs:

HIV ⊖

RPR NR

TSH 1.6

RUA ⊖

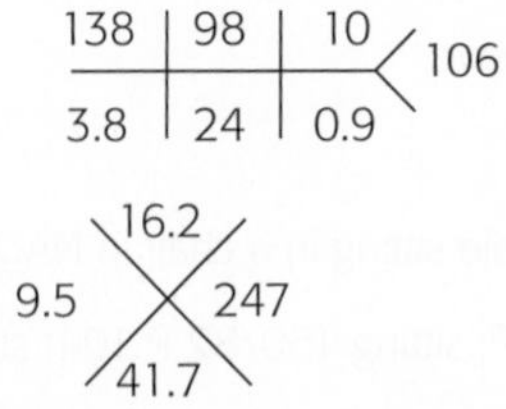

Assessment: The assessment and plan below were discussed with [attending doctor or senior resident].

TM is a 20-year-old male with a 3-year h/o depressive and paranoid symptoms, noncompliant with Zyprexa, now with 2 weeks of increasing isolation and auditory hallucinations. The patient is exhibiting key features of psychosis of the paranoid type, including a h/o hallucinations and delusions for approximately 3 years. He is also showing concurrent features of a depressive episode, including lack of interest in normal activities, reduced appetite, and reduced sleep. TM's biological risk factors for mental illness include a family history of depression, a personal history of being diagnosed with schizophrenia, cocaine and alcohol abuse, and medication noncompliance. His psychological risk factors include the recent stress of failing a college class and poor coping skills. Social risk factors include isolation from any support beyond that of his parents. These factors all likely contribute to his current presentation. At this time, it is unclear if he is suffering from a 1° psychotic disorder or from a mood disorder with psychosis; further information on concentration, level of energy, and overall mood (patient now denies being depressed) must be explored. At the moment, given the patient's current symptoms, he requires inpatient admission for safety, containment, and continued management of his mental illness.

Axis I: Schizophrenia of paranoid type with depressive features—

- R/o MDD with psychotic features.
- R/o BAD vs. SAD.
- R/o substance-related/induced mood d/o.

Polysubstance abuse.

Axis II: Deferred.

Axis III: None.

Axis IV: Poor social support, substance dependence, lives at home, has difficulty holding jobs.

Axis V: GAF 35–40.

Plan:

- Start olanzapine 5 mg PO QAM and QHS for psychotic symptoms, with monitoring of changes in his symptoms of auditory hallucinations. We will begin with this medication given its previous efficacy.
- Start Cogentin 1 mg PO BID PRN for signs and symptoms of EPS.
- Consider Wellbutrin in the future if patient presents with symptoms of depression.
- Ativan 1 mg PO q 4 h PRN anxiety.
- Tylenol 650 mg PO q 6 h PRN headache, fever, or pain.
- Colace 100 mg PO BID, PRN constipation.
- Monitor sleep, food intake, and activity level.
- Encourage milieu participation and attendance at all groups.
- Involve social work in planning outpatient rehab and a family meeting.

THE BIOPSYCHOSOCIAL FORMULATION

You might have noticed that the "Assessment" section of the admit note above incorporates the patient's particular biologic, psychological, and social risk factors for mental illness. Students sometimes struggle with which elements to include within such a formulation. However, documentation of these factors can help you, the writer, enhance your understanding of the patient while also allowing other members of the team to get a "snapshot" of the patient's overall situation. Common biologic, psychological, and social risk factors are as follows:

- **Biologic:**
  - A family history of mental illness and substance dependence/abuse.
  - A personal history of a mood, anxiety, or psychotic disorder.
  - Any concurrent medical disorder that might place the patient at greater risk for mental illness, including neurologic illness or a history of traumatic brain injury.
  - Any congenital or developmental problems.
  - Concurrent substance use issues.
  - Disabilities or handicaps.
  - Medication use and noncompliance.
- **Psychological:**
  - Precipitating events or stressors.
  - A history of trauma or loss.
  - Adequacy/maturity of coping mechanisms in dealing with stressors.
  - Personality traits that may affect the ability to cope with stressors.
- **Social:**
  - Family and social supports.
  - Employment and financial status.
  - Housing situation or homelessness.
  - Legal difficulties.

The incorporation of a biopsychosocial formulation for mental illness connects the current acute presentation to the patient's life in general. The inclusion of such a formulation in write-ups and presentations may both aid and impress the rest of the treatment team, whose effectiveness often depends on the breadth of medical students' knowledge of their patients' circumstances.

KEY PROCEDURES

The mental status exam (MSE) is the single most important procedure medical students must learn. Like the physical examination, the MSE provides a way to objectively document mental function and behavior. Although most often used in psychiatry, some form of MSE should be a part of all medical examinations. It is therefore helpful to create an MSE template that can be filled in during the interview (see Table 8-1). Always rule out organic causes of mental illness when evaluating psychiatric disorders.

> **KEY FACT**
>
> Memorize the MSE as soon as possible in your rotation.

WHAT DO I CARRY IN MY POCKETS?

You will want to carry a psychiatry handbook (see Top-Rated Review Resources) as well as your drug guide. Having a stethoscope, a penlight, and a reflex hammer available can be useful for medical clearance or neurologic examinations on admission.

High-Yield Clinical Topic Checklist

Read about these topics before you start the rotation. Most are discussed in this chapter. A full list of topics can be found at the end of this chapter.

- ❑ **Mental status exam, Mini-Mental Status Exam,** 5 axes.
- ❑ **Mood disorders:** Major depressive disorder, bipolar disorder.
- ❑ **Psychotic disorders:** Schizophrenia, schizoaffective disorder.
- ❑ **Anxiety disorders:** Generalized anxiety disorder, panic disorder, social phobia, obsessive-compulsive disorder, posttraumatic stress disorder.
- ❑ **Substance abuse, dependence, withdrawal, alcoholism.**
- ❑ **Adjustment disorder.**
- ❑ **Eating disorders:** Anorexia nervosa, bulimia nervosa.
- ❑ **Suicidality and risk assessment.**

TABLE 8-1. Mental Status Exam

COMPONENT	COMMENTS
Appearance	Alertness, gender, whether patient appears stated age, grooming, appropriateness of dress, level of distress (if any), any notable features (eg, piercings, tattoos).
Behavior	The way the patient interacts with the interviewer (eg, cooperative, hostile); level and consistency of eye contact.
Psychomotor	Psychomotor agitation; psychomotor retardation or slowing; tremor, posturing, mannerisms.
Speech/language	Rate, tone and volume, fluency, enunciation, clarity, amount, abnormalities (eg, aphasia).
Mood	Can be quoted directly based on what the patient reports.
Affect	Range and quality of emotion that the patient exhibits (eg, anxious, fearful, flat, blunted or restricted, full, expansive) and whether or not this appeared mood congruent or mood incongruent.
Thought process	The form of expression of a patient's thought, including quality, quantity, associations, and fluency of speech. Abnormalities include circumstantiality, tangentiality, flight of ideas, thought blocking, echolalia, neologisms, clanging, loosening of associations, and perseveration.
Thought content	The content of a patient's thoughts, including suicidal ideation, homicidal ideation, delusions, paranoia, major themes, preoccupations, obsessions, ideas of reference, and poverty of thought.
Perception	Hallucinations or illusions.
Cognition	Evaluation of various brain functions, level of consciousness (eg, alert, drowsy, stuporous, comatose), and level of alertness and orientation (eg, to person, place, time/date, reason for hospitalization). Includes the MMSE or other cognitive testing.
Abstraction	Can the patient think abstractly? Ask the patient about similarities between objects. Example: "What is the similarity between a watch and a ruler?" Answer: "They are both used to measure something."
Judgment	Does the patient understand the consequences of his or her actions? Does the patient appear capable of making healthy (or avoiding unhealthy) decisions?
Insight	How aware is the patient of his or her illness, its etiology, and treatment options?
Impulsiveness	Does the patient's interview or history appear to raise concern for impulsive and potentially harmful behavior?

Mental Status Exam and Mini-Mental Status Exam

Table 8-1 briefly outlines the key components of a complete MSE. You may want to use this table as a guide in creating a template. You should, however, refer to a text or manual for a complete treatment of this subject. You should also gain a familiarity with the Mini-Mental Status Exam (MMSE), which is rapidly administered, reliable, and both sensitive and specific for diagnosing dementia and delirium in hospitalized patients. With the guidance of your seniors, learn to perform MSEs both accurately and quickly.

KEY POINT

MINI-MENTAL STATUS EXAM

Orientation:

1. What is the year, month, date, day of the week, season? (5 points)
2. Where are we? Country, state, city, hospital, floor? (5 points)

Registration:

1. Name 3 objects and ask the patient to repeat the 3 objects. Repeat until the patient learns all 3, and record the number of trials. (1 point each)

Attention and calculation:

1. Serial 7's: Start with 100 and subtract 7; stop after 5 answers. (1 point each)
2. Spell *world* backward (an alternative that should be used only if the patient has a low educational level; not a substitute if the patient is uncooperative).
3. Alternatively, the interviewer says a string of letters and the patient taps his or her fingers every time a certain letter (eg, "D") is spoken.

Recall:

1. Recall the 3 objects that the patient repeated earlier. (1 point each)

Language:

1. Name 2 objects the interviewer points out. (naming, 2 points)
2. Repeat the phrase "No ifs, ands, or buts." (repetition, 1 point)
3. Follow a 3-step command: "Take a paper in your right hand, fold it in half, and put it on the floor." (3 points)
4. Read and obey the command "Close your eyes." (1 point)
5. Write a sentence. (1 point)

Visual/spatial:

1. Copy a design (eg, interlocking pentagons). (1 point)

Total score:

24–30 = normal

18–23 = mild/moderate cognitive impairment

0–17 = severe cognitive impairment

Note: Validity is questionable if the patient has less than an eighth-grade education, is hearing impaired, or is not a fluent English speaker.

Mood Disorders

Mood disorders are composed of episodes, each with a certain set of symptoms representing the patient's dominant mood state. These episodes—major depressive episode (MDE), mania, hypomania, and mixed (both manic and depressed) presentations—are not themselves diagnostic. However, they are used by psychiatrists to help make the diagnosis of a mood disorder.

MAJOR DEPRESSIVE DISORDER (MDD)

MDD is the most prevalent psychiatric disorder, with a lifetime risk of 15–20%. The female-to-male ratio is 2:1, with an average age of onset in the mid-20s. Chronic illness and stress ↑ the risk of MDD, and concurrently, MDD can complicate the treatment of chronic disease. Left untreated, MDEs typically last > 4 months, and the recurrence rate is > 50% after 1 episode.

- Although it has recently fallen into disfavor, the most widely known theory regarding the etiology of MDD is the biogenic amine theory, which holds that depression is due to low levels of amine neurotransmitters (eg, norepinephrine and serotonin [5-HT]) in the synaptic cleft.
- This theory has been supported by evidence that antidepressants ↑ the functional quantity of amine neurotransmitters that can bind postsynaptic receptors in the CNS.

SIGNS AND SYMPTOMS

The signs and symptoms of MDD are outlined in the mnemonic **SIG E CAPS.**

DIFFERENTIAL

The differential diagnosis for a patient with mood symptoms is as follows:

- **Psychiatric:** MDD, bipolar I or II disorder, schizoaffective disorder, substance-induced mood disorder, dementia, mood disorder due to a general medical condition, delirium, bereavement, adjustment disorder with depressed mood.

KEY POINT

MAJOR DEPRESSIVE DISORDER VS. GRIEF

- Normal bereavement begins immediately or a few months after the loss of a loved one.
- The symptoms of bereavement are similar to those of MDD, but the latter is not diagnosed unless **symptoms persist beyond 2 months** or if **excessive depressive symptoms** (eg, suicidal ideation, excessive guilt, or preoccupation with worthlessness) are present.
- Note that some form of auditory hallucination, such as intermittently hearing the voice of a lost loved one, can be a normal part of bereavement rather than part of a true mood or psychotic disorder.
- Bereavement may vary by culture.

MNEMONIC

Symptoms of depression–

SIG E CAPS

Sleep–↑ or ↓
Interest–anhedonia (loss of interest or pleasure)
Guilt or worthlessness
Energy–↓
Concentration–difficult or disturbed
Appetite–↑ or ↓
Psychomotor changes
Suicidal ideation

KEY FACT

In diagnosing MDD, it is important to rule out hypothyroidism, as this condition is both common and treatable. Always check a TSH level.

KEY FACT

An ↑ risk of suicide has been reported immediately following the initiation of pharmacotherapy for MDD, especially among young adults. This population should therefore be closely monitored after antidepressant treatment is started.

KEY FACT

Consider mirtazapine for patients with poor appetite and weight loss—eg, elderly patients with depression and failure to thrive (FTT), in whom it may boost appetite and weight.

KEY FACT

Treat TCA overdose with sodium bicarbonate.

KEY FACT

Discontinue SSRIs 5 weeks before starting MAOIs and vice versa given the risk of serotonin syndrome, which presents with **fever, myoclonus, and mental status changes** and may lead to cardiovascular collapse.

- **Organic:** Hypothyroidism, AIDS, MS, Parkinson's disease, Addison's disease, Cushing's disease, anemia (especially pernicious anemia), infectious mononucleosis, neuroborreliosis, influenza, malnutrition, malignancies (eg, pancreatic cancer).
- **Pharmacologic:** OCPs, cimetidine, steroids, some β-blockers, withdrawal from medications or side effects from newly initiated medications (eg, antidepressants, some of which can transiently ↑ suicidality).

Workup

- DSM-IV criteria for the diagnosis of MDD are as follows:
  - At least 5 symptoms of depression, at least 1 of which must be one of the "big 2": depressed mood or anhedonia.
  - Symptoms must persist for at least 2 weeks; must lead to significant social or occupational dysfunction; and must not be caused by drugs, medications, medical conditions, or bereavement.
- Distinguishing bereavement from MDD may be difficult in patients with a normal response lasting > 2 months.

Treatment

- A combination of pharmacotherapy and psychotherapy is the most effective approach. Antidepressants often take a minimum of 2–3 weeks to take effect, so do not discontinue or assume inefficacy until at least 8 weeks of treatment have elapsed (for most antidepressants).
- SSRIs and other antidepressants (bupropion, venlafaxine, mirtazapine, trazodone) are well tolerated and are considered first-line therapy for depression. The 2006 results of the Sequenced Treatment Alternatives to Relieve Depression (STAR*D) trial supported beginning treatment with an SSRI and maximizing the effective dose over several weeks before considering switching classes of medication or augmenting with a different medication.
- Alternative medical agents include TCAs and MAOIs, which are less frequently used because of the higher risk of side effects. Electroconvulsive therapy (ECT) is usually reserved for refractory or catatonic depression. ECT is generally considered safe with few contraindications and has even been approved for use in pregnant women.
- Psychoanalytically oriented (psychodynamic) and supportive therapies are perhaps the most commonly used psychological modalities, but cognitive-behavioral therapy (CBT) and interpersonal therapy are also effective.

Complications

- MDD is associated with high recurrence rates—50% after 1 episode, 70% after 2 episodes, and 90% after 3 episodes.
- Side effects of antidepressants are as follows:
  - **SSRIs: Sexual side effects,** insomnia, headache, tremor, GI upset, sleep and appetite disturbances, changes in mood.
  - **SNRIs and other antidepressants:** Characterized by a relative lack of sexual side effects, but can cause sedation, weight changes, a ↓ **seizure threshold** (bupropion), and **priapism** (trazodone). Discuss the details of individual drug profiles with your residents and attendings.
  - **TCAs:** Can be lethal in overdose and can lead to prolonged QRS intervals on ECG.
  - **MAOIs:** Less frequently used because they can lead to hypertensive crisis if taken with high-tyramine foods (eg, aged cheese, wine).

KEY POINT

KEY ANTIDEPRESSANT MEDICATIONS

Selective serotonin reuptake inhibitors (SSRIs):

- **Drugs:** Fluoxetine (Prozac), sertraline (Zoloft), paroxetine (Paxil), fluvoxamine (Luvox), citalopram (Celexa), escitalopram (Lexapro).
- **Mechanism:** 5-HT-specific reuptake inhibitors.
- **Clinical use:** Endogenous depression in adults. SSRIs have been associated with an ↑ suicide risk in children and adolescents in the early stages of treatment. Currently, only fluoxetine is approved for use in children (must be ≥ 8 years of age).
- **Side effects:** GI upset, sleep and appetite disturbances, sexual dysfunction, agitation, neuromuscular restlessness (akathisia), anorexia, and multiple drug interactions, including serotonin syndrome (restlessness, confusion, hyperthermia, muscle rigidity, cardiovascular collapse, death) when used with other serotonergic medications (eg, MAOIs).
- **Pros:** Relatively well tolerated, so you can usually start at the therapeutic dose. Safer in overdose relative to other drug classes, with fewer side effects than TCAs. Citalopram and sertraline are commonly used in patients with multiple comorbid conditions, as they have very few drug interactions and are helpful for anxiety commonly associated with depression.
- **Cons:** Sexual dysfunction is very common and is often the cause of noncompliance. Like all antidepressants, SSRIs take 2–3 weeks to have an effect.

Tricyclic antidepressants (TCAs):

- **Drugs:** Amitriptyline (Elavil), imipramine (Tofranil), desipramine (Norpramin), clomipramine (Anafranil), nortriptyline (Pamelor), doxepin (Sinequan).
- **Mechanism:** Block reuptake of norepinephrine and 5-HT.
- **Clinical use:** Endogenous depression, bedwetting (imipramine), OCD (clomipramine), chronic pain.
- **Side effects:** Anticholinergic effects (dry mouth, blurred vision, constipation, urinary retention, delirium, worsening glaucoma), sedation, α-blocking effects (orthostatic hypotension), cardiac arrhythmias (widened QRS, prolonged PR and QTc, potential for SVT/VT/VF), seizures, respiratory depression, confusion, hallucinations in the elderly. 3° TCAs (imipramine, amitriptyline) have more anticholinergic side effects and sedation than do 2° TCAs (nortriptyline). Desipramine is the least sedating.
- **Pros:** Inexpensive, well studied, and effective in severe depression; occasionally used for patients with concurrent chronic pain issues.
- **Cons:** Poor compliance owing to side effects. Lethal in overdose, so must titrate slowly. The **"3 C's"** of TCA toxicity are **C**onvulsions, **C**oma, and **C**ardiac arrhythmias.

- **Labs:** Check an ECG before starting, after a few days, and at the therapeutic dose (look particularly for QRS prolongation). Check blood levels if no response is obtained, excessive side effects occur, or there is suspected noncompliance.

Monoamine oxidase inhibitors (MAOIs):

- **Drugs:** Selegiline (EMSAM patch), phenelzine (Nardil), tranylcypromine (Parnate), isocarboxazid (Marplan).
- **Mechanism:** Nonselective MAO inhibition.
- **Clinical use:** Atypical depression, anxiety, hypochondriasis.
- **Side effects:** Hypertensive crisis ("tyramine reaction" or "wine and cheese reaction"; avoid aged cheeses, red wine, cured foods, yeast extracts, meperidine, and common sympathomimetic "cold and pain" drugs); headache, dizziness, insomnia, orthostatic hypotension, weight gain.
- **Pros:** Inexpensive; efficacious; highly effective for atypical depression.
- **Cons:** Dietary restrictions and poor tolerability of side effects. Contraindicated for use with β-agonists, SSRIs, or meperidine.

Common second-line antidepressants attempted after SSRIs:

- **Venlafaxine (Effexor):** Inhibits norepinephrine and 5-HT reuptake. Can also be used in GAD. Side effects include stimulant effects (insomnia, anxiety, agitation, headache, and nausea) and ↑ diastolic BP. BP must be monitored.
- **Duloxetine (Cymbalta):** Acts as a multiple reuptake inhibitor with strong norepinephrine action. Also useful in diabetics with peripheral neuropathic pain. In particular, it may improve symptoms of apathy and fatigue. Associated with a risk of interaction with thioridazine; requires slow taper to prevent withdrawal syndrome. Avoid in renal failure.

Atypical/heterocyclic antidepressants:

Second- and third-generation antidepressants have varied mechanisms of action.

- **Bupropion (Wellbutrin):** Also used in smoking cessation (as Zyban). Rarely lethal in overdose and has few sexual side effects. Other side effects include tachycardia, agitation, dry mouth, anxiety, aggravation of psychosis, and a tendency to lead to seizures.
- **Mirtazapine (Remeron):** An α_2-antagonist (↑ norepinephrine and 5-HT neurotransmission) and a potent 5-HT_2 receptor antagonist. Has fewer sexual side effects, although it leads to marked sedation, ↑ appetite, and weight gain (which could be of use in underweight patients with depression or in elderly patients with FTT).
- **Nefazodone (Serzone)/trazodone (Desyrel):** Primarily inhibit serotonin reuptake by a mechanism different from that of the SSRIs. Both have short half-lives. Side effects include sedation (especially trazodone), postural hypotension, and priapism (trazodone only). Because of the side effect of sedation, trazodone in combination with another antidepressant may be effective in depressed patients with insomnia.

KEY POINT

ELECTROCONVULSIVE THERAPY (ECT)

Despite its infamous reputation, ECT is safe and effective for use in MDD. Patients usually require 6–12 treatments. ECT can be done on an outpatient basis and can be lifesaving for refractory or catatonic depression. It can also be used in bipolar disorder (for mania and depression) and acute psychosis.

- **Pre-ECT evaluation:** Conduct a history and physical (H&P); obtain an ECG, electrolytes, CBC, LFTs, UA, TFTs, CXR, a spinal x-ray series, and a head CT. Alert anesthesiology in advance. Informed consent is required.
- **Procedure:** The patient signs a consent form after discussion with a psychiatrist and is generally evaluated by anesthesiologists as well. The patient is kept NPO for at least 8 hours. If possible, any medications with antiepileptic activity are held in the morning (eg, benzodiazepines, gabapentin). A short-acting barbiturate (methohexital) is given for anesthesia. Prior to the induction of muscle paralysis with succinylcholine, a tourniquet is placed around an extremity to prevent paralysis in that area in order to monitor the seizure. Unipolar leads are preferred to bipolar leads, and these administer increasing amounts of current to achieve a seizure. The patient's vital signs are closely monitored throughout the process and are generally monitored closely afterward during recovery from anesthesia.
- **Contraindications:** Very few contraindications; include recent MI, recent stroke, and intracranial mass. However, these are sometimes bypassed given the severity of psychiatric symptoms. ECT is also a relative contraindication in patients who are a high anesthesia risk.
- **Side effects:** Postictal confusion, arrhythmias, headaches (resolve in hours), retrograde amnesia (usually no longer than 6 months), sore muscles. Some patients find that side effects diminish with subsequent treatments.

Other somatic treatments include deep brain stimulation (DBS), transmagnetic stimulation (TMS), and vagus nerve stimulation (VNS). There is an increasing evidence base showing the efficacy of these treatments for treatment-resistant depression and other diagnoses. It may be useful to discuss this issue with residents and attendings who have experience with each modality.

DYSTHYMIC DISORDER

Has a 6% lifetime prevalence and a twofold greater incidence among females than males. Patients have chronic depression of > 2 years' duration that is not severe enough to meet the criteria for MDD. Dysthymic disorder lacks psychotic features, does not lead to social or occupational dysfunction, and does not require hospitalization.

KEY FACT

Dysthymia is the presence of at least 2 years of chronic depression that is not severe enough to meet the criteria for major depression.

Differential

Similar to that of MDD.

WORKUP

To meet DSM-IV criteria for dysthymic disorder, in addition to depressed mood more days than not, a patient must exhibit **2 or more** of the following 6 symptoms **for more days than not over a period of at least 2 years:**

- ↑ or ↓ appetite
- ↑ or ↓ sleep
- ↓ energy or fatigue
- ↓ self-esteem
- Difficulty concentrating or disturbed concentration
- Hopelessness

TREATMENT

Antidepressants that are effective in treating MDD may also be effective in dysthymic disorder. Supportive psychotherapy and psychoeducation (teaching patients and their families about this illness) are helpful as well.

BIPOLAR DISORDER

Bipolar I Disorder

Bipolar I disorder, or manic-depression, is an affective disorder with a 0.5–1.5% lifetime prevalence. Men and women are affected equally, and the average age of onset is 21 years. As in MDD, there is a strong genetic component, with a 70% concordance in monozygotic twins. The recurrence rate after 1 manic episode is 90%, and 10–15% of patients will commit suicide.

SIGNS AND SYMPTOMS

- DSM-IV criteria for the diagnosis of a manic episode include the presence of an elevated, expansive, or irritable mood with at least 3 (or 4 if the mood is irritable) signs and symptoms from the **DIG FAAST** mnemonic.
- Symptoms of a **manic** or **mixed** episode (ie, one that meets the criteria for both an MDE and a manic episode) must be present for at least 1 week (or less if hospitalization was required).
- Only a single manic episode is required for diagnosis. Suspect bipolar disorder in any patient who presents with a history of a manic episode.
- Patients may initially present with depression.
- More commonly associated with substance abuse than other psychiatric disorders.

DIFFERENTIAL

- **Psychiatric:** MDD, schizophrenia, schizoaffective disorder, substance-induced mood disorder, cyclothymia, borderline personality disorder, ADHD.

MNEMONIC

Signs and symptoms of mania—

DIG FAAST

Distractibility
Insomnia—↓ need for sleep
Grandiosity—inflated self-esteem
Flight of ideas
↑ in goal-directed **A**ctivity; psychomotor **A**gitation
Pressured **S**peech
Thoughtlessness—seeks pleasure without regard for consequence (eg, substance abuse, hypersexual behavior, shopping sprees)

KEY POINT

BIPOLAR I SUBTYPES

- **Rapid cycling:** Some 20% of bipolar I patients suffer from rapid cycling, in which at least 4 mood episodes (MDE, mania, hypomania, or mixed) occur in 12 months. This subtype carries a poorer prognosis.
- **Bipolar I with psychotic features:** Can feature mood-congruent or mood-incongruent delusions or hallucinations.

- **Organic:** Brain tumors, CNS syphilis, encephalitis, metabolic disorders, hyperthyroidism, MS.
- **Pharmacologic:** Cocaine, amphetamines, corticosteroids, anabolic steroids, phenylpropanolamine, INH, captopril, antidepressants.

Treatment

- Assess patients for suicidal and homicidal ideation and the need for hospitalization. Treat with a combination of pharmacotherapy and psychotherapy.
  - **Acute mania:** Give mood stabilizers (eg, lithium, valproic acid, carbamazepine). Since mood stabilizers can take some time to take effect, low-dose antipsychotics may be required for stabilization. Olanzapine and risperidone are often used in treatment-naïve patients, as is haloperidol. Antipsychotic medication is particularly helpful if the patient has psychosis associated with mania. Benzodiazepines or other anxiolytics may be useful in refractory agitation.
  - **Bipolar depression:** Use mood stabilizers +/– an antidepressant. Start mood stabilizers first to avoid inducing mania with an antidepressant. Antidepressants alone can also precipitate rapid cycling.
- **Prophylaxis and maintenance:**
  - Lifelong prophylaxis with a mood stabilizer is warranted after the second episode, after a first episode that is severe or life threatening, or in the presence of a strong family history.
  - Lithium and valproic acid are considered first-line therapy; carbamazepine and lamotrigine are second-line agents if first-line treatments fail.
  - ECT is effective but is reserved for patients who are refractory to pharmacotherapy or when a more immediate treatment response is required.
  - Psychotherapy focuses on helping patients understand and accept their illness, cope with its consequences, and maintain medication compliance.
  - Patients with bipolar I disorder are statistically at higher risk for suicide than those with major depression, a fact that clinicians should keep in mind during management.

Bipolar II Disorder

Patients must have at least 1 MDE and 1 hypomanic episode to be diagnosed with bipolar II disorder; mixed and manic episodes are absent. Has a lifetime prevalence of 0.5%, with an incidence that is slightly greater for women.

Signs and Symptoms

- DSM-IV criteria require at least 4 days of abnormally elevated, expansive, or irritable mood **and** at least 3 signs and symptoms (or 4, if the mood is irritable) from the **DIG FAAST** mnemonic.
- Changes due to hypomania are not severe enough to require hospitalization, cause psychotic features, or lead to social or occupational dysfunction. However, depressive episodes can occasionally prove as severe as those of bipolar I disorder.
- Can also show rapid cycling.

Treatment

Similar to that of bipolar I disorder.

KEY FACT

Unlike adults, who show well-defined, distinct episodes of depression and mania, children with bipolar disorder may present with both classes of symptoms within the same day.

KEY FACT

If a young woman being treated for bipolar disorder presents with ataxia, coarse tremor, and nystagmus and appears dehydrated, think lithium toxicity leading to nephrotoxicity (eg, nephrogenic DI).

KEY FACT

Bipolar II disorder requires the presence of at least 1 MDE and 1 hypomanic episode.

Q

A 29-year-old woman presents to the ED with days of irritable mood, poor sleep, and rapid speech and threatens others by claiming that she "knows people in high places." She yells and bangs on the walls of the room. The patient has no known allergies. What medication can be used for her agitation?

KEY MOOD STABILIZERS

Lithium:

- **Clinical use:** The mainstay of treatment for bipolar disorder and mania (acute episodes and prophylaxis). Also has mild antidepressant effects.
- **Side effects:** Fine tremor, nausea, acne, weight gain, benign leukocytosis, arrhythmias, other ECG cardiac changes (flattened T waves or T-wave inversion), hypothyroidism, nephrogenic DI (lithium is an ADH antagonist), CKD, teratogenesis.
- **Pros:** Inexpensive and well studied for long-term use.
- **Cons:** Regular lab studies are required because long-term renal damage is possible. Dosage must be titrated owing to the narrow therapeutic index; aim for a level of 0.8–1.2 mEq/L in acute mania and 0.6–1.0 mEq/L for maintenance. Note, however, that the dose is sometimes titrated to a patient's symptoms rather than to serum level. NSAIDs, ACEIs, and diuretics (when first started) ↑ plasma lithium level and should be avoided if possible.
- **Signs of toxicity:** Coarse tremor, arrhythmias, dysarthria, ataxia, nausea, diarrhea, nystagmus (level of 1.5 mEq/L); seizures and coma (2.5 mEq/L); and death (≥ 3 mEq/L). Patients may require dialysis.

Valproate/valproic acid (Depakote):

- **Clinical use:** As effective as lithium in bipolar disorder and better in mixed mania, substance abuse, and rapid cycling. Can be used for acute episodes and prophylaxis.
- **Side effects:** Carries a black-box warning for hepatotoxicity. GI distress, sedation, hepatotoxicity (eg, rare hepatitis, ↑ LFTs, ↑ ammonia), pancreatitis (rare), thrombocytopenia (rare).
- **Pros:** Well tolerated, broad therapeutic index, and relatively benign in overdose. Patients can start at the therapeutic dose, and fewer blood tests are required once the dosage is established. Useful in patients suspected of having an underlying epileptic condition.
- **Cons:** LFTs, platelets, and valproic acid levels should be checked at regular intervals.

Carbamazepine (Tegretol):

- **Clinical use:** A second-line agent used in patients who do not respond to lithium.
- **Side effects:** Rare but serious side effects include Stevens-Johnson syndrome, agranulocytosis, aplastic anemia, and hepatitis.
- **Cons:** A CBC is needed before starting and should be obtained on a monthly basis for the first 3–6 months and then once every 3–6 months.
- **Signs of toxicity:** Ataxia, confusion, tremors.

A

Antipsychotic medication for acute mania.

CYCLOTHYMIA

A mild form of bipolar disorder consisting of recurrent mood disturbances alternating between hypomania and dysthymia. Some 30% of patients have a family history of bipolar disorder.

Signs and Symptoms

- DSM-IV criteria require at least 2 years of cycling hypomanic and dysthymic episodes without major depressive, manic, or mixed episodes. The patient must not be symptom free for > 2 months at a time.
- Symptoms are less severe than those of bipolar I and II disorders but may cycle more rapidly.
- Patients may also have borderline personality disorder; one-third to one-half will develop a mood disorder (usually bipolar II).

Treatment

The treatment of choice is a mood stabilizer. Antidepressants alone may precipitate manic episodes in some cases.

Psychotic Disorders

Psychotic disorders are defined by the presence of psychosis, which is a "gross impairment in reality testing," or disorganization of thought or behavior.

SCHIZOPHRENIA

A psychotic disorder that is characterized by a disruption in thought, affect, volition, social behavior, and motor activity in which the patient becomes increasingly preoccupied with his or her internal environment. Its prevalence is approximately 1%, and the male-to-female ratio is 1:1. Peak onset in men is earlier (15–25 years as opposed to 25–35 years in women) and is of greater severity. In general, patients exhibit a chronic and progressive course. Risk factors and etiologies are as follows:

- In the United States, an ↑ prevalence of the disease has been observed among lower socioeconomic classes, likely due to a "downward drift" of these patients into the lower classes as a result of impairment from their disease.
- Dizygotic twins and children of a single schizophrenic parent have a 12% prevalence of schizophrenia, and the prevalence ↑ to 40% and 47% with 2 parents with schizophrenia or a monozygotic twin, respectively.
- Various neurotransmitter abnormalities have also been identified in association with schizophrenia.
  - An imbalance of dopamine (the "dopamine hypothesis"), the most widely favored theory, posits that ↑ dopamine activity and receptors in some parts of the brain correlate with the ⊕ symptoms of the disease, whereas ↓ dopamine activity in others correlates with ⊖ symptoms.
  - This hypothesis is supported by the observation that dopamine receptor antagonists (antipsychotic medications) alleviate psychotic symptoms, while dopamine agonists (eg, cocaine and amphetamines) may induce such symptoms.

KEY FACT

Approximately 10–15% of patients with schizophrenia die by suicide, while 40–50% of patients make a suicide attempt.

Q

A 43-year-old man presents to the ED with command auditory hallucinations and is given a dose of PO risperidone before being admitted to the inpatient unit. Two hours later he complains of stiffness and discomfort of his right arm and the right side of his neck. What medication should he be given?

KEY POINT

FOUR IMPORTANT DOPAMINE PATHWAYS

1. **Mesolimbic:** Associated with ⊕ symptoms.
2. **Mesocortical:** Associated with ⊖ symptoms (remember that **"C"** in "**C**ortical" = **"C"** in "**C**atatonia").
3. **Nigrostriatal pathway:** Associated with extrapyramidal symptoms (EPS) and tardive dyskinesia.
4. **Tuberoinfundibular:** Associated with hyperprolactinemia.

- More recently, the neurotransmitter glutamate has been implicated in the pathogenesis of schizophrenia; research in this field is ongoing. Early studies indicate that glutamate plays an important role in the upstream regulation of dopamine pathways (particularly the mesocortical and mesolimbic pathways). It may be useful to read more about this, although pharmacotherapy making use of this mechanism remains forthcoming.

MNEMONIC

Evolution of EPS–

4 and A

4 hours: **A**cute dystonia
4 days: **A**kinesia
4 weeks: **A**kathisia
4 months: Tardive dyskinesia (often permanent)

KEY FACT

Always consider the possibility of delirium and organic causes of mental status change in patients who present with perceptual changes suggesting psychosis.

A

Benztropine or diphenhydramine for dystonia.

Signs and Symptoms

- According to the DSM-IV, patients must present with at least 2 of the following signs and symptoms for at least 6 months:
  - ⊕ **symptoms:** The presence of unusual thought, behaviors, or perceptions, including hallucinations (usually auditory or visual), delusions, bizarre behavior (eg, echolalia, echopraxia, odd dress), and disordered thought (eg, ideas of reference, tangentiality, loose associations).
  - ⊖ **symptoms:** Lack of normal social and/or mental function, including flat affect, poverty of thought and/or speech, apathy, anhedonia, and lack of purposeful actions. May progress to the point of catatonia.
- These symptoms must lead to social and/or occupational dysfunction. Depression, if present, is brief in comparison to the duration of the illness.

Differential

- **Psychiatric:** Other psychotic disorders (eg, schizoaffective, schizophreniform), mood disorders (eg, bipolar disorder, severe melancholia, mood disorder with psychotic features), delusional disorder, delirium, dementia, Cluster A personality type, developmental disorders (eg, Asperger's syndrome, autism).
- **Organic:** Early Huntington's disease, early Wilson's disease, complex partial seizures (eg, temporal lobe epilepsy), frontal or temporal lobe tumors, early MS, early SLE, acute intermittent porphyria, electrolyte imbalances, hepatic encephalopathy, HIV encephalopathy, viral encephalitis, neurosyphilis, endocrine abnormalities (eg, Cushing's disease, calcium imbalance, thyroid dysfunction, hypoglycemia).
- **Pharmacologic:** Substance abuse (eg, amphetamines, cocaine, PCP), medications (eg, digoxin, ACTH, INH, L-dopa).

Workup

- According to the DSM-IV, the criteria for the diagnosis of schizophrenia include the presence of 2 or more of the above signs and symptoms for a period of at least 1 month, with continuous evidence of social and/or occupational dysfunction 2° to psychiatric disturbance for at least 6 months.

KEY PSYCHIATRIC TERMS

- **Affect:** The outward expression, including facial expression, of the patient's internal emotional state.
- **Circumstantiality:** Indirect speech that is delayed in reaching the point but does eventually reach the desired goal (ie, the ability to "get from point A to point B" after some period of time).
- **Clanging:** Association of words with similar sounds but not similar meaning.
- **Compulsions:** Conscious, stereotyped behaviors or thoughts that the patient manifests to prevent the distress or anxiety induced by an obsession.
- **Delusions:** Fixed false beliefs that are not consistent with the patient's cultural background and cannot be altered by reasoning.
- **Depersonalization:** A state in which the self is felt to be unreal or detached from reality.
- **Derealization:** Perception of the world around a person as unreal.
- **Echolalia:** Persistent repetition of the words or phrases of another person.
- **Flight of ideas:** Rapid, continuous use of words with constant shifting between connected ideas.
- **Hallucinations:** False sensory perceptions without a basis in external stimuli (as opposed to illusions; see below).
- **Ideas of reference:** A patient's belief that an object (eg, a radio or television) is referring to him or her.
- **Illusions:** Misinterpretations of actual stimuli.
- **Loosening of associations:** Flow of thought with random shifting of ideas from one subject to another.
- **Mood:** The patient's subjective, internal emotional state in their own words.
- **Neologisms:** New words, often created by combining syllables of other words.
- **Obsessions:** Recurrent, intrusive thoughts, impulses, or images that lead to anxiety and that the patient attempts to suppress or neutralize in order to ↓ anxiety.
- **Perseveration:** Persistent response to a previous stimulus when a new stimulus is presented; obsessive rumination or "getting stuck" on a certain topic.
- **Poverty of thought:** Having only a few thoughts, which lack variety and richness.
- **Pressured speech:** Rapid speech that is ↑ in amount and is difficult to understand or interrupt.
- **Tangentiality:** Inability to have goal-directed thought (ie, inability to "get from point A to point B" at all), going off on partially relevant topics.
- **Thought blocking:** Abrupt interruption in a train of thought before the thought or idea is completed.
- **Thought broadcasting:** Belief that one's thoughts are being transmitted to others.

KEY POINT

SCHIZOPHRENIA AND RELATED DISORDERS

- **Schizophrenia:** At least 6 months of psychotic features.
- **Schizophreniform disorder:** Requires 1–6 months of psychotic features.
- **Brief psychotic disorder:** One day to 1 month of psychotic features.
- **Schizoaffective disorder:** Combines symptoms of schizophrenia with a major affective disorder (MDD or bipolar disorder).

- These symptoms cannot be due to a preexisting medical condition, a substance-related condition, or another psychiatric condition. Subtypes of schizophrenia are outlined in Table 8-2.
- Imaging studies are not necessary, although schizophrenic brains may show abnormal findings such as enlarged ventricles and cortical atrophy.

TREATMENT

- Treatment consists primarily of antipsychotic (neuroleptic) medications. The side effects of typical antipsychotics include EPS, hyperprolactinemia, and anticholinergic effects.
- Psychosocial intervention includes supportive treatment such as vocational rehabilitation and arranged social support in the community.
- Hospitalization may be required, especially during psychotic episodes.

KEY FACT

If medication is discontinued, the 2-year relapse rate for schizophrenia approaches 75–80%.

TABLE 8-2. Schizophrenia Subtypes

SUBTYPE	COMMENTS
Paranoid	Delusions or hallucinations (frequently auditory). Lacks disorganized speech, disorganized or catatonic behavior, and ⊖ symptoms. Relatively good self-care. Has the best prognosis—relatively good preservation of thought, personality, and function over time.
Disorganized	Prominent disorganized speech, disorganized behavior (poor personal appearance), and flat/inappropriate affect (eg, disinhibited). Does not involve catatonic behavior. Associated with the worst prognosis.
Catatonic	Diagnosis requires at least 2 the following: ▪ Motor immobility (rigidity) ▪ Excessive motor activity ▪ Extreme negativism or mutism ▪ Peculiar voluntary movement and bizarre posturing (waxy flexibility) ▪ Echolalia or echopraxia
Undifferentiated	Has characteristics of > 1 subtype.
Residual	The patient meets the criteria for schizophrenia in the past but now lacks delusions and hallucinations. The patient has residual ⊖ symptoms or attenuated hallucinations, delusions, and other thought disorders.

SCHIZOPHRENIFORM DISORDER

The prevalence of schizophreniform disorder is slightly less than that of schizophrenia (0.2%). This diagnosis has fallen out of favor because many patients eventually develop schizophrenia while others develop a mood disorder.

Signs and Symptoms

- Patients with schizophreniform disorder meet the criteria for schizophrenia, except that the **duration of illness is > 1 month but < 6 months** (instead of > 6 months as in schizophrenia).
- Social and/or occupational function may or may not be impaired.
- Males and females are affected equally.

Treatment

Methods of psychotherapy, family and social-vocational therapies, and pharmacotherapy used in schizophrenia may all be considered in schizophreniform disorder.

BRIEF PSYCHOTIC DISORDER

This diagnosis carries a better prognosis than schizophrenia.

Signs and Symptoms

Patients exhibit 1 or more of the following symptoms for 1 day to 1 month: delusions, hallucinations, disorganized speech, grossly disorganized behavior, and catatonic behavior.

Differential

- Since the differential diagnosis of an acute psychotic episode is broad and this disorder is rare, it is critical to rule out other causes.
- The disorder can occur with or without the presence of stressors, including parturition (episode within 4 weeks of giving birth).

Treatment

- Brief hospitalization if necessary.
- A short course of neuroleptics or benzodiazepines may prove useful.

KEY POINT

KEY ANTIPSYCHOTIC MEDICATIONS

Antipsychotic medications are usually divided into "typical" and "atypical" medications. Atypicals produce fewer EPS, have a better side effect profile, and do not ↑ prolactin levels but are very expensive.

Typical antipsychotics:

- **Drugs:** Can be divided into high, medium, and low potency.
  - **High:** Haloperidol (Haldol), fluphenazine (Prolixin), thiothixene (Navane), droperidol (Inapsine).

- **Medium:** Trifluoperazine (Stelazine), perphenazine (Trilafon).
- **Low:** Thioridazine (Mellaril), chlorpromazine (Thorazine).

- **Mechanism:** Block dopamine receptors (mostly D_2 and D_4 subtypes).
- **Clinical use:** Most effective in treating ⊕ symptoms.
- **Side effects:** Similar for all typical agents. Higher-potency drugs have more EPS, while lower-potency drugs have more anticholinergic, sedative, and orthostatic hypotensive effects.
  - **EPS:**
    - **Acute dystonia:** Early, sudden-onset twisting of the neck or rolling of the eyes (torticollis and oculogyric crisis, respectively), occurring mainly in young men after 10–14 days of treatment. Can also present as painful, slow muscle movements elsewhere. Treat with IM anticholinergics such as benztropine (Cogentin), diphenhydramine (Benadryl), or trihexyphenidyl (Artane).
    - **Akathisia:** A subjective sense of inner restlessness in the legs that may or may not lead to objective manifestations of restlessness (eg, walking around or difficulty remaining still). Treat with β-blockers (eg, propranolol) or benzodiazepines (eg, clonazepam, diazepam).
    - **Parkinsonism:** Resting tremor, cogwheel rigidity, bradykinesia, shuffling gait, and masklike facies. Treat with oral anticholinergics and possibly amantadine (a dopamine-releasing agent).
    - **Tardive dyskinesia:** Involuntary, abnormal lip smacking, tongue protrusion, and writhing movements of the limbs or trunk. Occurs in 10–30% of long-term neuroleptic users (especially elderly patients, women, and patients with mood disorders). Treatment involves withdrawing neuroleptics or changing to clozapine. Often irreversible.
  - **Neuroleptic malignant syndrome:** Fever, rigidity, autonomic instability, clouding of consciousness. Can give rise to rhabdomyolysis, myoglobinuria, and renal failure; in this case, CK is usually markedly ↑. The condition is uncommon but life threatening (20% mortality). Treat by withdrawing neuroleptics, by initiating supportive measures, and sometimes by administering dantrolene, bromocriptine, or amantadine. Occasionally difficult to distinguish from serotonin syndrome (see "Antidepressants"), for which these treatments should be avoided.
  - **Hyperprolactinemia:** Causes amenorrhea, galactorrhea, and gynecomastia. A pituitary tumor must be ruled out.
  - **Anticholinergic effects:** Include dry mouth, urinary retention, and constipation.
  - **Other:** Orthostatic hypotension, weight gain, sedation, seizures, ECG changes or arrhythmias (eg, conduction delays).

Atypical antipsychotics:

- **Drugs:**
  - **Risperidone (Risperdal):** Side effects include a low incidence of EPS (although it is the mostly likely of atypical antipsychotics to cause EPS) as well as hyperprolactinemia, fatigue, tachycardia, sedation, orthostatic hypotension, and weight gain.
  - **Olanzapine (Zyprexa):** Particularly effective in treating ⊖ symptoms and in treating more agitated patients. Has a low incidence of EPS; the most common side effects are drowsiness, akathisia, weight gain, insomnia, and dry mouth. No hepatotoxicity. Generally avoided in patients at risk for obesity, metabolic syndrome, and hyperlipidemia.
  - **Quetiapine (Seroquel):** Has a very low incidence of EPS. Side effects include somnolence and orthostasis. Usually dosed more than once daily. Generally considered one of the more sedating antipsychotics; often dosed at nighttime.
  - **Ziprasidone (Geodon):** Side effects include QT prolongation, insomnia, and restlessness. Must be taken with food in order to be effective.
  - **Aripiprazole (Abilify):** A D_2 and 5-HT_{1A} partial agonist and an HT_{2A} antagonist with rapid onset of action and a lower rate of weight gain than other medications, together with a very low rate of hyperprolactinemia and cardiotoxicity. Because it is a partial agonist/antagonist, some literature has suggested that it may influence the efficacy of other concurrent antipsychotic medications.
  - **Paliperidone (Invega):** Side effects include sedation, weight gain, and a low risk of EPS similar to that of other atypical antipsychotics.
  - **Clozapine (Clozaril):** A second-line treatment thought to be more effective for treatment-resistant schizophrenia and ⊖ symptoms. A dangerous side effect is **agranulocytosis,** which occurs in 0.5–1.0% of patients, thus mandating a weekly CBC for the first 6 months of treatment and every other week thereafter. Also requires monitoring of serum clozapine level. Other side effects include severe sedation, anticholinergic effects, orthostatic hypotension, vertigo, weight gain, seizures, arrhythmias, and eosinophilia.
- **Mechanism:** All medications of this class have some degree of 5-HT_2 receptor antagonism, but each has a different combination of receptor blockade.
- **Clinical use:** Atypical antipsychotics have fewer anticholinergic symptoms and EPS. Because of this, they are currently used as first-line drugs in newly diagnosed schizophrenia. These agents can be effective in treating patients with ⊕ and ⊖ symptoms as well as those who are refractory to typical antipsychotics.
- **Side effects:** These drugs do not lead to agranulocytosis but may be less effective than clozapine in treatment-resistant patients. Key side effects of the atypicals as a class include weight gain, type 2 diabetes mellitus (DM), and QT prolongation on ECG.

SCHIZOAFFECTIVE DISORDER

Unlike schizophrenia and schizophreniform disorder, schizoaffective disorder is said to be present when a patient concurrently meets the criteria for schizophrenia and for MDE, manic episode, or mixed episode. The lifetime prevalence is 0.5–0.8%, with a peak age of onset in the late teens and early 20s.

Workup

- Mood symptoms must be present for a significant portion of the disease, but acute psychotic symptoms (eg, delusions, hallucinations) must be present for at least 2 weeks in the absence of mood symptoms. This disorder also has bipolar and depressive subtypes.
- Schizoaffective disorder can be difficult to distinguish from a mood disorder with psychotic features, and therefore the patient history and clinician experience are crucial in making the diagnosis.

Treatment

- Give a combination of an antipsychotic and a mood stabilizer.
- Antidepressants and possibly ECT may be indicated for acute depressive types.

DELUSIONAL DISORDER

Like schizophrenia, delusional disorder is chronic. Unlike schizophrenia, however, its hallmark feature is nonbizarre (or plausible) delusions. Its prevalence is 0.03%, with males and females equally affected. The age of onset is variable but generally peaks in the 40s.

Workup

- To fulfill DSM-IV criteria, delusions must be present for at least 1 month in the absence of hallucinations, disorganized speech, disorganized behavior, or ⊖ symptoms.
- The subtypes of delusional disorder are defined by the predominant delusional content and are as follows:
  - **Persecutory:** Delusions that the individual is being harassed or malevolently treated.
  - **Grandiose:** Delusions that the individual possesses exaggerated power, money, or knowledge.
  - **Erotomanic:** Delusions that another person, usually of higher status, is in love with the individual.
  - **Somatic:** Delusions that the individual has a physical defect or a medical condition.
  - **Jealous:** Delusions that the individual's partner is unfaithful.
  - **Mixed:** Delusions that are of > 1 type.
  - **Unspecified.**

Treatment

Effective treatment is difficult, as most patients are refractory to neuroleptics. Long-term psychotherapy and pharmacologic treatment of concurrent psychiatric illness may provide some benefit.

KEY FACT

Some 10–15% of cases of delusional disorder resolve over time, whereas 40–55% worsen and 30–50% do not change.

Anxiety Disorders

A group of disorders in which anxiety—the presence of a sense of impending doom or threat—is the prominent feature. The patient's anxiety is poorly based in reality, is out of proportion to the actual threat, and is vague or poorly defined. The anxiety disorders are the most prevalent of all psychiatric disorders and are also most commonly comorbid with mood disorders.

GENERALIZED ANXIETY DISORDER (GAD)

Has a prevalence of nearly 5%, with a female-to-male ratio of 2:1. GAD commonly coexists with other psychiatric disorders. Patients may report excessive worry as adolescents, but the disorder generally becomes prominent when patients reach their 20s.

Signs and Symptoms

- The defining symptom is **chronic, excessive anxiety or worry** about a number of actual life events.
- Somatic manifestations are common and include palpitations, lightheadedness, dizziness, clammy hands, dry mouth, dysphagia, ↑ urinary frequency, difficulty breathing, abdominal pain, and diarrhea.

Differential

- **Psychiatric:** Other anxiety disorders (eg, panic disorder, OCD, social phobia, hypochondriasis), mood disorders (eg, depression, dysthymia), psychotic disorders.
- **Organic:** Hyperthyroidism; pheochromocytoma; abnormalities of calcium, glucose, or phosphate.
- **Pharmacologic:** Substance-induced anxiety disorder (eg, intoxication with caffeine, cocaine, or amphetamines); substance withdrawal (eg, benzodiazepines, alcohol).

Workup

According to DSM-IV criteria, the patient must have excessive anxiety on more days than not for 6 or more months, along with at least 3 of the 6 following symptoms:

- Restlessness or a feeling of being "on edge"
- Easy fatigability
- Difficulty concentrating or "mind going blank"
- Irritability
- Muscle tension
- Sleep disturbance (insomnia)

Treatment

- Combination pharmacotherapy and psychotherapy.
- External stressors (eg, caffeine, nicotine, sleep disturbances) should be eliminated.
- First-line pharmacotherapy includes SSRIs, venlafaxine, and buspirone. Avoid benzodiazepines in patients dealing with substance abuse.
- SSRIs and TCAs may be used for the treatment of GAD with depressive symptoms.
- CBT, with a focus on relaxation techniques, is a useful adjunct.

KEY ANTIANXIETY MEDICATIONS

Benzodiazepines:

- **Drugs (by half-life):**
  - **Long (> 100 hours):** Clonazepam (Klonopin), clorazepate (Tranxene), chlordiazepoxide (Librium), diazepam (Valium), flurazepam (Dalmane).
  - **Intermediate (10–20 hours):** Alprazolam (Xanax), lorazepam (Ativan), temazepam (Restoril).
  - **Short (3–8 hours):** Oxazepam (Serax), triazolam (Halcion).
- **Mechanism:** Bind to $GABA_A$ receptors (↑ GABA-binding affinity and ↑ the frequency of chloride channel opening). Remember that GABA is an inhibitory neurotransmitter, so this functions to ↑ inhibition.
- **Clinical use:** Used for a broad spectrum of anxiety disorders (eg, GAD, social phobia, panic disorder) and sleep disorders (eg, insomnia) as well as for alcohol detoxification, seizures, catatonia, and mood/adjustment/psychotic disorders with anxiety components. Also used as muscle relaxants.
- **Side effects:** Sedation, slurred speech, ataxia, dizziness, tolerance, cross-tolerance, dependence, anterograde amnesia, respiratory depression (especially with other sedatives or in COPD patients).
- **Pros:** Lorazepam, oxazepam, and temazepam are not metabolized by the liver and are safe to use in patients with hepatic dysfunction.
- **Cons:**
  - The potentiation of alcohol and other CNS depressants ↑ the risk of sedation and respiratory depression. **There is a high risk of dependence and abuse even in patients without a history of substance abuse.** Generally not indicated for long-term treatment of anxiety disorders because of the increasing tolerance and dependence with which they are associated. SSRIs and other psychotropic drugs are better suited for long-term management of anxiety.
  - P-450 inhibitors (eg, cimetidine, fluoxetine, INH, estrogen) ↑ levels, while drugs such as carbamazepine and rifampin ↓ levels.
  - Lorazepam and oxazepam are predominantly metabolized in the kidneys and may be preferable in patients with liver disease, such as those with a history of alcohol abuse.
  - Chlordiazepoxide and diazepam are predominantly metabolized in the liver and may be preferable in patients with renal failure.
  - Lorazepam, alprazolam, and diazepam are most frequently abused in patients with a history of alcohol and drug abuse.
  - Withdrawal symptoms are more severe and abrupt with shorter-acting agents.

- **Buspirone (BuSpar):**
  - **Mechanism:** Partial agonist for 5-HT_{1A} receptors.
  - **Clinical use:** GAD. Not useful in panic disorder. Can augment antidepressant treatment in MDD or OCD.
  - **Side effects:** Infrequent sedation, dizziness, headache, GI upset.
  - **Pros:** Safe and without the tolerance, dependence, withdrawal, and respiratory depression of benzodiazepines. Favored in patients with a history of substance abuse.
  - **Cons:** Slow onset of action. Thus, it is **not** useful in panic disorder. Less reliable than benzodiazepines in the treatment of anxiety disorders.

PANIC DISORDER

Characterized by unexpected, discrete periods of terror (panic attacks) as well as by anticipatory anxiety about future attacks. The lifetime prevalence is 1.5–3.5%, and females have a threefold ↑ in risk compared to males. The peak age of onset is in the mid-20s, and the disorder rarely presents after age 45.

SIGNS AND SYMPTOMS

- The DSM-IV has 2 criteria for the diagnosis of panic disorder: recurrent, unexpected panic attacks that begin suddenly, peak in intensity within 10 minutes, and include a sensation of intense fear along with at least 4 of the following symptoms:
  - Palpitations or ↑ heart rate, sweating, trembling, shaking, shortness of breath, or a feeling of choking.
  - Chest pain or discomfort; nausea or abdominal distress; dizziness or lightheadedness.
  - Derealization or depersonalization.
  - Fear of losing control or "going crazy"; fear of dying.
  - Paresthesias, chills, hot flashes.

KEY POINT

ACUTE PHARMACOTHERAPY FOR GENERALIZED ANXIETY DISORDER

- Like most psychiatric medications, SSRIs and SNRIs require several weeks to show a significant clinical effect. In the interim, patients may be given a benzodiazepine-buspirone combination.
- Benzodiazepines with longer half-lives are used, including clonazepam and diazepam. These medications take effect immediately but lead to dependence and withdrawal with > 2–3 weeks of use.

KEY FACT

Patients with panic disorder should be screened for 2 major comorbid conditions: MDD (50%) and agoraphobia (50%).

- At least 1 attack must be followed for 1 month or more by 1 of the following:
  - Persistent worry about additional attacks (anticipatory anxiety).
  - Worry about the implications of the attack.
  - A change in baseline function 2° to the attack.
- Agoraphobia (ie, fear and avoidance of places or situations where escape might be embarrassing or difficult) is present in 30–50% of cases.

DIFFERENTIAL

- **Psychiatric:** GAD, social phobia, OCD, PTSD.
- **Pharmacologic:** Substance-induced anxiety disorder (eg, caffeine, cocaine, amphetamines).
- **Organic:** Pheochromocytoma, arrhythmia, pulmonary embolism, hypoxia, angina, hyperthyroidism.

TREATMENT

- Treat with combination pharmacotherapy and psychotherapy.
- The most effective psychotherapy is CBT with a focus on relaxation techniques and reversal of symptom misinterpretation.
- SSRIs are first-line treatment; TCAs and MAOIs are second-line choices and are rarely used for this indication. MAOIs are more effective than TCAs, although they are limited in use owing to their side effects.
- Benzodiazepines (often alprazolam and clonazepam) may be used for immediate relief, but long-term use of these drugs should be avoided in some patients in light of their addiction potential and risk in the context of overdose.
- Buspirone is **not** effective in panic disorder.

SOCIAL PHOBIA

Defined as at least 6 months of persistent, intermittent fear of a social or public situation in which the patient is exposed to unfamiliar persons or to situations in which his or her performance will be scrutinized.

- Affects 3–13% of the population, with a female-to-male ratio of 1:1.
- Onset is usually in adolescence and is preceded by childhood shyness.

SIGNS AND SYMPTOMS

- Can be **situational** (most commonly public speaking or meeting new people) or **generalized** (fear of nearly all social situations). Phobic situations usually provoke a panic attack and impair social or occupational functioning.
- Patients recognize that their fear is excessive and irrational.

TREATMENT

- CBT with relaxation techniques.
- Pharmacotherapy consists of MAOIs, SSRIs, and occasionally β-blockers (eg, for stage fright). Benzodiazepines are indicated if SSRIs are not effective.

OBSESSIVE-COMPULSIVE DISORDER (OCD)

OCD has a lifetime prevalence of 2–3%. Although men and women are equally affected, men tend to develop OCD at an earlier age. The disorder usually begins during adolescence or early adulthood and shows a gradual progression. Issues complicating treatment and diagnosis are concomitant depression, reluctance to discuss symptoms, and substance abuse.

SIGNS AND SYMPTOMS

- The DSM-IV requires that the patient have either obsessions or compulsions and that **the patient recognize them as excessive and irrational.**
  - **Obsessions: Persistent, unwanted,** and **intrusive ideas, thoughts, impulses, or images** that lead to significant anxiety or distress. Common obsessions include cleanliness, contamination, or a fear of harm to self or loved ones.
  - **Compulsions: Repeated mental acts or behaviors** that neutralize anxiety from obsessions—eg, excessive cleaning (hands may be chafed 2° to frequent washing), elaborate rituals for conducting ordinary tasks (eg, walking through the doorway), or excessive checking (eg, multiple trips back home to check that the door is locked).
- Obsessions and compulsions must be time consuming (ie, they must take up > 1 hour per day), must be associated with marked distress, and must interrupt normal social or occupational function.

DIFFERENTIAL

- **Psychiatric:** GAD, specific phobia, trichotillomania, body dysmorphic disorder, obsessive-compulsive personality disorder (OCPD) (which, in comparison, is ego syntonic and lacks separate obsessions and compulsions), Tourette's syndrome, schizophrenia (which can include obsessions and compulsions, but with hallucinations and delusions), MDD (usually with obsessive rumination).
- **Organic:** Brain tumor or temporal lobe epilepsy.
- **Drugs:** Substance-induced anxiety disorder (eg, cocaine, amphetamines, caffeine).

> **KEY FACT**
>
> - OCD is **ego dystonic**—patients know their behavior is problematic.
> - OCPD is **ego syntonic**—symptoms are part of a person's personality, and patients are usually unaware of their problematic perfectionist behavior.

TREATMENT

- SSRIs are effective first-line treatment and are usually given at higher doses than those used for MDD. Fluvoxamine (Luvox) may be particularly helpful with obsessive symptoms and is one of the few drugs that has actually been studied for this indication. Clomipramine may also be of benefit.
- Behavioral therapy involves exposure-response prevention, thought stopping, and flooding.

POSTTRAUMATIC STRESS DISORDER (PTSD)

PTSD can occur after an individual is exposed to a traumatic event that is associated with intense fear or horror and that involves actual or threatened harm. Its lifetime prevalence is roughly 8% and is highest among young adults. In populations exposed to combat or assault, however, its prevalence approaches 60%.

SIGNS AND SYMPTOMS

- Presentation includes the following:
  - **Reexperiencing of traumatic events** through intrusive thoughts, flashbacks, and nightmares. These symptoms may occasionally be confused with visual or auditory hallucinations when in fact they stem from the reexperiencing of traumatic events.
  - Persistent **avoidance** of stimuli associated with the trauma.
  - A **numbing of responsiveness** as indicated by at least 3 of the following symptoms: anhedonia, amnesia, restricted affect, and detachment.

- ↑ **arousal** as indicated by 2 of the following: hypervigilance, insomnia, ↑ startle response, poor concentration, and irritability.
- Associated symptoms include survivor guilt, personality change, dissociation, aggression, depression, substance abuse, and suicidality.
- Symptoms **must be present for > 1 month** and are classified according to their duration:
  - **Acute:** Symptoms present for < 3 months.
  - **Chronic:** Symptoms present for > 3 months.
  - **Delayed onset:** Symptoms start > 6 months after the traumatic event.

KEY FACT

Acute stress disorder is similar to PTSD, but symptoms occur within 1 month of the traumatic event and last 2 days to 1 month.

DIFFERENTIAL

Acute stress disorder, MDD, OCD, anxiety disorder, adjustment disorder, malingering, borderline personality disorder.

TREATMENT

- SSRIs and mood stabilizers are first-line therapy (higher-than-normal doses of antidepressants are required). Buspirone is occasionally helpful.
- Anxiolytics such as β-blockers, benzodiazepines, and α_2-agonists may be used if first-line treatment fails. Benzodiazepines are generally less effective but may be helpful in the early stages; however, their use must be balanced against the high risk of addiction and abuse potential.
- CBT and support groups are also effective.

Personality Disorders

KEY FACT

Personality disorders are pervasive, persistent, maladaptive patterns of behavior that are best managed with long-term psychotherapy.

Personality disorders (see Table 8-3) are maladaptive patterns of perceiving, relating to, and thinking about oneself, other people, and the environment. They typically begin in childhood, crystallize by late adolescence, and affect all facets of the personality, including cognition, mood, behavior, and interpersonal style. However, they are not diagnosed in individuals < 18 years of age. Personality disorders are coded on Axis II and often coexist with, and affect the treatment of, acute psychiatric illnesses (Axis I).

MNEMONIC

Features of personality disorders—

MEDIC

Maladaptive
Enduring
Deviates from norm
Inflexible
Causes impaired social functioning

SIGNS AND SYMPTOMS

- Characterized by a stable, enduring pattern of experiences and behaviors that deviates markedly from cultural expectations.
- Behaviors are persistent, inflexible, and maladaptive, leading to significant impairment in social or occupational function. Hallmark features are summarized in the mnemonic **MEDIC.**

DIFFERENTIAL

- Normal variants of an individual's personality or environmental stressors.
- Substance abuse.
- Axis I psychiatric disorders (eg, schizophrenia, MDD, bipolar disorder, delusional disorder, anxiety disorders).

KEY FACT

Personality disorders are typically ego syntonic, and patients therefore have little insight into their disorders.

TREATMENT

Long-term psychotherapy is usually the treatment of choice. Pharmacotherapy with anxiolytics and/or low-dose antipsychotics may be necessary for anxiety or agitation.

TABLE 8-3. Classes of Personality Disorders

EXAMPLE	CHARACTERISTICS	CLINICAL DILEMMA	COPING STRATEGY
		CLUSTER A: "WEIRD"	
Paranoid	Persistent distrust and suspicion that others are harming or deceiving the patient. Patients are reluctant to confide in others and perceive attacks on character that are not apparent to others.	Patients are suspicious of physicians and do not trust them. Patients rarely visit the physician.	Use a clear, honest attitude and a noncontrolling, nondefensive approach. Avoid humor and maintain distance. Patients' defense mechanisms are projection and fantasy.
Schizoid	Social isolation and restricted emotional range (cold and detached). Patients lack close friends, lack interest in sexual experiences, and are indifferent to praise.	Same.	Same.
Schizotypal	Odd beliefs, speech, behavior, or appearance; magical thinking, ideas of references, and unusual "out-of-body" perceptual experiences.	Same.	Same.
		CLUSTER B: "WILD"	
Borderline	Marked impulsivity; unstable sense of self and interpersonal relationships; recurrent suicidal ideation. Inability to control mood lability and chronic feelings of emptiness.	Patients will change the rules on the physician. They are clingy, demand attention, and feel that they are special. Patients may manipulate the physician and staff such that conflict arises ("splitting").	**Be firm:** Stick to the treatment plan. **Be fair:** Do not be punitive or derogatory. **Be consistent:** Do not change the rules. **Be a team:** Encourage clear communication on where/when the patient is "splitting" as well as a clear division of responsibilities. Treat with dialectic behavioral therapy. Patients' defense mechanisms are dissociation, denial, splitting, and acting out.
Histrionic	Excess emotionality and attention seeking with a constant need to be the "center of attention." Inappropriate sexual or provocative behavior, self-dramatization, and suggestibility.	Same.	Same.
Narcissistic	Persistent grandiosity about self and accomplishments; need for excessive admiration; sense of entitlement, envy of others, and lack of empathy.	Same.	Same.

(continues)

TABLE 8-3. Classes of Personality Disorders *(continued)*

Example	Characteristics	Clinical Dilemma	Coping Strategy
	Cluster B: "Wild" *(continued)*		
Antisocial	Blatant disregard for the rights of others with failure to conform to social norms and lawful behavior. Impulsivity, deceitfulness, and lack of remorse. Disregard for the safety of self and others, aggression, and irresponsibility.	Patients may be manipulative or seductive and show a range of risky behavior. They must fit the criteria for conduct disorder before adulthood to meet the criteria for antisocial personality disorder, although opinions vary on this definition.	Same.
	Cluster C" "Worried and Wimpy"		
Obsessive-compulsive	Preoccupation with details, cleanliness, order, and control over all aspects of life. Perfectionism is evident in excessive devotion to work over leisure. Patients may present with inflexibility in morals and values, an inability to discard objects, miserliness, and rigidity.	Patients may subtly sabotage their own treatment. They are very controlling, and words are not necessarily consistent with actions.	Avoid power struggles. Passive wins over active. Give clear treatment recommendations, but do not push patients into a decision. Patients' defense mechanisms are hypochondriasis, passive aggression, and isolation.
Avoidant	Social inhibition; feelings of inadequacy; excessive shyness and hypersensitivity to rejection. Avoidance of activities and relationships for fear of being disliked or ridiculed.	Same.	Same.
Dependent	Submissive and clinging behavior; a need to be "taken care of"; difficulty making decisions, expressing disagreement, and initiating projects. Uncomfortable with being alone.	Same.	Same.

Substance Abuse and Dependence

KEY FACT

The highest prevalence of alcoholism is found among males 21–34 years of age.

Substance abuse and dependence have a 13% lifetime prevalence in the United States, and alcohol is the most commonly abused substance (excluding tobacco and caffeine). Alcohol abuse and dependence have a lifetime prevalence of 6% in the general U.S. population. Males are affected nearly 4 times more frequently than females, but the incidence of alcoholism in women is increasing. Like anxiety, substance abuse and dependence are commonly comorbid with mood disorders.

SIGNS AND SYMPTOMS

- **Substance dependence:** Defined as at least 3 of the following for at least 1 year:
  - **Tolerance:** Using progressively larger amounts to obtain the same effect.
  - **Withdrawal:** Symptoms occur when not taking the substance.
  - Persistent desire or attempts to cut down.
  - Considerable time and energy spent trying to obtain the substance, use the substance, or recover from its effects.
  - Important social, occupational, or recreational activities given up or reduced because of substance use.
  - Continued use despite awareness of the problems that it causes.
- **Substance abuse:** Defined as > 1 of the following for at least 1 year (see also Table 8-4):
  - Failure to fulfill major obligations at work, school, or home.
  - Recurrent substance use in physically hazardous situations.
  - Recurrent substance-related legal problems.
  - Continued use despite problems caused by use.

DIFFERENTIAL

Delirium, Axis I disorders (schizophrenia, MDD, bipolar disorder, anxiety disorders).

WORKUP

- A complete history is key. It is often necessary to consult collateral sources (eg, family, friends), as substance use is often denied or underreported.
- Use the **CAGE** questionnaire (see mnemonic) to screen for alcoholism.
  - Ask follow-up questions, including the frequency of use of each substance and the time and amount of last use.
  - Ask about any history of withdrawal symptoms (particularly seizures, cardiac issues, and DTs) and inpatient detoxifications.

MNEMONIC

CAGE questions:

1. Have you ever felt the need to **C**ut down on your drinking?
2. Have you ever felt **A**nnoyed by criticism of your drinking?
3. Have you ever felt **G**uilty about drinking?
4. Have you ever had to take a morning **E**ye-opener?

More than one "yes" answer makes alcoholism likely.

KEY POINT

ALCOHOL WITHDRAWAL SYNDROMES

- **Uncomplicated withdrawal:** Occurs within several hours (usually 6–8 hours) after cessation of drinking; characterized by tremulousness, tachycardia, hypertension, diaphoresis, anxiety, nausea, insomnia, hypervigilance, hyperreflexia, weakness, tinnitus, blurred vision, paresthesias, and numbness.
- **Alcoholic hallucinosis:** Occurs within 2 days after cessation of or ↓ in drinking; characterized by auditory hallucinations that persist after the withdrawal symptoms have disappeared. The sensorium is clear (no delirium). Delusions or paranoid ideation may be present.
- **DTs:** Occur approximately 1–8 days after cessation of drinking (most often within **24–72 hours after cessation**) and can be life threatening (has an untreated mortality of 15–20%). DTs are characterized by disorientation, fever, agitation, tremor, delusions, seizures, memory deficits, insomnia, visual and tactile hallucinations, and autonomic instability and should be promptly treated with benzodiazepines and close monitoring of vital signs.

TABLE 8-4. Signs and Symptoms of Substance Abuse

Drug	Receptor/Mechanism	Intoxication	Withdrawal
Alcohol	$GABA_A$ and glutamate	Disinhibition, emotional lability, incoordination, slurred speech, ataxia, coma, blackouts (retrograde amnesia).	Tremor, tachycardia, hypertension, malaise, nausea, seizures, DTs, tremulousness, agitation, hallucinations.
Opioids	Opioid receptor (μ, δ, κ) agonism	CNS depression, nausea and vomiting, constipation, pupillary constriction, seizures, respiratory depression (overdose is life threatening).	Anxiety, insomnia, anorexia, sweating, fever, rhinorrhea, piloerection, nausea, stomach cramps, diarrhea.
Amphetamines (dextroamphetamine, methamphetamine)	Norepinephrine, dopamine, and 5-HT release and reuptake inhibition	Psychomotor agitation, impaired judgment, pupillary dilation, hypertension, tachycardia, euphoria, prolonged wakefulness and attention, cardiac arrhythmias, delusions, hallucinations, fever.	Postuse "crash," including anxiety, lethargy, headache, stomach cramps, hunger, severe depression, dysphoria, fatigue, and insomnia/hypersomnia.
MDMA ("Ecstasy")	5-HT release and reuptake inhibition, dopamine reuptake inhibition	Euphoria; excessive empathy, trust, and sociability; anorexia, hyperthermia.	"Serotonin dip" (dysphoria, fatigue, memory problems, ↓ libido).
Cocaine	Norepinephrine, acetylcholine, 5-HT, and dopamine reuptake inhibition	Euphoria, psychomotor agitation, impaired judgment, tachycardia, pupillary dilation, hypertension, hallucinations (including tactile), paranoid ideations, angina, hyperthermia, arrhythmias, respiratory depression, convulsions, death.	Hypersomnolence, fatigue, depression, malaise, suicidality, irritability.
Phencyclidine piperidine (PCP)	NMDA and acetylcholine antagonism	Altered ability to differentiate between self and nonself; belligerence, impulsiveness, fever, psychomotor agitation, vertical and horizontal nystagmus, tachycardia, ataxia, homicidality, psychosis, delirium.	Recurrence of symptoms due to reabsorption from lipid stores; sudden onset of severe violence.
Lysergic acid diethylamide (LSD)	$5\text{-}HT_2$ agonism	Marked anxiety or depression, delusions, visual hallucinations, flashbacks.	None.

TABLE 8-4. Signs and Symptoms of Substance Abuse *(continued)*

DRUG	RECEPTOR/MECHANISM	INTOXICATION	WITHDRAWAL
Marijuana	Opioid, acetylcholine, norepinephrine, and dopamine release	Euphoria, anxiety, paranoid/persecutory delusions, slowed sense of time, impaired judgment, social withdrawal, ↑ appetite, dry mouth, conjunctival injection, hallucinations, amotivation.	None.
Barbiturates	$GABA_A$ agonism	Respiratory depression (major).	Anxiety, seizures, delirium, life-threatening cardiovascular collapse.
Benzodiazepines	$GABA_A$ agonism	Alcohol interactions, amnesia, ataxia, sleep, respiratory depression.	Rebound anxiety, seizures, tremor, insomnia, hypertension, tachycardia.
Caffeine	Adenosine antagonism, norepinephrine release	Restlessness, insomnia, diuresis, muscle twitching, arrhythmias.	Headache, lethargy, depression, weight gain.
Nicotine/tobacco	β-subunit acetylcholine agonism, dopamine release	Restlessness, insomnia, anxiety, arrhythmias.	Irritability, headache, anxiety, weight gain, tachycardia.

- Toxicology screen, CBC, electrolytes, LFTs, and a Breathalyzer or serum ethanol level.
- Always offer HIV and hepatitis testing to substance abusers (especially IV drug abusers), as they often engage in high-risk behaviors.

TREATMENT

- Treatment depends on the substance abused and the context in which it is used (see Table 8-5). The first goal is usually abstinence/detoxification; the rehabilitation process then targets the patient's physical, psychological, and social well-being.
- The treatment of alcohol withdrawal includes the following:
  - Rule out any medical complications (eg, hepatic dysfunction, Wernicke's encephalopathy) by physical examination and laboratory tests.
  - Start a benzodiazepine taper (eg, chlordiazepoxide) for withdrawal symptoms. Lorazepam, temazepam, or oxazepam should be used if the patient has liver dysfunction.
  - Monitor patients on the appropriate scale for symptoms of withdrawal (varies by institution), and dose medications appropriately.
  - Give multivitamins with thiamine (before glucose) and folate. Correct any electrolyte abnormalities.
  - Check vital signs and give fluid replacement if necessary.
  - For patients with an alcohol seizure history, give anticonvulsants. Avoid neuroleptics, which ↓ seizure threshold.
  - Alcohol dependence can be treated with group therapy (Alcoholics Anonymous).
  - Although disulfiram and naltrexone were previously used, these drugs have fallen out of favor owing to common side effects that ↓ patient tolerability and compliance.

KEY FACT

↑ GGT and ↑ MCV suggest chronic alcohol abuse (GGT from liver damage; MCV from folate or B_{12} deficiency, leading to macrocytic anemia).

Q

A 52-year-old man with alcohol dependence and depression grows distracted, flushed, diaphoretic, and tremulous during physical examination. His blood alcohol level is 315, but his labs and toxicology studies are otherwise unremarkable. He has a heart rate of 125 bpm and a BP of 165/108 mm Hg. He grows more confused as the examination progresses. What medications should you give immediately?

TABLE 8-5. Management of Intoxication

Drug	Management
Hallucinogens (eg, LSD)	If severe, give benzodiazepines or traditional antipsychotics; otherwise, provide reassurance.
Cocaine	Severe agitation is treated with haloperidol, benzodiazepines, antiemetics, antidiarrheals, and NSAIDs (for muscle cramps).
PCP	If severe, benzodiazepines; otherwise, provide reassurance.
Amphetamines	Same as that for cocaine.
Opioids	Naloxone/naltrexone block opioid receptors, reversing their effects. Beware of the antagonist being cleared before the opioid, particularly with longer-acting opioids such as methadone.

Complications

- ↑ risk of accidental and traumatic injuries, especially motor vehicle accidents.
- IV drug abusers are at ↑ risk of acquiring HIV, HBV, HCV, endocarditis, cellulitis (especially among "skin poppers"), and STIs.
- Substance abusers are often exceptionally destructive both to themselves and to their families. Always ask about the care of their children (you may need to contact child protection agencies) and how they obtain their drug money (this may give you clues to other potential medical and legal problems).

Childhood and Adolescent Disorders

Many of these disorders are more common in boys and often coexist with other conditions. In addition, childhood disorders can persist into adulthood or parallel similar disorders in adults. In many cases, the combination of gender, maladaptive interactions between the child and the environment, and unconscious or conscious prompting by parents can play a role in these disorders. Interviewing a child poses a unique dilemma; pictures, role playing, play therapy, and storytelling are techniques that can be used to facilitate the interview.

ATTENTION-DEFICIT HYPERACTIVITY DISORDER (ADHD)

A

A fast-acting benzodiazepine for alcohol withdrawal.

A disorder of attention that occurs almost 9 times more often in boys than in girls, with 7% of school-age children and an estimated 4% of adults in the United States affected. ADHD generally presents in children between 3 and 13 years of age and typically manifests as poor performance in school. There is a genetic predisposition to this condition.

Signs and Symptoms

- Characterized by inattention in work/school/play, hyperactivity, distractibility, and/or impulsivity that lead to significant impairment in academic and social function.
- Many children also have associated learning disabilities.

DIFFERENTIAL

- **Psychiatric:** Learning disability, major depression, bipolar disorder, cyclothymic disorder, anxiety disorders, intermittent explosive disorder, oppositional defiant disorder.
- **Organic:** Head trauma.
- **Pharmacologic:** Bronchodilators and sedatives (sleeping pills may elicit a paradoxic stimulant effect in children).
- **Other:** Normal active child.

WORKUP

- Diagnosis requires 6 or more symptoms of inattention or 6 or more symptoms of hyperactivity and impulsivity (listed below) in at least 2 settings that lead to clinically significant impairment in social and academic functioning. In order to make a firm diagnosis, it is often necessary to obtain information from collateral sources such as a school or a day-care center to supplement the parents' reports.
- Symptoms cannot be accounted for by another Axis I disorder and must present before age 7.
- ADHD is classified as (1) predominantly inattentive type, (2) predominantly hyperactive/impulsive type (more common in boys), or (3) combined.
  - **Inattentive:**
    - Makes careless mistakes owing to an inability to pay attention to detail.
    - Has difficulty maintaining attention in schoolwork or at play.
    - Has difficulty listening even when spoken to directly.
    - Fails to follow instructions or complete tasks or schoolwork.
    - Has difficulty organizing tasks and activities.
    - Avoids or dislikes tasks requiring concentration or sustained mental effort.
    - Loses items necessary for the completion of school tasks (eg, pencils, paper, books).
    - Is easily distracted by external stimuli.
    - Is forgetful in daily activities.
  - **Hyperactive/impulsive:**
    - Is fidgety (eg, squirms in seat).
    - Unexpectedly leaves desk in classroom.
    - Runs about excessively in inappropriate situations.
    - Has difficulty playing quietly.
    - Is often "on the go" or acts as if "driven by a motor."
    - Talks excessively.
    - Blurts out answers before questions have been completed.
    - Has difficulty waiting his or her turn.
    - Often interrupts or intrudes on others.

TREATMENT

- First-line treatment for ADHD is conservative. Address associated learning disabilities and maladaptive family behavior patterns. Behavior modification techniques are often useful.
- Pharmacologic treatment is used for cases in which impairment is significant and is not improved by conservative measures.
  - **Psychostimulants:** Methylphenidate (has abuse potential); dextroamphetamine. Side effects include insomnia, ↓ appetite, tic exacerbation, and ↓ growth velocity. These drugs have high abuse potential and high street value. Amphetamines may also have long-term effects on neural development.
  - **Other:** Antidepressants and α_2-agonists can also be used.

KEY FACT

Nearly 40% of children with ADHD show symptom resolution by adulthood.

KEY FACT

The diagnosis and treatment of ADHD are controversial, particularly in adults. This may stem from the use of behavior to diagnose a cognitive problem that does not always significantly impair functioning.

KEY FACT

Recent studies do not show any evidence of an ↑ risk of cardiovascular events such as MI, sudden cardiac death, or stroke with the use of ADHD psychostimulant medications.

KEY ADHD MEDICATIONS

Psychostimulants:

- **Drugs:** Methylphenidate (Ritalin, Concerta), dextroamphetamine (Dexedrine), pemoline (Cylert), dextroamphetamine + racemic amphetamine (Adderall).
- **Clinical use:** Treatment of ADHD in children and adolescents.
- **Side effects:** Insomnia, ↓ appetite, irritability, tachycardia, hypertension, exacerbation of tics, ↓ growth velocity.
- **Pros:** Long history of clinical use.
- **Cons:** Methylphenidate is a schedule II controlled substance.

Nonstimulants—atomoxetine (Strattera):

- **Mechanism:** SNRI.
- **Clinical use:** Treatment of ADHD in children, adolescents, and adults.
- **Side effects:** GI distress, nausea, dry mouth, severe liver injury (rare). Avoid MAOIs.
- **Pros:** Minimal anorexia; QD or BID dosing; no abuse potential.

Antidepressants:

- **Drugs:** Nortriptyline, imipramine, bupropion.

α_2-agonists:

- **Drugs:** Clonidine, guanfacine (better for hyperactivity and impulsivity than for inattention).

KEY FACT

Nearly 75% of autistic children have comorbid mental retardation, and approximately 25% have seizures.

KEY FACT

Contrary to some popular media reports, extensive research has concluded that childhood vaccination does **not** lead to autism.

AUTISM SPECTRUM DISORDERS

Autism spectrum disorders are severe, persistent impairments in developmental areas (eg, communication, social interaction) or stereotypical, repetitive behaviors or interests. They encompass a number of disorders, including autism, Asperger's syndrome, pervasive developmental disorder—not otherwise specified (PDD-NOS), Rett syndrome, and childhood disintegrative disorder.

- Autism, like schizophrenia, involves a preoccupation with the internal world.
- Autism has an incidence of 2–6 in 10,000 live births, frequently presents before age 4, and is 3–4 times more common in males. It is organic in nature, **not** a reaction to a cold and distant mother, and is associated with familial transmission, tuberous sclerosis, and fragile X syndrome.

Signs and Symptoms

- Autism generally presents with 3 hallmark features: deficiencies in social interaction, communication, and behavior. Impairing symptoms and restricted activities/interests should be evident before age 3.
  1. **Impaired social interaction:** Failure to develop nonverbal communication skills such as a social smile; impaired ability or desire to create relationships (with parents or peers) or show enjoyment.

KEY POINT

OTHER PERVASIVE DEVELOPMENTAL DISORDERS

- **Asperger's syndrome:** An autism-like disorder without marked language or cognitive delays.
- **Rett syndrome:** A genetic neurodegenerative disorder with progressive impairment (language, coordination) after several months of normal development. Associated with stereotypical hand-wringing or hand-washing gestures. More commonly seen in females.
- **Childhood disintegrative disorder:** Severe developmental regression after < 2 years of normal development. More commonly seen in males.
- **PDD-NOS:** A diagnosis for people who are well described by the "PDD" label but cannot be categorized by any other disorder.

2. **Communication deficiencies:** Impaired language development, inability to start or sustain a conversation, and use of repetitive or idiosyncratic language (eg, echolalia, pronoun reversals, abnormalities in speech quality).
3. **Behavioral deficiencies:** Represent patients' fixation on the internal world. Patients may show ritualized behaviors (eg, staring at the flushing toilet), stereotyped motor movements (eg, body rocking), and preoccupation with a restricted area of knowledge (eg, sports trivia). They may also show self-injurious behavior (eg, biting oneself) and compulsive behavior (eg, arranging objects in a certain way).

- The American Academy of Pediatrics recommends that all children be screened for autism at well-child checks at 18 and 24 months. Key points to note include no babbling by 12 months, no gesturing by 12 months, no single words by 16 months, no 2-word spontaneous phrases by 24 months, and any loss of language/social skills at any age.

DIFFERENTIAL

- **Psychiatric:** Mental retardation, childhood psychosis, language disorders, OCD, Tourette's syndrome, other pervasive developmental disorders.
- **Organic:** Congenital deafness or blindness, congenital CMV, hepatic encephalopathy, fragile X syndrome.

WORKUP

- Obtain a complete history and an MSE.
- Monitor developmental milestones and delays.
- Evaluate vision and hearing for any underlying pathology that may lead to abnormal presentations.

TREATMENT

- Provide a highly structured educational setting to help patients learn communication and living skills.
- Behavioral management to help reduce stereotyped behaviors.
- Psychotherapy may be of benefit both to the parents and to the patient.
- Unless a comorbid disorder is present, medications are rarely useful. Neuroleptics may be given for aggressive and self-injurious behaviors, and anticonvulsants may be used for concurrent seizure disorder.

CONDUCT DISORDER

Defined as a repetitive and persistent pattern of inappropriate conduct for 6 months or more in which patients < 18 years of age ignore or violate the rights of others. Patients frequently have comorbid ADHD or learning disorders. Note that a patient must fit the diagnosis for conduct disorder early in life in order to meet the criteria for antisocial personality disorder as an adult.

Signs and Symptoms

- Behavior can be aggressive (eg, violence, destruction, theft) or nonaggressive (eg, violation of rules, lying).
- Patients may or may not form social bonds, but if they do, bonding with a loyal group often manifests in gang formation.
- If behavior continues as an adult, it is defined as antisocial personality disorder.

KEY FACT

Patients with oppositional defiant disorder do not show blatant disregard for the rights of others but demonstrate disruptive, annoying behavior inappropriate for their mental age.

Treatment

- Individual and family therapy is necessary to address emotional conflicts and sociocultural factors.
- Pharmacotherapy may include medications for the management of anxiety or agitation.

MENTAL RETARDATION

Defined as intellectual functioning significantly below that expected for a child's developmental stage, with cognitive performance below the third percentile of the general population. Mental retardation has a prevalence of 1–2% and is 2 times more common in males than in females. Causes include genetic disorders, congenital infections, teratogens, and disease acquired after birth. Down syndrome and fragile X syndrome are common causes.

KEY FACT

Fragile X syndrome is the most common heritable form of mental retardation. Fetal alcohol syndrome is the most common potentially preventable cause of mental retardation.

Signs and Symptoms

- IQ (defined as mental age divided by chronological age) ≤ 70 (see Table 8-6).
- Concurrent deficiencies in multiple areas of adaptive functioning (eg, social skills, self-hygiene, communication).
- Onset of symptoms before the age of 18.

TABLE 8-6. Levels of Mental Retardation

Level	IQ Score	Educational Potential
Mild	50–69	Educable
Moderate	35–49	Trainable
Severe	20–34	Limited
Profound	< 20	Very limited

DIFFERENTIAL

Learning disorders, depression, seizure disorders, ADHD, schizophrenia.

WORKUP

Steps involved in diagnosis are as follows:

1. Physical examination (including neurologic examination).
2. IQ testing. Levels of severity are as noted in Table 8-6.
3. Brain imaging and EEG (if seizure disorder is suspected).

TREATMENT

Management depends on severity. Family counseling and support, speech and language therapy, occupational/physical therapy, behavioral therapy, and educational assistance may all be useful.

- **Mild:** Patients may be able to function in society and maintain employment.
- **Moderate:** Patients should be able to perform activities of daily living and live in a group home.
- **Severe:** Patients are unable to care for themselves and usually suffer a premature death.

LEARNING DISORDERS

Learning disorders are relatively common, affecting roughly 5% of school-aged children. Males are at a two- to fourfold greater risk than females. Such disorders are also more common in those of low socioeconomic status (SES). Diagnosis is usually made around the fourth or fifth grade.

SIGNS AND SYMPTOMS

- There are 3 categories of learning disorders: reading, mathematics, and written expression.
- In comparison to mental retardation, learning disorders are deficiencies in a particular area that place the child below the expected performance for his or her chronological age, intelligence, and education (often measured by standardized test achievement).

DIFFERENTIAL

Mental retardation, communication disorders, ADHD, depression, anxiety disorders (eg, school phobia), physical disorders (eg, abnormal hearing or sight), cultural factors (eg, language barriers), poor education.

WORKUP

Involves intelligence and subject-specific achievement testing.

TREATMENT

Management involves learning strategies to overcome deficits, academic remediation, and, if possible, teaching in environments that support patients.

Miscellaneous Disorders

ADJUSTMENT DISORDER

A state in which emotional ideas and actions are the result of a particular stressor.

- The disorder **must arise within 3 months** of experiencing the stressor and, unless the stressor is chronic, must resolve within 6 months.
- To qualify as an adjustment disorder, Axis I or bereavement criteria must not be met.

ANOREXIA NERVOSA

> **KEY FACT**
>
> Mortality rates approach 10–15% for patients who have been hospitalized for anorexia nervosa.

An eating disorder affecting 0.5–1.0% of females, with a female-to-male ratio of nearly 20:1. The peak ages of onset are 14 and 18, although the disorder has been diagnosed in much younger girls. Nearly two-thirds of patients have a history of a depressive episode.

Signs and Symptoms

- Characterized by a body weight < 85% of ideal body weight (for age and height).
- Patients have a distorted body image (patients perceive themselves, incorrectly, as fat) and an intense fear of gaining weight.
- Patterns of dieting include **restricting** (eg, fasting, dieting, or exercising excessively) or engaging in **binge-eating and purging** behavior (eg, vomiting, laxative abuse, excessive exercise).
- Amenorrhea (absence of 3 consecutive cycles) and ↓ sexual activity/interest are common.
- Patients may exhibit lanugo, dry skin, bradycardia, lethargy, hypotension, electrolyte disturbances (eg, metabolic acidosis due to vomiting and/or metabolic alkalosis due to laxatives), cold intolerance, anemia and leukopenia, osteoporosis, nephrolithiasis, and low thyroid function.
- A rigid personality, obsessive-compulsive features (eg, counting calories), and a need to control the social environment are also seen.

Differential

- **Psychiatric:** MDD, social phobia, OCD, bulimia nervosa, body dysmorphic disorder.
- **Organic:** AIDS, malignancies, superior mesenteric ischemia (all of which lead to vomiting or weight loss without a distorted body image), Addison's disease, DM, hyperthyroidism, drug abuse.

Workup

- Conduct a complete H&P and psychiatric evaluation with attention to any comorbid disorders.
- Obtain height and weight measurements.
- Labs/studies include CBC, serum albumin (↓), electrolytes (hypocalcemia, hypokalemia, hyponatremia, hypomagnesemia, and hypophosphatemia), endocrine tests, and an ECG.

TREATMENT

- Early treatment involves monitoring caloric intake to stabilize weight and achieve weight gain.
- In severe cases, hospitalization may be required to restore nutritional status and/or to correct electrolyte imbalances.
- Later treatment includes individual, family, and/or group psychotherapy.
- SSRIs may help treat comorbid depression.

BULIMIA NERVOSA

Bulimia nervosa has a prevalence of 1–3% in young females and 0.1–0.3% in males. It is characterized by recurrent episodes of bingeing (eating excessive amounts of food in a 2-hour period) during which the patient feels a lack of self-control. Most patients have a history of dieting, and many have coexisting personality or impulse-control disorders.

> **KEY FACT**
>
> Unlike patients with anorexia, bulimic patients generally maintain a normal weight but may still suffer from medical complications (eg, dangerous electrolyte abnormalities).

SIGNS AND SYMPTOMS

- Presents with dental enamel erosion (from vomiting), enlarged parotid glands, and scars on the dorsal surfaces of the hands (from inducing vomiting).
- Menstrual irregularities are also seen.
- Emetic abuse can lead to cardiomyopathy, and laxatives can damage GI mucosa.

WORKUP

- To fulfill DSM-IV criteria for bulimia, bingeing and compensatory behavior must occur at least twice a week for 3 months.
- Binge eating takes place rapidly and secretly. Bulimic patients tend to be more disturbed by and ashamed of their behavior than anorexic patients.
- Patients try to compensate for binge behaviors through vomiting, excessive exercise, or laxatives in order to prevent weight gain.
- Electrolyte abnormalities (hypochloremic hypokalemic metabolic alkalosis 2° to vomiting) may be seen.

TREATMENT

- Psychotherapy and CBT are the most effective treatments and focus on behavior and body self-image modification.
- Antidepressants such as fluoxetine, imipramine, and desipramine are effective in both depressed and nondepressed patients.

SOMATOFORM AND RELATED DISORDERS

The principal characteristics of somatoform and related disorders are outlined in Tables 8-7 and 8-8.

SUICIDALITY

Suicide is the eighth leading cause of death in the United States and is the second leading cause of death (after accidents) in people between the ages of 15 and 24. In general, women are more likely to attempt suicide than men,

TABLE 8-7. Somatoform Disorders

Disorder	Comments
Somatization disorder (Briquet's syndrome)	A history of many physical complaints beginning before age 30 and occurring over a period of several years. Affects up to 1% of the population, with a 5:1 female-to-male predominance. Individual symptoms must include 4 pain symptoms, 2 GI symptoms, 1 sexual symptom, and 1 pseudoneurologic symptom. Symptoms cannot be explained by organic causes and are in excess of examination findings. Patients may have had multiple procedures or surgeries and often "doctor shop." Psychotherapy and regular, planned, brief primary care visits may be beneficial.
Conversion disorder	One or more **neurologic** complaints (eg, paralysis, paresthesia, blindness, pseudoseizures) that cannot be explained by a medical disorder. Psychological factors must be associated with symptom onset in order for the diagnosis to be made. Patients often show a characteristic lack of concern (*"la belle indifférence"*). Conversion is most common in women, usually affecting adolescents and young adults. Men have been noted to experience this disorder after battlefield trauma. May spontaneously remit, but anxiolytics may help. Symptoms are not intentionally produced or feigned.
Hypochondriasis	Preoccupation with and fear of having a serious disease leading to significant psychological distress and/or impaired social or occupational functioning for > 6 months. Based on misinterpretation of bodily symptoms. Men and women are equally affected; onset is most common between 20 and 30 years of age. Group therapy and frequent reassurance from the physician are necessary for treatment.
Body dysmorphic disorder	Preoccupation with an imagined physical defect or abnormality (eg, facial features, hair, body build) or, if a defect is present, excessive concern about that defect. The preoccupation must lead to significant distress or impaired social and occupational functioning. Patients often present to dermatologists or plastic surgeons. Women are affected slightly more often than men, with an average onset at 15–20 years of age. May be associated with depression. Patients with body dysmorphic disorder have high suicide rates. Antidepressants such as SSRIs and clomipramine may be effective.

but men are more likely to complete suicide. Men are also more likely to commit suicide by violent means such as firearm use; women are more likely to commit suicide by drug ingestion. Risk factors include the following (see also the mnemonic **SAD PERSONS**):

- A previous suicide attempt.
- Male gender.
- Increasing age.

TABLE 8-8. Nonsomatoform Disorders

Disorder	Comments
Malingering	Occurs when a patient intentionally feigns illness for 2° gain (eg, financial compensation, avoiding work, obtaining food or shelter). It differs from factitious disorder (defined below) in that what is sought is concrete and is usually related to material gain.
Factitious disorder (Munchausen syndrome)	Conscious simulation or creation of psychiatric or physical symptoms or illness for 1° gain in order to play the sick role and receive attention from medical personnel or special consideration. It is most common in men and among health care personnel. **Munchausen by proxy** involves simulation of illness in another person, usually in a child by a parent.

- Depression (depressed patients are 30 times more likely to commit suicide than the general population) or other psychiatric illness; recent recovery from suicidal depression (since patients have regained the energy to kill themselves) or recovery from a first episode of schizophrenia (since patients have developed insight).
- Alcohol or substance abuse.
- The presence of rational thought or an organized plan.
- A family history of suicide.
- Access to firearms and other weapons.
- A recent severe stressor (eg, bereavement, job loss, examinations).
- A history of impulsive behavior.
- Chronic medical conditions or illnesses (eg, terminal cancer, HIV).
- Divorced parents, unmarried status, poor social support.
- **Other demographics:** Caucasians commit suicide more frequently than do African Americans; Protestants have a higher suicide rate than do Catholics. Police officers and physicians have a higher suicide rate than that of any other occupation.

Workup

- Ask the patient about a ⊕ family history, a previous attempt, ambivalence about death, and feelings of hopelessness. Ask specifically about suicidal ideation, intent, and plan.
- Assess if the patient has an available means of committing suicide.
- Perform a complete MSE.

Treatment

- Patients who express the desire to kill themselves, or who you believe may do so, require emergent inpatient hospitalization even if it is against their wishes. The actively suicidal patient needs intensive monitoring, close contact, and ongoing assessment.
- When the patient is stable, identification of the underlying stressor/disorder is necessary. Patients frequently require intensive psychotherapy and hospitalization as well as antidepressant and/or antipsychotic medication.
- ECT may be used as a second-line treatment for actively suicidal patients who are refractory to medications and psychotherapy. Severely depressed patients are often at greatest risk for suicide in the first few weeks after starting an antidepressant, as their energy may return before the depressed mood lifts.

MNEMONIC

Suicide risk factors–

SAD PERSONS

Sex (male)
Age
Depression
Previous attempt
Ethanol
Rational thought
Sickness
Organized plan
No spouse
Social support lacking

Other key risk factors are a family history of suicide, a history of self-injury, and access to weapons (particularly firearms).

KEY FACT

Asking the patient about suicide will **not** "plant" the idea in the patient's thoughts.

SEXUAL AND PHYSICAL ABUSE

Most frequently affect women < 35 years of age, although men are also frequent victims. Many of those affected have a partner who is a substance abuser and/or abuse substances themselves, or have a restraining order against a current or previous spouse or significant other. Women who are abused are also often experiencing marital discord, are of low SES, or are pregnant. Victims of childhood abuse are more likely to be abused as adults and are at risk of becoming abusers.

Signs and Symptoms

- Characterized by frequent ED visits with multiple somatic complaints, bruising, unexplained injuries, and delayed medical treatment.
- Look for unequal power in interactions between victim and partner.
- Patients may act afraid or hostile, deny abuse, and avoid eye contact.
- Children may present with premature sexual behavior, genital or anal trauma, STIs, UTIs, and psychiatric trauma.

Treatment

- Provide emotional support and counseling.
- Administer medical care.
- Provide information to the patient about available support services, and encourage them to contact such services. Document the encounter.

Common Clerkship Topics

The following is a list of core topics that you are likely to encounter in the course of your psychiatry rotation and on a shelf examination:

- **Mental status exam, Mini-Mental Status Exam, 5 axes**
- **Mood disorders:**
  - Major depressive disorder
  - Dysthymic disorder
  - Bipolar disorder
- **Psychotic disorders:**
  - Schizophrenia
  - Brief psychotic disorder
  - Schizoaffective disorder
  - Delusional disorder
- **Anxiety disorders:**
  - Generalized anxiety disorder
  - Panic disorder
  - Social phobia
  - Obsessive-compulsive disorder
  - Posttraumatic stress disorder
- **Personality disorders**
- **Substance abuse, dependence, withdrawal**
- **Childhood and adolescent disorders:**
  - Attention-deficit hyperactivity disorder
  - Pervasive developmental disorders—autism
  - Conduct disorder
  - Mental retardation
  - Learning disorders
  - Tourette's syndrome
- **Miscellaneous disorders:**
  - Adjustment disorder
  - Anorexia nervosa
  - Bulimia nervosa
  - Somatoform and factitious disorders
  - Suicidality
  - Sexual and physical abuse
  - Dementia
  - Delirium
  - Pathologic grief

CHAPTER 9

SURGERY

Ward Tips

Your general surgery rotation will likely be one of the most challenging experiences of medical school. Success on this rotation will hinge on your ability to integrate a great deal of clinical information, become a valuable team member, and perform floor work as needed. This can be a challenge given the significant demands made on your time and energy. Surgery is a unique field, and your basic rotation may help you make the big career decision of "medicine or surgery." In either case, most students emerge from this rotation with a broad fund of knowledge, greater confidence in their clinical and procedural skills, and, inevitably, a newfound appreciation for food and sleep.

WHAT IS THE ROTATION LIKE?

The surgery clerkship is designed to expose students to the principles of basic surgical management, including the evaluation of patients to determine the need for surgery; pre- and postoperative care; and hands-on experience in basic bedside procedures, sterile technique, and operating room (OR) tasks. The structure of the rotation will vary from service to service depending on the patient population served, the nature of the surgical illnesses managed, and the specific emphases of the attendings on a given service. As with your other rotations, your experience in surgery will be heavily influenced by the team of residents and attendings with whom you work. The following outline summarizes the nature and responsibilities of the clerkship:

- **Clinical experience:**
  - Inpatient and ambulatory experiences in general surgery.
  - Trauma/emergency service.
  - Surgical subspecialties, often including otolaryngology, cardiothoracic, urologic, orthopedic, neurosurgical, transplantation, vascular, pediatric, and plastic surgery.
- **Didactic instruction:**
  - Departmental grand rounds, weekly multidisciplinary conferences, and lectures organized by the faculty for students.
  - Weekly service conferences where house staff present details of the patient census, operative and perioperative complications (morbidity and mortality conferences), and patient cases that illustrate interesting clinical issues. Remember that these topics are protected by HIPAA, so be sure not to discuss them in public areas.
  - Informal teaching sessions from the house staff as time permits.
  - **Independent reading** in the little free time left, as you will need sufficient preparation for the shelf test. This may include material in subspecialties you may not have had a chance to rotate in. You should try to develop a **routine daily reading plan.**
- **Responsibilities:**
  - Prerounding on all patients.
  - Presenting patients on ward rounds.
  - Writing the admission history and physical (H&P) for new patients.
  - Writing notes (preoperative, operative, postoperative) on the patients whose surgeries you are involved with.
- **Tips for success:**
  - Try to follow patients throughout their stay—from their admission to surgery to postoperative care. This will allow you not only to cultivate a better relationship with your patients but also to observe the complete picture.

- Keep in mind that competence is only half the story; knowing your patients will impress not only the patients themselves but your residents and attendings as well.
- Plan out which surgery you want to participate in the next day, and then read up on the procedure and relevant anatomy. Be sure to **learn about the patient's history and presentation,** if only by briefly reading his or her chart prior to starting the case.
- Try to attend multiple clinics with 1 or 2 attendings, as this is a great way to spend one-on-one time with attendings without a lot of residents present.
- Practice some basic suturing and knot-tying skills in the event that you are given the opportunity to help close an incision. You can use unopened suture at the end of the case while waiting for the patient to awaken from anesthesia. This is a perfect opportunity to ask for pointers from your resident!
- Learn some of the medical jargon common to surgeries, and be willing to **ask questions** pertaining to the technique involved. Be familiar with the names of common surgical instruments.
- Be ready to **answer questions** about the basic anatomy, surgical procedure, and prognosis of the surgery being performed.
- Strive to create a **balanced experience**—one in which you spend enough time in the OR to understand sterile technique and get a basic understanding of intraoperative care, while also devoting some time to helping residents take care of patients on the floor, seeing patients in clinic, and reading relevant material. You will be a master at time management by the end of the rotation!

KEY FACT

Never go into an OR case blind!

WHO ARE THE PLAYERS?

Attendings. Every service is staffed by several attendings, each of whom has ultimate responsibility for patient management. The attending physicians have responsibility for the perioperative management of their patients as well as for what takes place during the surgery itself. At most teaching institutions, much of the operating is done by the appropriate-level resident under the guidance of the attending. The extent to which this is the case, however, depends on the nature of the service (ie, whether it is an elective general surgery service at a private hospital, a trauma service at a county hospital, or a vascular service at a VA) as well as on the nature of the surgical disease and the complexity of the surgery. Simple procedures such as hernia repairs and appendectomies, for example, are frequently performed by interns and junior residents, whereas complicated operations such as the Whipple procedure (pancreaticoduodenectomy for pancreatic cancer) are usually performed by the chief resident. As a general rule, an attending must be present for every surgery performed.

Chief resident. If the attending is the "chairman of the board" of the service, the chief resident functions as the chief executive officer, assuming responsibility for the management of the entire service as well as for the day-to-day running of the ward team. All patients on the service are managed by the chief resident, regardless of their individual attendings; therefore, the chief resident must be aware of every important issue affecting each patient on the service, including lab and x-ray results, plans for wound/dressing/line care, plans for advancing patients' diets, and dispositions. Since each attending on a service may have specific preferences for certain management issues (eg, staples out on day 5, advance from NPO to clear liquids vs. a soft diet), the chief must be well informed about these issues, as he or she must answer to the attendings if things go wrong.

Because culpability tends to roll downhill, it is in the best interest of all the residents and students to ensure that things function as smoothly as possible and that the chief is kept abreast of any problems that may arise. Chiefs spend most of their time in the OR, although they often have significant administrative and didactic responsibilities as well. They are generally in charge of arranging patient presentations for conferences and may schedule teaching sessions for the students on their service. They also arrange admissions and oversee consultations to other services. As a student, you may find that the chief resident bears significant responsibility for your evaluation. The onus is therefore on you to **ensure that your efforts do not go unnoticed by your chief.**

KEY FACT

Surgery fosters a more formal pecking order.

Senior resident(s). On a given surgery service, there may be 1 or 2 senior residents (residents in their third or fourth clinical year) who assist the chief resident in the management of the service. Typically, the senior resident is responsible for running rounds in the morning and updating the service for the chief, since the chief may or may not walk on rounds with the team each morning. Also, when issues come up during the day that cannot easily be managed by the interns and junior residents, the senior resident may be called on to assume responsibility, as the chief may be busy operating. Of course, senior residents do their fair share of operating as well, handling less complex cases such as bowel resections for cancer and mastectomies. You may find yourself working more closely with your senior resident than with your chief on a daily basis. If this is the case, your senior(s) will play a critical role in your ultimate evaluation.

KEY FACT

If you have a question, start at the bottom. Never page the attending unless told to do so.

Interns and junior residents. Interns and second-year residents are responsible for the minutiae of patient care—eg, writing notes, checking labs, writing and dictating discharge summaries, checking wounds, and changing dressings. They also respond to pages from the nursing staff when patients are crashing. They are thus harried and get little sleep, so part of your job is to make their days easier.

KEY FACT

Help your interns!

Subinterns ("sub-I's"). Sub-I's, also known as acting interns or advanced clerks, are fourth-year medical students who typically plan to complete a surgical residency and are taking on the role of an intern. This means that sub-I's will be working hard to function at an intern level and to shine in the eyes of their chiefs and attendings. As a third-year student, you may be intimidated by the idea of working on a service with sub-I's and being compared to them. Bear in mind, however, that the expectations of a third-year student's performance differ greatly from those of a sub-I. Also keep in mind that you are more than likely capable of performing most of the tasks that the sub-I's do; you're just on a steeper portion of the learning curve. A typical sub-I will be expected to take call on a schedule comparable to that of an intern (again, services vary in their expectations), will assume some responsibility for evaluating patients on consults or in the ER, will take on a fair amount of daily scut work, and will try to squeeze into the OR whenever they can. As acting interns, however, sub-I's should also assume some responsibility for the education of the service, particularly for the third-year students.

KEY FACT

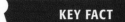

Use your sub-I as a resource! They can advise you on how to do well on the rotation.

HOW IS THE DAY SET UP?

On OR days, the chief/senior residents and attendings will spend most of the day in surgery. Although some of the surgical cases may be simple outpatient procedures such as breast biopsies and hernia repairs, most will be procedures in which patients are admitted for postoperative care that can last up to several days. On clinic days, new patients are seen for their referred problems, established patients are worked up for their preoperative evaluations, and postoperative patients are seen for follow-up. On both operative and clinic days, the entire inpatient service will need to be rounded on, and most teams will try to write all the progress notes on morning rounds before heading off to the OR or to clinic. This, of course, means that the workday starts especially early on a surgery service—usually anywhere from 5:00 to 6:00 A.M. Here is the overall structure of a typical OR day on a general surgery service:

5:00–6:00 A.M.	Prerounds
6:00–7:00 A.M.	Morning rounds
7:00–7:30 A.M.	OR preoperative preparation of patients
7:30 A.M.–6:00 P.M.	Surgery or floor work
6:00–7:30 P.M.	"Afternoon" rounds
7:30 P.M.–?	Postrounds floor work

On clinic days, the morning schedule is usually similar, as rounds must be completed before the start of clinic. The evening schedule may be lighter depending on whether clinic is scheduled in the afternoon and on how many patients need to be worked up or admitted for surgery the next day. On days in which there is not a great deal of scut work, the intern/residents on call may offer to complete the work so that the rest of the team can leave for the day.

On operative days, the senior and chief residents will usually be tied up in the OR, so the responsibility for scut work, consults, and procedures will fall to the junior resident(s), intern(s), and students. You may therefore find yourself shuttling from the OR to the floor between cases to help the interns write orders, check labs, change dressings, see consults, get films read, and so on. Because your role in the OR is usually minimal, you may be expected to spend the bulk of your time doing scut work, especially if you are on a scut-heavy service with a high census (eg, vascular surgery). In the OR, you may be able to participate in a case or you may find yourself relegated to observing from outside the surgical field, depending on the attendings' and residents' preferences, your own interest in getting hands-on surgical experience, and the need for your help in taking care of patient issues on the floor.

KEY FACT

Balance your time between the OR and the wards.

WHAT DO I DO DURING PREROUNDS?

Your day on a surgery service begins with prerounding. Your responsibilities will vary depending on your team's expectations. The team may expect you to preround only on patients you are following, which on average will be 2–3 patients. Keep in mind that interns will also follow these patients in order to check your work, but you will have the responsibility of presenting them during rounds.

On other services, you may not have assigned patients and will instead be expected to do a modified prerounds, which includes skeletonizing the day's progress note prior to the start of rounds. For this, you will write down vitals, intake and output (I/Os), and labs for every patient on the service prior to rounding. There is no need to see the patient during prerounding, as the team will see each patient as a group. In this case, your role during formal rounds will often consist of reading the information in your skeletonized note to the team.

As a rule, the following information should be updated during prerounds each morning:

- **Basic information:** The patient's diagnosis, surgical procedure, hospital day number, and postoperative day number.
- **Subjective data:** Any overnight events (respiratory distress, nausea/vomiting, bleeding)? How is the patient's pain control (on a scale of 1 to 10)? Has he or she passed gas or had a bowel movement? (This is relevant for postoperative feeding.) Is the patient tolerating PO?
- **Vital signs:** Maximum and current temperature, BP, heart rate, respiratory rate, O_2 saturation, and weight. Some chiefs may want the 24-hour ranges as well.
- **I/Os:** Record the total intake and output for the prior day and since midnight. Divide intake into PO (NPO, clear liquids, or solid food?) and IV fluids (type and rate of fluid repletion, boluses given). Divide output into urine output (Foley or spontaneous void?), stool output, emesis, NG output, and output of indwelling drains.
- **Other data:** What lines does the patient have in place? What type and amount of pain medication is the patient getting? Is he or she on a patient-controlled analgesia (PCA) device or receiving boluses of pain meds from the nurses? Which antibiotic is the patient taking, and how many days remain in the regimen? Are any other significant medications being given (eg, steroid taper, antiemetics, promotility agents)? Is the patient diabetic, and if so, how high has his or her blood glucose been running, and how much insulin does he or she require?
- **Physical examination:** You should perform a focused, directed examination based on the patient's presenting problem. In general, all patients should receive a brief respiratory, cardiac, and abdominal examination in addition to a global assessment of mental status every morning. In addition, postoperative patients will require an assessment of urinary status (look at the Foley bag), drain output, and wound healing. Look at the dressing/wound and ask yourself the following questions: Is there wound drainage? Purulent exudate? Excessive peri-incisional tenderness or erythema? Do the sutures or staples need to come out? Is there any sign of wound dehiscence?
- **Assessment and plan (A&P):** You should construct an A&P for rounds even if it is incorrect. It shows that you have been thinking. Things to consider include diet, antibiotics, wound care, and ultimate disposition.

KEY FACT

Keep a running checklist during rounds of scut work to be done. It will impress your interns!

HOW DO I EXCEL IN SURGERY?

Your role on the surgery service will be a hodgepodge of scut work, reading, and simply being with the team. The following are some guidelines for excelling on this service:

- **Never whine or complain.**
- **Always show up on time.**
- **Communicate frequently.**

- **Be visible.** Expect to stay late for evening rounds (unless you are excused by your chief). Your residents may expect you to follow 2–3 patients closely and take primary responsibility for their management with direct supervision from the intern(s). Alternatively, a "team approach" may be taken wherein the entire team shares responsibility for each patient—in which case you won't be expected to know as much detail about every patient but may have more information to keep track of.
- **Become a "Highly Absorbent Information Sponge."** Reading about perioperative care, the pathophysiology of surgical illnesses, the basics of trauma evaluation, and the like will occupy a significant portion of your time, but necessarily so.
- **Know the expectations.** It is wise to ask your attending or chief resident to sit down with you early in the clerkship to discuss his or her expectations with regard to third-year students on the service. You may be expected to participate in many intern-level tasks, which may include performing preoperative H&Ps in clinic, checking labs and x-rays, following patients' I/Os, taking out sutures and staples postoperatively, writing discharge paperwork, evaluating patients in the ED, placing and changing arterial and venous lines, assisting in the OR, writing medication orders, and giving presentations on rounds and in conferences. The balance of these activities will depend on your own initiative and on the demands of your service.
- **Work quickly, independently, and efficiently.** Remain focused, organized, and brief when presenting each patient.
- **Be assertive.** Ask thoughtful questions (you should know something about the subject matter before asking the questions), know other patients on the service (for your own learning and in case you are asked to fill in), take the initiative to ask for demonstrations of procedures, volunteer for drawing blood (you need to practice anyway), and **ask for feedback** from your residents and chiefs both at the midpoint of the rotation and at the end.
- **Be a team player.** Be helpful to your interns and residents. This may require that you do a little extra scut work on other patients for some "quid pro quo" teaching from the interns, but it will be well worth your while. In general, you will have a successful surgery experience if you **show interest,** accept responsibility eagerly and fulfill it competently, make your interns' lives easier, **laugh and smile** a lot, follow your patients closely, give crisp and succinct oral presentations, and **make an extra effort** to read and present interesting issues to the rest of the team. Do anything less and you will almost certainly pass the rotation but may get overshadowed by overly enthusiastic classmates or by solicitous sub-I's. **Unless policies are being broken, never complain about the workload.** Hard work, after all, is what surgery is all about.
- **Get feedback** early in the rotation and often.

KEY FACT

Efficiency, efficiency, efficiency!

KEY FACT

Try not to ask simple questions that you can easily look up later.

KEY NOTES

You will often be responsible for writing notes that your intern or resident can cosign. Below are descriptions of common notes.

SOAP note. This note includes **S**ubjective data, **O**bjective data, **A**ssessment, and **P**lan. The SOAP note is the daily progress note and will need to be completed for each patient on the service during rounds. These should follow the format given in the boxed item below.

KEY FACT

When reading off labs, always read them in order!

SAMPLE SOAP NOTE: BLUE SURGICAL SERVICE

55 yo WM admitted for perforated peptic ulcer, HD#3, POD#2 s/p Graham patch.

S: Pt ambulating. Pain well controlled on PCA. c/o peri-incisional pain (3/10 this A.M.), no drainage. No flatus or bowel movements. Good use of incentive spirometer (↑ 1500 cc). No other overnight issues.

O: VS T_m 38^3 / T_c 38^1 BP 110/63 P 86 RR 16 SpO_2 99% 2 L NC.

I/O: Net +800/+200. IN 2000/420 (NPO, D5 ½ NS + 20 KCl at 84 cc/hr). OUT 1200/220 (UOP 800/150, NGT 200/20, JP 200/50).

Gen: WD/WN male in NAD, A&O × 3.

CV: RRR, nl S1/S2, no M/R/G.

Pulm: CTAB, no W/R/R.

Abd: Hypoactive BS, soft, NT/ND, dressing C/D/I, no induration/erythema, JP drain holding suction with serosanguinous output.

Labs:

140 | 100 | 8 < 92
3.5 | 24 | 0.8

(stable from 12.5)
8.4 > 12.3 / 37.2 < 280

Sputum Cx pending; CXR unremarkable and unchanged from prior.

Lines: Right RAL (day 3), Foley catheter (day 3).

A/P: 55 yo WM POD#2 s/p Graham patch for perforated peptic ulcer, doing well. Low-grade temperature most likely 2° to atelectasis.

1. Continue abx regimen. Ancef (day 1/5), Flagyl (day 1/5).
2. Encourage OOB, ambulation, and incentive spirometry.
3. Consider D/C PCA; switch to oral analgesics.
4. Switch to oral meds, but keep NPO except meds for now; will advance diet to clear liquids when flatus passed.
5. D/C JP drain, D/C Foley.

Admission H&P. If this is a preoperative H&P for an elective surgery, you should include a succinct history of present illness (HPI), a brief past medical history (PMH) with particular attention paid to illnesses that have significance for perioperative management (eg, a history of atrial fibrillation, COPD, or diabetes), and information on medications and allergies. Your examination should be comprehensive but should focus on the particular organ system involved (eg, a thorough abdominal examination for GI cases and a detailed peripheral vascular examination for vascular cases) and should always include a rectal examination.

Operative note. This is a note that is entered into the chart at the completion of a surgical procedure documenting the findings and events of the case. It is usually a brief summary and should include pertinent data regarding the participants, the pre- and postoperative diagnoses (which are usually the same but are sometimes different, particularly in exploratory cases), total fluid exchange, disposition, and any complications. Ask the anesthesiologist for fluid totals, and consult your resident to resolve any other questions.

Key:

A&O × 3 = alert and oriented to person, place, and time
A/P = assessment and plan
abx = antibiotics
BS = bowel sounds
C/D/I = clean, dry, and intact
c/o = complains of
CTAB = clear to auscultation bilaterally
Cx = culture
D/C = discontinue
HD = hospital day
JP = Jackson-Pratt drain
M/R/G = murmur/rubs/gallops
NAD = no acute distress
NC = nasal cannula
NGT = nasogastric tube
nl = normal
NPO = nothing by mouth
NS = normal saline
NT/ND = nontender and nondistended
O = objective data
OOB = out of bed
P = pulse rate
POD = postoperative day
RAL = radial arterial line
RR = respiratory rate
RRR = regular rate and rhythm
S = subjective data
s/p = status post
SpO_2 = oxygen saturation
T_c = current temperature
T_m = maximum temperature
UOP = urine output
VS = vital signs
WD/WN = well developed and well nourished
WM = white male
W/R/R = wheezes/rhonchi/rales

BRIEF OPERATIVE NOTE: BLUE SURGICAL SERVICE

Pre-op Dx: Biliary colic.

Post-op Dx: Cholelithiasis.

Procedure: Laparoscopic cholecystectomy + intraoperative cholangiography.

Surgeons: Attending, resident (PGY-5), intern (PGY-1), med student (MS-3).

Anesthesia: GETA.

Fluids: 1400 cc LR.

EBL: 200 cc.

UOP: 400 cc.

Drains: None.

Intraoperative findings: Distended GB with slightly thickened wall, multiple stones within GB, no CBD stones by IOC.

Specimens: GB to path (no cultures taken).

Complications: None.

Disposition: To PACU in stable condition, awake and extubated.

Key:

CBD = common bile duct

Dx = diagnosis

EBL = estimated blood loss

GB = gallbladder

GETA = general endotracheal anesthesia

IOC = intraoperative cholangiogram

LR = Lactated Ringer's solution

PACU = postanesthesia care unit

KEY FACT

To remember the components of the operative note, think **PPP SAFE U DISC.**

Postoperative orders. Interns and sub-I's are normally responsible for writing postoperative orders. If you are comfortable writing such orders, **this is an area in which you can shine.** A sample set of postoperative orders is shown below.

KEY FACT

To remember the components of a postoperative order, think **ADC VAAN DDIML.**

POSTOPERATIVE ORDERS

Admit to: 3-West, General Surgery; Attending: Dr. Jones; Interns Lee (×46789) and Smith (×97850); MS-3 Stone (×57689).

Diagnosis: Perforated peptic ulcer.

Condition: Stable.

Vitals: Per routine.

Allergies: NKDA.

Activity: As tolerated, OOB TID.

Nursing orders: Strict I/Os Q4H with Foley catheter to gravity. NG to suction. IS 10 times/hr when awake.

DVT prophylaxis: Heparin 5000 units SQ Q12H, TEDs/SCDs.

Diet: NPO.

IV fluids: NS to run at 84 cc/hr.

Key:

CBC = complete blood count

CHO = call house officer

DVT = deep venous thrombosis

IS = incentive spirometry

NKDA = no known drug allergies

PRN = as needed

Q4H = every 4 hours

SCD = sequential compression device

SQ = subcutaneous

TED = thromboembolic deterrent stockings

TID = 3 times daily

UA = urinalysis

Medications: Cefotaxime 1 g IV × 1 dose. Fentanyl PCA.

(Remember to list all the patient's preoperative and PRN medications.)

Labs: CBC, chem-7, UA in A.M. CXR in A.M.

CHO if: HR > 100 or < 60; BP > 180/100 or < 90/60; RR > 25 or < 12; or temp > 39.5.

MNEMONIC

Causes of postoperative fever (> 38.5°C)–

The 5 W's

Wind: Atelectasis, pneumonia.
Water: UTI.
Wound: Infection.
Walking: Pulmonary embolus arising from a DVT.
Wonder drug: Drug fever.

KEY FACT

The most common cause of fever on the first postoperative day is atelectasis.

MNEMONIC

How to remove a drain–

The 3 S's

Stitch cut
Suction off
Steady pull

KEY FACT

Remember that drain diameter ↑ with lower gauge and higher French measurements.

Postoperative check. Generally, patients will need to be seen 2–4 hours after surgery to be evaluated for immediate complications (eg, hypotension, hemorrhage, dyspnea), adequacy of urine output, level of comfort, and the like. A brief postoperative note—presented again in the standard SOAP format—should then be written. The subjective section of the note should primarily address the patient's postoperative pain control; the objective portion should include vital signs, intraoperative and postoperative blood loss and fluid intake, urine output, wound drainage, appearance of the incision and dressings, postoperative lab results from the recovery room, and any significant abnormalities on physical examination. Always communicate abnormal findings and/or laboratory values to your team.

Procedure note. Frequently, surgical patients will undergo other procedures, such as central line insertion, chest tube placement/removal, extubation, incision and drainage of abscesses, thoracentesis, paracentesis, lumbar puncture, and suturing of lacerations. When these are done as bedside procedures, they should be documented in the medical chart with an appropriate procedure note. This procedure note should follow the standard format. Remember to get informed consent and document having done so in the chart.

KEY PROCEDURES

Because surgery is principally an intervention-oriented specialty, you should gain hands-on experience with procedures that may be relevant to you in other specialties. These include suturing lacerations (including learning techniques of local anesthesia), knot tying and suture cutting, gowning and gloving in sterile fashion, arterial line placement, starting IVs, ABGs, paracentesis, thoracentesis, chest tube placement, incision and drainage of abscesses, staple and suture removal, dressing changes, Foley catheterization, NG tube insertion, central venous cannulation, and drain pulling (see the boxed item below). You should also become familiar with the process of patient preparation and transfer to and from the operating suite. Surgical knots are best learned from a resident and then practiced at home. Of course, you'll get plenty of practice at retraction in the OR. Do not kill yourself trying to do all of these procedures, but make use of the opportunities that present themselves. Remember, if you fall in love with surgical procedures, you can always do a subinternship in your fourth year.

OPERATING ROOM ETIQUETTE

One of the most challenging (and often frustrating) concepts that you must learn during your surgical ward rotation is the maintenance of a sterile field in the OR. This includes making sure you are not contaminating the operating field (or yourself) and staying out of the way of other team members in the OR (eg, the residents, scrub nurse, circulating nurse, and x-ray technicians).

KEY POINT

TUBES AND DRAINS

- **Closed-suction drain (ie, Jackson-Pratt [JP], Blake, or Hemovac drains):** Used to drain surgical wounds and to keep bacteria and blood from building up; drains are usually attached to bulb suction. You will see the resident "strip" or milk these tubes, which means pulling along the length of the clear tube filled with blood to prevent clotting.
- **Penrose drain:** A hollow tube that is usually used to drain large abscesses or infected surfaces. No suction.
- **Negative-pressure wound therapy:** A vacuum dressing (or VAC) used to promote healing in acute and chronic wounds.
- **NG tube:** A tube leading from the nasopharynx to the stomach; used to drain the stomach of fluids (gastric decompression). It can also be used for feeding when the patient's GI tract starts working after surgery.
- **G-tube or gastrostomy tube:** Goes from the stomach to the outside; resembles a permanent NG tube used for feeding patients with an obstruction above the stomach, or for decompression in patients with pyloric outlet obstruction.
- **J-tube or jejunostomy tube:** Primarily used for feeding.
- **GJ-tube/Moss tube:** Has 2 ports: 1 to the stomach and the other to the jejunum. Acts like 1 G-tube and 1 J-tube. J- and GJ-tubes are often used in patients at high risk for aspiration.
- **T-tube:** A biliary tube shaped like a "T."
- **Chest tube:** Drains blood, pus, fluid, or air from the thorax.
- **Foley catheter:** Routinely placed in the OR for drainage of the bladder or for strict monitoring of I/Os.
- **Central line:** Provides central access to the venous vasculature; often required for administration of vasopressors. Typically placed in the internal jugular, subclavian, or femoral veins.

Since you will probably be the least experienced member of the group, it is important to know some of the points of etiquette associated with working in the OR. These include the following:

- **Introduce yourself** both to the OR circulating nurse and to the scrub nurse when you first enter the OR, and tell them that you will be scrubbing in on the case. If there is a white board in the room with everyone's names, write yours down as well. Tell the circulating nurse what size gown you will need. Pull your gloves and give them to the scrub nurse yourself! Be sure to ask the scrub nurse whether you should place the gloves on the tray with sterile technique or leave them on the side. If you don't know your glove size, follow this general guideline: size 6 = small; size 7 = medium; size 8 = large.
- Remember to **double-glove** to protect yourself against needlesticks. In double-gloving, many people prefer that the outer set of gloves be a half size smaller than the inner set to maximize dexterity.

- Ask the circulating nurse or resident if he or she needs any help in moving or positioning the patient on the operating table or "prepping" the patient for surgery (including clipping hair and placing the Foley catheter). In some hospitals, the nurses will prep the patient; in other facilities it may be up to you (ask your resident or sub-I prior to your first OR case).
- Before scrubbing, place your beeper on one of the nonsterile side tables with a piece of paper attached to it giving your name. This will not only allow the circulating nurse to return your pages but also help you find the beeper if you accidentally leave it in the OR after the case is over.
- Remember to **take off any jewelry** (eg, rings, bracelets, watches, earrings) and put on your mask, cap, and safety eyewear before you start scrubbing.
- Although there is no specific rule on how long to scrub, a good rule of thumb is to scrub for 5 minutes prior to the first case of the day. For subsequent cases, be sure to scrub **1–2 minutes longer than your attending** so that he or she won't be able to criticize you for not scrubbing thoroughly enough. Some hospitals use sterile gel after the first case, but be sure to follow your attending's preferences.
- Offer to help with the draping of the patient after you are gowned. If no help is needed, quietly stand out of the way of others who are doing so.
- Try to **keep your hands above your waist and below your shoulders.** Place your hands on the drapes during the surgery to ensure that your gloves remain sterile.
- Do not reach over or pass any instrument unless you are specifically instructed to do so.
- When the surgeon is using the bovie (electrocautery device) to incise fat, muscle tissue, and fascia, use the suction device to suck up the smoke and noxious odor associated with it.
- When you return needles or blades back to the scrub nurse, always announce out loud the presence of any sharps on the field that are being returned to the instrument tray (eg, "needle down" or "knife back"). This is extremely important for patients who are HIV or hepatitis ⊕. It is also helpful to announce when the initial incision has been made so that the anesthesiologist knows when the surgery has started and can document the time of incision. He or she will also appreciate knowing if irrigation is being done to adequately keep track of fluid losses. At the end of the case, ask the anesthesiologist for the estimated blood loss and how much fluid the patient received intraoperatively at a convenient time (this information is then recorded on the operative note).
- Try to **make yourself helpful** by paying attention to minor details such as providing adequate retraction, adjusting the overhead lights, and suctioning excess blood from the area of dissection. These measures will allow the surgeon to have good visualization of the operative field. If you have seen the procedure before, try to anticipate the next step and have necessary instruments in hand (eg, hold suture scissors and be ready to cut excess suture when the resident or attending finishes tying).
- Those of you who wear eyeglasses should be aware that the easiest way to contaminate yourself is to accidentally adjust your glasses with your sterile glove. Work to avoid that habit in the OR! A tip is to use a strip of tape over the bridge of your nose and mask to prevent your glasses from fogging up.
- If you do end up contaminating your gown, glove, or sleeve, step out of the operating field and let the scrub nurse know so that he or she can replace the contaminated parts and help ensure that you do not end up contaminating anything else.

KEY FACT

If in doubt, ask! It is better to ask than to contaminate the surgical instruments.

KEY FACT

If you get stuck with a needle, be sure to inform your team immediately so that you can take the necessary precautions.

- If you follow these basic principles of OR etiquette, you are likely to find your OR experience more enjoyable and far less stressful. One last thing: Don't forget to **carry a pen in the pocket of your scrubs** so that you can write the operative note and postoperative orders when the case is complete.

HOW TO SUTURE LIKE A PRO

One way to get more out of your OR experience is to become highly proficient at suturing and surgical knot tying. Unfortunately, the only way to do so is to **practice, practice, practice!** The best way to sharpen your suturing technique is to go to the ED/OR supply room and obtain the following:

- **Sutures of different types and sizes:** The most common sutures with which to practice surgical knot tying are 3–0 silk suture ties. Ideally, however, you should try to become proficient in suturing with many different types of sutures, such as 5–0 nylon (most commonly used when suturing up the skin), 1–0 Vicryl (most commonly used when suturing up deep fascia and muscle layers), and 4–0 Vicryl (most commonly used when closing up the subcutaneous layer). It is also helpful to remember which sutures are absorbable as opposed to nonabsorbable (see Table 9-1).
- **A "laceration tray" from the ED:** Specific instruments you will need include a needle driver, a pair of pickups, and a pair of suture scissors. Laceration trays usually have many of these instruments in varying sizes.
- **A box of gloves:** Remember that when you are suturing on a patient, you should be double-gloved to protect against needlesticks. It would thus make sense to practice suturing and surgical knot tying with 2 sets of gloves on so that the process won't prove to be too awkward when you work on an actual patient.
- **A suture removal kit:** This should include a pair of forceps as well as a fine-pointed pair of scissors for taking out sutures.

KEY FACT

Don't take instruments or suture from the OR itself, as these are contaminated. Get fresh material from the supply room or on the floor.

KEY FACT

Tapered suture needles are used for fascia and subcutaneous tissues, whereas cutting needles are used for the skin only.

The next step is to find a fourth-year medical student (eg, a sub-I) or an intern (ideally one who is not very busy) who would be willing to show you how to suture and tie surgical knots. The types of suture methods that you should learn include the following:

- Simple interrupted sutures (most commonly used to close up skin lacerations)
- Vertical mattress sutures (used to close skin that is under tension)
- Horizontal mattress sutures (also used to close skin that is under tension)
- "Buried" (subcutaneous) sutures (used to close surgical incisions)
- Figure-of-eight sutures (used to tie off a bleeding vessel)
- Running sutures (used to quickly close deep fascial layers)

TABLE 9-1. Types of Sutures

Absorbable	Nonabsorbable
Vicryl	Nylon
Polydioxanone (PDS)	Silk[a]
Dexon	Stainless steel
Chromic	Prolene
Catgut[a]	

[a] Natural material.

As for surgical knot tying, focus on learning how to tie surgical knots by the "instrument tie" and the 2-handed tie before progressing to the more advanced 1-handed surgical knot tie. Good materials to practice suturing on include pigs' feet (for the classic diehard surgeon-to-be), chicken breast, orange peels, banana peels, and 2-sided sponges.

WHAT DO I CARRY IN MY POCKETS?

As with any rotation, surgery has its necessary gear. Unlike most residents, however, surgery residents try to carry as little extraneous material as possible with them, as they tend to shift rapidly from OR to clinic to ward to cafeteria and must therefore remain as unencumbered as possible. As a student, you should adopt this minimalist stance as well. This means not carrying around too many handbooks and not wearing a fanny pack laden with tuning forks, otoscopes, and the like. The main requirements for the surgery rotation include the following:

- **White coat:** Always wear one on the first day. Find out if you're expected to wear it daily or just in clinic.
- **Stethoscope:** Essential on any rotation. However, be aware of the fact that many surgeons frown on wearing the stethoscope as a necklace ("dog collar"), as this signals that you are an internal medicine resident. To be safe, carry your stethoscope in the pocket of your white coat.
- **Penlight:** Critical for its common uses (checking pupils) and for examining wounds and the like.
- **Pens:** Residents often use (and lose) your pens, so keep a good stash.
- **Extra suture:** This is great for practicing tying knots when you have a free moment.
- **Trauma scissors:** Trauma scissors, or surgical shears, are a pair of heavy-duty scissors that are used primarily to cut through a patient's clothing during an acute trauma situation or to cut through bulky dressings on rounds. These handy, all-purpose scissors will prove useful during both your general surgery and your ED rotations. To score points with your chief/senior resident, cut your patients' dressings open when you preround so that they can be easily and quickly removed on rounds.
- **Index cards/clipboard/patient data sheets:** You will need something portable to manage information (eg, lab data) on each patient. Figure out which method works most effectively and efficiently for you, and then stick with it and abandon extraneous gear. Keep in mind that clipboards can and often do get lost.
- **Wound care accessories:** It is helpful to carry spare gauze (Kerlix rolls and 4 × 4 cotton gauze pads), surgical tape, fine-pointed scissors, alcohol pads, flushes, and other wound care accessories for rapid dispensing at the request of your chief resident on rounds. Keep these in your pockets or carry a pack during rounds.
- **Surgery handbook:** There are a number of useful, concise pocket guidebooks for surgery students and residents. Some of the more popular handbooks are reviewed in the Top-Rated Review Resources section.

KEY FACT

Check with your resident on your service's protocol for checking dressings. Oftentimes, they will want to keep the dressing intact for 24–48 hours to allow for epithelialization.

You should probably purchase the above items if you don't already own them. Most will come in handy for other rotations, and a good pocket handbook is great to have as a quick reference before conferences or teaching (pimping) rounds.

High-Yield Clinical Topic Checklist

Read about these topics before you start the rotation. Most are discussed in this chapter. A full list of common clerkship topics can be found at the end of this chapter.

- ❑ Acute abdomen
- ❑ GI bleeding
- ❑ Small and large bowel obstruction/ileus
- ❑ Colorectal cancer
- ❑ Gallbladder disease
- ❑ Pancreatic cancer
- ❑ Hernias (direct, indirect, hiatal)
- ❑ Abdominal aortic aneurysm
- ❑ Lung cancer
- ❑ Breast cancer
- ❑ Prostate cancer

General Postoperative Care

FLUID MANAGEMENT

The calculation of maintenance fluid requirements can be done using 2 simple rules:

- **100/50/20 rule:** Fluid requirements for a 24-hour period are calculated as 100 cc/kg for the first 10 kg, 50 cc/kg for the next 10 kg, and 20 cc/kg for every kilogram over 20 kg.
- **4/2/1 rule:** Hourly fluid requirements are calculated as 4 cc/kg for the first 10 kg, 2 cc/kg for the next 10 kg, and 1 cc/kg for every kilogram over 20 kg.

KEY FACT

The minimal urine output for an adult patient is 0.5 cc/kg/hr.

KEY POINT

THIRD SPACING

- Fluid often accumulates in the interstitium of tissues and can manifest as tachycardia and ↓ urine output.
- Treatment is with IV hydration with isotonic fluids. But beware, as third-spaced fluids will mobilize back to the intravascular space around POD #3 and can result in fluid overload.

Gastrointestinal Disease

ACUTE ABDOMEN

The workup of a patient with an acute abdomen is a diagnostic challenge as well as a key component of the surgical rotation. Early diagnosis is critical, as early intervention is required to prevent significant morbidity and mortality.

Signs and Symptoms

A thorough H&P is indispensable in making the diagnosis of acute abdomen and should include the following information:

- HPI:
  - Onset, duration, and progression of the pain (eg, maximal at onset, sudden or gradual onset, intermittent, constant, worsening).
  - Aggravating and alleviating factors.
  - Quality (burning, cramping, sharp, aching) and severity of the pain.
  - Location of the pain both at onset and at presentation, and radiation of the pain.
  - GI complaints (nausea, vomiting, anorexia, hematemesis, hematochezia, melena, or change in bowel function).
  - Gynecologic complaints and last menstrual period.
  - Similar episodes in the past.
- PMH:
  - CAD, heart failure, hernias, gallstones, EtOH abuse, PUD, STIs.
  - Metabolic or endocrine disease (eg, diabetes, Addison's disease, porphyria).
  - Prior surgical history (eg, cholecystectomy, appendectomy, hysterectomy).
- **Medications** (in particular, note any NSAID use).
- **Physical examination:** Begin with general observation. How ill is the patient? Is he or she writhing in pain or lying motionless?
  - **Abdominal examination: Inspect** (distention, symmetry, scars, trauma); **auscultate** (absent or hypoactive bowel sounds can indicate ileus, high-pitched sounds or tinkles can indicate obstruction, and bruits can point toward aneurysm); **palpate** (look for tenderness to palpation, rebound tenderness, referred pain, voluntary or involuntary guarding, flank tenderness, masses, and hernias); and **percuss** (shifting dullness or a fluid wave indicates ascites).
  - **Rectal examination:** Look for occult blood, mass lesions, tenderness, sphincter tone, and the presence or absence of stool in the rectal vault.
  - **Pelvic examination:** Check for adnexal tenderness, masses, cervical discharge, cervical motion tenderness, and uterine size and consistency.

MNEMONIC

Assessment of pain–

OPQRST

Onset
Precipitating or **P**alliative factors
Quality
Radiation
Severity
Timing

KEY FACT

All female patients with an acute abdomen need a pelvic examination, a pregnancy test, and ultrasound to rule out PID, ectopic pregnancy, ovarian torsion, and the like.

KEY FACT

Remember the 6 causes of abdominal pain that cause patients to crump:

- Abdominal aortic aneurysm
- Aortic dissection
- Tension pneumothorax
- MI
- Cardiac tamponade
- Pulmonary embolism

Differential

See Figures 9-1 and 9-2 for a limited differential diagnosis of acute abdomen by abdominal quadrant. Below is a more comprehensive differential by system:

- **GI:** Small or large bowel obstruction, paralytic ileus, volvulus, viscus perforation, PUD/gastritis, appendicitis, diverticulitis, acute cholecystitis/cholangitis, pancreatitis, splenic rupture.
- **GU:** Obstructive uropathy, pyelonephritis, nephrolithiasis, ovarian torsion or cyst, ruptured ectopic pregnancy, PID.

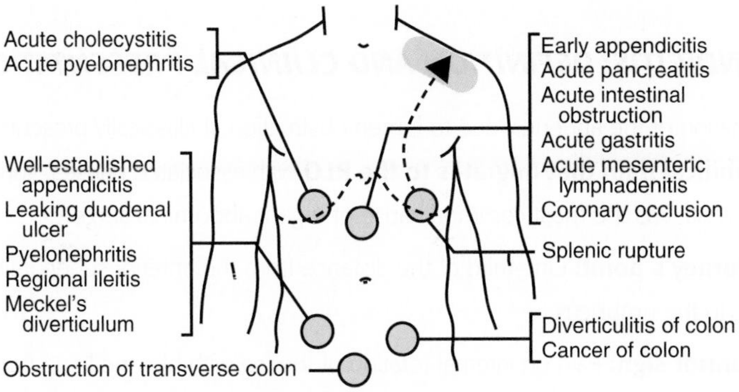

FIGURE 9-1. Common locations of acute abdominal pain. (Reproduced with permission from LeBlond RF et al. *DeGowin's Diagnostic Examination,* 9th ed. New York: McGraw-Hill, 2009, Fig. 9-19.)

- **Cardiac:** Pericarditis, angina, MI.
- **Pulmonary:** Pneumonia, pleurisy, empyema, pulmonary embolism (PE).
- **Vascular:** Abdominal aortic aneurysm (AAA), mesenteric ischemia.
- **Hematologic:** Acute intermittent porphyria, sickle cell crisis (can cause ischemic hepatitis).
- **Endocrine:** DKA, addisonian crisis, uremic crisis.
- **Autoimmune:** SLE.
- **Toxins:** Lead, venom.

WORKUP

- **Labs:** CBC, electrolytes, LFTs, amylase, lipase, lactate, UA, urine microscopic examination, urine culture, hCG in women.
- **Imaging:** CXR and AXR to look for free air; kidneys, ureters, and bladder (KUB); CT of the abdomen/pelvis; RUQ ultrasound.

KEY FACT

Free air under the diaphragm on CXR or AXR is highly suggestive of a ruptured viscus, especially perforated peptic ulcer.

KEY FACT

The only time air under the diaphragm is acceptable is after laparoscopic surgery or laparotomy.

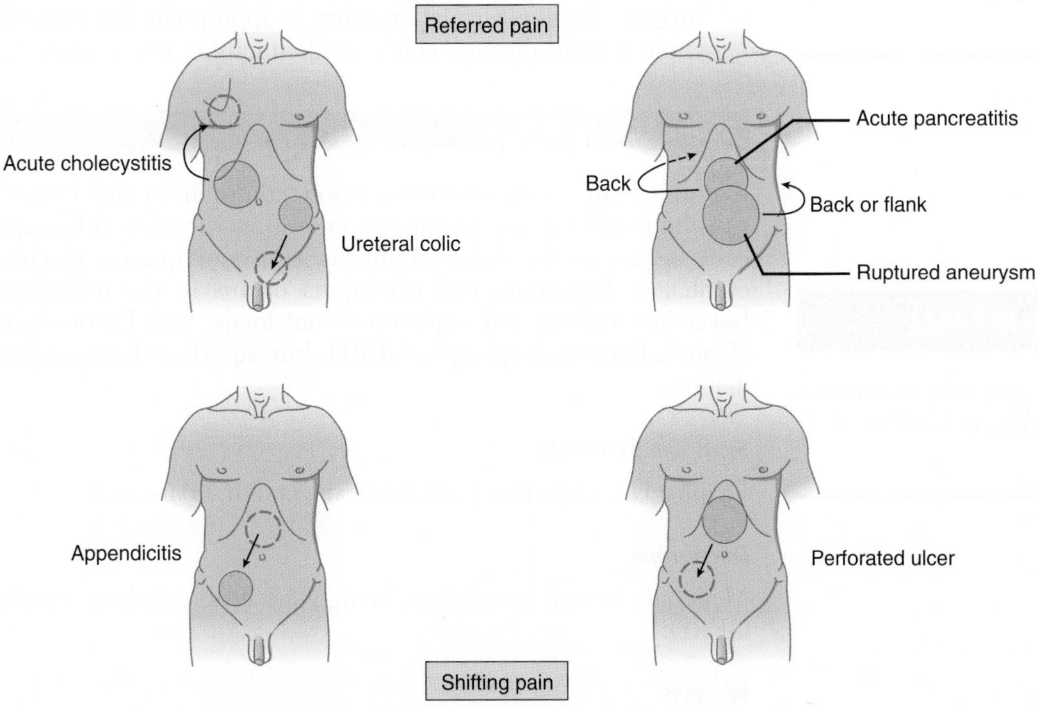

FIGURE 9-2. Referred pain and shifting pain in the acute abdomen. Solid circles indicate the site of maximal pain; broken lines indicate sites of lesser or referred pain. (Reproduced with permission from Doherty GM. *Current Diagnosis & Treatment: Surgery,* 13th ed. New York: McGraw-Hill, 2010, Fig. 21-2.)

APPENDICITIS: DEFINITION AND CLIINICAL PRESENTATION

Inflammation of the appendix due to lumen obstruction. It classically presents as **periumbilical pain that migrates to the RLQ** with associated nausea, vomiting, and anorexia. It is the most common cause of urgent abdominal surgery.

- **McBurney's point:** One-third of the distance from the anterior superior iliac spine to the umbilicus.
- **Obturator sign:** Pain on internal rotation of the leg with hip and knee flexed.
- **Psoas sign:** Pain on extension of the hip with the knee in full extension, or pain on flexing the hip against resistance.
- **Rovsing's sign:** Palpation of the LLQ results in pain in the RLQ.

TREATMENT

- First determine if the condition represents a surgical abdomen (ie, an abdomen in need of emergent surgical treatment) or if it can be treated with expectant management.
- **Expectant management:**
  - NPO.
  - NG suction in cases of nausea and vomiting, hematemesis, or suspected GI tract obstruction.
  - Aggressive IV fluid hydration and correction of electrolyte abnormalities.
  - Monitoring of vital signs and serial abdominal examinations.
  - Foley catheterization to evaluate fluid status and response to rehydration therapy if the patient is unable to urinate independently.
  - Serial labs, including CBC and electrolytes.
- **Surgery: Exploratory laparotomy** is appropriate for unstable patients in whom a surgically correctable or identifiable cause is suspected.

> **KEY FACT**
>
> Always try to minimize the use of Foley catheters in floor patients to minimize the risk of UTI.

ESOPHAGEAL CANCER

Includes both adenocarcinoma (most common in the United States) and squamous cell carcinoma (most common worldwide). Adenocarcinoma typically occurs in the distal esophagus as a consequence of chronic Barrett's esophagus. Squamous cell carcinoma occurs in the mid-esophagus and is linked to smoking and ingestion of hot foods. Risk factors include tobacco, alcohol, Barrett's esophagus, GERD, hot liquids or burns, achalasia, and radiation.

> **KEY FACT**
>
> Esophageal cancer is often symptomatic only after it has blocked two-thirds of the lumen.

SIGNS AND SYMPTOMS

Dysphagia, weight loss, pain, cachexia, cough, hoarseness.

DIFFERENTIAL

Metastatic tumor, lymphoma, benign stricture, achalasia, esophageal spasm, GERD.

WORKUP

- Endoscopy with biopsy; barium swallow/upper GI series.
- Imaging for staging includes CXR, CT of the chest/abdomen/pelvis, endoscopic ultrasound, and bronchoscopy.

TREATMENT

Most tumors are malignant and often are advanced, as there is no serosa. Treatment includes surgery if in an early stage; otherwise multimodality therapy can be considered.

GI BLEEDING

Upper GI Bleeding (UGIB)

Defined as bleeding proximal to the ligament of Treitz, which includes the esophagus, stomach, and duodenum. Risk factors include alcohol, smoking, a history of PUD or bleeding disorders, burn injuries, trauma, and medication use (eg, NSAIDs, anticoagulants, steroids). Etiologies include the following:

- Peptic ulcer (45%)
- Gastric erosions (23%)
- Varices (10%)
- Mallory-Weiss tear (7%)
- Esophagitis/duodenitis (6%)

SIGNS AND SYMPTOMS

- **Hematemesis:** Vomiting of bright red blood or coffee-ground emesis (blood exposed to gastric acid).
- **Melena:** Black, tarry stools (usually due to an upper GI bleeding source).
- **Hematochezia:** Bright red blood per rectum (BRBPR). May be seen in cases of vigorous upper GI bleeding.
- Dehydration (pallor, tachycardia, orthostasis, syncope), shock, epigastric discomfort, and guaiac-⊕ stools are commonly seen.

> **KEY FACT**
>
> Be aware that some medications, such as Pepto-Bismol, can cause dark stools that can be mistaken for melena.

DIFFERENTIAL

In addition to the disease entities listed above, consider gastric cancer, splenic vein thrombosis, epistaxis, and hemoptysis.

WORKUP

- **Labs:** CBC, electrolytes, LFTs, coagulation studies, type and cross 4–6 units of packed RBCs (PRBCs).
- NG lavage; stool guaiac.
- **Imaging:** Upright AXR; upper endoscopy (EGD).

TREATMENT

- **Assess fluid status** and **resuscitate** with 2 L NS or LR followed by PRBCs until the patient is hemodynamically stable. Be sure the patient has at least 2 large-bore IVs (16–18 gauge).
- Assess the magnitude of hemorrhage using vital signs, urine output, serial hemoglobins, O_2 saturation, and evidence of active bleeding.
- Correct any underlying coagulopathy with FFP/vitamin K. Give platelets for severe thrombocytopenia.
- **Identify the bleeding source:**
  - **NG lavage:** If aspiration yields bright red blood or coffee grounds, perform saline lavage of the GI tract to remove blood clots until clear fluid returns. A nonbloody bilious aspirate suggests lower GI bleeding.
  - **EGD:** Identify the site of bleeding and coagulate the bleeding vessels. Always biopsy any ulcers or masses found, and test for *H pylori*.
  - **Angiography:** If GI bleeding is to be identified with angiography, the rate of bleeding must be > 0.5 cc/min. If a source is identified, perform embolization.

> **Q**
>
> A 47-year-old man presents to the ED with orthostasis and is found to have guaiac-⊕ stools. What is the first step in management?

INDICATIONS FOR SURGICAL TREATMENT OF UPPER GI BLEEDING

- In 80–85% of cases, bleeding will stop spontaneously; approximately 20% will require surgery.
- In general, surgery is indicated if patients require **6 or more units of blood** in the first 24 hours or if they rebleed while receiving maximal medical therapy.
- Other indications for surgery are as follows:
  - **Esophageal variceal bleeding despite medical measures:** Consider performing a transjugular intrahepatic portosystemic shunt (TIPS) procedure to decompress portal hypertension.
  - **Perforation.**
  - **Gastric outlet obstruction.**

- Control bleeding:
  - Sclerotherapy or embolization should be used during the localization procedure.
  - Vasopressin is often used to improve hemodynamic stability by decreasing flow to varices. Bear in mind that in addition to vasoconstricting the enteric circulation, vasopressin will also cause coronary vasoconstriction. Therefore, it is commonly given with nitroglycerin to ↓ the risk of MI.
  - Balloon tamponade can be used as a temporary measure (< 48 hours) in cases of refractory variceal hemorrhage.

KEY FACT

Large-gauge peripheral lines are better than central lines for rapid resuscitation because they are "short and fat" tubes.

Lower GI Bleeding (LGIB)

Defined as bleeding distal to the ligament of Treitz, including the jejunum, ileum, colon, and rectum. Most cases occur in the colon. Etiologies include the following:

- **Acute:** Diverticulosis, angiodysplasia (AVM, telangiectasia), IBD, ischemic colitis, intussusception, volvulus, UGIB, Meckel's diverticulum (in children).
- **Chronic:** Colorectal cancer, hemorrhoids, anal fissures.

KEY FACT

The most common cause of LGIB is UGIB. The next most common causes are diverticulosis in adults and angiodysplasia in children.

SIGNS AND SYMPTOMS

Hematochezia (BRBPR) or melena, abdominal pain, anorexia, fatigue, syncope, change in bowel habits.

WORKUP

- **Labs:** CBC, electrolytes, PT/PTT, type and cross 4–6 units of PRBCs, stool guaiac.
- **Imaging:** Colonoscopy, tagged RBC scan, angiography, Meckel's scan (ie, Tc-99m pertechnetate scintigraphy to detect pancreatic/gastric mucosa in Meckel's diverticulum).

KEY FACT

Diverticulosis is the most common cause of LGIB in patients > 40 years of age.

A

Fluid resuscitation with 2 L NS or LR, followed by transfusion of PRBCs through 2 large-bore peripheral IVs.

TREATMENT

- **Resuscitate:** Guidelines are the same as those for UGIB. In 90% of cases, bleeding will stop spontaneously following 2 units of transfusion.
- **Identify the bleeding source:**
  - NG lavage yields bilious GI contents in the case of LGIB.
  - DRE, anoscopy, and/or sigmoidoscopy to rule out hemorrhoids or polyps.
- **Colonoscopy:** Direct visualization of the colon by a gastroenterologist.
- **RBC scintigraphy:** A technetium-labeled RBC scan is sensitive for slow bleeds (0.1 cc/min) but is less specific than angiography.
- **Angiography:** As with UGIB, brisk bleeding (> 0.5 cc/min) is required to make the diagnosis.
- **Control the bleeding source:**
  - Embolization is often performed during angiography.
  - Laser coagulation or electrocoagulation can be used.
- **Surgical indications** include the following:
  - Persistent bleeding despite angiographic or endoscopic therapy.
  - Segmental colectomy if the bleeding site is well localized.
  - If it is not possible to localize the bleeding site, consider total colectomy with ileorectal anastomosis.

SMALL BOWEL DISEASE

Small Bowel Obstruction (SBO)

Defined as blocked passage of bowel contents through the duodenum, jejunum, or ileum. Fluid and gas build up proximal to the obstruction, leading to fluid and electrolyte imbalances and significant abdominal discomfort. The obstruction can be complete or partial and may be dangerous if strangulation of the bowel occurs. Etiologies are as follows:

- Adhesions from a prior abdominal surgery (60%)
- Hernias (10–20%)
- Neoplasm (10–20%)
- Intussusception
- Gallstone ileus
- Stricture from IBD

SIGNS AND SYMPTOMS

- **Cramping abdominal pain:** A recurrent crescendo-decrescendo pattern at intervals of 5–10 minutes (see Figure 9-3).
- **Vomiting:** Nonfeculent in the setting of proximal obstruction; feculent in the presence of distal obstruction. Keep in mind that feculence is 2° to bacterial overgrowth, not actual emesis of feces.
- **Obstruction:** Suspect complete obstruction if no flatus or stool is passed; suspect partial obstruction with continued passage of flatus but no stool.
- Fever, hypotension, and tachycardia due to hypovolemia are also seen.
- Examination reveals **abdominal distention,** high-pitched and hypoactive bowel sounds, tympany to percussion, abdominal tenderness, and masses or hernias.

DIFFERENTIAL

Acute appendicitis; **postoperative ileus** due to abdominal surgery, hypokalemia, or medications; large bowel obstruction; IBD; mesenteric ischemia; carcinoid tumor; renal colic.

KEY FACT

Adhesions are the leading cause of SBO in adults; hernias are the leading cause in children.

KEY FACT

Be able to distinguish SBO from ileus. In SBO there is a clear transition point on imaging. In ileus the bowel is diffusely distended.

KEY FACT

The presence of radiopaque material at the cecum and pneumobilia is suggestive of gallstone ileus.

Q

A 60-year-old woman is POD #2 status post ventral hernia repair. She complains of abdominal pain and distention. She has been passing flatus and small amounts of stool. Examination reveals hypoactive bowel sounds. What is the diagnosis and treatment?

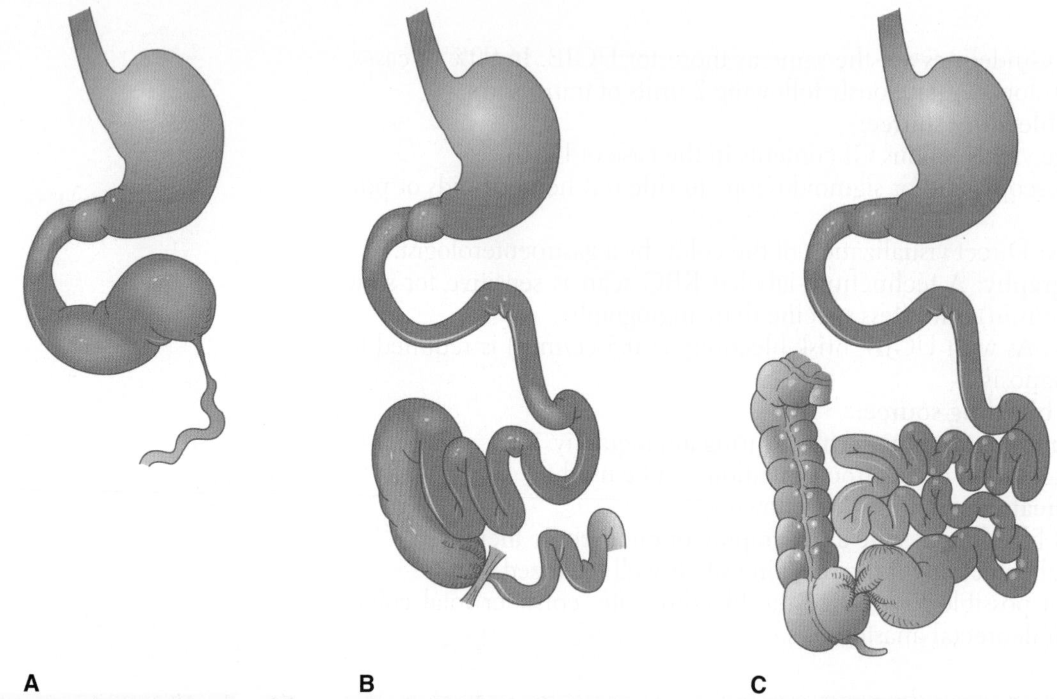

FIGURE 9-3. Small bowel obstruction by level of blockage. (A) **High.** Characterized by frequent vomiting, no distention, and intermittent pain that is not of the classic crescendo type. (B) **Middle.** Typically presents with moderate vomiting, moderate distention, and intermittent pain (crescendo, colicky) with free intervals. (C) **Low.** Marked by late, feculent vomiting, marked distention, and variable pain that may not be of the classic crescendo type. (Reproduced with permission from Doherty GM. *Current Diagnosis & Treatment: Surgery,* 13th ed. New York: McGraw-Hill, 2010, Fig. 29-4.)

KEY FACT

Nonstrangulated SBO carries a total mortality of roughly 2%, whereas the risk of death from strangulated SBO ↑ in proportion to time from diagnosis to operative therapy, with a peak of ~ 25%.

A

This is likely postoperative ileus, although you should consider a possible obstruction as well. Start with conservative treatment, including NPO, NG decompression, and IV hydration.

Workup

- **Labs:** CBC (leukocytosis = strangulation), **electrolytes** (patients often have K^+ and Na^+ abnormalities due to dehydration or metabolic alkalosis due to vomiting).
- **Imaging:** Upright KUB shows a **stepladder** pattern of **dilated small bowel loops** and **air-fluid levels** (see Figure 9-4). It is possible to see an **absence of colon gas** as well. CT of the abdomen/pelvis is often used to find the etiology of SBO.

Treatment

- **Medical management:** Appropriate for partial SBO in stable patients. Includes NPO, NG tube decompression, IV hydration, correction of electrolyte abnormalities, and pain management.
- **Surgical management:**
  - Appropriate for complete SBO, vascular compromise, hemodynamic instability, or SBO of > 3 days' duration without resolution.
  - Exploratory laparotomy may be performed with lysis of adhesions, resection of necrotic bowel, and running the bowel (inspection of the entire length of bowel) with evaluation for stricture, tumor, IBD, and hernias.

LARGE BOWEL DISEASE

Diverticular Disease

Prevalent in 35–50% of the general population; more common in the elderly and in industrialized nations. Risk factors include a low-fiber diet, chronic

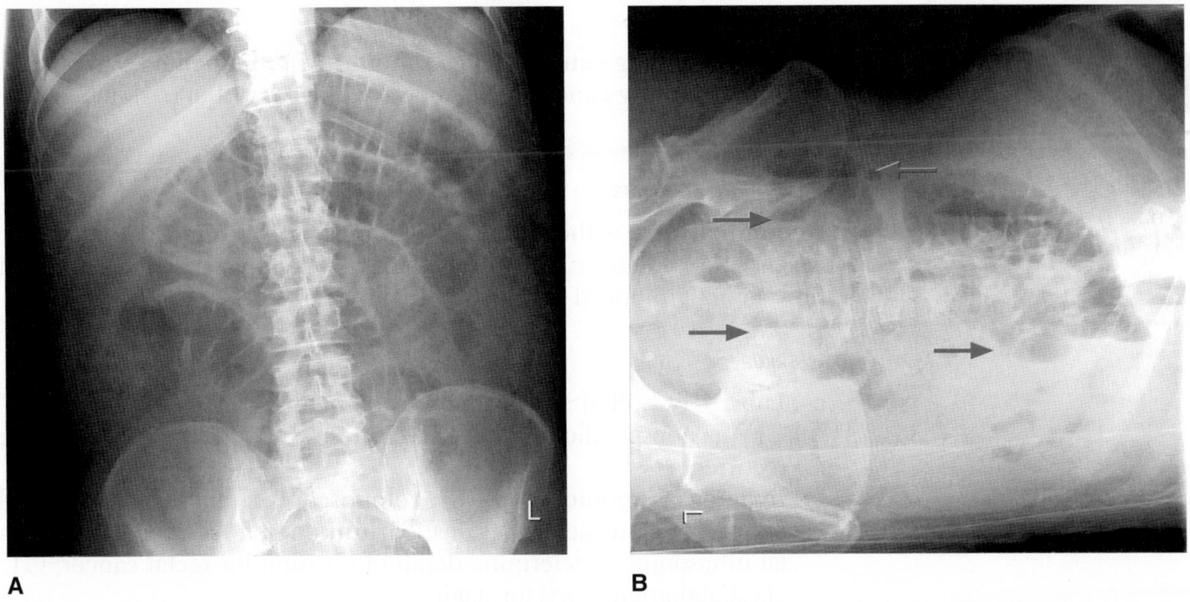

FIGURE 9-4. Complete small bowel obstruction. (A) Supine AXR shows dilated air-filled small bowel loops with relatively little gas in the colon. (B) Left lateral decubitus film on the same patient demonstrates multiple air-fluid levels (arrows) at different levels. (Reproduced with permission from Doherty GM. *Current Diagnosis & Treatment: Surgery,* 13th ed. New York: McGraw-Hill, 2010, Fig. 29-5.)

constipation, and a ⊕ family history. Distinguished as follows (see also Table 9-2):

- **Diverticulosis:** Herniation of the mucosa and submucosa through the muscular layer, forming **false, or pulsion, diverticula.** Caused by weakness in the bowel wall at areas where blood vessels enter and leave the colon as well as by ↑ intraluminal pressure. Most commonly found in the **sigmoid portion** (95%) with sparing of the rectum.
- **Diverticulitis:** Inflammation of a diverticulum that may lead to perforation and typically results in peritonitis.

KEY FACT

Massive LGIB is common with diverticulosis but rare with diverticulitis. Colonoscopy and barium enema are contraindicated in diverticulitis in light of the risk of perforation.

TABLE 9-2. Diverticulosis vs. Diverticulitis

VARIABLE	DIVERTICULOSIS	DIVERTICULITIS
Symptoms	Often **painless** (80%); presents with rectal bleeding.	**LLQ pain;** constipation or diarrhea; fever, chills, anorexia, nausea/vomiting.
Workup	↓ hematocrit due to bleeding. Barium enema and/or colonoscopy.	↑ WBC count. AXR reveals ileus, air-fluid levels, or free air if perforated. CT is the study of choice. **Barium enema/colonoscopy are contraindicated.**
Treatment	**High-fiber diet;** stool softeners; resuscitation in the presence of massive bleeding.	**Mild:** IV fluids; bowel rest; broad-spectrum antibiotics. **Severe:** If emergent, resection of bowel and creation of colostomy and a Hartmann pouch. If elective, resection of bowel and a 1° anastomosis. **Surgery should be considered after the second episode in light of the high recurrence rate.**

Colorectal Cancer

The **third leading cause of cancer mortality** in the United States after breast, prostate, and lung cancer. Incidence ↑ with age, with a peak incidence at 70–80 years.

KEY FACT

The 3 most common causes of cancer incidence in the United States are breast cancer (women) and prostate cancer (men), lung cancer, and colorectal cancer.

Signs and Symptoms

Abdominal pain is the most common presenting complaint, although in the absence of screening, colorectal cancer typically presents symptomatically only after a prolonged period of silent growth (see Figure 9-5 and Table 9-3).

Workup

- **Labs:** CBC often shows microcytic anemia; stool is ⊕ for occult blood; CEA is nonspecific but is useful for follow-up after treatment to screen for recurrence.
- **Imaging: Sigmoidoscopy or colonoscopy** should be performed with biopsy of all suspicious lesions; **barium enema** (see Figure 9-6); transrectal ultrasound to determine depth of invasion for rectal cancer; CT of the chest/abdomen/pelvis for staging.

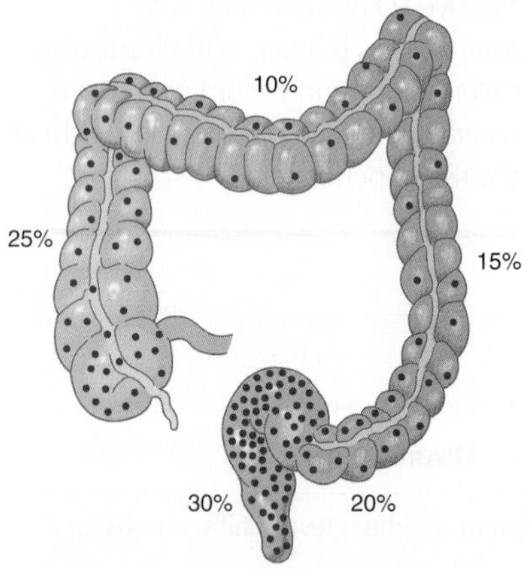

FIGURE 9-5. Distribution of cancer of the colon and rectum. (Reproduced with permission from Doherty GM. *Current Diagnosis & Treatment: Surgery,* 13th ed. New York: McGraw-Hill, 2010, Fig. 30-7.)

KEY POINT

RISK FACTORS AND SCREENING FOR COLORECTAL CANCER

- **Risk factors:**
  - **Age.**
  - **Hereditary syndromes: Familial adenomatous polyposis** (100% risk), hereditary nonpolyposis colorectal cancer (HNPCC).
  - **Family history.**
  - **IBD:** Ulcerative colitis >> Crohn's disease.
  - **Adenomatous polyps:** Villous polyps progress more often than tubular polyps, and sessile more often than pedunculated.
  - A past history of colorectal cancer.
  - A high-fat, low-fiber diet.
- **Methods of screening:**
  - A **DRE with a fecal occult blood test (FOBT)** should be performed yearly after age 50. Up to 10% of lesions are palpable with a finger, and up to 50% of guaiac-⊕ tests are due to colorectal cancer.
  - **Flexible sigmoidoscopy** should be performed every 5 years after age 50. It is possible to visualize and biopsy 50–75% of lesions with sigmoidoscopy.
  - **Colonoscopy** is indicated every 10 years starting at age 50.
  - For patients with multiple risk factors or a ⊕ family history, **screening may need to be done at an earlier age.**

TABLE 9-3. Presenting Symptoms of Colorectal Cancer by Location

Location of Lesion	Mass Characteristics	Common Presenting Symptoms
Right-sided lesions	Bulky, fungating, ulcerating masses.	**Anemia** from chronic occult blood loss. Weight loss, anorexia, weakness. Obstruction is rare.
Left-sided lesions	**"Apple-core"** obstructing mass (see Figure 9-6).	Obstruction, since feces in the left colon are more solid and the wall is less distensible. Change in bowel habits.
Rectal lesions	Can coexist with hemorrhoids.	**BRBPR.** Rectal pain, tenesmus.

- **Metastatic workup:** LFTs, CXR, CT of the chest/abdomen/pelvis, brain MRI. Metastases may arise from the following:
  - **Hematogenous spread:** Blood-borne metastases commonly go to the liver (40–50% of cases), lungs, bone, and brain.
  - **Lymphatic spread:** Pelvic lymph nodes are often affected.
  - **Direct extension:** Local viscera.
  - **Peritoneal spread.**

TREATMENT

- **Colonic lesions:**
  - Surgical resection of the lesion with 3- to 5-cm bowel margins.
  - Resection of the lymphatic drainage and mesentery at the origin of the arterial supply.
  - 1° anastomosis of bowel can usually be performed.
- **Rectal lesions:**
  - **Abdominoperineal resection:** For **low-lying lesions** near the anal verge, remove the rectum and anus, and provide a permanent colostomy.

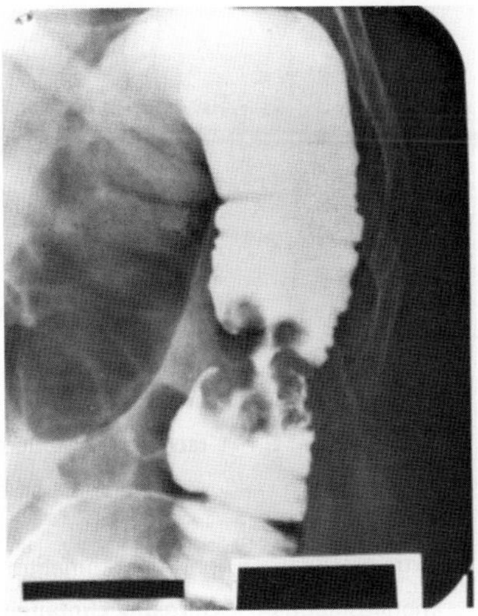

FIGURE 9-6. Colorectal cancer. Barium enema x-ray shows the classic "apple-core" lesion of an encircling carcinoma in the descending colon. Note the loss of mucosal pattern and the "hooks" at the margins of the lesion due to undermining. (Reproduced with permission from Way LW, Doherty GM. *Current Surgical Diagnosis & Treatment,* 11th ed. New York: McGraw-Hill, 2003.)

KEY POINT

DUKES' STAGING (ASTLER-COLLER MODIFICATION)

Dukes' staging has been supplanted by TNM staging but is still a favorite pimp topic.

Stage	Description	Five-Year Survival
A	Tumor limited to submucosa	> 90%
B1	Tumor invades into muscularis propria	70–80%
B2	Tumor invades through muscularis propria	50–65%
C1	B1 plus nodes	40–55%
C2	B2 plus nodes	20–30%
D	Distant metastasis/unresectable local spread	< 5%

KEY FACT

The most common metastatic locations for colorectal cancer are liver, lungs, and bone.

KEY FACT

Any lesion > 3 cm must be removed!

- **Low anterior resection:** For **proximal lesions,** perform a 1° anastomosis of the colon to the rectum.
- **Wide local excision:** For small, low-stage, well-differentiated tumors in the lower one-third of the rectum.
- **Adjuvant therapy:**
  - Chemotherapy is indicated in cases of colon cancer with ⊕ lymph nodes.
  - In contrast to its role in rectal cancer, radiation has proven ineffective for colon cancer.
- **Follow-up:** LFTs, serial CEA levels, colonoscopy, CXR, CT of the chest/abdomen/pelvis (for metastases).

TABLE 9-4. Crohn's Disease vs. Ulcerative Colitis

VARIABLE	ULCERATIVE COLITIS	CROHN'S DISEASE
Site of involvement	The **rectum** is always involved. May extend proximally in a **continuous fashion.** Inflammation and ulceration are **limited to the mucosa and submucosa.**	May involve **any portion** of the GI tract, particularly the **ileocecal region,** in a discontinuous pattern ("skip lesions"). The rectum is often spared. **Transmural** inflammation.
Signs and symptoms	**Bloody diarrhea,** lower abdominal cramps, tenesmus, urgency. Examination may reveal orthostatic hypotension, tachycardia, abdominal tenderness, frank blood on rectal examination, and extraintestinal manifestations.	Abdominal pain, abdominal mass, low-grade fever, weight loss, watery diarrhea. Examination may reveal fever, abdominal tenderness or mass, **perianal fissures, fistulas,** and extraintestinal manifestations.
Extraintestinal manifestations	Aphthous stomatitis, episcleritis/uveitis, arthritis, **1° sclerosing cholangitis, toxic megacolon,** erythema nodosum, pyoderma gangrenosum.	Same as ulcerative colitis, as well as nephrolithiasis and **fistulas** to the skin, biliary tract, or urinary tract or between bowel loops.
Workup	CBC, AXR, stool cultures, O&P, stool assay for *C difficile.* Colonoscopy can show diffuse and continuous rectal involvement, friability, edema, and **pseudopolyps.** Definitive diagnosis can be made with biopsy.	Same laboratory workup as ulcerative colitis. Colonoscopy may show aphthoid, linear, or stellate ulcers, strictures, **"cobblestoning,"** and **"skip lesions."** "Creeping fat" may also be present. Definitive diagnosis can be made with biopsy.
Treatment	**Sulfasalazine** or **5-ASA** (mesalamine); corticosteroids and immunosuppressants for refractory disease. **Total colectomy is curative** for long-standing or fulminant colitis or toxic megacolon. Symptoms can actually improve with **smoking,** but don't recommend this to your patients!	**Sulfasalazine;** corticosteroids and immunosuppression are indicated if no improvement is seen. Surgical resection may be necessary for suspected perforation, stenosis, fistula, abscess, or severe bleeding. **May recur** anywhere in the GI tract.
Incidence of cancer	**Markedly ↑ risk of colorectal cancer** in long-standing cases. Monitor with frequent FOBTs and colonoscopy after 8 years of disease.	The incidence of 2° malignancy is much lower than in ulcerative colitis.

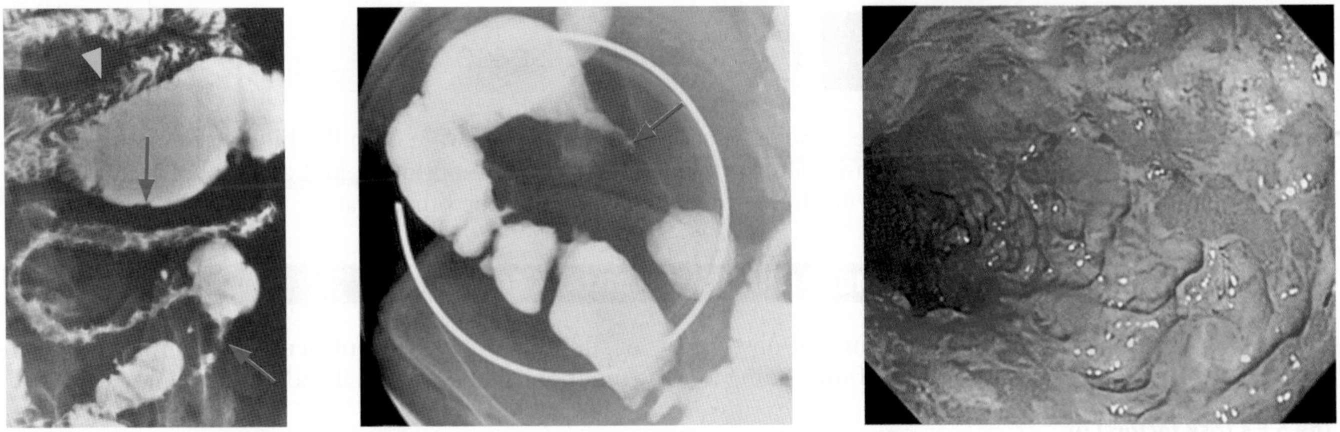

A B C

FIGURE 9-7. Crohn's disease. (**A**) Small bowel follow-through (SBFT) barium study shows skip areas of narrow small bowel with nodular mucosa (arrows) and ulceration. Compare with normal small bowel (arrowhead). (**B**) Spot compression image from SBFT shows "string sign" narrowing (arrow) due to stricture. (**C**) Deep ulcers in the colon of a patient with Crohn's disease, seen at colonoscopy. (Image A reproduced with permission from Chen MY et al. *Basic Radiology,* 1st ed. New York: McGraw-Hill, 2004, Fig. 10-30. Image B reproduced with permission from USMLERx.com. Image C reproduced with permission from Fauci AS et al. *Harrison's Principles of Internal Medicine,* 17th ed. New York: McGraw-Hill, 2008, Fig. 285-4B.)

INFLAMMATORY BOWEL DISEASE (IBD)

A chronic, often progressive inflammatory disease of the small bowel, colon, and rectum. The 2 principal disorders, Crohn's disease and ulcerative colitis, differ in their histologic and clinical manifestations, their natural course, and their modes of therapy (see Table 9-4 and Figures 9-7 and 9-8).

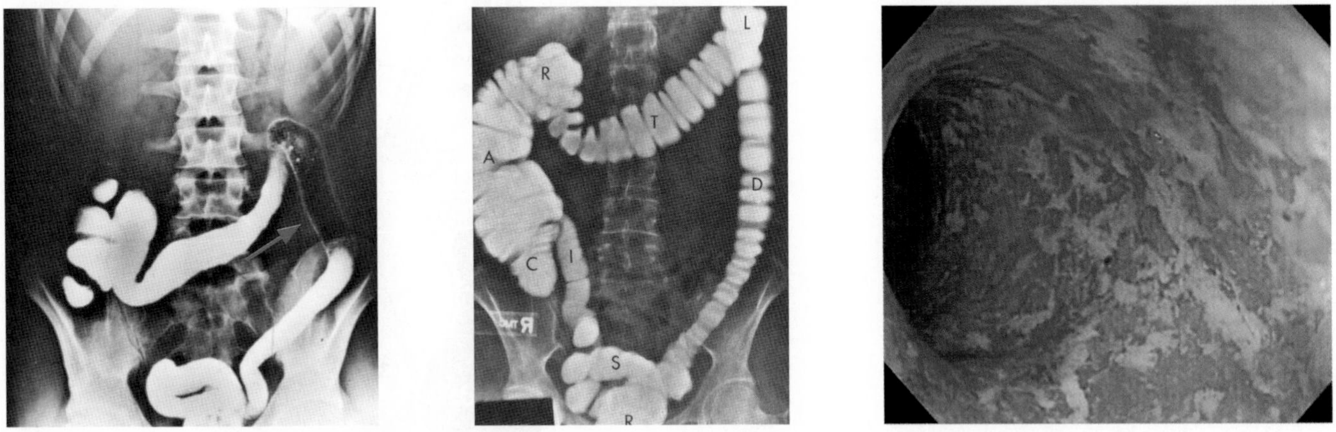

A B C

FIGURE 9-8. Ulcerative colitis. (**A**) Radiograph from a barium enema showing a featureless "lead pipe" colon with small mucosal ulcerations (arrow). (**B**) Compare with normal haustral markings. (**C**) Diffuse mucosal ulcerations and exudates at colonoscopy in chronic ulcerative colitis. (Image A reproduced with permission from Doherty GM. *Current Diagnosis & Treatment: Surgery,* 13th ed. New York: McGraw-Hill, 2010, Fig. 30-17. Image B reproduced with permission from Chen MY et al. *Basic Radiology,* 1st ed. New York: McGraw-Hill, 2004, Fig. 10-10A. Image C reproduced with permission from Fauci AS et al. *Harrison's Principles of Internal Medicine,* 17th ed. New York: McGraw-Hill, 2008, Fig 285-4A.)

Hepatobiliary Disease

The 4 major disease processes to be aware of in the biliary system are cholelithiasis, acute cholecystitis, choledocholithiasis, and acute cholangitis. Figure 9-9 illustrates the basic anatomy of the biliary tract.

CHOLELITHIASIS AND BILIARY COLIC

Transient obstruction of the cystic duct **without acute inflammation or infection** leading to recurrent bouts of postprandial abdominal pain.

Signs and Symptoms

- **Postprandial abdominal pain** (usually in the RUQ) radiating to the right subscapular area or epigastrium. Pain is typically abrupt in onset with gradual relief and is self-limited but recurrent.
- Nausea and vomiting.
- Fatty food intolerance, dyspepsia, bloating, and flatulence are also common.
- Gallstones may be **asymptomatic in up to 80%** of patients.

Differential

Acute cholecystitis, PUD, pancreatitis, GERD, appendicitis, hepatitis, MI.

MNEMONIC

The 5 F's (risk factors) of cholelithiasis:

Female
Fat
Fertile
Forty
Flatulent

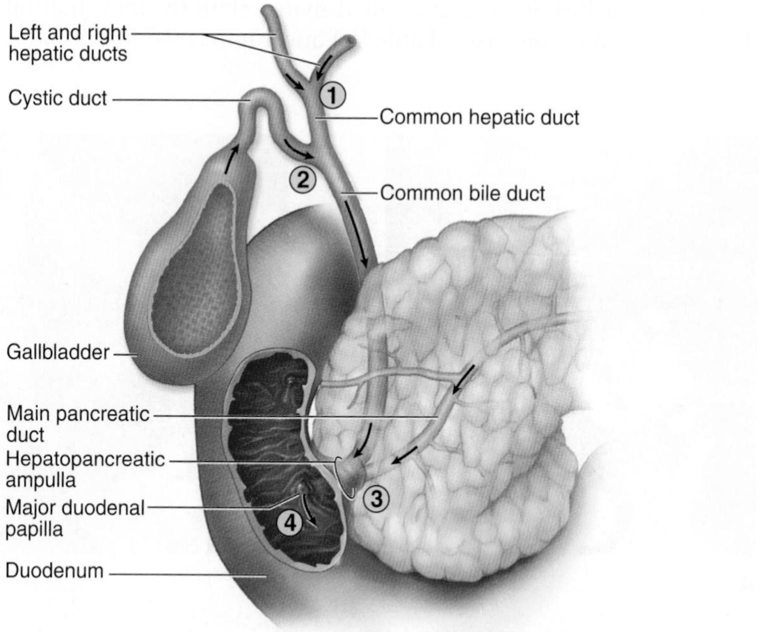

FIGURE 9-9. Anatomy of the biliary tract. Bile leaves the liver in the left and right hepatic ducts, which merge (1) to form the common hepatic duct, which connects to the cystic duct serving the gallbladder. The 2 ducts merge (2) to form a common bile duct (CBD). The main pancreatic duct merges with the CBD at the hepatopancreatic ampulla (3), which enters the wall of the duodenum. Bile and pancreatic juices are secreted from the major duodenal papilla into the duodenal lumen (4). (Reproduced with permission from Mescher AL. *Junqueira's Basic Histology: Text and Atlas,* 12th ed. New York: McGraw-Hill, 2010, Fig. 16-20.)

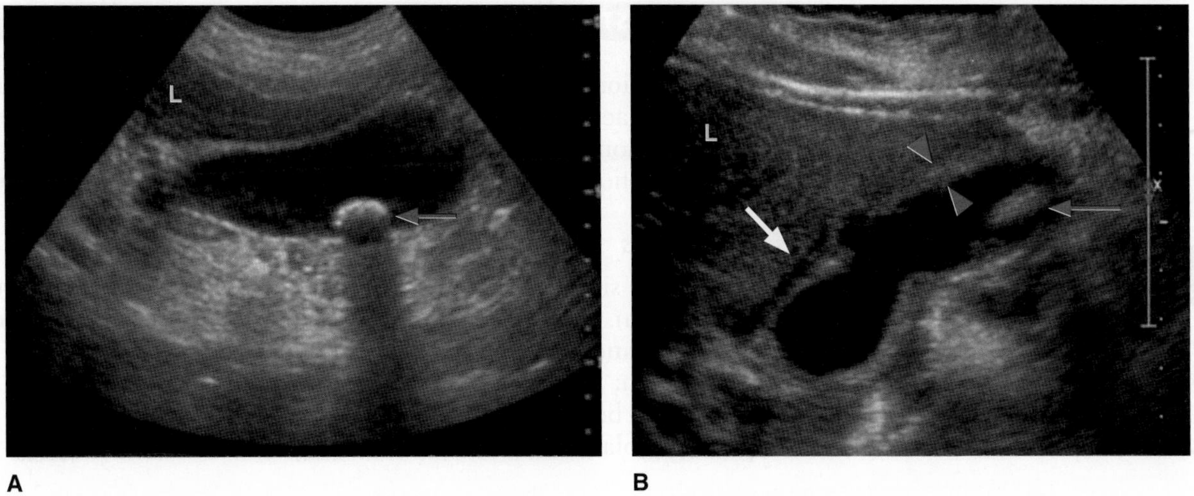

FIGURE 9-10. Gallstone disease. (A) **Cholelithiasis.** Ultrasound image of the gallbladder shows a gallstone (arrow) with posterior shadowing. (B) **Acute cholecystitis.** Ultrasound image shows a gallstone (red arrow), a thickened gallbladder wall (arrowheads), and pericholecystic fluid (white arrow). L = liver. (Reproduced with permission from USMLERx.com.)

Workup

- **Labs:** CBC, electrolytes, amylase, lipase, LFTs, bilirubin.
- **Imaging: RUQ ultrasound** may show gallstones (90% sensitive), a dilated bile duct, and thickness of the gallbladder wall (see Figure 9-10A). Plain x-rays are rarely diagnostic (only 10–15% of stones are radiopaque).
- CXR and ECG to rule out cardiopulmonary processes.

Treatment

- Dietary modification (avoid triggering substances such as fatty foods).
- Ursodiol (Actigall) desaturates the bile, impairing cholesterol nidus formation. Effective in only 15% of patients; reserved for patients who are not surgical candidates.
- Lithotripsy uses extracorporeal shock waves to break up stones and is followed by dissolution therapy of the small fragments.
- **Cholecystectomy** (usually laparoscopic) represents definitive and curative therapy.

KEY POINT

ESSENTIALS OF GALLSTONES

Stone formation requires (1) imbalance of the ratio of cholesterol/lecithin/bile salts, (2) a nucleating nidus, and (3) stasis. Subtypes include:

- **Cholesterol stones (80%):** Radiolucent and arise when bile becomes supersaturated with cholesterol, leading to cholesterol precipitation.
- **Pigmented stones (20%):** Radiopaque.
  - **Black stones:** Contain calcium bilirubinate and are caused by hyperbilirubinemia due to chronic hemolysis or cirrhosis.
  - **Brown stones:** Associated with biliary tract infection and may have gram-⊖ bacteria in their core.

KEY FACT

Only 10–15% of gallstones are radiopaque.

Q

A 42-year-old obese woman with a history of multiple prior gallstones presents with postprandial abdominal pain and jaundice. CT imaging shows a rim of calcification along the gallbladder. What does this signify?

ACUTE CHOLECYSTITIS

Acute inflammation of the gallbladder caused by stone impaction in the cystic duct. May be accompanied by sepsis, gallbladder necrosis, or abscess formation. Obstruction of the cystic duct leads to gallbladder distention, inflammation, and infection.

Signs and Symptoms

- Symptoms are similar to those of biliary colic but are more severe and of longer duration. These include nausea/vomiting, RUQ pain and **abdominal guarding and/or rebound tenderness** +/– fever/chills, and jaundice.
- **Murphy's sign:** Inspiratory arrest with subcostal palpation (30–98% sensitive). Can also be elicited during ultrasound.
- **Palpable gallbladder.**

KEY FACT

Murphy's sign is arrest of inspiration while palpating or placing an ultrasound probe on the RUQ.

Differential

Biliary colic, cholangitis, pancreatitis, PUD, GERD, hepatitis, appendicitis, renal colic, MI, pneumonia.

Workup

- **Labs:** CBC (leukocytosis), electrolytes, amylase, lipase, **LFTs, bilirubin** (often with mild hyperbilirubinemia).
- **Imaging: RUQ ultrasound** often shows stones, biliary sludge, pericholecystic fluid, and a thickened gallbladder wall (see Figure 9-10B).
- **HIDA scan** to assess the patency of the cystic duct and, after cholecystokinin (CCK) administration, gallbladder ejection fraction (normal > 35%). A ⊕ HIDA usually indicates cholecystitis.

KEY FACT

Ultrasound is the gold standard for the diagnosis of gallstones. Ultrasound and physical examination are the gold standards for cholecystitis. HIDA or CT is used when ultrasound is equivocal.

Treatment

- NPO, IV fluids.
- **IV antibiotics** (often piperacillin/tazobactam, ampicillin/sulbactam, or meropenem). Commonly associated bacteria include *E coli*, *Bacteroides fragilis*, *Klebsiella*, *Enterococcus*, and *Pseudomonas*.
- **Cholecystectomy** (commonly laparoscopic) should be done after the 1° inflammation has subsided, typically within 72 hours.

Complications

Abscess formation (15–20%), sepsis/perforation, gallbladder gangrene, gallstone ileus.

CHOLEDOCHOLITHIASIS

The presence of gallstones in the **common bile duct** can lead to cholangitis, pancreatitis, biliary colic, and/or jaundice.

Signs and Symptoms

RUQ pain, abdominal tenderness, biliary colic, jaundice.

Workup

- **Labs:** CBC, electrolytes, amylase, lipase, LFTs (may show only ↑ **alkaline phosphatase**), bilirubin.
- **Imaging: RUQ ultrasound** often shows bile duct dilatation but is only 15–30% sensitive for demonstrating common bile duct stones. **MRCP** and CT are also useful diagnostic modalities.

A

This is indicative of porcelain gallbladder, which is highly associated with malignancy. Treatment includes surgical cholecystectomy and wedge resection of the liver adjacent to the gallbladder.

TREATMENT

- **ERCP** with sphincterotomy and stone removal (both diagnostic and therapeutic).
- Mechanical lithotripsy.
- Extracorporeal shock wave lithotripsy.

ACUTE CHOLANGITIS

A potentially **life-threatening** infection caused by gallstone or biliary sludge blockage of the common bile duct; can lead to severe septic shock without early intervention. Etiologies include the following:

- **Obstruction** due to common bile duct stones, stricture, or neoplasm.
- **Infection** by gram-⊖ bacteria (*E coli, Klebsiella, Pseudomonas, Enterobacter, Proteus, Serratia*).

SIGNS AND SYMPTOMS

- **Charcot's triad:** RUQ pain, fever, and jaundice (the complete triad is present in only 20% of patients).
- **Reynolds' pentad:** Charcot's triad plus shock and altered mental status.

> **KEY FACT**
>
> Charcot's triad consists of RUQ pain, fever, and jaundice and is pathognomonic for acute cholangitis.

DIFFERENTIAL

Cholecystitis, pancreatitis, hepatitis, sepsis.

WORKUP

- **Labs:** CBC (leukocytosis), electrolytes, amylase, lipase, LFTs (↑ **alkaline phosphatase**), ↑ **bilirubin** (direct >> indirect). Blood cultures are ⊕ in ~ 50% of cases.
- **Imaging: Ultrasound** reveals ductal dilatation and gallstones (95% sensitivity). **MRCP** can best visualize the common bile duct.

TREATMENT

- IV hydration, electrolyte repletion, antibiotics.
- Bile duct decompression via endoscopic sphincterotomy, percutaneous transhepatic drainage, or operative decompression.

HEPATOCELLULAR CARCINOMA (HCC)

Formerly known as **hepatoma,** HCC is the most common 1° malignancy of the liver. Risk factors include HBV and HCV, cirrhosis, aflatoxin from *Aspergillus flavus*, hemochromatosis, liver fluke infection, and anabolic steroid use.

SIGNS AND SYMPTOMS

Presents with dull RUQ abdominal pain, **painful hepatomegaly,** weight loss, ascites, jaundice, consequences of portal hypertension, fever, and anemia.

DIFFERENTIAL

Metastatic disease, hepatocellular adenoma, hemangioma, cirrhosis.

WORKUP

- **Labs:** CBC, electrolytes, LFTs, **elevated α-fetoprotein** (AFP).
- **Imaging:** Ultrasound, CT, and MRI are all commonly used for initial diagnosis and follow-up.

KEY FACT

The most common site of metastasis for HCC is the lungs.

- Often treated without tissue diagnosis. Can be treated clinically if the patient is cirrhotic or has hepatitis, the patient has an elevated AFP, and imaging is consistent with HCC.

TREATMENT

- **Surgical** options include resection (ie, lobectomy) or liver transplantation.
- If the patient is not a surgical candidate, other treatment choices include **percutaneous** (ethanol injection, radiofrequency ablation, cryoablation) and **intra-arterial** (embolization +/– chemotherapy) techniques.

Pancreatic Disease

ACUTE PANCREATITIS

MNEMONIC

Causes of acute pancreatitis–

I GET SMASHED

Idiopathic
Gallstones (can obstruct pancreatic outflow—40%)
Ethanol (30%)
Trauma
Steroids
Mumps and other viruses (EBV, CMV)
Autoimmune disease (SLE, polyarteritis nodosa)
Scorpion sting, **S**nake or **S**pider bites
Hypercalcemia, **H**yperlipidemia, **H**yperparathyroidism
ERCP
Drugs (NSAIDs, diuretics, estrogens)

Acute inflammation of the pancreas. Etiologies are described in the mnemonic **I GET SMASHED.**

SIGNS AND SYMPTOMS

- **Epigastric abdominal pain** often **radiating to the back** (present in 90% of cases), nausea/vomiting, fever.
- Dehydration, hypovolemia, tachycardia, tachypnea, hypotension, and shock.
- An **abdominal mass** may be suggestive of a pseudocyst, abscess, or phlegmon.
- Dullness over the left lower lung suggests a pleural effusion or pseudocyst.
- **Grey Turner's sign:** Ecchymotic discoloration of the flank from pancreatic hemorrhage; seen in 1–2% of cases.
- **Cullen's sign:** Ecchymosis of the periumbilical area from pancreatic hemorrhage; seen in 1–2% of cases.

KEY FACT

The 2 most common causes of acute pancreatitis are gallstones and alcohol.

DIFFERENTIAL

Perforated peptic ulcer, cholecystitis, appendicitis, mesenteric ischemia, SBO, hepatitis, nephrolithiasis, pyelonephritis, MI, ruptured AAA.

KEY FACT

Lipase is more specific than amylase.

KEY FACT

There is no evidence to support daily measurement of amylase and lipase!

WORKUP

- **Labs:** CBC (moderate leukocytosis), electrolytes, LFTs, PT/PTT, **serum amylase and lipase levels typically 3 times the upper limit of normal.**
- **Imaging:**
  - **CT:** Indicated in severe cases to monitor for complications, such as pancreatic necrosis, abscesses, and pseudocysts. This should be done 2–3 days after admission.
  - **CXR:** Shows basilar atelectasis indicative of a pleural effusion.
  - **AXR:** Shows sentinel loop or colon cutoff signs (a distended colon to the midtransverse colon with no air distally).
  - **Ultrasound:** Good for identifying pseudocyst, abscess, gallstones, and bile duct dilatation.

TREATMENT

Can be operative or nonoperative depending on the severity of the disease and on the presence of operable complications such as hemorrhage, pancreatic necrosis, or pseudocyst formation.

- **Medical management:**
  - NPO. Consider NG suction in cases with abdominal distention and/or emesis.
  - Fluid and electrolyte repletion.
  - **Pain control:** Meperidine (Demerol) may cause less spasm of the sphincter of Oddi than morphine (controversial) but is not typically used.
  - **Nutrition:** Patients may require TPN if they are to be NPO for more than several days.
  - Initiate **alcohol withdrawal prophylaxis** (benzodiazepines) if indicated.
  - There is no benefit to using antibiotics except in cases of pancreatic necrosis/abscess or sepsis.
- **Surgical management:**
  - **Pancreatic necrosis:** Surgical debridement.
  - **Noninfected pseudocysts:** Operative drainage via cystogastrostomy, cystojejunostomy, or cystoduodenostomy is performed if the patient is symptomatic. Otherwise, they are often left alone.
  - **Infected pseudocysts:** Must drain externally.
  - **Pancreatic hemorrhage:** Operative hemostasis or angiographic embolization.
  - **Gallstone pancreatitis:** ERCP and sphincterotomy with stone extraction followed by interval cholecystectomy (done after pancreatitis has resolved).

COMPLICATIONS

- The mortality rate for acute pancreatitis is 10–20%. The prognosis worsens with a higher **Ranson's score** (see Table 9-5) or coexistent hemorrhage, respiratory failure, or severe persistent hypocalcemia.
- Complications include pseudocyst (10%); DIC/hemorrhage; sepsis, ARDS, and renal failure; and pleural effusion.

TABLE 9-5. Ranson's Criteria[a]

On Admission	48 Hours After Admission
Age > 55 years	Hematocrit fall > 10%
WBC count > 16,000/mm^3	BUN rise > 5 mg/dL
SGOT (AST) > 250 IU/dL	Serum Ca^{2+} < 8 mg/dL
Serum LDH > 350 IU/L	Arterial Po_2 < 60 mm Hg
Blood glucose > 200 mg/dL	Estimated fluid sequestration > 6 L
	Base excess > 4 mEq/L

[a] The risk of mortality is 20% with 3–4 signs, 40% with 5–6 signs, and 100% with ≥ 7 signs.

Q

A 48-year-old woman presents with abdominal pain, fatigue, and unintentional weight loss. Imaging shows a hilar tumor at the junction of the left and right hepatic bile ducts. What is the diagnosis?

CHRONIC PANCREATITIS

Chronic inflammation of the pancreas with damage to the parenchyma, resulting in **endocrine and exocrine dysfunction.** Etiologies are outlined in the discussion of acute pancreatitis.

KEY FACT

The most common cause of chronic pancreatitis in the United States is alcohol abuse (70–80%).

Signs and Symptoms

Recurrent epigastric pain that often radiates to the back, weight loss, **steatorrhea** due to lipase insufficiency from destruction of the exocrine pancreas, **diabetes** due to insulin insufficiency from destruction of the endocrine pancreas.

Workup

- **Labs:** CBC, electrolytes, LFTs, PT/PTT, **amylase, lipase.**
- **Imaging: CT** is the preferred diagnostic test. KUB may reveal calcifications; ERCP/MRCP may show ductal dilatation and strictures ("chain of lakes" pattern).

Treatment

- **Medical management:** Similar to that of acute pancreatitis, plus insulin and pancreatic enzyme replacement in light of endocrine and exocrine dysfunction.
- **Surgical management:** Indicated after failure of medical therapy as well as failed ERCP with pancreatic sphincterotomy and endostent placement. Can include pancreatectomy or **pancreaticojejunostomy** for decompression of the pancreatic ducts.

PANCREATIC CANCER

Most often characterized by adenocarcinoma arising from the **duct cells.** Tumors are most often found in the **head of the pancreas.** The prognosis is very poor for these patients, with only a 15–25% 5-year survival rate. Risk factors include male gender, age > 65 years, smoking, diabetes, alcohol abuse, high-fat and high-protein diets, African American ethnicity, and industrial exposure.

Signs and Symptoms

- **Painless jaundice,** pruritus, dark urine, light stools, anorexia, weight loss, midepigastric abdominal pain, back pain.
- **Courvoisier's sign:** A nontender, distended gallbladder (50% of pancreatic cancer patients).

Workup

- **Labs:** CBC, electrolytes, LFTs, PT/PTT, amylase and lipase (often normal), **CEA, CA 19-9.**
- **Imaging:** CT, ERCP or MRCP, endoscopic ultrasound, staging laparoscopy or laparotomy.

A

This is a cholangiocarcinoma, or Klatskin's tumor. These uncommon tumors become symptomatic late in their development and often have a poor prognosis.

TREATMENT

- **Whipple procedure** (pancreaticoduodenectomy): For tumors in the head of the pancreas.
- **Distal pancreatectomy with splenectomy:** For tumors of the body and tail of the pancreas.
- **Unresectable disease:** Palliation of biliary obstruction with endoprosthesis, percutaneous catheter, or biliary bypass (hepaticojejunostomy or choledochojejunostomy).

Hernias

Defined as abnormal protrusions of structures through the tissues that normally contain them. Hernias are the most common surgical disease in men and are 8–9 times more common in males than in females.

INGUINAL HERNIA

Protrusion of abdominal contents (usually the small intestine) into the inguinal region through a weakness or defect in the inguinal floor or internal ring. Defined as direct or indirect according to their relationship to the inguinal anatomy (see Table 9-6).

> **KEY FACT**
>
> The most common hernia in both men and women is an indirect inguinal hernia.

COMPLICATIONS

- The recurrence rate after repair is 1–3% when mesh reinforcement is used.
- Risk factors for recurrence include excessive suture line tension, use of an absorbable suture, failure to properly identify the hernia sac, postoperative wound infection, and chronic conditions that ↑ intra-abdominal pressure (eg, constipation, morbid obesity, prostatism, chronic cough).

> **KEY FACT**
>
> Inguinal hernias occur much more often in men than in women.

TABLE 9-6. Direct vs. Indirect Inguinal Hernia

VARIABLE	DIRECT INGUINAL HERNIA	INDIRECT INGUINAL HERNIA
Definition	Herniation of abdominal contents through the **floor of Hesselbach's triangle** (see Figure 9-11).	Herniation of abdominal contents through the **internal inguinal ring** of the inguinal canal.
Defect	Acquired defect in the **transversalis fascia** from mechanical breakdown.	Congenital **patent processus vaginalis.**
Risk factors	Age.	The **most common hernia** in both men and women.
Characteristics	Does not traverse the internal inguinal ring. Herniates directly through the abdominal wall; contained within the aponeurosis of the external oblique muscle.	Traverses the external inguinal ring and ends up in the scrotum.
Treatment (surgical unless medically contraindicated)	Reduction or ligation of the hernia sac with repair of the defect in the transversalis fascia with Bassini repair, McVay repair, or, most commonly, mesh repair.	Isolation and high ligation of the hernia sac with repair or enlarged internal ring.

INGUINAL HERNIA ANATOMY AND KEY TERMS

- **Anatomy:**
  - **Layers of the abdominal wall:** Skin, subcutaneous fat, Scarpa's fascia, external oblique muscle, internal oblique muscle, transversus abdominis muscle, transversalis fascia, and peritoneum.
  - **Inguinal (Poupart's) ligament:** The thickened lower border of the aponeurosis of the external oblique muscle, which runs from the anterior superior iliac spine to the pubic tubercle on each side.
  - **Inferior epigastric artery:** The branch of the external iliac artery that supplies the lower portion of the abdominal wall.
  - **Hesselbach's triangle:** An area formed by the inguinal ligament inferiorly, the lateral border of the rectus abdominis muscle medially, and the inferior epigastric vessels laterally (see Figure 9-11).
  - **Superficial (external) inguinal ring:** A defect in the external oblique aponeurosis through which the spermatic cord or round ligament passes en route to the scrotum/labia majora.
  - **Deep (internal) inguinal ring:** A defect in the transversalis fascia lateral to Hesselbach's triangle through which the spermatic cord emerges from the peritoneal cavity.
- **Key terms:**
  - **Reducible hernia:** The contents of the hernia sac return to the abdomen with manual pressure.
  - **Incarceration:** The hernia cannot be reduced by external manipulation. Go to the OR urgently.
  - **Strangulation:** The blood supply to the contents of an incarcerated hernia is compromised, leading to ischemia. Go to the OR emergently!

KEY FACT

Femoral hernias occur more often in women than in men.

FEMORAL HERNIA

An abnormal protrusion of abdominal contents **through the femoral canal** medial to the femoral vein. More common in women (85%). Carries the **highest risk of incarceration and strangulation** owing to the narrow and unforgiving femoral canal, which is bordered superiorly by the inguinal ligament.

HIATAL HERNIA

Present in 80% of patients with **GERD.** Subtypes are as follows:

- **Type I: Sliding hiatal hernias** (> 90%):
  - The gastroesophageal junction and the fundus of the stomach are displaced into the mediastinum.

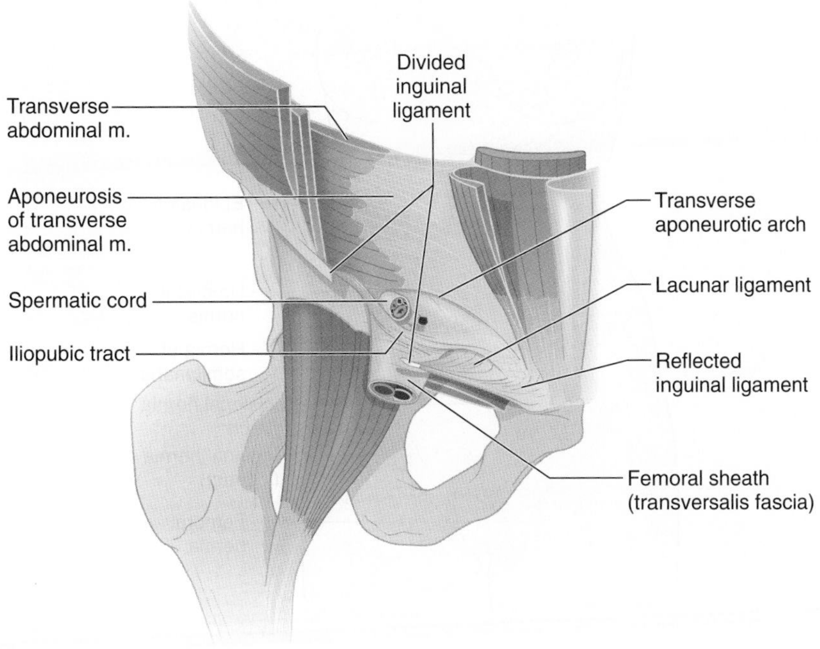

FIGURE 9-11. Hesselbach's triangle. (Reproduced with permission from Schwartz SI et al. *Principles of Surgery,* 7th ed. New York: McGraw-Hill, 1999: 1588.)

- **Signs/Sx:** Reflux, dysphagia, and esophagitis are common, but patients can be asymptomatic.
- **Tx:** Antacids, small meals, head elevation.

- **Type II: Paraesophageal hernias** (< 5%):
  - The fundus herniates alongside the esophagus while the gastroesophageal junction remains in a normal position.
  - **Tx/Cx:** Incarceration and strangulation are common complications, and surgical repair is therefore indicated.

OTHER HERNIAS

Figure 9-12 shows the location of other common hernias.

- **Ventral hernia:** Commonly occurs along the midline of the abdominal wall.
- **Incisional hernia:** Ventral hernias that occur at the site of previous abdominal surgery.
- **Umbilical hernia:** Occur beneath or near the navel. Do not repair in children < 3 years of age, as 90% will spontaneously close.
- **Sliding hernia:** One wall of the inguinal hernia sac is formed by a viscus (cecum or sigmoid colon).
- **Pantaloon hernia:** A combination of a direct and an indirect inguinal hernia.
- **Richter's hernia:** Only one wall of the bowel (antimesenteric) lies within the hernia sac.
- **Spigelian hernia:** A ventral hernia occurring at the junction of the semilunar line and the lateral edge of the rectus muscle.
- **Littre's hernia:** The hernia sac contains Meckel's diverticulum.

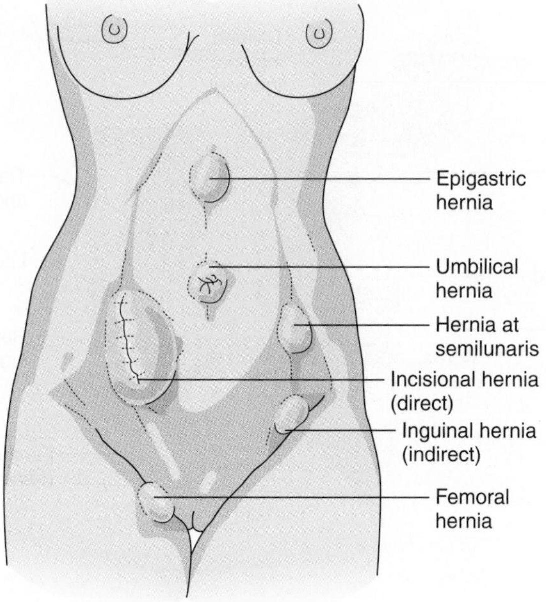

FIGURE 9-12. Locations of hernias. (Reproduced with permission from DeCherney AH, Nathan L. *Current Diagnosis & Treatment: Obstetrics & Gynecology,* 10th ed. New York: McGraw-Hill, 2007, Fig. 2-10.)

Vascular Surgery

ABDOMINAL AORTIC ANEURYSM (AAA)

Abnormal dilation of the abdominal aorta that develops from weakness or a defect in the wall of the vessel. Most AAAs are infrarenal. Risk factors include atherosclerosis, hypertension, smoking, age > 60 years, and male gender.

> **KEY FACT**
>
> The most common cause of AAA is atherosclerosis.

SIGNS AND SYMPTOMS

Often asymptomatic. May present with **abdominal pain radiating to the back** or a **pulsatile abdominal mass** in the midepigastrium or LUQ. Hypotension is also seen with rupture.

DIFFERENTIAL

Aortic dissection, MI, pancreatitis, diverticulosis, renal colic.

WORKUP

- AXR may demonstrate a calcified outline of the AAA.
- **Ultrasound** is the best test for screening and follow-up of known small AAAs.
- CT is appropriate only for **hemodynamically stable patients.** Contrast allows full evaluation of aneurysmal size and possible dissection.
- ECG and tests of renal and pulmonary function to evaluate the risk of surgical repair.

> **KEY FACT**
>
> Risk of rupture with AAA:
> - **5 cm:** 5% per year
> - **6 cm:** 7% per year
> - **7 cm:** 15–20% per year

TREATMENT

- **Ruptured AAAs are surgical emergencies.**
- **Medical management:** BP control, IV access with 2 large-bore IVs, type and cross, supplemental O_2.

- **Surgical management:** Elective surgical repair to prevent rupture is indicated if the AAA is > **5 cm.** This is now more commonly done with endovascular stent graft placements rather than with traditional open prosthetic graft placement.
- The operative mortality rate for nonruptured AAAs is < 5%, whereas that for ruptured AAAs is > 50%.

PERIPHERAL VASCULAR DISEASE

Caused by occlusive atherosclerotic plaques in the lower extremities. The most commonly involved artery is the **superficial femoral artery** in the adductor (Hunter's) canal. Risk factors include atherosclerosis, hyperlipidemia, diabetes, smoking, and hypertension.

Signs and Symptoms

- **Claudication:** Reproducible leg pain on ambulation, with relief of the pain on resting. Rest pain represents a more severe progression of peripheral vascular disease.
- Absent pulses, impaired sensation, bruits, muscular atrophy, ↓ hair growth, impotence, tissue infection.

Workup

- The **ankle-brachial index (ABI)** measures the ratio of systolic BP at the ankle to that of the arm.
  - **ABI 1.0–1.2:** Normal.
  - **ABI 0.4–0.9:** Moderate arterial obstruction, often associated with claudication.
  - **ABI < 0.4:** Advanced ischemia.
  - **Note:** ABI is falsely elevated in DM owing to arterial calcification.
- **Doppler ultrasound.**

Treatment

- Exercise and dietary modification. **Smoking cessation** is critical to the long-term success of any vascular reconstruction.
- Treatment of hypertension; use of statins.
- Pentoxifylline can improve circulation by decreasing blood viscosity.
- If severe, treat with **bypass graft** (autologous vein or prosthetic), stent, or angioplasty. Consider **amputation** if all else fails.

ACUTE ARTERIAL OCCLUSION

Insufficient arterial blood flow to meet the metabolic demands of tissue can lead to limb-threatening ischemia. The most common site of occlusion is the common femoral artery. Etiologies include embolism, vascular trauma, and thrombosis of an atherosclerotic lesion.

Signs and Symptoms

Presents with the **"6 P's"** (see mnemonic) plus ischemic ulcers and limb gangrene.

Workup

ABI, Doppler ultrasound, CT angiography, MRI angiography.

KEY FACT

Rest pain typically occurs with an ABI < 0.4.

MNEMONIC

The 6 P's of acute arterial occlusion:

Pain
Paralysis
Pallor
Paresthesia
Poikilothermia
Pulselessness

Q

A 70-year-old man with a long-standing history of atrial fibrillation presents to the ED with postprandial abdominal pain. On examination, the physician notes that he has "pain out of proportion to the exam." What is the diagnosis and treatment?

TREATMENT

- Anticoagulation (ie, IV heparin).
- **Surgical thrombectomy/embolectomy or arterial bypass.** Compartment syndrome is a possible sequela to revascularization; check compartment pressures and perform fasciotomy if > 30 mm Hg. If this is clinically suspected, perform fasciotomy despite or even without pressure readings.
- Amputation.

KEY FACT

The most common cancer in women is breast cancer.

Breast Disease

BREAST CANCER

The most common cancer and the second most frequent cause of cancer death in women (next to lung cancer). Approximately 10% of women in the United States will be diagnosed with breast cancer during their lifetime. Although women are most commonly affected, a small number of men get breast cancer as well. Risk factors include the following:

KEY FACT

The most common cause of cancer death in women is lung cancer; breast cancer is the second leading cause.

- Female gender, increasing age, postmenopausal obesity.
- Early menarche (before age 12), late menopause (after age 50), nulliparity, first pregnancy after age 30.
- A previous history of breast cancer, ductal carcinoma in situ (DCIS), and/or lobular carcinoma in situ (LCIS).
- A history of ovarian/endometrial cancer.
- A ⊕ family history of breast cancer.
- BRCA 1/2 genes.

SIGNS AND SYMPTOMS

- A breast mass that does not change in size with menstrual cycle.
- Breast mass **tenderness.**
- Nipple discharge or retraction.
- A change in breast appearance, contour, or symmetry.

DIFFERENTIAL

- **Benign masses:** Well circumscribed, mobile, and tender; change in size with the menstrual cycle.
  - **Fibrocystic change (the most frequent breast lesion): Painful** (↑ before menses); fluctuate in size; often multiple/bilateral. Associated with an ↑ breast cancer risk only in the presence of ductal/atypical hyperplasia.
  - **Fibroadenomas:** Firm, round, mobile, and **nontender (the most common breast mass in women < 30 years of age).**
  - **Intraductal papilloma:** The most common cause of bloody nipple discharge.
  - **Other:** Lipoma, breast abscess, fat necrosis, mastitis.
- **Malignant masses:** Hard, irregular, and fixed; associated with nipple retraction, dimpling of the skin, edema, and lymphadenopathy (see Figure 9-13).
  - **Ductal carcinoma:** The **most common** breast malignancy (75% of breast cancer cases).
  - **Lobular carcinoma:** Approximately 8–10% of cases.

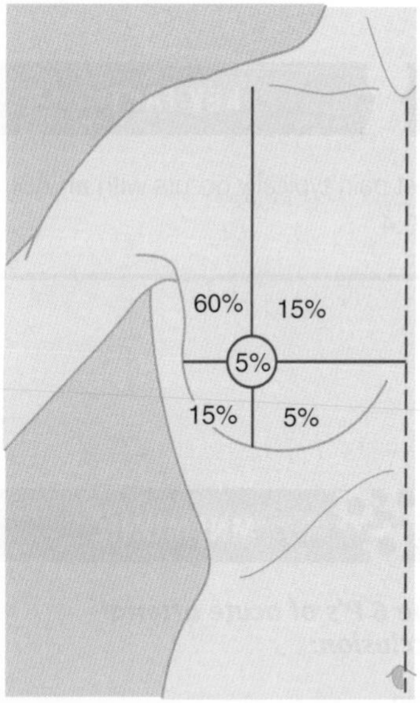

FIGURE 9-13. Frequency of breast cancer at various anatomic sites. (Reproduced with permission from McPhee SJ et al. *Current Medical Diagnosis & Treatment 2012.* New York: McGraw-Hill, 2012, Fig. 17-2.)

A

This is a classical presentation of acute mesenteric ischemia, which can be confirmed by angiography. Treatment includes papaverine vasodilation via angiography, embolectomy, and surgical bowel resection.

KEY POINT

BREAST CANCER SCREENING RECOMMENDATIONS

- Yearly **mammogram** starting at age 40.
- **Clinical breast examination** every 3 years for women 20–39 years of age; yearly for women ≥ 40 years of age.
- Women can optionally perform monthly breast self-examinations starting at age 20.

Note that these are the **American Cancer Society** guidelines, which differ slightly from those of the U.S. Preventive Services Task Force (USPSTF).

- **Paget's carcinoma:** Infiltrating ductal carcinoma in the nipple. Symptoms include itching/burning of the nipple with **superficial ulceration** or erosion.
- **Inflammatory carcinoma:** The most aggressive lesion; poorly differentiated and rapidly lethal. Symptoms include diffuse induration, warmth, erythema, edema, and axillary lymphadenopathy. **Peau d'orange,** or "orange peel" skin, is often seen.

KEY FACT

↑ exposure to estrogen, ↑ risk of breast cancer.

WORKUP

- Clinical breast examination.
- Diagnostic **mammography.**
- Ultrasound to further evaluate palpable masses.
- If the lesion is cystic on ultrasound, fluid aspiration with or without ultrasound guidance may be performed. If the lesion contains solid components, **fine-needle aspiration** (FNA) is performed.
- If FNA is nondiagnostic, perform **core needle biopsy.** This modality is far superior to FNA in that it provides histology of the mass (FNA provides only cytology).
- Excisional biopsy should be done only if FNA or core needle biopsy pathology is equivocal.
- Ductography and cytology are often performed for nipple discharge.

KEY FACT

Work up **all** breast nodules!

TREATMENT

- **Wide local excision (lumpectomy) plus radiation of remaining breast tissue:** Complete excision of the tumor with margins and axillary node dissection, followed by radiotherapy. Contraindicated in any of the following conditions:
  - A large cancer or a small breast.
  - Inability to obtain a ⊖ margin.
  - Diffuse microcalcifications.
  - Previous radiation to the breast.
- **Simple mastectomy:** Removal of the breast and nipple only. Can be used as prophylaxis, but does not represent adequate treatment of breast cancer.
- **Modified radical mastectomy:** Removal of the breast and nipple with axillary node dissection (spares the chest wall muscles).
- **Radical mastectomy:** Removal of the breast, nipple, axillary nodes, and chest wall muscles. No longer commonly used to treat breast cancer.
- **Adjuvant therapy:** Carried out to eliminate micrometastases responsible for late recurrence. Often depends on estrogen receptor (ER) status (see Table 9-7).

TABLE 9-7. Adjuvant Therapy in Breast Cancer

ER STATUS	≤ 1 CM WITHOUT NODES	> 1 CM WITHOUT NODES	⊕ NODES
ER ⊕	None	Tamoxifen + chemotherapy	Chemotherapy (+ tamoxifen if postmenopausal)
ER ⊖	None	Chemotherapy	Chemotherapy

Endocrine Disease

PHEOCHROMOCYTOMA

A tumor of the adrenal medulla that produces excess catecholamines. It follows the **rule of 10's** (see mnemonic). Risk factors include a ⊕ family history, MEN 2 syndrome, von Recklinghausen's disease, and von Hippel–Lindau disease.

MNEMONIC

Pheochromocytoma rule of 10's:

10% are malignant
10% are extra-adrenal
10% are bilateral
10% are familial

SIGNS AND SYMPTOMS

Presents with uncontrolled hypertension, palpitations, headache, episodic diaphoresis, flushing, and anxiety.

DIFFERENTIAL

Renovascular hypertension, carcinoid syndrome, hyperthyroidism, anxiety disorder.

WORKUP

- **Labs: Urine vanillylmandelic acid (VMA) and metanephrines;** urine and serum epinephrine and norepinephrine levels.
- **Imaging:** CT, MRI, and **MIBG scan** to highlight norepinephrine analog.

TREATMENT

Surgical resection with **perioperative α-blockade** (ie, phenoxybenzamine or prazosin) to ↓ catecholamine-induced vasoconstriction.

KEY POINT

MULTIPLE ENDOCRINE NEOPLASIA (MEN) SYNDROMES

- **MEN 1: P**arathyroid hyperplasia, **P**ancreatic islet cell tumors, **P**ituitary adenomas.
- **MEN 2A:** Thyroid medullary carcinoma, pheochromocytoma, parathyroid hyperplasia.
- **MEN 2B:** Thyroid medullary carcinoma, pheochromocytoma, mucosal neuromas, body habitus (thick lips, kyphosis, pectus excavatum).

Urologic Disease

PROSTATE CANCER

The most common visceral malignant neoplasm affecting U.S. males, with the risk of disease approximating 1 in 5 in that population. The mortality rate is decreasing, with a current annual risk of approximately 3%. Roughly 95% of masses are adenocarcinomas. Risk factors include increasing **age** (85% of diagnoses are made in patients > 65 years of age), African American ethnicity, a family history of prostate cancer, and dietary polyunsaturated fats.

Workup

- Localized prostate cancer rarely causes symptoms at earlier stages, as the disease usually occurs at the periphery of the gland away from the urethra.
- Conflicting data exist regarding the efficacy of early screening, so the decision to pursue testing should be made on an individual basis.
  - The American Urological Association recommends getting a **baseline PSA level and DRE starting at age 40.**
  - However, the USPSTF does not recommend using the PSA for screening in patients of any age, as the harms are viewed as outweighing the benefits.
- Abnormalities on DRE (nodularity, induration) or an elevated PSA (> 4 ng/mL) can prompt the use of prostate biopsy for histologic diagnosis.
- **Grading and staging:**
  - **Tumor grade:** Elucidated from prostate biopsy. The **Gleason grading system** classifies cancers by describing the low-magnification architecture of the biopsy specimen. The Gleason score is considered predictive of prognosis and disease extent.
  - **Tumor stage:** Most often classified by means of the TNM staging system; can be either clinical (using pretreatment parameters) or pathologic (determined following prostate removal and careful histologic analysis).

Treatment

- **Radical prostatectomy:** The gold standard for clinically localized disease, although there is some current debate. Usually performed by the retropubic approach.
  - Involves complete removal of the prostate gland and seminal vesicles along with modified pelvic lymph node dissection. Anatomic nerve-sparing dissection is performed if the surgeon is comfortable with the technique and disease is limited.
  - Complications include bleeding, impotence, incontinence, and rectal injury.
- **Radiation therapy:** Can be delivered by an external beam or through implantation of radioactive seeds **(brachytherapy).** Complications include functional urinary complaints, impotence, hematuria, strictures, and rectal complaints.
- **Androgen ablation:** Usually reserved for extraprostatic disease, cases of refractory disease, or patients who do not seek other modalities of treatment. Often used as neoadjuvant therapy in conjunction with surgery or radiation for T2 disease or as nonadjuvant 1° therapy for more progressive disease.

> **KEY FACT**
>
> Orthopedic emergencies:
> - Open fractures and dislocations.
> - Vascular or neural compromise.
> - Compartment syndrome.
> - Osteomyelitis and septic arthritis.
> - Hip dislocation with subsequent avascular necrosis.

> **KEY FACT**
>
> Pelvic fractures have the highest mortality.

> **KEY FACT**
>
> Common orthopedic injuries:
> - **Anterior shoulder dislocation:** Axillary nerve.
> - **Supracondylar humeral fracture:** Median nerve and brachial artery.
> - **Posterior knee dislocation:** Popliteal artery.
> - **Distal radius fracture:** Median nerve.
> - **Fibular neck fracture:** Common peroneal nerve.

> **KEY FACT**
>
> In melanoma, a poor prognosis is associated with lesions > 0.75 mm; lesions on the back, arms, neck, and scalp; and female gender.

Orthopedic Surgery

OPEN FRACTURES

Defined as fractures that are in continuity with the outside environment through some type of wound and are thus at high risk of infection. This is compared to a **closed fracture,** where there is intact skin over the site of fracture.

WORKUP

Radiographs with 2 views, including the **joints above and below the fracture.** Perform neurologic and vascular examinations.

TREATMENT

- Prophylactic antibiotics (typically cefazolin) and surgical debridement.
- **Open reduction** and stabilization though external fixation if needed.

Plastic Surgery

MELANOMA

The leading cause of death from skin disease. Risk factors include a personal or family history, fair skin, red or blond hair, a tendency to burn, a large number of benign nevi, and UV radiation.

SIGNS AND SYMPTOMS

Remember the mnemonic ABCDE:

- Asymmetry
- Border irregularity
- Color variation
- Diameter > 6 mm
- Evolution or Elevation

WORKUP

Full-thickness skin biopsy.

TREATMENT

Surgical resection with adequate margins (see Table 9-8).

TABLE 9-8. Staging of Melanoma and Surgical Margins

STAGE	DESCRIPTION	SURGICAL MARGINS
Tis	Tumor confined to epidermis	5 mm
T1	Tumor depth ≤ 1 mm	1 cm
T2	Tumor depth 1.01–2 mm	1–2 cm
T3	Tumor depth 2.01–4 mm	2 cm
T4	Tumor depth > 4 mm	> 2 cm

Common Clerkship Topics

The third-year surgery clerkship often involves time not only in general surgery but also in some of the surgical specialties. The following questions can help you focus on the specific topics at hand:

- What is the natural history and appropriate evaluation of the current surgical problem?
- How do surgeons make the decision to intervene and prioritize the various therapeutic options?
- How do surgeons evaluate the risks and benefits of those therapeutic options in the context of a patient's problems, overall status, and life expectancy?

Given these considerations, the following list outlines common diseases and key topics that you are likely to encounter in the course of your surgery rotation.

- **Gastrointestinal disease:**
  - Acute abdomen
  - Esophageal disorders (achalasia, esophageal varices, esophageal rupture, esophageal cancer)
  - Stomach disorders (gastritis, gastroenteritis, gastric cancer, GERD [see Internal Medicine], peptic ulcer disease [see Internal Medicine])
  - Upper and lower GI bleeding
  - Small bowel disease (small bowel obstruction)
    - Benign neoplasms (adenomas, hemangiomas, leiomyomas, lipomas)
    - Malignant neoplasms (adenocarcinoma, carcinoid, lymphoma, metastatic)
  - Large bowel disease (colitis, diverticular disease)
    - Fistulas
    - Hemorrhoids
    - Intussusception (see Pediatrics)
    - Colorectal cancer
    - Inflammatory bowel disease (Crohn's vs. ulcerative colitis)
    - Appendicitis (see Emergency Medicine)
- **Hepatobiliary disease:**
  - Cholelithiasis and biliary colic
  - Acute cholecystitis
  - Choledocholithiasis
  - Acute cholangitis
  - Hepatocellular carcinoma
- **Pancreatic disease:**
  - Acute pancreatitis
  - Chronic pancreatitis
  - Pancreatic pseudocysts and necrosis
  - Pancreatic cancer
  - Splenic rupture
- **Hernias:**
  - Inguinal hernia
  - Femoral hernia
  - Hiatal hernia
  - Other hernias

- **Vascular surgery:**
  - Abdominal aortic aneurysm
  - Carotid vascular disease, carotid endarterectomy (see Neurology)
  - Peripheral vascular disease, diabetic vascular disease, acute arterial occlusion, deep venous thrombosis, varicose veins, lymphedema
- **Cardiothoracic surgery:**
  - Coronary artery disease (see Internal Medicine)
  - Congenital and valvular heart disease (see Internal Medicine)
  - Lung cancer (see Internal Medicine)
  - Pulmonary emboli (see Internal Medicine)
  - Potentially life-threatening injuries and their treatment (pneumothorax, tamponade [see Emergency Medicine])
- **Breast disease (also see OB/GYN):**
  - Breast cancer
  - Fibrocystic disease
  - Fibroadenoma
- **Endocrine disease:**
  - Pheochromocytoma
  - MEN syndromes
- **Urology:**
  - Benign prostatic hyperplasia
  - Incontinence
  - Prostate cancer
  - Renal and ureteral stones
  - Testicular torsion
- **Orthopedic surgery:**
  - Fractures and trauma
  - Osteomyelitis and other infections
  - Bone tumors
- **Neurosurgery:**
  - Head bleeds
- **Plastic surgery:**
  - Melanoma
- **Otolaryngology:**
  - Head and neck tumors
  - Hyperthyroidism
  - Hyperparathyroidism
- **Other:**
  - Anesthesiology (intubation)
  - Burns (see Emergency Medicine)
  - Fluids and acid-base balance (see Practical Information for All Clerkships)
  - Wound healing/surgical infection
  - Trauma and shock (see Emergency Medicine)

SECTION 3

TOP-RATED REVIEW RESOURCES

HOW TO USE THE DATABASE

This section is a database of recommended books and study guides for use during wards rotations. For each book, we list the **Title** of the book, the **First Author** (or editor), the **Current Publisher,** the **Copyright Year,** the **Edition,** the **Number of Pages,** the **ISBN Code,** and the **Approximate List Price** of the book. Entries also include Summary Comments that describe the various books' style and utility for study and review. Finally, each book receives a **Rating.** The books are sorted into a general section as well as into sections corresponding to the seven clinical rotations (emergency medicine, internal medicine, neurology, OB/GYN, pediatrics, psychiatry, and surgery). Also included are review sections devoted to apps/smartphones; pocket drug references; ECG books; resources on fluids, electrolytes, and acid-base physiology; and radiology books. Within each section, books are arranged first by Rating, then by Author, and finally by Title.

For this fifth edition of *First Aid for the Wards*, the database of review books has been completely revised, with in-depth summary comments. A letter rating scale with six different grades reflects detailed student evaluations. Each book receives a rating as follows:

A+	Excellent for the wards.
A A–	Very good for the wards; choose among the group.
B+ B B–	Good, but use only after exhausting better sources.

The **Rating** is meant to reflect the overall usefulness of the book. This is based on a number of factors, including the following:

- The cost of the book
- The readability of the text
- The appropriateness and accuracy of the book
- The quality and appropriateness of the illustrations (eg, graphs, diagrams, photographs)
- The length of the text (longer is not necessarily better)
- The quality and number of other books available in the same discipline

Many books with low ratings are well written and informative but are not ideally suited to the wards experience. We have also avoided listing or commenting on the wide variety of general textbooks available in the clinical sciences.

Evaluations are based on the cumulative results of formal and informal surveys of hundreds of medical students from medical schools across the country. The summary comments and overall ratings represent a consensus opinion, but there may have been a large range of opinions or limited student feedback on any particular book.

Please note that the data listed are subject to change because:

- Publishers' prices change frequently.
- Individual bookstores often charge an additional markup.
- New editions come out frequently, and the quality of updating varies.
- The same book may be reissued through another publisher.

We actively encourage medical students and faculty to submit their opinions and ratings of these books so that we may update our database (see "How to Contribute," p. xiii). In addition, we ask that publishers and authors submit review copies of clinical science resources, including new editions and books not included in our database, for evaluation. We also solicit reviews of new books or suggestions for alternate modes of study that may be useful for the wards, such as flash cards, computer-based tutorials, and Internet Web sites.

DISCLAIMER/CONFLICT-OF-INTEREST STATEMENT

No material in this book, including the ratings, reflects the opinion or influence of the publisher. All errors and omissions will gladly be corrected if brought to the attention of the authors through the publisher.

GENERAL

A+ ***Bates' Pocket Guide to Physical Examination and History Taking*** **$51.95**

Bickley

Lippincott Williams & Wilkins, 2009, 6th ed., 453 pages, ISBN 9780781780667

A concise yet thorough overview of the physical exam, written in full color with numerous illustrations and organized into 2 columns for rapid reference. A compact version of *Bates' Guide,* the book is probably all one needs to master the physical exam from children to pregnant women.

A+ ***Sapira's Art & Science of Bedside Diagnosis*** **$113.00**

Orient

Lippincott Williams & Wilkins, 2010, 4th ed., 678 pages, ISBN 9781605474113

A text on the physical exam, written in an artful storytelling style. Describes methods in step-by-step detail, with clinical pearls, vignettes, practical clinical experience, personal history, explanations of the physiologic significance of findings, and extensive discussions of evidence-based medicine. A great home-reference text for students aiming to excel at the physical exam.

A ***Boards and Wards*** **$46.50**

Ayala

Lippincott Williams & Wilkins, 2009, 4th ed., 578 pages, ISBN 9780781787437

Written in a succinct, high-yield outline style, this boards-format question-and-answer book provides an excellent overview of nearly every topic tested on the Step 2 CK exam. The book is easy to read and allows for a quick review of large topics but is not thorough enough to be used for the boards. Best for a quick read-through of each section prior to clerkship rotations.

A ***DeGowin's Diagnostic Examination*** **$48.95**

LeBlond

McGraw-Hill, 2009, 9th ed., 914 pages, ISBN 9780071478984

A classic handbook divided into physical exam, lab tests, and common disease patterns. Gives clear explanations of pathophysiology and provides differentials for nearly every physical finding imaginable. Includes brief discussions of the pathophysiology of abnormal lab values. The section on diagnostic clues highlights signs and symptoms along with abnormal labs associated with specific diseases. Much too big to carry in the pocket; ideally used as a supplement to *Bates' Guide* or another more basic exam book.

A ***Textbook of Physical Diagnosis: History and Examination*** **$99.95**

Swartz

Elsevier, 2010, 6th ed., 902 pages, ISBN 9781416062035

An excellent introductory physical exam textbook geared toward medical students, offering abundant color photographs. Focuses on the "how" but does not contain enough of the "why," an element that is more thoroughly discussed in physical exam textbooks such as *Sapira's.*

A⁻ ***Clinician's Pocket Reference*** ***$43.95***
GOMELLA
McGraw-Hill, 2007, 11th ed., 722 pages, ISBN 9780071454285

A good overall wards orientation that makes excellent use of tables, graphs, and diagrams to explain concepts. Provides an effective reference for procedures, and includes useful algorithms, protocols for medical emergencies, interpretations of abnormal lab values, and a chapter on commonly used drugs with dosages and contraindications. Practical sections on basic ECG reading and critical care medicine are also provided. Does not emphasize pathophysiology or differential diagnoses. General and light on coverage of diseases; fits tightly in most coat pockets. Most beneficial for students entering the wards.

A⁻ ***Maxwell's Quick Medical Reference*** ***$7.95***
MAXWELL
Maxwell Publishing, 2006, 5th ed., 32 pages, ISBN 9780964519138

Popular, compact, spiral-bound fact cards detailing ACLS algorithms, various in-house notes, normal lab values, basic formulas, the H&P, and the psychiatric and neurologic exams. Especially important at the beginning of the clinical years, but not as critical toward the end, when students have become better acquainted with the wards. The most frequently used features are the common lab values, formulas, and sample notes. Great for quick reference, and small enough to fit in any pocket.

A⁻ ***Pocket Guide to Diagnostic Tests*** ***$45.95***
NICOLL
McGraw-Hill, 2008, 5th ed., 518 pages, ISBN 9780071489683

A concise and useful reference for common diagnostic tests in quick-flip tabular format. Discusses physiologic bases for and interpretation of lab results. Includes useful sections focusing on microbiology, drug monitoring, ECG interpretation, and diagnostic radiology. The text fits in the pocket but is relatively heavy, so students may want to carry it in a backpack for quick reference when needed.

A⁻ ***Images from the Wards: Diagnosis and Treatment*** ***$54.95***
STUDDIFORD
Elsevier, 2010, 1st ed., 305 pages, ISBN 9781416063834

A compendium of the 500-plus most common and important clinical images one will encounter, organized in a boards-style multiple-choice question format to support the learning and review process. An extremely useful book to use during the third year of medical school.

A⁻ ***Wallach's Interpretation of Diagnostic Tests*** ***$75.95***
WALLACH
Lippincott Williams & Wilkins, 2011, 9th ed., 1143 pages, ISBN 9781605476674

A text that is organized by organ system with summaries of available tests for most diseases. Discusses the interpretation of abnormal labs and differentials, and includes tables comparing test results from similar diseases. Similar to *Pocket Guide to Diagnostic Tests* but larger and more comprehensive, with excellent, encyclopedic coverage. Will not fit in the pocket; best used as a reference.

B+ ***On Call Procedures*** **$54.95**
Adams
Elsevier, 2006, 2nd ed., 300 pages, ISBN 9781416024446

A quick, concise resource on basic and advanced procedures, including endotracheal intubation, central line placement, and fluid taps. Includes indications, contraindications, precautions, step-by-step techniques, complications, and guidelines for removal. Good diagrams are provided for anatomy and approach. Although there is no substitute for actual hands-on experience, the book provides a clear picture of the invasive medical and surgical procedures one is likely to encounter on the wards.

B+ ***On Call Principles and Protocols*** **$42.95**
Marshall
Elsevier, 2011, 5th ed., 592 pages, ISBN 9781437723717

A practical guidebook designed for the intern or resident on call. Not as useful for third-year medical students, but may come in handy for subinterns. Attempts to cover a broad range of problems, which makes it superficial in its scope. Most useful for internal medicine and surgery. Divided into phone-call management, elevator thoughts, threats to life, and bedside care.

B+ ***Differential Diagnosis of Common Complaints*** **$49.95**
Seller
Elsevier, 2007, 5th ed., 468 pages, ISBN 9781416029069

A detailed discussion of 36 common complaints or problems and their associated diagnoses, including ways to differentiate between them. Best used for patients with common complaints but complicated clinical pictures or for reviewing the general management of common complaints.

B ***Saint-Frances Guide to Clinical Clerkships: The Answer Book*** **$40.95**
Wiese
Lippincott Williams & Wilkins, 2006, 1st ed., 531 pages, ISBN 9780781737548

An all-purpose approach toward success in the clinical clerkships. One-third of the text offers general tips for medical clerkships, from charting to navigating the hospital environment to communicating and gathering information. A third is devoted to a detailed review of the physical exam. The final third of the text describes specific tips and characteristics of the individual clerkships. Designed to help students succeed on the wards, the book is of limited utility for more advanced students but is ideal for those about to enter their first clerkship.

B- ***Ferri's Differential Diagnosis*** **$25.95**
Ferri
Elsevier, 2011, 2nd ed., 540 pages, ISBN 9780323076999

A pocket-sized book that presents differential diagnoses, organized by sign and symptom as well as by disorder. May be of limited use for beginning third-year medical students, as it does not include explanations for the differentials presented or information on how to tease out diagnostic and management clues. More useful for subinterns or for those with a good foundation of knowledge.

B- ***Review 2 Rounds: Visual Review and Clinical Reference*** **$30.95**
Gallardo
Elsevier, 2010, 1st ed., 452 pages, ISBN 9781437701692

A spiral-bound book presented in a 2-color tabular format with some useful illustrations, graphs, and tables. Not the most beneficial text for beginning third-year medical students. Lacks detailed explanations for differentials and management.

APPS/SMARTPHONE

Rating	Resource	Price
A+	***DynaMed*** http://dynamed.ebscohost.com A point-of-care reference tool that is updated daily and contains more than 3000 clinically organized summaries based on evidence medicine. Organized in an outline/bulleted format that makes for easy reading. Does not read like a textbook. Includes excellent references at the end, allowing ambitious students to look up the primary literature in order to excel on clerkship rotations. Check to see if it can be accessed for free through your institution's subscription.	***$99.95***
A+	***UpToDate*** www.uptodate.com A comprehensive collection of clinical summaries, recommendations, and treatment information based on the latest clinical evidence. Best used as a textbook-like reference. Some sections contain expert opinions and recommendations that may not be based on true evidence-based literature. Check to see if it can be accessed for free through your institution's subscription.	***$195.00***
A	***Calculate by QxMD*** www.qxmd.com An easy-to-use collection of useful clinical calculators and clinical supporting tools.	***Free***
A	***Epocrates Rx*** www.epocrates.com A quick, accurate, and comprehensive resource on drugs, labs, and disease information that is updated continually. Provides accurate and up-to-date information on clinical indications, adult and pediatric dosing, contraindications, adverse reactions, mechanisms of action, forms of administration, potential interactions, and prices for virtually any pharmaceutical product. Additional references and features are available at a cost.	***Free***
A	***MedCalc*** http://medcalc.medserver.be/ An easy-to-use collection of more than 200 relevant formulas, classifications, scores, and scales.	***Free***
A–	***Eponyms (for students)*** www.eponyms.net A collection of more than 1700 common and obscure medical eponyms and their meaning.	***Free***
B+	***AQRH ePPS*** www.uspreventiveservicestaskforce.org/index.html A useful tool with which to identify appropriate preventive services based on risk factors. Of particular interest to those seeking a quick review of preventive screening as they begin their ambulatory medicine or family medicine rotation.	***Free***
B+	***Outlines in Clinical Medicine*** www.skyscape.com Offers 850 separate succinct summaries of topics encountered in general internal medicine, internal medicine subspecialties, emergency medicine, and family practice. Not comprehensive enough for detailed discussion of certain topics.	***Free***

POCKET DRUG REFERENCES

A ***The Sanford Guide to Antimicrobial Therapy*** **$16.75**

GILBERT

Antimicrobial Therapy, 2011, 41st ed., 220 pages, ISBN 9781930808652

The gold-standard pocket antimicrobial reference guide, updated yearly. Includes dosage, coverage, sensitivities, length of therapy, renal dosing, and drugs of choice for common and uncommon infections. Presented in tabular format. The small print is sometimes difficult to read. Remember to determine if your own institution has its own guidelines or formulary. Otherwise, a pocket-worthy guide for any rotation.

A ***Tarascon Pocket Pharmacopoeia: Classic Shirt-Pocket Edition*** **$16.95**

HAMILTON

Jones & Bartlett Learning, 2011, 25th ed., 192 pages, ISBN 9780763793050

An excellent pocket reference book of drugs indexed by generic and trade names. Includes drug class, typical dosing, metabolism, safety in pregnancy and lactation, relative cost, tables, and conversion factors. Also includes a short summary of ACLS protocols, emergency drug infusions, and pediatric dosing. A must-have for the wards, especially for subinterns. Compact and inexpensive.

ECG BOOKS

A ***Rapid Interpretation of EKGs*** ***$38.00***

DUBIN

Cover Publishing, 2000, 6th ed., 368 pages, ISBN 9780912912066

Presented as a workbook, this classic reference facilitates the rapid acquisition of ECG fundamentals, emphasizing active learning with fill-in-the-blank exercises and visual aids on each page. Includes excellent quick-reference pages at the end that can be copied and placed in one's coat pocket. Can easily be read in a weekend. Although its content has not changed significantly in several years, this book is still considered a basic stepping stone for the junior student. However, it falls somewhat short on practice ECGs, and another book will likely be needed for more advanced ECG interpretation.

A ***The Only EKG Book You'll Ever Need*** ***$61.95***

THALER

Lippincott Williams & Wilkins, 2010, 6th ed., 326 pages, ISBN 9781605471402

A text that stresses basic electrophysiology and simple ECG interpretation, organized according to problem. Includes useful chapter summaries and a comprehensive review of important principles. Also offers case presentations, tables, graphs, and sample 12-lead ECGs. Concise and highly readable, but would benefit from more practice ECGs. Good for beginners looking for simple explanations and descriptions, but may be too superficial for those who seek to master ECG interpretation.

A⁻ ***The ECG Made Easy*** ***$37.95***

HAMPTON

Elsevier, 2008, 7th ed., 179 pages, ISBN 9780443068171

An extremely quick review of major ECG findings. Includes tables and a few rhythm strips, but does not offer practice problems or case discussions. Examples might be more informative if they showed an entire 12-lead ECG rather than just 1 lead and if arrows were used to point to the precise abnormalities. Can fit in a coat pocket.

A⁻ ***ECG Workout: Exercises in Arrhythmia Interpretation*** ***$49.95***

HUFF

Lippincott Williams & Wilkins, 2011, 6th ed., 378 pages, ISBN 9781451115536

A practical workbook with more than 500 actual ECGs. Includes updated ACLS guidelines. Emphasizes arrhythmias with no discussion of MI, ischemia, or hypertrophy. Includes good tables, illustrations, and self-assessment problems. Best used in conjunction with a primary ECG reference. Too advanced for third-year medical students seeking to learn the basics of ECG interpretation.

A⁻ ***150 Practice ECGs: Interpretation and Review*** ***$49.95***

TAYLOR

Blackwell Publishing, 2006, 3rd ed., 264 pages, ISBN 9781405104838

A spiral-bound workbook with sections dedicated to basic electrophysiology and practice. Excellent for medical students wishing to practice, but can be difficult to use, as reviews for the ECGs are randomly organized and some are highly advanced. Lacks thorough explanations of ECG pathology and physiology, but frequently focuses on clinical management.

A⁻ ***Marriott's Practical Electrocardiography*** ***$87.50***

WAGNER

Lippincott Williams & Wilkins, 2008, 11th ed., 468 pages, ISBN 9780781797382

A thorough ECG reference that includes normal and abnormal ECG findings. May be too detailed for third-year medical students. Includes illustrations, literature references, ECG tracings, and a glossary. Excellent for cardiology subinterns as well as for those who are interested in going to the next level of ECG interpretation.

FLUIDS, ELECTROLYTES, AND ACID-BASE

A ***Fluid, Electrolyte, and Acid-Base Physiology*** ***$69.95***

Halperin

Elsevier, 2010, 4th ed., 596 pages, ISBN 9781416024422

A well-written clinical approach toward recognizing, diagnosing, and treating common metabolic abnormalities. Presented in a case-based format with numerous clinical vignettes and clinically oriented questions. Good illustrations integrate basic science principles into the discussion of metabolic disorders. A highly comprehensive book for those who seek detailed information, but may be low yield for third-year students seeking a quick review.

A ***Acid-Base, Fluids, and Electrolytes Made Ridiculously Simple*** ***$22.95***

Preston

MedMaster, Inc., 2011, 2nd ed., 146 pages, ISBN 9780940780989

A concise, practical approach toward solving problems of acid-base, fluid, and electrolyte abnormalities. Easy to read and well organized with good use of tables, but more diagrams and figures would be of benefit, and some mnemonics are a stretch. Several questions with detailed explanations at the end of each section reinforce key principles. Reasonably priced in view of the amount and complexity of material covered.

RADIOLOGY

A+ ***Learning Radiology: Recognizing the Basics*** **$55.95**
HERRING
Elsevier, 2011, 2nd ed., 317 pages, ISBN 9780323074445

An excellent and concise text that discusses in detail a wide range of common and uncommon conditions based on imaging findings. Includes more than 700 images with excellent explanations of the diagnostic approach. Can easily be read cover to cover during a radiology clerkship rotation.

A ***Radiology 101: The Basics and Fundamentals of Imaging*** **$79.00**
ERKONEN
Lippincott Williams & Wilkins, 2010, 3rd ed., 376 pages, ISBN 9781605472256

A good overview of radiology with special emphasis on the normal anatomy of different organ systems. Contains numerous radiographic illustrations and easy-to-understand explanations for the clinical aspects of various imaging modalities. As its name suggests, the book is geared toward students who want to understand the fundamentals of reading films, but it is also useful in anatomy.

A− ***Clinical Radiology: The Essentials*** **$72.00**
DAFFNER
Lippincott Williams & Wilkins, 2007, 3rd ed., 544 pages, ISBN 9780781799683

Specifically designed for third- and fourth-year medical students, this book outlines basic information on different imaging modalities, organized by organ system. It discusses more pathology than *Radiology 101* but makes for heavier reading and includes fewer illustrations.

A− ***Squire's Fundamentals of Radiology*** **$111.50**
NOVELLINE
Harvard University Press, 2004, 6th ed., 638 pages, ISBN 9780674012790

The standard radiology textbook written for medical students. Comprehensive and better suited for those going into radiology. Not an easy read, and not appropriate for use as a high-yield text during a typical radiology clerkship rotation.

A− ***Lecture Notes on Radiology*** **$39.95**
PATEL
Wiley, 2010, 3rd ed., 324 pages, ISBN 9781405195140

A good general overview of diagnostic radiology, presented in a disease-specific manner. A double-page-spread format with radiographs of a specific disorder on 1 page and a succinct explanatory text on the other allows for immediate cross-reference. Covers the basic physics of the different radiographic forums as well as treatment options for radiographically detected diseases.

B+ ***Clinical Radiology Made Ridiculously Simple*** **$30.95**
OUELLETTE
MedMaster Inc., 2006, 2nd ed., 109 pages, ISBN 9780940780750

A good, concise introduction to the basics of radiology in easy-to-understand terms. Offers easy-to-read content that is ideally suited for use at the beginning of a rotation, covering the basics of CXRs, AXRs, bone films, and head CTs. However, the text is not comprehensive and omits many other important components of clinical radiology, including ultrasound, body CTs, MRIs, and angiograms. Offers fewer illustrations and figures than most radiology texts.

B+

Radiology Secrets Plus **$59.95**

PRETORIUS

Elsevier, 2011, 3rd ed., 562 pages, ISBN 9780323067942

A resource based on the case and question-and-answer approach toward learning radiology. Excellent as a means of quickly picking up radiologic pearls, but difficult to use as a general reference text.

B

Blueprints in Radiology **$43.50**

UZELAC

Lippincott Williams & Wilkins, 2006, 2nd ed., 170 pages, ISBN 9781405104609

A text review of radiologic findings for common diseases, organized by organ system (eg, thorax, abdomen) and by common disease processes associated with each. Includes a number of plain radiographs as well as ultrasound and CT images along with 25 questions at the end. A fairly superficial review of basic radiology topics; more useful as an overview than for test preparation.

EMERGENCY MEDICINE

HANDBOOK/POCKETBOOK

A− ***NMS Clinical Manual of Emergency Medicine*** **$30.95**

BIDDINGER

Lippincott Williams & Wilkins, 2002, 2nd ed., 283 pages, ISBN 9780781735513

A small, pocket-sized resource presented in a standardized format for common complaints, outlining key information, the patient history, the physical exam, the differential, lab tests, imaging, treatment, and disposition. The text walks readers through relevant details, making it ideal for use before seeing new patients or presenting to a resident or an attending. Information is organized by system, with each chapter subdivided alphabetically. Also includes numerous table and figures for easy reference. Some management algorithms may be slightly outdated.

A− ***Pocket Emergency Medicine*** **$52.50**

ZANE

Lippincott Williams & Wilkins, 2011, 2nd ed., 288 pages, ISBN 9781605477312

A concise pocket text organized by symptom-based presentation. Offers a quick and easy primer on pathophysiology, diagnostic, and treatment algorithms for use both before and after seeing a patient. Not as well referenced as its sibling, *Pocket Medicine.*

B+ ***Current Essentials of Emergency Medicine*** **$45.00**

STONE

McGraw-Hill, 2005, 1st ed., 520 pages, ISBN 9780071440585

Organized by organ system, this book contains a succinct summary of each disease, focusing on practical clinical information. One disease and pearl is offered on each page. Good for quick reference and review. Easy to read, although it would benefit from a more extensive discussion of pathophysiology.

B ***SOAP for Emergency Medicine*** **$31.95**

BOND

Lippincott Williams & Wilkins, 2005, 1st ed., 202 pages, ISBN 9781405104425

A thin pocketbook that presents information in a SOAP-note format. Organized by organ system, the book focuses heavily on clinical problems, not on diagnosis. The "S" (subject) section contains a helpful list of questions to ask when interviewing patients and writing notes. The book would be most useful in guiding day-to-day management and in formulating an assessment and plan for patients with a known diagnosis. Would benefit from some figures or diagrams.

REVIEW/MINI-REFERENCE

A — ***Emergency Management of the Trauma Patient: Cases, Algorithms, Evidence*** **$40.95**
BISANZO
Lippincott Williams & Wilkins, 2007, 1st ed., 180 pages, ISBN 9781405104876

Although not intended for boards review or fundamental wards preparation, this text would be of benefit for students who are interested in learning more about trauma management. Presents scenarios and then emphasizes the role of clinical judgment and the ACLS protocol in making appropriate management decisions.

A — ***Emergency Management of the Coding Patient: Cases, Algorithms, Evidence*** **$40.95**
SENECAL
Lippincott Williams & Wilkins, 2005, 1st ed., 170 pages, ISBN 9781405104555

Although not intended for boards review or fundamental wards preparation, this text would be of benefit for students who are interested in learning more about the management of a coding patient. Presents scenarios and then emphasizes the role of clinical judgment and the ACLS protocol in making appropriate management decisions.

A — ***First Aid for the Emergency Medicine Clerkship*** **$45.00**
STEAD
McGraw-Hill, 2011, 3rd ed., 542 pages, ISBN 9780071739061

A comprehensive overview of pertinent topics in emergency medicine, written in outline format with well-organized tables and helpful figures. Covers essential high-yield information and common procedures in a succinct, systematic manner. Also includes the appropriate breadth of topics, and the depth given to each topic is ideal both for wards preparation and for the clerkship shelf exam. Helpful descriptions of certain procedures are also included. Overall, an excellent review of the broad field of emergency medicine. This publication is not affiliated with the authors of *First Aid for the Wards*.

A− — ***Blueprints Clinical Cases in Emergency Medicine*** **$36.95**
SILVERS
Lippincott Williams & Wilkins, 2007, 2nd ed., 486 pages, ISBN 9781405104975

Organized by common presenting signs and symptoms, this book contains 60 symptom-based clinical cases followed by thought questions and a discussion. Also provided are 100 USMLE-style questions. A popular question book that is very high yield for both wards and shelf preparation.

B+ — ***In A Page Emergency Medicine*** **$43.50**
CATERINO
Lippincott Williams & Wilkins, 2003, 1st ed., 316 pages, ISBN 9781405103572

A concise review of more than 250 diseases, organized by organ system. Each disease pathology is explained in 1 page, from etiology to prognosis. Provides a big picture and high-yield information; best suited for quick review before seeing a patient or preparing for a pimp session. Thin enough to carry around everywhere but lacks figures and tables, so students will need to refer to other textbooks for more detailed information.

B+

Underground Clinical Vignettes: Emergency Medicine ***$30.95***

KIM

Lippincott Williams & Wilkins, 2007, 4th ed., 200 pages, ISBN 9780781768344

A well-organized review of clinical vignettes commonly encountered on the shelf and Step 2 CK exams. Includes a focused, high-yield discussion of pathogenesis, epidemiology, management, and complications. Black-and-white images are included where relevant. Also offers several "minicases" in which only key facts related to each disease are presented. An entertaining, easy-to-use supplement for studying during the clinical rotation. May benefit from increased coverage of surgical subspecialties, including ophthalmology, anesthesiology, and pediatric surgery.

B

Blueprints in Emergency Medicine ***$43.50***

MICK

Lippincott Williams & Wilkins, 2005, 2nd ed., 307 pages, ISBN 9781405104616

A text that covers the essentials of the field but does not go into extensive detail. Features boards-format questions and answers with explanations along with useful charts. Great for a general introduction to the field, but best used in conjunction with a more comprehensive text. Intended for clerkship preparation as well as for boards review.

B−

First Exposure to Emergency Medicine Clerkship ***$41.95***

HOFFMAN

McGraw-Hill, 2004, 1st ed., 467 pages, ISBN 9780071417167

Organized by symptom as well as by organ system, this book offers a thorough discussion of each emergency medicine topic at a level of detail that is probably appropriate for a month-long clerkship. Because of its prose style, it is not ideal for quick reference. Includes common procedures in the ED at the end. A comprehensive source of information, but would benefit from more tables and bulleted lists for easier reading.

QUESTION BOOKS

A⁻ ***Emergency Medicine Secrets*** ***$49.95***

MARKOVCHICK

Elsevier, 2011, 5th ed., 750 pages, ISBN 9780323071673

A concise, easy-to-read, and highly effective text with "key point" boxes and mnemonics, lists, and quick-reference tables. Fits in a lab coat pocket and allows for quick reference or review. Should not be used as a stand-alone book for the clerkship; must be supplemented with a general review book or textbook.

TEXTBOOK/REFERENCE

A

Current Diagnosis & Treatment: Emergency Medicine ***$80.00***

STONE

McGraw-Hill, 2011, 7th ed., 1009 pages, ISBN 9780071701075

A comprehensive text with discussions of common emergency problems one is likely to encounter on the clerkship. Focuses on practical clinical information, and includes problem-oriented cases. Also contains numerous illustrations that are helpful for the rotation.

A⁻

Introduction to Emergency Medicine ***$56.95***

MITCHELL

Lippincott Williams & Wilkins, 2005, 1st ed., 708 pages, ISBN 9780781732000

A resource that falls between a review book and a text in terms of its length and content. A few figures and tables interspersed throughout make it easier to understand. Organized by system and common presenting symptom; contains a series of questions at the end of some chapters with which students can prepare for the shelf and Step 2 CK exams. Geared toward medical students. May contain outdated management information.

A⁻

Emergency Medicine: A Comprehensive Study Guide ***$134.78***

TINTINALLI

McGraw-Hill, 2010, 7th ed., 2208 pages, ISBN 9780071388757

A classic, highly comprehensive textbook covering almost all aspects of medicine. Organized by organ system, the updated book is heavy on text with some evidence-based recommendations. However, the book may be too dense for a quick and easy read, and some readers have reported conflicting information.

INTERNAL MEDICINE

HANDBOOK/POCKETBOOK

A+ ***Pocket Medicine*** ***$61.95***
SABATINE
Lippincott Williams & Wilkins, 2010, 4th ed., 304 pages, ISBN 9781608319053

A small but essential pocketbook with great overviews of most diseases encountered in inpatient settings, along with the latest management approaches and up-to-date references to primary literature following each subject. Also includes handy tables, charts, and algorithms, although the small print may be a drawback. Note cards can easily be added to the ring-bound pocketbook, but pages can rip out of the binder. Limited in detail owing to its size and scope, but easy to carry everywhere. Great for a quick reference before and after seeing patients.

A ***Practical Guide to the Care of the Medical Patient*** ***$54.95***
FERRI
Elsevier, 2011, 8th ed., 585 pages, ISBN 9780323071581

A concise and well-organized pocketbook that covers common diseases through a discussion of etiology, differentials, diagnostic approach, and management. Written at an appropriate level for medical students. Includes excellent tables and algorithms that are useful on the wards.

A ***The Washington Manual of Medical Therapeutics*** ***$61.95***
FOSTER
Lippincott Williams & Wilkins, 2010, 33rd ed., 1048 pages, ISBN 9781608310036

An excellent handbook outlining the pathophysiology and diagnosis of common diseases. Contains highly detailed descriptions of various therapeutic options that help resolve specific questions. Aimed toward medical residents, but highly useful for medical students as well, especially subinterns. Fits tightly in most coat pockets. Contains references for the retrieval of primary sources.

A− ***Current Essentials of Medicine*** ***$40.00***
TIERNEY
McGraw-Hill, 2010, 4th ed., 593 pages, ISBN 9780071637909

A quick reference for wards and outpatient medicine, organized into bulleted lists covering the essentials of diagnosis, differentials, and treatment. Each medical disorder is presented on its own page along with clinical pearls and general primary references with the goal of highlighting crucial points of each disease. Does not include detailed discussions of pathophysiology, diagnosis, and management, limiting its usefulness.

B+ ***Harrison's Manual of Medicine*** ***$59.95***
FAUCI
McGraw-Hill, 2009, 17th ed., 1243 pages, ISBN 9780071477437

A "baby" pocket version of the parent book, this manual focuses on commonly encountered diseases, providing a wealth of information on pathophysiology, clinical manifestations, and therapeutics. Useful for quick reading on established diagnoses, although its dense copy and large blocks of text make it difficult to skim. Not as practical for day-to-day wards problems, as it lacks thorough explanations of the approach toward diagnosis and management. Great as a pocket reference book for reviewing diseases that students have encountered on the wards or are considering on their differential.

B+

Internal Medicine on Call ***$45.95***

HAIST

McGraw-Hill, 2005, 4th ed., 714 pages, ISBN 9780071439022

A quick-reference guidebook giving a step-by-step approach toward most commonly encountered medical "on-call" problems. Organized by common presenting symptoms, this book is most useful for formulating differential diagnoses and appropriate management plans when new patients are encountered on call. Includes sections on laboratory interpretation, procedures, fluids and electrolytes, ventilator management, and commonly used drugs. Would benefit from more diagrams and tables. Somewhat outdated.

B+

Tarascon Internal Medicine & Critical Care Pocketbook ***$19.95***

LEDERMAN

Jones & Bartlett Learning, 2011, 5th ed., 352 pages, ISBN 9781449620059

A small, inexpensive, pocket-sized book containing excellent tables, graphs, and algorithms for the workup and treatment of common emergency problems encountered in internal medicine. Occasionally too complex, as information is presented in a highly technical manner with little discussion; geared more toward those with prior knowledge of the highlighted diseases. More appropriate for subinterns. A section at the end is dedicated to a description of commonly used drugs in the critical care setting.

B−

SOAP for Internal Medicine ***$31.95***

UZELAC

Lippincott Williams & Wilkins, 2005, 1st ed., 178 pages, ISBN 9781405104364

A thin pocketbook that presents information in a SOAP-note format. Organized by organ system, the book focuses heavily on clinical problems, not diagnoses. The "S" (subject) section contains a helpful list of questions to ask when interviewing patients and writing notes. The book would be most useful in guiding day-to-day management and in formulating an assessment and plan for patients with a known diagnosis. Similar to *Internal Medicine on Call* in concept, but focuses more on treatment plans than on differentials. Would benefit from more figures and diagrams. Contains some errors.

REVIEW/MINI-REFERENCE

A+

Step-Up to Medicine **$54.95**

AGABEGI

Lippincott Williams & Wilkins, 2012, 3rd ed., 576 pages, ISBN 9781609133603

An excellent high-yield resource for the internal medicine clerkship as well as for the shelf and Step 2 CK exams. Well organized in an easy-to-read format with abundant pictures and diagrams, and presented at an optimal level of detail. Also includes ample information on epidemiology, diagnosis, presentation, and treatment, although the text does not prioritize treatments by effectiveness/side effect profile, and some chapters do not list the order in which tests should be performed. Also includes an excellent ambulatory care section.

A

First Aid for the Medicine Clerkship **$46.95**

KAUFMAN

McGraw-Hill, 2010, 3rd ed., 420 pages, ISBN 9780071633826

A good overview of pertinent topics in internal medicine, written in outline format and intended for the shelf and Step 2 CK exams. Covers essential high-yield information in a succinct and well-written manner. A quick and easy-to-read review book, although it may not be sufficiently detailed and lacks an extensive discussion of pathophysiology. Some illustrations are provided. Overall, an excellent and clinically relevant review of the broad field of internal medicine. This publication is not affiliated with the authors of *First Aid for the Wards.*

A

Case Files Internal Medicine **$34.95**

TOY

McGraw-Hill, 2009, 3rd ed., 580 pages, ISBN 9780071613644

An excellent pocket-sized casebook that offers an overview of cases commonly encountered on the internal medicine clerkship. Cases help readers think critically about differential diagnosis, workup, and management. Questions at the end of each case test the reader's understanding of the concept just reviewed. A useful companion for the clerkship, and a good source of practice cases for the shelf exam.

A−

In A Page Inpatient Medicine **$40.95**

PERKINS

Lippincott Williams & Wilkins, 2008, 1st ed., 239 pages, ISBN 9780781764995

A review of 200 diseases, organized by organ system. Each disease pathology, from etiology to prognosis, is explained in a 1- or 2-page list format. Provides a big picture and high-yield information; best suited for quick review before seeing a patient or preparing for a pimp session. Thin enough to carry around everywhere, but lacks sufficient detail to be used as a general review reference.

A−

Case Files Family Medicine **$34.95**

TOY

McGraw-Hill, 2009, 2nd ed., 608 pages, ISBN 9780071600231

A case-based book that makes good use of figures and tables and also includes algorithms for medical management with coverage of relevant topics in women's health and ambulatory internal medicine. Covers the epidemiology, etiology, prevention, presentation, diagnosis, treatment, and prognosis of disorders commonly encountered in an ambulatory setting. Also includes a comprehensive look at the diagnosis and treatment of virtually all important conditions in obstetrics and gynecology.

B+ ***Cecil Essentials of Medicine*** **$79.95**

ANDREOLI

Elsevier, 2011, 8th ed., 1282 pages, ISBN 9781416061090

A great condensed version of the parent book. Offers clear, detailed explanations of pathophysiology, but not as useful as a treatment reference or for differential diagnosis. More useful for reference than for practical wards work. Contains many effective tables and charts. Not portable.

B+ ***Blueprints Clinical Cases in Medicine*** **$36.95**

LI

Lippincott Williams & Wilkins, 2007, 2nd ed., 418 pages, ISBN 9781405104913

Organized by common presenting signs and symptoms, this book contains symptom-based clinical cases accompanied by 200 USMLE-style questions. The format is similar to that of the Case Files series but places less emphasis on discussions and greater focus on questions. May contain some errors.

B+ ***Internal Medicine Clerkship Guide*** **$54.95**

PAAUW

Elsevier, 2008, 3rd ed., 651 pages, ISBN 9780323045582

Designed specifically for medical students beginning their internal medicine clerkships, this text is divided into sections addressing the basic skills needed for the clerkship, common symptoms or signs, and common diseases. Provides practical core knowledge of common medical conditions along with basic questions and answers that help guide students in their transition to clinical thinking. Not useful for looking up detailed information, but an effective introduction to clinical problem solving and diagnosis.

B+ ***Blueprints in Medicine*** **$43.50**

YOUNG

Lippincott Williams & Wilkins, 2010, 5th ed., 381 pages, ISBN 9780781788700

A good review book that students can read early in the rotation to learn the fundamentals of internal medicine. Provides an easy-to-read overview, with good tables and charts to illustrate key points. The text is far too simplistic and may not be comprehensive enough for the clerkship shelf exam. Best when supplemented with a separate review book such as *Step-Up to Medicine* or the *Harrison's* series of texts.

B ***In A Page Signs & Symptoms*** **$40.95**

KAHAN

Lippincott Williams & Wilkins, 2009, 2nd ed., 377 pages, ISBN 9780781770439

Organized by common presenting signs and symptoms, this book focuses on differential diagnosis and workups. Like its counterpart, *In A Page Inpatient Medicine*, the book explains each symptom with lists in 1 page. Excellent for quick review, and a great companion to use while on call, providing guidelines on how to work up "fresh" patients.

B ***Underground Clinical Vignettes: Internal Medicine, Vol. 1*** **$29.95**

KIM

Lippincott Williams & Wilkins, 2007, 4th ed., 190 pages, ISBN 9780781768351

A well-organized review of clinical vignettes commonly encountered on the clerkship shelf exam. Includes focused, high-yield discussions of pathophysiology, epidemiology, management, and complications. Covers cardiology, endocrinology, gastroenterology, hematology, and oncology. An entertaining and easy-to-use supplement for studying during the clinical rotation. The only drawback lies in its slightly outdated management options.

B

Underground Clinical Vignettes: Internal Medicine, Vol. 2 **$29.95**

KIM

Lippincott Williams & Wilkins, 2007, 4th ed., 182 pages, ISBN 9780781768368

See the above review of *Underground Clinical Vignettes: Internal Medicine, Vol. 1.* This volume covers dermatology, infectious disease, nephrology, urology, pulmonary disease, and rheumatology.

B

Pathophysiology of Disease: An Introduction **$72.95**

MCPHEE

McGraw-Hill, 2009, 6th ed., 737 pages, ISBN 9780071621670

A concise, interdisciplinary reference text of the pathophysiology of common diseases, organized by system. Offers excellent explanations of disease processes. Not designed for the wards or for dealing with treatment and management issues, but useful as an adjunct to a more traditional textbook. Some students may find it more appropriate for pathophysiology classes during preclinical years.

B

High-Yield Internal Medicine **$30.95**

NIRULA

Lippincott Williams & Wilkins, 2006, 3rd ed., 219 pages, ISBN 9780781781695

Part of a popular USMLE Step 1 prep series that offers a review book for each clerkship. Typical of its format, the book contains high-yield information in a clear and concise outline format organized by organ system. Would benefit from more tables and figures. Useful for a quick review before the clerkship shelf exam.

B

NMS Medicine **$49.95**

WOLFSTHAL

Lippincott Williams & Wilkins, 2011, 7th ed., 712 pages, ISBN 9781608315819

A thorough and detailed text that is organized by system, with easy-to-read chapters presented in outline format. Includes questions at the end of each chapter to solidify concepts just learned as well as a comprehensive exam at the end. Geared toward studying for the shelf and Step 2 CK exams, but can also be used to review topics on the wards. Offers few diagrams, tables, and illustrations, and information is not always up to date. The inclusion of some esoteric information may make it difficult for readers to find the essentials.

B-

Color Atlas and Text of Clinical Medicine **$64.95**

FORBES

Elsevier, 2003, 3rd ed., 518 pages, ISBN 9780723431947

A sizable softcover text that offers a broad overview of medicine in an excellent, highly readable format. The text includes great illustrations and tables, but its strength lies in its more than 1500 color photos. Illustrations include physical signs of disease, radiographic images, and pathology slides. Not meant for in-depth review, but highly effective both as an introductory clinical text and as a visual encyclopedia. A good resource to use as a supplement to more traditional reference textbooks.

QUESTION BOOKS

A+

MKSAP for Students 5 **$54.95**

AMERICAN COLLEGE OF PHYSICIANS

American College of Physicians, 2011, 5th ed., 304 pages, ISBN 9781934465547

A must-have book both for the wards and for the shelf exam, and a great means of reviewing the essential content of the core internal medicine rotation. Contains more than 450 new patient-centered self-assessment questions and detailed answers that mimic the format of the end of the clerkship and the USMLE board exam. Questions provide good practice for the boards while also helping solidify information that one needs to know for the rotation. Case-based questions with explanations help hone readers' clinical reasoning, which will be needed both on the wards and on the exam.

A–

PreTest Internal Medicine **$32.00**

URBAN

McGraw-Hill, 2009, 12th ed., 421 pages, ISBN 9780071601627

A collection of 500-plus multiple-choice questions covering a wide range of topics in internal medicine. Includes clinical vignette–style questions, and offers detailed, paragraph-format explanations for each answer. Provides a quick preparation for the boards and the clerkship shelf exam, and the pocket-sized format allows readers to carry the book in their pocket and quickly review questions during downtime on the wards. Although some questions may be too basic, the text is probably the most widely used resource for shelf exam preparation.

B+

Medical Secrets **$39.95**

HARWARD

Elsevier, 2011, 5th ed., 624 pages, ISBN 9780323063982

A pocket-sized book in question-and-answer format that covers all common conditions and their treatment. Serves as a good companion to other review books. Bulleted lists, tables, and short answers make for a quick and easy read. Designed for surviving wards pimping sessions that contain useful and clinically relevant information. However, the format is not for all students.

B

Medicine Recall **$43.50**

BERGIN

Lippincott Williams & Wilkins, 2011, 4th ed., 809 pages, ISBN 9781605476759

A large yet portable book that is good for rapid review as well as for answering pimp questions. Follows the standard Recall-series question-and-answer format of high-yield information organized by medical specialty. Requires significant time commitment to complete. No images are provided, and some information is incorrect or out of date. Useful as a supplement to other resources.

B

Hospital Medicine Secrets **$54.95**

GLASHEEN

Elsevier, 2007, 1st ed., 649 pages, ISBN 9780323040877

A review of many critical topics in hospital medicine accompanied by discussions of issues such as patient safety, the subtleties of patient management, and evidence-based medicine. Highly useful for those interested in careers in medicine. Includes many helpful tips and equations for the effective use and interpretation of diagnostic tests. Also provides pertinent questions along with concise answers.

TEXTBOOK/REFERENCE

A+ ***Cecil Medicine*** ***$179.00***
GOLDMAN
Elsevier, 2011, 24th ed., 2569 pages, ISBN 9781437727883

One of the classic textbooks of medicine, written in an easy-to-read format. Not as comprehensive or detailed as *Harrison's*, but an excellent resource covering all the important diseases and concepts in internal medicine, supplemented by numerous tables and color illustrations. More appropriate than *Harrison's* for medical students and junior house staff.

A+ ***Harrison's Principles of Internal Medicine*** ***$199.00***
WEINER
McGraw-Hill, 2011, 18th ed., 4012 pages, ISBN 9780071748896

The gold-standard textbook for internal medicine. An excellent and comprehensive reference that includes tables, graphs, illustrations, and radiographs. Not a quick read, but an essential resource for those who seek in-depth information on specific topics. Requires serious concentration and reading time, and thus may not be appropriate for medical students starting out on the wards.

A ***Current Medical Diagnosis & Treatment*** ***$75.00***
MCPHEE
McGraw-Hill, 2011, 51st ed., 1867 pages, ISBN 9780071763721

A comprehensive, clinically oriented pocket reference book that is concise yet detailed and highly readable. Features well-organized text with excellent descriptions of pathophysiology, clinical findings, and treatment. The beginning of each section offers the essentials of diagnosis. The text is revised annually and thus offers useful tables and up-to-date references. Offers more thorough coverage of ambulatory care than that found in other pocketbooks.

A− ***The Merck Manual of Diagnosis & Therapy*** ***$65.00***
MERCK
Merck & Co., 2011, 19th ed., 3800 pages, ISBN 9780911910193

Offers clear discussions of a wide variety of diseases, but with limited tables, charts, or illustrations. Well organized, comprehensive, and well indexed. May be used as a reference book, but not as extensive as *Harrison's* or *Cecil*. Useful as an adjunctive, quick home-reference textbook.

NEUROLOGY

HANDBOOK/POCKETBOOK

A ***Pocket Neurology*** **$52.50**

Greer

Lippincott Williams & Wilkins, 2010, 1st ed., 288 pages, ISBN 9781608312566

A practical, comprehensive pocketbook guide presented in a concise bulleted format, supplemented by multiple tables and algorithms for commonly encountered inpatient and outpatient neurologic disorders. Contains primary literature references. A quick and easy read that can help users get up to speed before or after seeing a patient.

A ***Weiner and Levitt's Neurology (House Officer Series)*** **$50.00**

Rae-Grant

Lippincott Williams & Wilkins, 2008, 8th ed., 307 pages, ISBN 9780781781541

A clinically oriented pocketbook organized by signs and symptoms. Concise chapters offer clinically relevant material, although the text is somewhat short on tables and diagrams. Covers most topics thoroughly, but lacks detail. Written for interns and residents, but can also be useful for medical students during their initial patient encounters.

A- ***On Call Neurology*** **$54.95**

Marshall

Elsevier, 2007, 3rd ed., 505 pages, ISBN 9781416023753

A compact book addressing on-call neurologic issues a physician is likely to encounter. The structure of the book effectively models the process of working up a patient in a hospital setting: phone-call management (pertinent questions and orders), elevator thoughts (differential diagnoses), major threats to life, bedside management (neuro exam, labs), and management. Not high yield for studying for a shelf exam, but well designed (though a little large) as a pocket reference for students on a rotation or a subinternship.

A- ***Manual of Neurologic Therapeutics*** **$70.00**

Samuels

Lippincott Williams & Wilkins, 2010, 8th ed., 607 pages, ISBN 9781605475752

A spiral-bound pocketbook written in expanded outline format and patterned after the *Washington Manual.* Strikes an excellent balance between concise, practical information and reference-level detail. Better for clinical management than for review of pathophysiology. An appendix lists agencies that provide support and education for patients with specific neurologic problems.

A- ***Little Black Book of Neurology*** **$72.95**

Zaidat

Elsevier, 2008, 5th ed., 638 pages, ISBN 9780323039505

An alphabetically organized pocketbook with a format similar to that of a dictionary. Content is presented in essay form without an index or a table of contents, detracting from its utility as a quick reference. Written more for residents than for medical students. Best used for review by advanced neurology students.

B-

Merritt's Neurology Handbook ***$77.50***

MAZZONI

Lippincott Williams & Wilkins, 2006, 2nd ed., 707 pages, ISBN 9780781762700

A volume that follows its parent text, *Merritt's Neurology*, chapter by chapter, with an abbreviated text in a pocket-sized format. Accordingly, a wide range of topics is covered, but with little depth. No images of scans are included. Better as a quick reference for residents or attendings than for medical students.

REVIEW/MINI-REFERENCE

A ***Neurological Examination Made Easy*** **$44.95**

FULLER

Elsevier, 2008, 4th ed., 247 pages, ISBN 9780443069642

A review of the neurologic exam for medical students, written from the author's perspective of what to do, what one finds, and what it means. Excellent flow diagrams guide the reader through the process of examining the patient. Good for the non-neurologist who wishes to learn the neurologic exam extremely well, or for the serious neurology student who wants to start off with an excellent foundation.

A ***Clinical Neuroanatomy Made Ridiculously Simple*** **$24.95**

GOLDBERG

MedMaster, Inc., 2010, 4th ed., 95 pages, ISBN 9780940780927

A quick, easy-to-read review of the most relevant clinical neuroanatomy, featuring mnemonics, humor, and case presentations that one may encounter on the wards. Best used with a comprehensive review book or textbook for clinical management information.

A ***The Four-Minute Neurologic Exam*** **$13.95**

GOLDBERG

MedMaster, Inc., 2011, 2nd ed., 49 pages, ISBN 9780940780965

A quick, practical guide reviewing the fundamentals of the neurologic screening examination. Best used before or in the early part of the rotation. Can be read in a few hours to provide a good foundation for physical exam skills.

A ***Clinical Neurology*** **$59.00**

SIMON

McGraw-Hill, 2009, 7th ed., 408 pages, ISBN 9780071546447

A well-organized, clinically oriented reference that is extremely useful on the neurology clerkship. The text is comprehensive enough to serve as a primary resource for the medical student. Emphasizes essential information with excellent use of tables and diagrams. A great introductory neurology text for the motivated student. Highly useful appendices offer guides on how to perform an extensive neurologic exam.

A⁻ ***Neurology and Neurosurgery Illustrated*** **$97.95**

LINDSAY

Elsevier, 2004, 4th ed., 598 pages, ISBN 9780443070563

Offers extensive coverage of a wide variety of topics, with great line drawings illustrating key aspects of pathophysiology, clinical features, and treatment. Not for reading cover to cover during a short rotation, but can be used as a reference for the essential features of neurologic disease. Sections are organized both by presenting complaint and by specific disorder.

A⁻ ***Case Files Neurology*** **$34.95**

TOY

McGraw-Hill, 2008, 1st ed., 476 pages, ISBN 9780071482875

Written in a case-based format, this text offers 53 high-yield clinical cases of commonly encountered disorders. The ensuing discussions in each chapter help medical students think through the diagnosis and management algorithm. Best used as a supplement to a review book or textbook and during the clerkship to consolidate learning.

B+ ***Lecture Notes on Neurology*** **$39.95**

Ginsberg

Wiley, 2010, 9th ed., 200 pages, ISBN 9781405177221

A good, concise review of key points with great tables, figures, and illustrations. May be read from cover to cover during a short rotation. Organized primarily by pathology rather than by presenting complaint.

B+ ***Underground Clinical Vignettes: Neurology*** **$29.95**

Kim

Lippincott Williams & Wilkins, 2007, 4th ed., 186 pages, ISBN 9780781768375

A well-organized review of clinical vignettes commonly encountered on the shelf and Step 2 CK exams. Includes a focused, high-yield discussion of pathogenesis, epidemiology, management, complications, and associated diseases. Black-and-white images are included where relevant. Also contains several "minicases" in which only key facts related to each disease are presented. An entertaining, easy-to-use supplement for studying during the clinical rotation, although it is neither as comprehensive nor as relevant for day-to-day wards activities.

B+ ***Blueprints Clinical Cases in Neurology*** **$36.95**

Sheth

Lippincott Williams & Wilkins, 2007, 2nd ed., 390 pages, ISBN 9781405104944

Organized by common presenting signs and symptoms, this book contains symptom-based clinical cases accompanied by 200 USMLE-style questions. The format is similar to that of the Case Files series but places less emphasis on discussions and greater focus on questions.

B ***In A Page Neurology*** **$34.95**

Brillman

Lippincott Williams & Wilkins, 2005, 1st ed., 209 pages, ISBN 9781405104326

A dry review of more than 150 diseases, organized by type of neurologic condition. Each disease pathology is explained in 1 page, from etiology to prognosis, with lists. Provides a big picture and high-yield information; best suited for quick review before seeing a patient or preparing for a pimp session. Thin enough to carry around, but not pocket-sized. No figures or tables are included, and readers will need to refer to other textbooks for more detailed information.

B ***High-Yield Neuroanatomy*** **$30.95**

Fix

Lippincott Williams & Wilkins, 2009, 4th ed., 186 pages, ISBN 9780781779463

An outline review designed for USMLE Step 1 exam preparation. Best used for prerotation study for those interested in getting a head start. Not comprehensive, but some students consider it a good "minimalist" reference for short neurology rotations. Good for pathways and review of general pathophysiology, but lacks a discussion of management issues.

B ***Manter & Gatz's Essentials of Clinical Neuroanatomy and Neurophysiology*** **$39.95**

Gilman

F. A. Davis, 2003, 10th ed., 281 pages, ISBN 9780803607729

An extensive, in-depth review of neuroanatomy and neurophysiology that is too detailed for most medical students; would be difficult to read during the relatively brief neurology rotation. Offers excellent pathway diagrams. Only for the highly motivated student with a deep interest in the basic sciences.

QUESTION BOOKS

A⁻

PreTest Neurology **$26.95**

ANSCHEL

McGraw-Hill, 2009, 7th ed., 355 pages, ISBN 9780071597920

A collection of 500 multiple-choice questions covering a wide range of topics in neurology. Includes clinical vignette–style questions and provides detailed paragraph-format explanations for each answer. Probably the most widely used preparatory text for shelf exams. Good for last-minute review before the exam.

B+

Neurology Secrets **$54.95**

ROLAK

Elsevier, 2011, 5th ed., 470 pages, ISBN 9780323057127

A pocket-sized book in a question-and-answer format with bulleted lists, mnemonics, and practical tips from the authors. Features a 2-color page layout, "key point" boxes, and lists of useful Web sites. Provides a concise overview of essential material for a quick read during downtime on the wards. Should be supplemented with a good general review book or textbook.

B

Neurology Recall **$45.50**

MILLER

Lippincott Williams & Wilkins, 2003, 2nd ed., 377 pages, ISBN 9780781745888

A text written in a question-and-answer format typical of the Recall series. A good reference for students preparing for pimping on wards, it provides fast, easy-to-read reviews of disorders. Not as detailed as *Neurology Secrets*, so future neurologists will need another reference for in-depth discussion of disease.

TEXTBOOK/REFERENCE

Grade	Resource	Price
A	***Adams and Victor's Principles of Neurology*** ROPPER **McGraw-Hill, 2009, 9th ed., 1572 pages, ISBN 9780071499927** A comprehensive reference text with detailed discussions of disease from a clinical perspective. Uniquely organized, with chapters transitioning from a general patient approach to cardinal manifestations of neurologic disease to specific diseases. Tables and figures are somewhat sparse. Most appropriate for students considering neurology as a specialty.	***$175.00***
A⁻	***Neurology: An Illustrated Colour Text*** FULLER **Elsevier, 2010, 3rd ed., 136 pages, ISBN 9780702032240** An introductory-level text of common neurologic disorders with good, cartoon-style images illustrating how to evaluate different aspects of the neurologic exam. Includes more color line drawings than color photographs or radiographs of disease. May lack the level of detail necessary for use as a reference during the clinical rotation, particularly with respect to management.	***$64.95***
A⁻	***Netter's Concise Neurology*** MISULIS **Elsevier, 2007, 1st ed., 565 pages, ISBN 9781929007899** A full-color illustrated atlas that uses excellent, familiar Netter-style illustrations. A brief overview of each disease is supplemented by classic drawings. May be more suitable for premedical students than for medical students on rotation, but several useful tables and flowcharts are included.	***$59.95***
B⁺	***Merritt's Neurology*** ROWLAND **Lippincott Williams & Wilkins, 2010, 12th ed., 1172 pages, ISBN 9780781791861** A reference textbook that covers the entire spectrum of neurologic disease in depth, although not in as much detail as *Principles of Neurology*. Concise chapters are accompanied by a number of clinical radiographs.	***$149.95***

OBSTETRICS AND GYNECOLOGY

HANDBOOK/POCKETBOOK

A

Current Clinical Strategies: Gynecology and Obstetrics **$16.95**

CHAN

Current Clinical Strategies, 2011, 2nd ed., 208 pages, ISBN 9781934323298

A quick, readable pocketbook containing essential high-yield information. Its outline format includes signs and symptoms, differential, treatment, and complications. Inexpensive and remarkably compact; great for both management and quick review on the wards. Includes an excellent, concise oncology section with classifications.

B+

Manual of Obstetrics **$66.95**

EVANS

Lippincott Williams & Wilkins, 2007, 7th ed., 706 pages, ISBN 9780781796965

A good pocketbook presented in the same format as the *Washington Manual.* Offers a cursory discussion of pathophysiology, symptoms, and signs but more detailed coverage of diagnostic approach and therapeutics. Covers a broad range of topics in obstetrics; useful for quick review. More appropriate for subinterns than for junior medical students.

B

On Call Obstetrics and Gynecology **$49.95**

CHIN

Elsevier, 2005, 3rd ed., 428 pages, ISBN 9781416023944

A compact guide presented in a format similar to the rest of the On Call series, addressing common problems the on-call physician will encounter in obstetrics and gynecology. Although not comprehensive enough for study, the pocketbook guides students' clinical thinking and approach toward emergent issues. More for residents on call than for medical students.

B

Obstetrics & Gynecology (House Officer Series) **$29.95**

RAYBURN

Lippincott Williams & Wilkins, 2002, 4th ed., 429 pages, ISBN 9780781728553

A good pocketbook for quick reference as patients are seen in the hospital. Written in essay form, the text is sometimes difficult to sift through for the main points. Offers basic, broad coverage of most conditions encountered on the wards and in outpatient clinics.

B

SOAP for Obstetrics and Gynecology **$31.95**

UZELAC

Lippincott Williams & Wilkins, 2005, 1st ed., 143 pages, ISBN 9781405104357

A thin pocketbook that presents information in a SOAP-note format. Focuses heavily on clinical problems, not on the diagnosis. The "S" (subject) section contains a helpful list of questions to ask when interviewing patients and writing notes. The book would be most useful in guiding day-to-day management and in formulating an assessment and plan for patients with a known diagnosis. Would benefit from some figures or diagrams.

REVIEW/MINI-REFERENCE

A

Blueprints in Obstetrics & Gynecology ***$40.95***
CALLAHAN
Lippincott Williams & Wilkins, 2008, 5th ed., 401 pages, ISBN 9780781782494

A good, concise introductory review for the obstetrics and gynecology rotation. Offers an excellent and easy-to-read synopsis of major topics along with good figures and tables. Some students feel that this is the best of the Blueprints series. Also includes an excellent review test for the shelf and Step 2 CK exams, but students considering a career in obstetrics and gynecology will need to find a more detailed textbook as well. Contains a section on breast disease.

A

First Aid for the Obstetrics & Gynecology Clerkship ***$46.95***
KAUFMAN
McGraw-Hill, 2011, 3rd ed., 400 pages, ISBN 9780071634199

An excellent primary resource that students can use while getting oriented in the obstetrics and gynecology clerkship. Includes typical presentations of the most common pathologies encountered during the rotation. Contains easy-to-read overviews of the diagnosis, pathophysiology, workup, and treatment of pertinent topics within obstetrics and gynecology. May be supplemented with a comprehensive text for an in-depth discussion of pathophysiology. Few figures and photographs are provided. Overall, an excellent review for a busy clerkship. This publication is not affiliated with the authors of *First Aid for the Wards*.

A

Case Files Obstetrics & Gynecology ***$34.95***
TOY
McGraw-Hill, 2009, 3rd ed., 508 pages, ISBN 9780071605809

A highly useful book, particularly at the beginning of the rotation. Presents a concise review of the most common problems encountered in obstetrics and gynecology, including an excellent summary of the process by which one considers the symptoms, diagnosis, and treatment algorithm of each disease. A quick burst of review questions in each chapter consolidates the learning concepts presented. An excellent companion to another general review book or textbook.

B+

Blueprints Clinical Cases in Obstetrics & Gynecology ***$36.95***
CAUGHEY
Lippincott Williams & Wilkins, 2007, 2nd ed., 418 pages, ISBN 9781405104906

Organized by common presenting signs and symptoms, this book contains symptom-based clinical cases accompanied by 200 USMLE-style questions. The format is similar to that of the Case Files series but places less emphasis on discussions and greater focus on questions.

B+

High-Yield Obstetrics & Gynecology ***$30.95***
SAKALA
Lippincott Williams & Wilkins, 2006, 2nd ed., 194 pages, ISBN 9780781796309

An excellent pocket reference book written in a concise outline format arranged by organ system. Offers a quick overview of the diseases and situations most commonly encountered on the clerkship. Should be supplemented with a more comprehensive review book or textbook.

B

In A Page OB/GYN & Women's Health ***$34.95***
CARR
Lippincott Williams & Wilkins, 2004, 1st ed., 156 pages, ISBN 9781405103800

A dry review of more than 120 diseases, organized by a woman's life span (from adolescence to post-menopause). Each disease pathology is explained in 1 page, from etiology to prognosis, with lists. Provides a big picture and high-yield information; best suited for quick review before seeing a patient or preparing for a pimp session. The book is thin but not pocket-sized and also lacks figures and tables, so readers will need to refer to other textbooks for more detailed information.

B

Underground Clinical Vignettes: OB/GYN ***$29.95***
KIM
Lippincott Williams & Wilkins, 2008, 4th ed., 184 pages, ISBN 9780781768405

A well-organized review of clinical vignettes commonly encountered on the shelf and Step 2 CK exams. Includes a focused, high-yield discussion of pathogenesis, epidemiology, management, complications, and associated diseases. Black-and-white images are included where relevant. Also contains several "minicases" in which only key facts related to each disease are presented. An excellent, entertaining, and easy-to-use supplement for studying during the clinical rotation.

B

NMS Obstetrics and Gynecology ***$45.95***
PFEIFER
Lippincott Williams & Wilkins, 2008, 6th ed., 469 pages, ISBN 9780781770712

A comprehensive review presented in an outline format that may be too dense for regular use. Well organized, but discussions can be lengthy and boring. An excellent comprehensive exam at the end poses questions similar to those found on the shelf and Step 2 CK exams. Offers few tables and diagrams.

B⁻

Lecture Notes on Obstetrics and Gynaecology ***$42.95***
HAMILTON-FAIRLEY
Wiley, 2009, 3rd ed., 366 pages, ISBN 9781405178013

A mini–review text designed for medical students. Offers excellent coverage of basic science, etiology, and clinical presentation, but its discussion of differentials, diagnostic approach, and therapeutic options is only average, limiting its usefulness on the wards. Portable enough to carry around in the coat pocket if readers wish to use it to study for shelf and Step 2 CK exams.

QUESTION BOOKS

A-

PreTest Obstetrics and Gynecology **$32.00**

SCHNEIDER

McGraw-Hill, 2009, 12th ed., 335 pages, ISBN 9780071599795

A collection of 500 multiple-choice questions covering a wide range of topic in obstetrics and gynecology. Includes clinical vignette–style questions, and provides detailed paragraph-format explanations for each answer. Probably the most widely used preparatory text for shelf exams. Good for last-minute review before the exam.

B+

Blueprints Q&A Step 2 Obstetrics & Gynecology **$19.95**

TRAN

Lippincott Williams & Wilkins, 2005, 2nd ed., 153 pages, ISBN 9781405103909

A resource that contains more than 200 USMLE-style questions with explanations for both correct and incorrect answers. Explanations are not as detailed or well referenced as those in the PreTest series. Originally designed for Step 2 CK preparation, but since the format of the shelf exam is similar, this would be a useful companion for clerkship preparation as well. Thin enough to carry in the pocket, and could easily be read in a few days.

B

Lange Q&A: Obstetrics & Gynecology **$43.95**

VONTVER

McGraw-Hill, 2006, 8th ed., 388 pages, ISBN 9780071461399

A question-and-answer book with 1600 multiple-choice questions organized under different topics. Provides detailed, paragraph-length explanations for each answer. Questions tend to focus on details rather than following the shelf-exam format. A good review of the topics, but could be overwhelming if used for last-minute preparation.

B-

Obstetrics and Gynecology Secrets **$39.95**

BADER

Elsevier, 2005, 3rd ed., 428 pages, ISBN 9780323034159

A text presented in the question-and-answer format typical of the Secrets series, with good coverage of many high-yield, clinically relevant topics. Detailed, but contains no vignettes or images. Some explanations appear inadequate. Provides a good clinical context for quick self-testing, but does not serve as a formal topic review.

B-

Obstetrics and Gynecology Recall **$45.50**

BOURGEOIS

Lippincott Williams & Wilkins, 2008, 3rd ed., 673 pages, ISBN 9780781770699

A question-and-answer format in Recall-series style set in 2 columns, making it easy to use for self-quizzing. Reviews many high-yield concepts and facts. Questions emphasize individual facts but do not integrate concepts, and no vignettes or images are included. In addition, some topics are covered only sparingly. Useful as a review of selected material, but not a comprehensive source for wards or end-of-rotation examinations.

TEXTBOOK/REFERENCE

A ***Essentials of Obstetrics and Gynecology*** **$59.95**
HACKER
Elsevier, 2010, 5th ed., 475 pages, ISBN 9781416059400

A full-color text that is comprehensive yet concise. Provides an excellent overview of the evaluation, diagnosis, and management of a wide range of obstetric and gynecologic disorders encountered on the rotation. Offers practical clinical information with photos, charts, and illustrations. Also includes full online access of the text supplemented by an additional image gallery, case studies, and online note-taking capabilities via Student Consult.

A⁻ ***Obstetrics and Gynecology*** **$69.95**
BECKMANN
Lippincott Williams & Wilkins, 2010, 6th ed., 497 pages, ISBN 9780781788076

A detailed textbook intended for medical students on their core obstetrics and gynecology rotation, based on the Association of Professors of Gynecology and Obstetrics Instructional Objectives. Features a case-based approach with brief coverage of topics and many questions. Chapters are short enough to finish in a single sitting and include some helpful tables, figures, and diagrams. Some students state that the book does not contain enough high-yield information for the wards.

A⁻ ***Williams Obstetrics*** **$175.00**
CUNNINGHAM
McGraw-Hill, 2010, 23rd ed., 1385 pages, ISBN 9780071497015

The definitive book within its field, meant for the serious obstetrics and gynecology student. Organized by organ system; includes good use of graphics to highlight material. Offers more ultrasound pictures than the previous edition contained. Well referenced with updated guidelines and a strong, evidence-based approach. Its usefulness is diminished only by the need to find another reference for gynecology.

A⁻ ***Danforth's Obstetrics and Gynecology*** **$175.00**
GIBBS
Lippincott Williams & Wilkins, 2008, 10th ed., 1136 pages, ISBN 9780781769372

An excellent core text for residents and students considering careers in obstetrics and gynecology, but too detailed for most others. A well-organized and comprehensive reference for both obstetrics and gynecology, with numerous illustrations. Places increased emphasis on the latest advances, evidence-based medicine, and the most recent clinical guidelines. Also offers good, concise outlines of many diseases, although some key points are not highlighted as well as they should be in view of the book's extensive detail.

B+ ***Current Diagnosis & Treatment: Obstetrics & Gynecology*** **$75.00**
DECHERNEY
McGraw-Hill, 2007, 10th ed., 1118 pages, ISBN 9780071439008

A good overall reference book. Makes effective use of graphics and tables, but minimal emphasis is placed on differential diagnosis. A good value, but not very high yield or appropriate for those with less interest in the specialty, especially when compared to other reference textbooks.

PEDIATRICS

HANDBOOK/POCKETBOOK

A

The Harriet Lane Handbook **$54.95**

Tschudy

Elsevier, 2011, 19th ed., 1132 pages, ISBN 9780323079426

An excellent pocket-sized resource book that is ideally suited for use on the pediatrics wards. Includes a helpful review of pediatric diagnoses and workup plans as well as a complete index of pediatric drugs and dosing. A must-have for pediatric subinterns. Also includes full online access to the comprehensive pediatric drug formulary. May be too dense for a quick read.

A

Schwartz's Clinical Handbook of Pediatrics **$48.95**

Zorc

Lippincott Williams & Wilkins, 2012, 5th ed., 1040 pages, ISBN 9781608315789

An excellent pocket-sized reference book focusing on the diagnostic approach toward 80-plus commonly encountered pediatric problems. Contains an extensive differential diagnosis list along with discussions of presenting symptoms and diagnostic and treatment algorithms. Also includes easy-to-read tables, figures, and charts. An extremely useful resource for medical students and interns.

B+

Manual of Pediatric Therapeutics **$61.95**

Graef

Lippincott Williams & Wilkins, 2008, 7th ed., 716 pages, ISBN 9780781771665

A relatively comprehensive spiral-bound manual that adequately covers the general principles, management, and treatment of common pediatric diseases, presented in a concise outline format that makes good use of tables and charts. Includes updated guidelines and a focused drug formulary section. Appropriate for subinterns.

B+

Pocket Pediatrics **$54.50**

Prasad

Lippincott Williams & Wilkins, 2010, 1st ed., ISBN 9781605474960

A pocket-sized reference book featuring bulleted lists, tables, and algorithms that address commonly encountered pediatric problems. Good for a quick read before and after seeing a patient. Has useful pediatric dosing information, and includes primary literature references for key concepts. The index is not optimally organized for easy search of pediatric problems.

B

SOAP for Pediatrics **$31.95**

Polisky

Lippincott Williams & Wilkins, 2005, 1st ed., 167 pages, ISBN 9781405104340

A thin pocketbook that presents information in a SOAP-note format. Organized according to the visit setting (inpatient vs. outpatient), the book focuses heavily on clinical problems, not on diagnosis. The "S" (subject) section contains a helpful list of questions to ask when interviewing patients and writing notes. The book would be most useful in guiding day-to-day management and in formulating an assessment and plan for patients with a known diagnosis. Would benefit from some figures or diagrams.

B-

Practical Guide to the Care of the Pediatric Patient ***$54.95***

ALARIO

Elsevier, 2008, 2nd ed., 947 pages, ISBN 9780323036702

A spiral-bound, student-friendly pocket manual written in outline format with emphasis on high-yield clinical features, diagnostic evaluation, and management of pediatric diseases. Contains sections on the pediatric H&P, development, and routine health maintenance and preventive care. Offers more information on pathophysiology and differentials than does *Harriet Lane*, but not as useful for pharmacology.

B-

On Call Pediatrics ***$54.95***

NOCTON

Elsevier, 2006, 3rd ed., 452 pages, ISBN 9781416023937

A practical, portable guide to the pediatric problems one is likely to encounter on call. Takes a systematic approach that begins with the phone call and includes preliminary evaluation, differential diagnosis, workup, and initial management. Sections are well organized by common problems, but readers will need to look elsewhere for more detail. Limited in breadth; cannot replace other pocket manuals in pediatrics. Not useful for beginning medical students.

REVIEW/MINI-REFERENCE

A

Nelson Essentials of Pediatrics **$79.95**

MARCDANTE

Elsevier, 2011, 6th ed., 831 pages, ISBN 9781437706437

An excellent, concise, full-color resource that is more readable than its parent text. Contains high-yield tables and numerous images offering an overview of essential pediatric concepts. Also includes full online access. Would pair well with another case-based book or question book.

A

First Aid for the Pediatrics Clerkship **$45.00**

STEAD

McGraw-Hill, 2011, 3rd ed., 616 pages, ISBN 9780071664035

A good resource that offers a general overview of commonly encountered problems in the pediatric clerkship. Information is presented in an easy-to-read bulleted/outline format that is concise and to the point, supplemented by thorough summary/review charts. Excellent for the pediatrics clerkship, but lacks detail on pathophysiology, and contains few images. This publication is not affiliated with the authors of *First Aid for the Wards.*

A⁻

Case Files Pediatrics **$34.95**

TOY

McGraw-Hill, 2010, 3rd ed., 497 pages, ISBN 9780071598675

A easy-to-read, pocket-sized text covering the major bread-and-butter topics encountered on the pediatrics rotation, presented in a case-based format. Offers differential diagnosis and management algorithms with excellent explanations. Does not cover some uncommon topics that may be tested on the pediatric shelf exam. A good companion to a more comprehensive review book or textbook.

B+

Oski's Essential Pediatrics **$67.00**

CROCETTI

Lippincott Williams & Wilkins, 2004, 2nd ed., 764 pages, ISBN 9780781737708

A good, basic reference text organized by problem. Includes illustrations and tables. Easier to read than *Nelson* and provides a good overview of treatment and management, but lacks detail, and sections vary in their depth of coverage. Useful for the time-limited student. An interesting section at the end describes common syndromes with morphologic abnormalities, including line illustrations of distinctive facial phenotypes. The text is somewhat outdated.

B+

Underground Clinical Vignettes: Pediatrics **$29.95**

KIM

Lippincott Williams & Wilkins, 2007, 4th ed., 183 pages, ISBN 9780781768443

A well-organized review of clinical vignettes commonly encountered on the shelf and Step 2 CK exams. Includes a focused, high-yield discussion of pathogenesis, epidemiology, management, and complications. Black-and-white images are included where relevant. Also offers several "minicases" in which only key facts related to each disease are presented. An excellent, entertaining, and easy-to-use supplement for studying during the clinical rotation, but not meant to be used as a primary text.

B+

Blueprints Clinical Cases in Pediatrics **$36.95**

LONDHE

Lippincott Williams & Wilkins, 2007, 2nd ed., 426 pages, ISBN 9781405104920

Organized by common presenting signs and symptoms, this book contains 50 symptom-based clinical cases accompanied by 200 USMLE-style questions. The format is similar to that of the Case Files series but places less emphasis on discussions and greater focus on questions.

B+ ***Blueprints in Pediatrics*** ***$43.50***

MARINO

Lippincott Williams & Wilkins, 2009, 5th ed., 364 pages, ISBN 9780781782517

A handy resource book of high-yield information that is likely to appear on the shelf and Step 2 CK exams. Presents adequate coverage of the basics, and includes good charts, diagrams, and key points. Not comprehensive enough to be a complete review book; some sections are too detailed and others too simplistic. Offers a good overview of topics that students are most likely to encounter while on the rotation. Some chapters are verbose and difficult to read.

B+ ***Rudolph's Fundamentals of Pediatrics*** ***$89.00***

RUDOLPH

McGraw-Hill, 2002, 3rd ed., 919 pages, ISBN 9780838584507

An excellent, well-organized softcover reference book written at an appropriate level for students on their pediatric clerkship. The highly readable text makes good use of algorithms that summarize approaches toward common pediatric diseases. Suffices as a general home reference, but students going into pediatrics should consider a more detailed textbook such as the parent volume. Has not been updated in several years.

B ***NMS Pediatrics*** ***$46.50***

DWORKIN

Lippincott Williams & Wilkins, 2009, 5th ed., 470 pages, ISBN 9780781770750

A lengthy review book that offers a detailed discussion of disease management and covers most of the pediatric disorders found on the shelf and Step 2 CK exams. Although more comprehensive than the Blueprints series, the text is occasionally too verbose, presenting more information than one needs to know for the shelf exam. The outline format often lacks organization, and few tables and figures are included. Review questions are available at the end of each chapter, and a comprehensive test is included at the end of the book.

B ***In A Page Pediatrics*** ***$40.95***

KAHAN

Lippincott Williams & Wilkins, 2008, 2nd ed., 455 pages, ISBN 9780781770453

A dry review of more than 200 diseases, organized by organ system. Each disease pathology is explained in 1 page, from etiology to prognosis. Provides a big picture and high-yield information; best suited for quick review before seeing a patient or preparing for a pimp session. The book is thin but is not pocket-sized and also lacks figures and tables, so students will need to refer to other textbooks for more detailed information.

B ***Lecture Notes on Paediatrics*** ***$42.95***

NEWELL

Wiley, 2008, 8th ed., 295 pages, ISBN 9781405145091

A portable review book on the core knowledge and fundamentals of pediatric diseases. Offers a number of useful tables and figures. Unique sections are dedicated to describing the essentials of the pediatric clinical exam, and self-assessment questions have been added. Too superficial for practical wards use given its limited coverage of diagnostic approach and management, but useful as a supplement to other textbooks. Costly for the limited amount of material covered.

B

In A Page Pediatric Signs & Symptoms ***$40.95***

TEITELBAUM

Lippincott Williams & Wilkins, 2004, 1st ed., 255 pages, ISBN 9781405104272

Organized by common presenting signs and symptoms, this book focuses on differential diagnosis and workup. As with its counterpart, *In A Page Pediatrics*, each symptom is explained in 1 page with lists. Best used as a quick review, and a great companion to use while on call, providing guidelines on how to work up "fresh" patients.

B-

Berkowitz's Pediatrics: A Primary Care Approach ***$74.95***

BERKOWITZ

American Academy of Pediatrics, 2008, 3rd ed., 837 pages, ISBN 9781581102833

A comprehensive review text with sections focusing on a key symptom or general disease category followed by step-by-step guidelines on diagnostic approach and treatment strategies. Case vignettes and self-assessment questions are included, but the book makes inadequate use of tables and illustrations. The format is somewhat difficult to follow and is not useful for test preparation. Sufficiently broad to help students understand general pediatric issues, but specific treatment regimens must be found in another reference.

B-

BRS Pediatrics ***$43.50***

BROWN

Lippincott Williams & Wilkins, 2005, 1st ed., 649 pages, ISBN 9780781721295

A resource that is organized in the same manner as its counterpart USMLE prep series. Contains substantial information on pediatric disorders with accompanying questions at the end of each section, but the text is a bit too dry for review during the rotation and is not designed for use as a quick reference. Has not been updated recently.

QUESTION BOOKS

A	***PreTest Pediatrics*** YETMAN **McGraw-Hill, 2009, 12th ed., 403 pages, ISBN 9780071597906** A collection of 500-plus multiple-choice questions and answers covering a wide range of topics in pediatrics. Explanations are appropriately detailed and are organized in a way that helps readers differentiate between similar answers. Probably the most widely used preparatory text for shelf exams. Good for last-minute review before the clerkship shelf exam or during downtime on the wards.	***$32.00***
A⁻	***Pediatric Secrets*** POLIN **Elsevier, 2011, 5th ed., 739 pages, ISBN 9780323065610** An easy-to-read question-and-answer book organized by organ system with good use of tables, charts, and mnemonics. Designed to prepare students for pimping sessions. Best used for quick self-testing during downtime. Some questions are too specific and detailed. A good companion to a general review book or textbook.	***$39.95***
B⁺	***Blueprints Q&A Step 2 Pediatrics*** FOTI **Lippincott Williams & Wilkins, 2005, 2nd ed., 159 pages, ISBN 9781405103916** A resource that contains more than 200 USMLE-style questions with explanations for both correct and incorrect answers. Explanations are not as detailed and well referenced as those in the PreTest series. Originally designed for Step 2 CK preparation, but since the format of the shelf exam is similar, this would be a useful companion for clerkship preparation as well. Thin enough to carry in the pocket, and could easily be read in a few days.	***$19.95***
B⁻	***Pediatrics Recall*** MCGAHREN **Lippincott Williams & Wilkins, 2011, 4th ed., 542 pages, ISBN 9781605476766** Like the Secrets series, this book is meant for quick self-testing during free time, covering essential bare-bones issues of pediatric health and disease in a question-and-answer format. A bit smaller than previous versions, but still too bulky to carry around in the coat pocket.	***$40.95***

TEXTBOOK/REFERENCE

A

Nelson Textbook of Pediatrics **$150.00**

KLIEGMAN

Elsevier, 2011, 19th ed., 2610 pages, ISBN 9781437707557

An authoritative reference book that many consider the "gold standard" of pediatric textbooks. Well organized with clear explanations and comprehensive discussions on the diagnosis and treatment of pediatric disorders. Worth the investment for those pursuing pediatrics as a career; otherwise, best borrowed from the library. Great for preparing complete, detailed presentations. Too lengthy to read through on a typical pediatric clerkship rotation.

A

Rudolph's Pediatrics **$159.00**

RUDOLPH

McGraw-Hill, 2011, 22nd ed., 2488 pages, ISBN 9780071497237

A comprehensive reference book for serious pediatric students, featuring treatment algorithms and specialty-oriented topics. A worthy alternative to *Nelson*, but somewhat easier to read. Not useful as a high-yield quick read for the average medical student on a pediatric rotation, but a great reference for detailed explanations about specific topics.

A⁻

Pediatrics for Medical Students **$59.95**

BERNSTEIN

Lippincott Williams & Wilkins, 2011, 3rd ed., 717 pages, ISBN 9780781770309

An introductory text developed in collaboration with the American Academy of Pediatrics for third-year medical students doing their pediatric clerkship. Divided into common primary care problems and pediatric subspecialty problems with illustrations and tables. Also offers full online access to the text and an additional image data bank and test bank.

A⁻

Current Diagnosis & Treatment: Pediatrics **$75.00**

HAY

McGraw-Hill, 2011, 20th ed., 1382 pages, ISBN 9780071664448

An up-to-date, comprehensive reference book with excellent organization of disease entities. Provides clinical information on ambulatory and inpatient medical care from birth to adolescence. Makes excellent use of tables, graphs, and illustrations. High-yield information is presented as essentials of diagnosis at the beginning of each section. Overall, a useful book for home reference. Easier to read than the "classic" texts, but not as detailed.

A⁻

Oski's Pediatrics: Principles and Practice **$169.95**

MCMILLAN

Lippincott Williams & Wilkins, 2006, 4th ed., 2808 pages, ISBN 9780781738941

An authoritative and comprehensive textbook that has been around for many years. Although presented in black and white with few figures or tables, the book is still a great resource for motivated students.

A⁻

Atlas of Pediatric Physical Diagnosis **$179.00**

ZITELLI

Elsevier, 2007, 5th ed., 966 pages, ISBN 9780323048781

A comprehensive hardcover reference and pictorial book for serious pediatric students. Contains less text than *Nelson*, but places greater emphasis on illustrations. An excellent visual reference book, but too much information for the general clerkship student.

B ***Illustrated Textbook of Paediatrics*** ***$61.95***

LISSAUER

Elsevier, 2011, 4th ed., 533 pages, ISBN 9780723435655

A solid, easy-to-understand textbook written at a good introductory level for medical students. Makes excellent use of numerous color photographs, diagrams, case histories, and clinical tips. A good basic reference for learning and reviewing the fundamentals of pediatrics. However, some students felt that the text lacks a comprehensive discussion of certain pediatric topics.

PSYCHIATRY

HANDBOOK/POCKETBOOK

A

Current Clinical Strategies: Psychiatry **$12.95**

HAHN

Current Clinical Strategies, 2010, 4th ed., 122 pages, ISBN 9781934323250

A concise pocketbook designed for quick reference while on the wards. Contains DSM-IV diagnostic criteria, differential diagnoses, and current treatment guidelines. An excellent psychopharmacology section at the end of the book contains tables comparing drugs and their side effects. Also included is a brief overview of the mental status exam and sample admitting orders for common psychiatric disorders. A good value for its size and price.

A

Kaplan & Sadock's Pocket Handbook of Clinical Psychiatry **$61.95**

SADOCK

Lippincott Williams & Wilkins, 2010, 5th ed., 566 pages, ISBN 9781605472645

This staple quick-reference handbook discusses etiologies, epidemiology, clinical features, and therapeutic measures in a well-organized outline format. Contains up-to-date diagnostic criteria and pharmacologic guidelines along with cross-references to its parent book, *Kaplan & Sadock's Comprehensive Textbook of Psychiatry*. Also includes useful tables, color photographs of commonly used psychiatric drugs, and a general overview of the psychiatric examination. The small print makes it difficult to read.

A⁻

Practical Guide to the Care of the Psychiatric Patient **$54.95**

GOLDBERG

Elsevier, 2007, 3rd ed., 577 pages, ISBN 9780323036832

A concise, easy-to-read, spiral-bound handbook patterned after the growing Practical Care series. Offers thorough coverage of all major psychiatric areas with DSM-IV criteria and numerous comparative charts and tables. Not comprehensive, but contains the basic information that a medical student needs. Also includes an interesting section on P-450 drug interactions. A drug formulary at the end of the book for commonly prescribed psychiatric medications includes some out-of-place drugs such as allopurinol, INH, and procainamide.

A⁻

Psychiatry Clerkship Guide **$54.95**

MANLEY

Elsevier, 2007, 2nd ed., 520 pages, ISBN 9781416031321

A well-designed pocket guide with one section organized by presentation and a second section grouped by known diagnosis, allowing readers to use the reference in either manner. Information within each chapter is organized in a question-and-answer format, with answers given in paragraph style. Covers many questions that come up on rotations, but may not be the quickest on-the-go reference.

A⁻ ***The Massachusetts General Hospital/McLean Hospital Residency Handbook of Psychiatry*** ***$46.50***

Rosenquist

Lippincott Williams & Wilkins, 2010, 1st ed., 270 pages, ISBN 9780781795043

An oversized pocket handbook with succinct, practical, and accessible information on the diagnosis and treatment of psychiatric disorders, written in an outline format with boxes, tables, and lists to provide high-yield information at a glance. Best suited for subinterns or for psychiatry house staff, the book contains major topics commonly encountered in psychiatry along with topics in psychiatric emergencies, symptom-based diagnosis and treatment, special populations, and psychopharmacology.

B⁺ ***Psychiatry (House Officer Series)*** ***$49.95***

Tomb

Lippincott Williams & Wilkins, 2008, 7th ed., 309 pages, ISBN 9780781774529

A compact pocketbook of commonly encountered psychiatric disorders, written in essay format with highlighted key words and phrases to facilitate rapid review. Contains good references for further in-depth study, updated management guidelines, a number of useful tables, and a color guide of psychiatric medications. A basic review book that is not comprehensive enough for primary study.

B⁻ ***Quick Reference to the Diagnostic Criteria from DSM-IV-TR*** ***$60.00***

American Psychiatric Association

American Psychiatric Press, 2000, 4th ed., 370 pages, ISBN 9780890420263

A pocketbook best used for the review of diagnostic criteria rather than for general wards work or application to patient care. Offers comprehensive coverage of all DSM-IV-TR psychiatric diseases, but lacks a discussion of etiologies and therapies, thus negating its clinical usefulness. The same diagnostic criteria for major disorders can be found in other handbooks.

B⁻ ***On Call Psychiatry*** ***$54.95***

Bernstein

Elsevier, 2006, 3rd ed., 340 pages, ISBN 9781416025740

A compact guide presented in a format similar to that of the rest of the On Call series, addressing common problems the on-call physician will encounter in psychiatry. Not comprehensive enough for study, but reviews important basic concepts of clinical thinking. Geared more toward residents on call than toward medical students. Some sections are related less to psychiatry than to general inpatient care.

REVIEW/MINI-REFERENCE

A+

First Aid for the Psychiatry Clerkship **$45.00**
STEAD
McGraw-Hill, 2011, 3rd ed., 230 pages, ISBN 9780071739238

A highly comprehensive overview of pertinent topics in psychiatry written in an outline format. A stellar general reference book for the clerkship shelf exam, offering a quick review of everything you need to keep in mind both on the wards and on the boards. Offers excellent organization with good clarity. This publication is not affiliated with the authors of *First Aid for the Wards*.

A

Case Files Psychiatry **$34.95**
TOY
McGraw-Hill, 2009, 3rd ed., 493 pages, ISBN 9780071598651

A compilation of more than 60 case series accompanied by extended discussions of each case in an easy-to-read and well-organized format. Contains a basic pharmacology section. Best used with a general reference book and a question-and-answer book to consolidate your knowledge and ace the clerkship shelf exam.

A–

Blueprints Clinical Cases in Psychiatry **$38.95**
HOBLYN
Lippincott Williams & Wilkins, 2008, 2nd ed., 499 pages, ISBN 9781405104968

Consists of 60 cases divided into adult, geriatric, and child/adolescent categories. Each case is presented in a comprehensive manner, and the discussion sections are in paragraph form but thorough. Each case study is followed by a few brief questions. Questions are not thorough enough to use alone for shelf study, but the cases are for the most part interesting and readable. Includes 100 USMLE-style questions for review.

A–

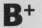

Clinical Psychopharmacology Made Ridiculously Simple **$15.95**
PRESTON
MedMaster, Inc., 2011, 7th ed., 83 pages, ISBN 9781935660057

A practical review of the pharmacologic treatment of psychiatric disease, written with a patient-oriented perspective. Numerous algorithms are provided on when and how to treat a patient as well as on common errors to avoid and advice to give to patients. May be best suited to residents prescribing treatment. Includes a limited discussion of mechanisms of action and adverse effects.

B+

Blueprints in Psychiatry **$36.95**
MURPHY
Lippincott Williams & Wilkins, 2007, 4th ed., 144 pages, ISBN 9781405105026

A brief review text of psychiatry designed for the shelf and Step 2 CK exams. Offers good coverage of high-yield topics with helpful tables, and the text is short, compact, and easily read within a few days. Lacks the detail necessary for rounds and the clinical clerkship, but remains a great resource for rapid review. The discussion of psychopharmacology is limited.

B+

NMS Psychiatry **$47.95**
THORNHILL
Lippincott Williams & Wilkins, 2011, 6th ed., 303 pages, ISBN 9781608315741

A highly detailed review book geared toward passing the shelf and Step 2 CK exams. Although the book is comprehensive, its dull, dry outline format makes it difficult to read. Multiple-choice questions are included after each chapter and at the end of the book, accompanied by lengthy explanations. Too detailed to be of use as a quick reference.

B ***Underground Clinical Vignettes: Psychiatry*** ***$30.95***

KIM

Lippincott Williams & Wilkins, 2007, 4th ed., 189 pages, ISBN 9780781768467

A well-organized review of clinical vignettes commonly encountered on the shelf and Step 2 CK exams. Includes 80 patient cases designed to take students from chief complaint through diagnostic workup and management. Black-and-white images are included where relevant, and the book provides a brief selection of USMLE-style questions. Offers a good discussion of differential diagnoses, but does not contain DSM-IV criteria. Overall, an entertaining, easy-to-use supplement for studying during the clinical rotation.

B ***DSM-IV-TR Casebook*** ***$89.00***

SPITZER

American Psychiatric Press, 2002, 1st ed., 576 pages, ISBN 9781585620593

This companion text to DSM-IV-TR consists of short clinical vignettes followed by a discussion of etiology, differentials, and treatment. The text is easy to read but is a long didactic tool for students interested in psychiatry. Geared more toward exam study than toward practical wards work; useful as a supplement to a more comprehensive review book.

QUESTION BOOKS

A

Lange Q&A: Psychiatry ***$45.00***

BLITZSTEIN

McGraw-Hill, 2011, 10th ed., 277 pages, ISBN 9780071703451

An excellent question-and-answer book to complement a general review book or textbook. Organized into easily readable sections with excellent explanations that tease out subtle differentials and management algorithms. Best used throughout the clerkship rotation.

A

PreTest Psychiatry ***$32.00***

KLAMEN

McGraw-Hill, 2009, 12th ed., 302 pages, ISBN 9780071598309

A collection of 500-plus multiple-choice questions covering a wide range of topics in psychiatry. Includes clinical vignette–style questions, and provides detailed paragraph-format explanations for each answer. Good for last-minute review before the exam, but less useful for general clerkship knowledge. Questions are neither too hard nor too easy, and explanations are detailed enough to allow readers to understand the topic without becoming low yield.

B+

Blueprints Q&A Step 2 Psychiatry ***$19.95***

MCLOONE

Lippincott Williams & Wilkins, 2005, 2nd ed., 85 pages, ISBN 9781405103923

A resource that contains 200 USMLE-style questions with explanations for both correct and incorrect answers, although the explanations are not as detailed and well referenced as those in the PreTest series. Originally designed for Step 2 CK preparation, but since the format of the shelf exam is similar, this would be a useful companion for clerkship preparation as well. Thin enough to carry in the pocket, and could easily be read in a few days.

B-

Psychiatry Recall ***$43.95***

FADEM

Lippincott Williams & Wilkins, 2004, 2nd ed., 210 pages, ISBN 9780781745116

Written in a quick question-and-answer format typical of the Recall series, this book reviews many high-yield facts that are covered on the shelf and Step 2 CK exams. Lacks clinical vignettes, and some of the topics covered can be obscure while others are not given enough attention. Useful as a quick-review supplement for another, more detailed text.

TEXTBOOK/REFERENCE

A ***Kaplan & Sadock's Concise Textbook of Clinical Psychiatry*** ***$79.00***
SADOCK
Lippincott Williams & Wilkins, 2008, 3rd ed., 738 pages, ISBN 9780781787468

An excellent, downsized version of *Kaplan & Sadock's Synopsis* that retains all the clinical psychiatry students need to know minus the behavioral science. Based on the DSM-IV and well organized, with practical chapters on psychopharmacology and laboratory tests. A nice addition to the bookshelf of the non-psychiatry-bound student.

A ***Kaplan & Sadock's Synopsis of Psychiatry*** ***$102.00***
SADOCK
Lippincott Williams & Wilkins, 2007, 10th ed., 1470 pages, ISBN 9780781773270

A comprehensive reference text pared down from its parent version. Not a good exam review book, as it is too detailed for shelf and Step 2 CK study. Offers solid tables, case studies, diagnostic coding tables, and instant online access, but information on some subjects is difficult to find. Provides good integration of information from the basic science and clinical years. A great reference for students going into psychiatry, but students may eventually want to consider *Kaplan & Sadock's Comprehensive Textbook* during residency and practice. Compare with *Kaplan & Sadock's Concise Textbook* for the amount of detail that is needed.

A⁻ ***Psychiatry*** ***$47.95***
CUTLER
Oxford University Press, 2010, 2nd ed., 636 pages, ISBN 9780195372748

An excellent introductory text written at an appropriate level for medical students. Discusses all major psychiatric disorders with numerous clinical vignettes to illustrate how each disorder may present. Contains good quick-reference tables of the DSM-IV criteria. Also includes chapters on the psychiatric interview, psychotherapy, and psychopharmacology.

A⁻ ***Kaplan & Sadock's Comprehensive Textbook of Psychiatry*** ***$399.95***
SADOCK
Lippincott Williams & Wilkins, 2009, 9th ed., 4520 pages, ISBN 9780781768993

The "gold standard" of psychiatric textbooks. Highly comprehensive, with interesting historical perspectives on psychiatric disease and treatment. Because of its size and hefty price, students should buy this text only as a long-term investment if they know they are going to pursue psychiatry. Even then, they may wish to wait and consider the more compact alternatives, as the text may still be too detailed. Available as a 2-volume set.

B⁺ ***Current Diagnosis & Treatment: Psychiatry*** ***$79.00***
EBERT
McGraw-Hill, 2008, 2nd ed., 739 pages, ISBN 9780071422925

A well-written text presented in a format consistent with that of the Current series. Offers a concise, easy-to-read reference, with each discussion of a disease beginning with the corresponding DSM-IV diagnostic criteria. Separately addresses psychiatry topics for children and adolescents, and includes a discussion of the psychological, biological, and sociological bases for disease. A good contender to *Kaplan & Sadock's Synopsis of Psychiatry*.

B

DSM-IV-TR ***$115.00***

American Psychiatric Association

American Psychiatric Press, 2000, 4th ed., 943 pages, ISBN 9780890420256

A comprehensive reference for psychiatric diagnostic criteria. Includes all existing psychiatric diseases defined by the American Psychiatric Association. Lacks a discussion of etiologic bases and treatment, detracting from its utility as a clinical resource. Not a worthwhile purchase unless one is considering psychiatry as a career. The newly updated DSM-V is slated to be published within the next 2 years.

SURGERY

HANDBOOK/POCKETBOOK

A

Surgery: A Competency-Based Companion **$39.95**
MANN
Elsevier, 2009, 1st ed., 772 pages, ISBN 9781416037477

An extremely high yield, pocket-sized book that covers essential surgical problems encountered on the surgical rotation. Well organized and clearly written, and offers a good overview of procedural and management issues that one typically confronts before going to the OR.

A⁻

Schwartz's Manual of Surgery **$63.95**
BRUNICARDI
McGraw-Hill, 2006, 8th ed., 1320 pages, ISBN 9780071446884

A highly detailed handbook whose essay format lends itself more to in-depth review than to quick reference while on the wards. Includes discussions of basic anatomy and physiology. Contains comprehensive coverage of surgical techniques, and offers more tables and illustrations than previous versions. A good supplement to the parent *Principles of Surgery* textbook. Too thick to fit in the coat pocket.

A⁻

Mont Reid Surgical Handbook **$61.95**
FISCHER
Elsevier, 2008, 6th ed., 947 pages, ISBN 9781416048954

A large pocketbook that is ideal for looking up information on rounds or at the spur of the moment. Sections are concise and clearly written. Not meant to be a desk reference, but comprehensive enough to more than cover the topics seen on the clerkship shelf exam.

A⁻

Pocket Surgery **$54.95**
GOLDFARB
Lippincott Williams & Wilkins, 2011, 1st ed., 352 pages, ISBN 9781451112962

An outline-format guide that follows the style of *Pocket Medicine*, featuring easily referenced information. A quick read before going to the OR.

A⁻

Washington Manual of Surgery **$61.95**
KLINGENSMITH
Lippincott Williams & Wilkins, 2008, 5th ed., 685 pages, ISBN 9780781774475

The counterpart to the *Washington Manual of Medical Therapeutics*, this text offers good coverage of basic general surgery as well as common problems in the surgical subspecialties. Also includes practical chapters on the day-to-day care of the surgical patient. True to its title as a manual, the text may be more appropriate for residents and subinterns, as it offers little description of etiology, pathophysiology, and clinical features. The fifth edition includes updates on evidence-based guidelines and minimally invasive surgical techniques.

B+ ***On Call Surgery*** **$49.95**

ADAMS

Elsevier, 2006, 3rd ed., 589 pages, ISBN 9781416024415

A compact guide presented in a format similar to that of *Surgery on Call*, addressing common problems surgeons confront while on call. Not comprehensive enough for wards preparation or study, but the text guides one's clinical thinking and approach toward emergent issues in a well-explained manner. Geared more toward residents on call than toward medical students.

B+ ***Pocket Companion to Sabiston Textbook of Surgery*** **$54.00**

TOWNSEND

Elsevier, 2005, 17th ed., 1176 pages, ISBN 9780721604824

A condensed version of the parent book written in a bulleted outline format, allowing for easy access to information. Would benefit from more illustrations, but serves as a good and quick reference resource. Size is an issue, however, as the book is a tight fit for the coat pocket. Consider carrying in a backpack instead.

B+ ***Current Clinical Strategies: Surgery*** **$12.95**

WILSON

Current Clinical Strategies, 2006, 6th ed., 113 pages, ISBN 9781929622573

A compact, quick-reference pocketbook that addresses common surgical problems in outline format. Includes sample admission orders and operative notes. Also offers good, high-yield descriptions of etiology, pathophysiology, clinical features, diagnostic procedures, and treatment. Contains few tables and no figures illustrating anatomy or surgical techniques. A good overall value for its size and price.

B ***Surgical Intern Pocket Survival Guide*** **$12.95**

CHAMBERLAIN

International Medical Publishing, 1993, 1st ed., 74 pages, ISBN 9780963406354

A practical pocketbook detailing the basic logistics of day-to-day surgical life. Written for the intern, but can serve as a guide for subinterns as well. Outlines the approach toward the medical management of surgical patients, including sample orders and notes. Some portions of the text may be too specific for beginning students, but most sections are useful. Some therapeutic measures are out of date. Sparse on topics other than common problems, but small, compact, and inexpensive.

B ***Surgery on Call*** **$43.95**

LEFOR

McGraw-Hill, 2006, 4th ed., 566 pages, ISBN 9780071402545

A practical, quick-reference handbook of common problems encountered by the physician on call. Provides guidelines for initial evaluation, formulation of differentials, diagnostic workup, and management. Offers limited discussion of pathophysiology, and sections are divided according to patient complaint. More useful for working up "fresh" patients than for general review.

B ***The Cleveland Clinic Guide to Surgical Patient Management*** **$47.00**

PONSKY

Elsevier, 2002, 1st ed., 441 pages, ISBN 9780323017091

A comprehensive pocket guide that addresses common surgical problems, with an emphasis on surgical operations. Disease pathophysiology, typical presentations, clinical findings, and therapy are described in detail along with sample preoperative, postoperative, and discharge orders. The absence of illustrations makes it difficult to visualize anatomy and procedures. Geared more toward intern- and resident-level education.

REVIEW/MINI-REFERENCE

A+

Cope's Early Diagnosis of the Acute Abdomen — ***$39.95***

SILEN

Oxford University Press, 2010, 22nd ed., 299 pages, ISBN 9780199730452

A classic, brief surgical textbook that every serious student of surgery should read. Offers an excellent exposition on differential diagnosis and physical examination, and uses a readable, personable approach to help students focus on the clinical skills they need to diagnose an acute abdomen. A great text for knowledge and patient management, but not high yield for boards review.

A

First Aid for the Surgery Clerkship — ***$46.95***

KAUFMAN

McGraw-Hill, 2009, 2nd ed., 543 pages, ISBN 9780071448710

A highly comprehensive overview of pertinent topics in surgery, written in outline format and intended for shelf and Step 2 CK exam study. Covers essential high-yield information in a succinct, systematic manner. Includes well-organized tables as well as helpful figures. High-yield mnemonics and clinical scenarios are provided in the margins. Overall, an excellent review of the broad field of surgery. This publication is not affiliated with the authors of *First Aid for the Wards*.

A

Case Files Surgery — ***$34.95***

TOY

McGraw-Hill, 2009, 3rd ed., 510 pages, ISBN 9780071598972

An excellent review of 60 conditions commonly seen on the surgical rotation, presented in a case-based format. Useful as a companion to a general reference book to help consolidate the core concepts of the surgery rotation.

A−

NMS Surgery Casebook — ***$46.50***

JARRELL

Lippincott Williams & Wilkins, 2008, 5th ed., 647 pages, ISBN 9780781759014

A great companion to any review book, with sections organized by organ system. Each section starts with case scenarios and is followed by a series of questions that prompt readers to think about the next step. Includes a detailed explanation for each case as well as figures and tables. Easy to read, and perfect for self-directed learning.

B+

In A Page Surgery — ***$40.95***

KAHAN

Lippincott Williams & Wilkins, 2004, 1st ed., 288 pages, ISBN 9781405103657

A dry review of more than 150 diseases, organized by organ system. Each disease pathology is explained in 1 page, from etiology to prognosis, with lists. Provides a big picture and high-yield information; best suited for quick review before seeing a patient or preparing for a pimp session. The book is thin but is not pocket-sized and also lacks figures and tables, so students will need to refer to other textbooks for more detailed information.

B+

Underground Clinical Vignettes: Surgery — ***$29.95***

KIM

Lippincott Williams & Wilkins, 2007, 4th ed., 185 pages, ISBN 9780781768474

A well-organized review, with 76 cases following the typical clinical vignette format seen in this series. Includes a focused, high-yield discussion of pathogenesis, epidemiology, management, and complications. Black-and-white images are included where relevant. Insufficient for use for clinical rotations or test preparation, but an easy-to-use supplement for either.

B+ ***Blueprints Clinical Cases in Surgery*** **$36.95**

Li

Lippincott Williams & Wilkins, 2007, 2nd ed., 304 pages, ISBN 9781405104937

Organized by common presenting signs and symptoms, this book contains 60 symptom-based clinical cases accompanied by 200 USMLE-style questions. The format is similar to that of the Case Files series but places less emphasis on discussions and greater focus on questions.

B+ ***General Surgery Review*** **$105.00**

Makary

Ladner-Drysdale, 2008, 2nd ed., 575 pages, ISBN 9780976066224

A comprehensive review text with an easy-to-follow case-based format that makes use of more than 1000 clinical scenarios. Topics are nicely summarized without superfluous information, and exam pearls are interspersed throughout. Includes general as well as all major subspecialty reviews. Great for shelf as well as wards review.

B ***Blueprints in Surgery*** **$36.44**

Karp

Lippincott Williams & Wilkins, 2008, 5th ed., 253 pages, ISBN 9780781788687

A brief but well-organized text review of general surgery with good, clear tables and diagrams. Easy to read, but with uneven coverage of high-yield topics. Includes a brief question-and-answer section at the end of the text. Because it is geared toward study for the shelf and Step 2 CK exams, some of the information presented is oversimplified, especially with regard to surgical operations and procedures. Excellent for the basics, but students will need a more detailed reference for the rotation. Some students feel it is among the weaker review books of the Blueprints series.

B ***High-Yield Surgery*** **$26.95**

Nirula

Lippincott Williams & Wilkins, 2006, 2nd ed., 149 pages, ISBN 9780781776561

Part of a popular USMLE Step 1 prep series that offers a review book for each clerkship. Contains high-yield information in a clear and concise outline format, organized by organ system. May be too concise for shelf exam preparation; best used for a quick preview before the rotation.

B ***Netter's Surgical Anatomy Review P.R.N.*** **$35.95**

Trelease

Elsevier, 2011, 1st ed., 420 pages, ISBN 9781437717921

An illustration-based book offering a review of anatomy, vessels, lymphatics, and clinical correlates for most common surgical procedures seen in the surgical rotation. Useful for a quick review before stepping into the OR.

B− ***Colour Guide to Surgical Signs*** **$23.51**

Campbell

Elsevier, 1999, 2nd ed., 146 pages, ISBN 9780443061455

Concise text descriptions with associated radiographs and color photographs of manifestations of surgical disease. Contains good illustrations, but the text is not complete, limiting its usefulness on the wards.

QUESTION BOOKS

A

Surgical Recall **$49.95**

Blackbourne

Lippincott Williams & Wilkins, 2011, 6th ed., 807 pages, ISBN 9781608314218

A practical and useful adjunct to a reference text, presented in a question-and-answer format typical of the Recall series. Excellent for wards pimping preparation and great to use in spare moments, especially before entering the OR. Covers a wide range of topics in the form of very high yield surgical pearls. Although its format makes for quick, easy reading, the text is insufficient for the shelf and board exams, as it covers topics superficially. Also available in an audio version as downloadable MP3 files. Highly recommended for junior students seeking to survive the common pimp questions of a difficult rotation.

A⁻

Abernathy's Surgical Secrets **$54.95**

Harken

Elsevier, 2009, 6th ed., 517 pages, ISBN 9780323057110

A question-and-answer-style book with useful bulleted lists and tables describing the most commonly encountered surgical procedures and techniques. A useful reference for a quick review prior to going into the OR.

B⁺

Lange Q&A: Surgery **$44.95**

Cayten

McGraw-Hill, 2007, 5th ed., 332 pages, ISBN 9780071475662

A question-and-answer book with more than 1000 questions organized under different topics. Provides detailed explanations of each answer, and includes a comprehensive practice exam with 100 questions at the end. Questions tend to focus on details. Best used as a supplement to the topic review books during the rotation.

B⁺

PreTest Surgery **$32.00**

Kao

McGraw-Hill, 2009, 12th ed., 373 pages, ISBN 9780071598637

A collection of 500 multiple-choice questions covering a wide range of topics in surgery. Includes clinical vignette–style questions, and provides detailed paragraph-format explanations for each answer. Considered one of the weaker question books of the PreTest series.

B⁺

Blueprints Q&A Step 2 Surgery **$19.95**

Nelson

Lippincott Williams & Wilkins, 2005, 2nd ed., 169 pages, ISBN 9781405103930

A resource that contains more than 200 USMLE-style questions with explanations for both correct and incorrect answers, although the explanations are not as detailed and well referenced as those in the PreTest series. Originally designed for Step 2 CK preparation, but since the format of the shelf exam is similar, this would be a useful companion for clerkship preparation as well. Thin enough to carry in the pocket, and could easily be read in a few days.

TEXTBOOK/REFERENCE

Rating	Resource	Price
A	***Schwartz's Principles of Surgery*** BRUNICARDI **McGraw-Hill, 2009, 9th ed., 1866 pages, ISBN 9780071547697** A reference textbook for the serious surgery student, and probably the most widely used of the surgical textbooks. Well organized and comprehensive, with a good discussion of surgical disease processes and in-depth, complex explanations of the diagnosis and treatment of surgical problems. Expensive and requires considerable reading time, but a great investment for those considering a surgical career. A valuable reference for presentations and in-depth study. This edition features a new focus on oncologic surgery and has strengthened the section on basic science.	***$189.00***
A⁻	***Greenfield's Surgery: Scientific Principles and Practice*** MULHOLLAND **Lippincott Williams & Wilkins, 2011, 5th ed., 2074 pages, ISBN 9781605473550** An excellent reference with a heavy emphasis on integrating the principles of basic science with a discussion of surgical disease. Similar in style to *Sabiston Textbook of Surgery*. Contains good photos and diagrams.	***$219.00***
A⁻	***Gowned and Gloved Surgery: Introduction to Common Procedures*** ROSES **Elsevier, 2009, 1st ed., 247 pages, ISBN 9781416053569** A well-written book with excellent illustrations and images of commonly encountered OR procedures and relevant anatomy. A great text to use before going into the OR. Best used as a companion to a general review reference book or textbook with more comprehensive management details.	***$39.95***
A⁻	***Sabiston Textbook of Surgery*** TOWNSEND **Elsevier, 2008, 18th ed., 2353 pages, ISBN 9781416036753** An excellent reference book and a good read for medical students entering a surgical career. Not quite as readable as *Principles of Surgery*, but places greater emphasis on basic science, and features a more extensive discussion of normal anatomy and physiology. Well organized with good coverage of surgical disease.	***$216.00***
B⁺	***Current Surgical Therapy*** CAMERON **Elsevier, 2011, 10th ed., 1353 pages, ISBN 9781437708233** A highly detailed and technical surgical textbook designed for the practicing surgeon, with emphasis placed on evidence-based medicine. Highly comprehensive, with many high-yield images. Too detailed even for the dedicated surgical student, although those going into surgery may consider buying it later in their careers.	***$195.00***
B⁺	***Current Surgical Diagnosis & Treatment*** DOHERTY **McGraw-Hill, 2006, 12th ed., 1453 pages, ISBN 9780071423151** A clinically practical, easy-to-read reference book that is geared toward residents but should also be useful for students considering surgery. Offers well-written explanations of the major diagnostic approaches toward and treatment options for surgical problems, but little information is given on operative procedures. The most recent edition offers more illustrations but is still heavy on text. Includes chapters on most surgical subspecialties.	***$69.95***

B+

Essentials of General Surgery **$59.95**

LAWRENCE

Lippincott Williams & Wilkins, 2006, 4th ed., 613 pages, ISBN 9780781750035

A basic introductory text to surgery that is written at the level of the junior medical student. Definitely an easy read, making it possible to cover the entire text within this busy rotation. Offers good pictorial and text reviews of pertinent anatomy and physiology, but lacks detail and depth in many areas. Weaker in its discussion of treatment and management, and does not cover subspecialties. Good questions and information on oral exam preparation are included at the end of each section. Appropriate as an introductory text for general surgery and for those who are not considering surgery as a career.

B+

Essentials of Surgical Specialties **$59.95**

LAWRENCE

Lippincott Williams & Wilkins, 2006, 3rd ed., 613 pages, ISBN 9780781750042

A text presented in the same format as *Essentials of General Surgery*, except that this version discusses different surgical subspecialty topics. Refer to the review above for a more detailed evaluation.

APPENDIX

ABBREVIATIONS

Abbreviation	Meaning
A&O × 3	alert and oriented to person, place, and time
A&O × 4	alert and oriented to person, place, time, and situation
A&P	assessment and plan
A-a	alveolar-arterial (oxygen gradient)
AAA	abdominal aortic aneurysm
AAP	American Academy of Pediatrics
Ab	antibody
ABCs	airway, breathing, circulation
ABG	arterial blood gas
ABI	ankle-brachial index
abx	antibiotics
ACA	anterior cerebral artery
ACC	American College of Cardiology
ACEI	angiotensin-converting enzyme inhibitor
ACG	American College of Gastroenterology
AChR	acetylcholine receptor
ACLS	advanced cardiac life support (protocol)
ACS	acute coronary syndrome, American Cancer Society
ACTH	adrenocorticotropic hormone
AD	Alzheimer's disease
ADA	adenosine deaminase, American Diabetes Association
ADH	antidiuretic hormone
ADHD	attention-deficit hyperactivity disorder
AF	atrial fibrillation
AFI	amniotic fluid index
AFOSF	anterior fontanelle open, soft, and flat
AFP	α-fetoprotein
AG	anion gap
AHA	American Heart Association
AI	aortic insufficiency
AIDS	acquired immunodeficiency syndrome
ALC	absolute lymphocyte count
ALL	acute lymphocytic leukemia
ALS	amyotrophic lateral sclerosis
ALT	alanine transaminase
ANA	antinuclear antibody
ANCA	antineutrophil cytoplasmic antibody
AOM	acute otitis media
AP	anteroposterior
APAP	acetaminophen
APD	afferent pupillary defect
aPTT	activated partial thromboplastin time
ARB	angiotensin receptor blocker
ARDS	acute respiratory distress syndrome
ARF	acute renal failure
AROM	artificial rupture of membranes
ARR	absolute risk reduction
AS	aortic stenosis
ASA	acetylsalicylic acid
5-ASA	5-aminosalicylic acid
ASCUS	atypical squamous cells of undetermined significance
ASD	atrial septal defect
ASO	antistreptolysin O
AST	aspartate transaminase
AV	arteriovenous, atrioventricular
AVM	arteriovenous malformation
AXR	abdominal x-ray
AZT	azidothymidine
BAD	bipolar affective disorder
BAL	2,3-dimercaptopropanol (dimercaprol)
BAS	balloon atrial septostomy
BCG	bacille Calmette-Guérin
BID	twice a day
BMI	body mass index
BMP	basic metabolic panel
BMT	bone marrow transplantation
BNP	B-type natriuretic peptide
BP	blood pressure
BPH	benign prostatic hypertrophy
bpm	beats per minute
BPP	biophysical profile
BPPV	benign paroxysmal positional vertigo
BR	bathroom
BRBPR	bright red blood per rectum
BS	bowel sounds
BSO	bilateral salpingo-oophorectomy
BUN	blood urea nitrogen
BV	balloon valvuloplasty
BW	birth weight, body weight
c̄	with

Abbreviation	Meaning
CABG	coronary artery bypass grafting
CAD	coronary artery disease
CAM	Confusion Assessment Method
CAP	community-acquired pneumonia
CBC	complete blood count
CBD	common bile duct
CBT	cognitive-behavioral therapy
CC	chief complaint
CCB	calcium channel blocker
C/C/E	clubbing/cyanosis/edema
CCK	cholecystokinin
CCP	cyclic citrullinated peptide
CD	cluster of differentiation
CDC	Centers for Disease Control and Prevention
C/D/I	clean, dry, and intact
CEA	carcinoembryonic antigen
CF	cystic fibrosis
CFTR	cystic fibrosis transmembrane regulator
CGD	chronic granulomatous disease
CHD	congenital heart disease
CHF	congestive heart failure
CHO	call house officer
CIDP	chronic inflammatory demyelinating polyneuropathy
CK	creatine kinase
CKD	chronic kidney disease
CK-MB	creatine kinase, MB isoenzyme
CLO	*Campylobacter*-like organism
CMP	complete metabolic panel
CMT	cervical motion tenderness
CMV	cytomegalovirus
CN	cranial nerve
CNS	central nervous system
c/o	complains of
COMT	catechol-O-methyltransferase
COPD	chronic obstructive pulmonary disease
COX	cyclooxygenase
CPAP	continuous positive airway pressure
CPP	cerebral perfusion pressure
CPR	cardiopulmonary resuscitation
CrCl	creatinine clearance
CRP	C-reactive protein
CSF	cerebrospinal fluid
CT	computed tomography
CTA	computed tomographic angiography
CTAB	clear to auscultation bilaterally
CV	cardiovascular, curriculum vitae
CVA	cerebrovascular accident, costovertebral angle
CVID	common variable immunodeficiency
CVS	chorionic villus sampling
c/w	consistent with
Cx	culture
CXR	chest x-ray
D&C	dilation and curettage

Abbreviation	Meaning
DBS	deep brain stimulation
d/c	discharge
D/C	diarrhea/constipation, discontinue
DCIS	ductal carcinoma in situ
ddC	dideoxycytidine
DDH	developmental dysplasia of the hip
ddI	dideoxyinosine
DES	diethylstilbestrol
DFA	direct fluorescent antibody
DHEAS	dehydroepiandrosterone sulfate
DIC	disseminated intravascular coagulation
DKA	diabetic ketoacidosis
DL_{CO}	diffusion capacity for carbon monoxide
DM	diabetes mellitus
DMARD	disease-modifying antirheumatic drug
DMSA	dimercaptosuccinic acid
DNA	deoxyribonucleic acid
DNase	deoxyribonuclease
DNR	do not resuscitate
d/o	disorder
DOA	day of admission
DOC	differential of consequence
DOE	dyspnea on exertion
DPP	dipeptidyl peptidase
DRE	digital rectal exam
dsDNA	double-stranded DNA
DSM	*Diagnostic and Statistical Manual*
D4T	didehydrodeoxythymidine
DT	diphtheria and tetanus (vaccine)
DTaP	diphtheria, tetanus, acellular pertussis (vaccine)
DTRs	deep tendon reflexes
DTs	delirium tremens
DUB	dysfunctional uterine bleeding
DVT	deep venous thrombosis
DWI	diffusion-weighted imaging
EBL	estimated blood loss
EBV	Epstein-Barr virus
ECG	electrocardiogram
ECT	electroconvulsive therapy
ED	emergency department
EDC	estimated date of confinement
EDD	estimated date of delivery
EDTA	ethylenediamine tetraacetic acid
EEG	electroencephalogram
EF	ejection fraction
EFW	estimated fetal weight
EGD	esophagogastroduodenoscopy
EGDT	early goal-directed therapy
ELISA	enzyme-linked immunosorbent assay
EM	emergency medicine
EMG	electromyogram
EOM	extraocular movement
EOMI	extraocular movements intact
EPS	extrapyramidal symptoms
ER	estrogen receptor

Abbreviation	Meaning
ERCP	endoscopic retrograde cholangiopancreatography
ESR	erythrocyte sedimentation rate
ESRD	end-stage renal disease
EtOH	ethanol
Ext	extremities
FAST	focused abdominal sonography for trauma
F/C/S	fever/chills/sweating
Fe_{Na}	excreted fraction of filtered sodium
$FeSO_4$	ferrous sulfate
FEV_1	forced expiratory volume in 1 second
FFP	fresh frozen plasma
FH	family history
FHR	fetal heart rate
FHT	fetal heart tracing
FiO_2	fraction of inspired oxygen
FISH	fluorescence in situ hybridization
FLAIR	fluid attenuation inversion recovery
FLM	fetal lung maturity
FM	fetal movement
FNA	fine-needle aspiration
FOBT	fecal occult blood test
FSH	follicle-stimulating hormone
FT	fine touch
FTA-ABS	fluorescent treponemal antibody—absorbed
FTN	finger to nose
FTT	failure to thrive
FUO	fever of unknown origin
FVC	forced vital capacity
G6PD	glucose-6-phosphate dehydrogenase
GA	gestational age
GABA	gamma-aminobutyric acid
GABHS	group A β-hemolytic streptococcus
GAD	generalized anxiety disorder, glutamic acid decarboxylase
GAF	Global Assessment of Functioning
GB	gallbladder
GBM	glioblastoma multiforme
GBS	group B streptococcus, Guillain-Barré syndrome
GC	gonorrhea culture
GCS	Glasgow Coma Scale
GERD	gastroesophageal reflux disease
GETA	general endotracheal anesthesia
GFR	glomerular filtration rate
GGT	gamma-glutamyltransferase
GI	gastrointestinal
GIP	gastric inhibitory peptide
GLP	glucagon-like peptide
GN	glomerulonephritis
GNR	gram-negative rod
GnRH	gonadotropin-releasing hormone
GU	genitourinary
H&P	history and physical
HA	headache

Abbreviation	Meaning
HAART	highly active antiretroviral therapy
HACEK	*Haemophilus, Actinobacillus, Cardiobacterium, Eikenella, Kingella*
HAV	hepatitis A virus, hepatitis A vaccine
Hb	hemoglobin
HBsAg	hepatitis B surface antigen
HBV	hepatitis B virus, hepatitis B vaccine
HC	head circumference
HCC	hepatocellular carcinoma
hCG	human chorionic gonadotropin
HCV	hepatitis C virus
HD	hospital day
HDL	high-density lipoprotein
HDV	hepatitis D virus
HEENT	head, eyes, ears, nose, and throat
HELLP	hemolysis, elevated liver (enzymes), low platelets
HEV	hepatitis E virus
HHNK	hyperosmolar hyperglycemic nonketotic coma
HHV	human herpesvirus
Hib	*Haemophilus influenzae* type b (vaccine)
HIDA	hepato-iminodiacetic acid (scan)
HIPAA	Health Insurance Portability and Accountability Act
HIV	human immunodeficiency virus
HLA	human leukocyte antigen
HNPCC	hereditary nonpolyposis colorectal cancer
h/o	history of
HOCM	hypertrophic obstructive cardiomyopathy
hpf	high-power field
HPI	history of present illness
HPO	hypertrophic pulmonary osteoarthropathy
HPV	human papillomavirus
HR	heart rate
HRT	hormone replacement therapy
HSM	hepatosplenomegaly
HSP	Henoch-Schönlein purpura
HSV	herpes simplex virus
5-HT	5-hydroxytryptamine (serotonin)
HTLV	human T-cell lymphotropic virus
HTN	hypertension
HTS	heel to shin
HUS	hemolytic-uremic syndrome
HVA	homovanillic acid
Hx	history
IBD	inflammatory bowel disease
IBS	irritable bowel syndrome
ICP	intracranial pressure
ICU	intensive care unit
ID	identification
Ig	immunoglobulin
IM	intramuscular
INH	isoniazid
INR	International Normalized Ratio
I/O	intake/output

Abbreviation	Meaning
IOC	intraoperative cholangiogram
IPV	inactivated polio vaccine
IS	incentive spirometry
ITP	idiopathic thrombocytopenic purpura
IUD	intrauterine device
IUGR	intrauterine growth retardation
IUP	intrauterine pregnancy
IV	intravenous
IVC	inferior vena cava
IVDU	intravenous drug use
IVIG	intravenous immunoglobulin
JIA	juvenile idiopathic arthritis
JP	Jackson-Pratt (drain)
JVD	jugular venous distention
JVP	jugular venous pressure
KCl	potassium chloride
KOH	potassium hydroxide
KUB	kidney, ureter, bladder
KVO	keep vein open
L&D	labor and delivery
LAA	left atrial abnormality
LAD	lymphadenopathy
LBBB	left bundle branch block
LBO	large bowel obstruction
LCIS	lobular carcinoma in situ
LDH	lactate dehydrogenase
LDL	low-density lipoprotein
LEEP	loop electrosurgical excision procedure
LES	lower esophageal sphincter
LFT	liver function test
LGIB	lower gastrointestinal bleeding
LH	luteinizing hormone
LLE	left lower extremity
LLQ	left lower quadrant
LLSB	left lower sternal border
LMN	lower motor neuron
LMP	last menstrual period
LMWH	low-molecular-weight heparin
LOC	loss of consciousness
LP	lumbar puncture
LR	lactated Ringer's solution
L/S	lecithin-to-sphingomyelin (ratio)
LUE	left upper extremity
LUQ	left upper quadrant
LVEDP	left ventricular end-diastolic pressure
LVH	left ventricular hypertrophy
MAE	moves all extremities
MAOI	monoamine oxidase inhibitor
MAP	mean arterial pressure
MAR	medication administration record
MCA	middle cerebral artery
MCTD	mixed connective tissure disorder
MCV	mean corpuscular volume
MCV4	meningococcal conjugate vaccine
MDD	major depressive disorder
MDE	major depressive episode

Abbreviation	Meaning
MDI	metered-dose inhaler
MELD	Model for End-Stage Liver Disease (score)
MEN	multiple endocrine neoplasia
MHA-TP	microhemagglutination assay—*Treponema pallidum*
MI	myocardial infarction
MIBG	metaiodobenzylguanidine (scan)
MIBI	methoxyisobutyl isonitrile (stress test)
MMM	mucous membranes moist
MMR	measle, mumps, rubella (vaccine)
MMSE	mini-mental status exam
6-MP	6-mercaptopurine
MPO	myeloperoxidase
MPTP	1-methyl-4-phenyl-tetrahydropyridine
MR	mitral regurgitation
MRA	magnetic resonance angiography
MRCP	magnetic resonance cholangiopancreatography
M/R/G	murmurs/rubs/gallops
MRI	magnetic resonance imaging
MRSA	methicillin-resistant *Staphylococcus aureus*
MS	mental status, mitral stenosis, multiple sclerosis, musculoskeletal
MS-1, 2, etc.	medical student (and year)
MSAFP	maternal serum α-fetoprotein
MSE	mental status examination
MuSK	muscle-specific kinase
MVI	multivitamin infusion
MVP	mitral valve prolapse
NABS	normoactive bowel sounds
NAD	no acute distress
NADPH	nicotinamide adenine dinucleotide phosphate
NAG	non–anion gap
NBME	National Board of Medical Examiners
NBNB	nonbilious, nonbloody
NC	nasal cannula
NC/AT	normocephalic/atraumatic
ND	nondistended
NDDG	National Diabetes Data Group
NG	nasogastric
NICU	neonatal intensive care unit
NIH	National Institutes of Health
NKDA	no known drug allergies
nl	normal
NMDA	N-methyl-D-aspartate
NNT	number needed to treat
NOS	not otherwise specified
NPO	nil per os (nothing by mouth)
NR	normal range
NS	normal saline
NSAID	nonsteroidal anti-inflammatory drug
NSCLC	non–small cell lung carcinoma
NSF	nephrogenic systemic fibrosis
NST	nonstress test
NSTEMI	non-ST-elevation myocardial infarction

Abbreviation	Meaning
NSVD	normal spontaneous vaginal delivery
NT	nontender
N/V	nausea/vomiting
NYHA	New York Heart Association
O&P	ova and parasites
OCD	obsessive-compulsive disorder
OCP	oral contraceptive pill
OCPD	obsessive-compulsive personality disorder
OME	otitis media with effusion
OOB	out of bed
O/P	oropharynx
OR	operating room
o/w	otherwise
P	pulse
PA	posteroanterior
$Paco_2$	partial pressure of carbon dioxide in arterial blood
PACU	postanesthesia intensive care unit
Pao_2	partial pressure of oxygen in arterial blood
PAo_2	alveolar oxygen pressure
PAPP-A	pregnancy-associated plasma protein A
PCA	patient-controlled analgesia, posterior cerebral artery
PCI	percutaneous coronary intervention
Pco_2	partial pressure of carbon dioxide
PCOS	polycystic ovarian syndrome
PCP	phencyclidine (“angel dust”), *Pneumocystis carinii* (now *jiroveci*) pneumonia
PCV	pneumococcal conjugate vaccine
PDA	patent ductus arteriosus
PDD	pervasive developmental disorder
PDS	polydioxanone (sutures)
PE	physical examination, pulmonary embolism
PEF	peak expiratory flow
PERC	pulmonary embolism rule-out criteria
PERRL	pupils equal, round, and reactive to light
PET	positron emission tomography
PFT	pulmonary function test
PG	plasma glucose, prostaglandin
PGY	postgraduate year
PID	pelvic inflammatory disease
PIV	parainfluenza virus
PMH	past medical history
PMI	point of maximal impulse
PML	progressive multifocal leukoencephalopathy
PMN	polymorphonuclear (leukocytes)
PNL	prenatal labs
PNV	prenatal vitamins
PO	per os (by mouth)
Po_2	partial pressure of oxygen
PO_4	phosphate
POD	postoperative day
PP	pin prick
ppd	pack per day

Abbreviation	Meaning
PPD	postpartum day, purified protein derivative (of tuberculin)
PPI	proton pump inhibitor
PPROM	premature preterm rupture of membranes
PPV	pneumococcal polysaccharide vaccine
PR	per rectum
PRBC	packed red blood cell
PRN	pro re nata (as needed)
PSA	prostate-specific antigen
PSH	past surgical history
PT	prothrombin time
PTA	prior to admission
PTCA	percutaneous transluminal coronary angioplasty
PTHrP	PTH-related peptide
PTSD	posttraumatic stress disorder
PTT	partial thromboplastin time
PUD	peptic ulcer disease
PVM	pulmonary vascular marking
QAM	every morning
QD	every day
QHS	every night
QID	four times a day
RA	rheumatoid arthritis, room air
RAA	right atrial abnormality
RAD	right axis deviation
RAE	right atrial enlargement
RAL	radial arterial line
RAM	rapid alternating movements
RBBB	right bundle branch block
RBC	red blood cell
RDS	respiratory distress syndrome
RF	radio frequency, rheumatoid factor
RLE	right lower extremity
RLQ	right lower quadrant
RNA	ribonucleic acid
r/o	rule out
ROM	range of motion, rupture of membranes
ROS	review of systems
RPR	rapid plasma reagin (test)
RR	red reflex, respiratory rate
RRR	regular rate and rhythm, relative risk reduction
RRT	renal replacement therapy
RSV	respiratory syncytial virus
RTA	renal tubular acidosis
RUA	routine urinalysis
RUE	right upper extremity
RUQ	right upper quadrant
RV	residual volume
RVH	right ventricular hypertrophy
SAAG	serum-ascites albumin gradient
SAB	spontaneous abortion
SAD	schizoaffective disorder
SAH	subarachnoid hemorrhage
Sao_2	arterial oxygen saturation

Abbreviation	Meaning
SBO	small bowel obstruction
SBP	systolic blood pressure
SCD	sequential compression device
SCFE	slipped capital femoral epiphysis
SCLC	small cell lung carcinoma
SCID	severe combined immunodeficiency
SCM	sternocleidomastoid
SEM	systolic ejection murmur
SES	socioeconomic status
SH	social history
SIADH	syndrome of inappropriate secretion of ADH
SIDS	sudden infant death syndrome
SIRS	systemic inflammatory response syndrome
SLE	systemic lupus erythematosus
SOAP	subjective (data), objective (data), assessment, and plan
SOB	shortness of breath
s/p	status post (postoperative)
SPEP	serum protein electrophoresis
SQ	subcutaneous
SSE	sterile speculum exam
SSRI	selective serotonin reuptake inhibitor
STEMI	ST-elevation myocardial infarction
STI	sexually transmitted infection
SVC	superior vena cava
SVR	systemic vascular resistance
T	temperature
TAB	therapeutic abortion
TAH	total abdominal hysterectomy
TB	tuberculosis
TBSA	total body surface area
TBW	total body water
3TC	dideoxythiacytidine
Tc	technetium
T_c	current temperature
TCA	tricyclic antidepressant
TED	thromboembolic deterrent (stockings)
T/E/D	tobacco/EtOH (alcohol)/drugs
TEE	transesophageal echocardiography
TFT	thyroid function test
TIA	transient ischemic attack
TIBC	total iron-binding capacity
TID	three times a day
TIPS	transjugular intrahepatic portosystemic shunt
TLC	total lung capacity
TM	tympanic membrane
T_m	maximum temperature
TMJ	temporomandibular joint
TMP-SMX	trimethoprim-sulfamethoxazole

Abbreviation	Meaning
TMS	transmagnetic stimulation
TN	trigeminal neuralgia
TNF	tumor necrosis factor
TNM	tumor, node, metastasis (staging)
TOA	tubo-ovarian abscess
TOC	test of cure
Toco	tocometer
ToRCHeS	toxoplasmosis, rubella, cytomegalovirus, herpes simplex, syphilis
tPA	tissue plasminogen activator
TPAL	term, preterm, abortion, living
TPN	total parenteral nutrition
TSH	thyroid-stimulating hormone
TTE	transthoracic echocardiography
TTP	thrombotic thrombocytopenic purpura
UA	urinalysis
UC	uterine contraction
UGIB	upper gastrointestinal bleeding
UMN	upper motor neuron
UOP	urine output
UPEP	urine protein electrophoresis
URI	upper respiratory infection
USMLE	United States Medical Licensing Examination
USOH	usual state of health
USPSTF	United States Preventive Services Task Force
UTD	up to date
UTI	urinary tract infection
VA	Department of Veterans Affairs
VB	vaginal bleeding
VC	vital capacity
VCUG	voiding cystourethrogram
VDRL	Venereal Disease Research Laboratory (test)
VF	ventricular fibrillation
VIP	vasoactive intestinal peptide
VMA	vanillylmandelic acid
VNS	vagus nerve stimulation
VOR	vestibulo-ocular reflex
V/Q	ventilation-perfusion (ratio)
VS	vital signs
VSD	ventricular septal defect
VT	ventricular tachycardia
VZIG	varicella-zoster immune globulin
VZV	varicella-zoster virus
WBC	white blood cell
WD/WN	well developed and well nourished
WHO	World Health Organization
W/R/R	wheezes/rhonchi/rales

INDEX

I

P

Q

R

NOTES

NOTES

NOTES

NOTES

About the Authors

Tao Le, MD, MHS

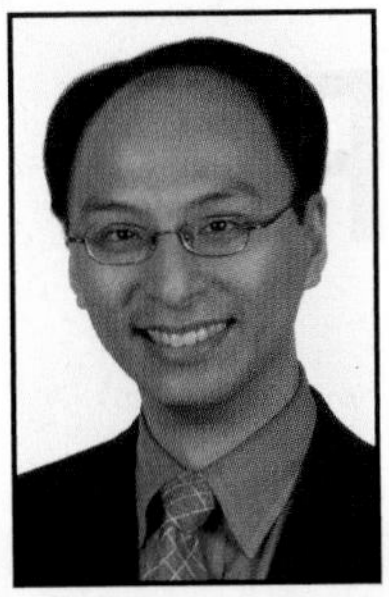

Tao developed a passion for medical education as a medical student. He currently edits more than 15 titles in the *First Aid* series. In addition, he is the founder of the *USMLERx* online video and test bank series as well as a cofounder of the *Underground Clinical Vignettes* series. As a medical student, he was editor-in-chief of the University of California, San Francisco (UCSF) *Synapse*, a university newspaper with a weekly circulation of 9000. Tao earned his medical degree from UCSF in 1996 and completed his residency training in internal medicine at Yale University and fellowship training at Johns Hopkins University. At Yale, he was a regular guest lecturer on the USMLE review courses and an adviser to the Yale University School of Medicine curriculum committee. Tao subsequently went on to cofound Medsn, a medical education technology venture, and served as its chief medical officer. He is currently conducting research in asthma education at the University of Louisville.

Vikas Bhushan, MD

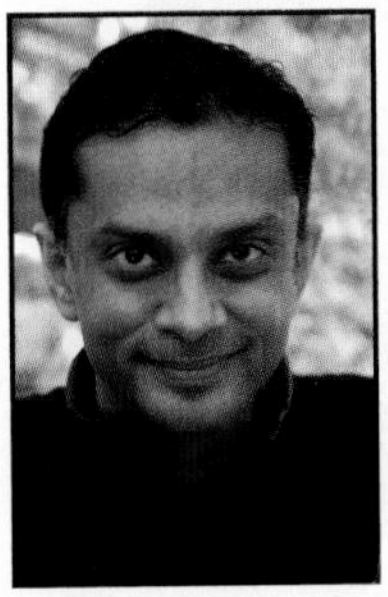

Vikas is an author, editor, entrepreneur, and teleradiologist. In 1990 he conceived and authored the original *First Aid for the USMLE Step 1*. His entrepreneurial adventures include a successful software company, a medical publishing enterprise (S2S), an e-learning company (Medsn), and an ER teleradiology service (24/7 Radiology). His eclectic interests include medical informatics, independent film, humanism, Urdu poetry, world music, South Asian diasporic culture, and avoiding a day job. A dilettante at heart, he coproduced a music documentary on qawwali music and coproduced and edited *Shabash 2.0: The Hip Guide to All Things South Asian in North America*. Vikas completed a bachelor's degree in biochemistry from the University of California, Berkeley; an MD with thesis from the University of California, San Francisco; and a radiology residency from the University of California, Los Angeles.

James S. Yeh, MD

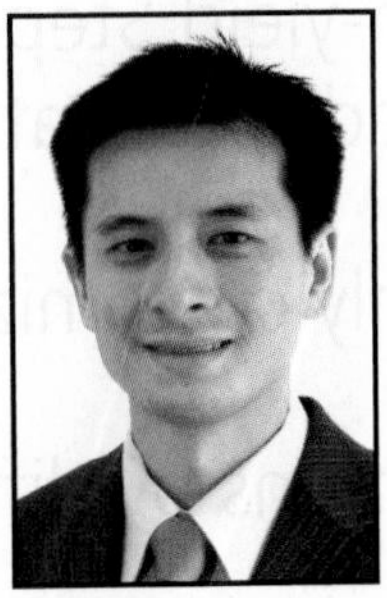

James is a resident physician at Cambridge Health Alliance and a clinical fellow in medicine at Harvard Medical School, where he has received multiple teaching awards in recognition of his work with medical students. He is a graduate of Boston University School of Medicine. While at Boston University School of Medicine, he was an Albert Schweitzer Fellow and was awarded the Henry J. Bakst Award in Community Medicine. He completed his undergraduate and graduate work at the University of California, Berkeley and at Harvard University. James has worked as author and editor on a number of projects in the *First Aid* series, including *First Aid for the USMLE Step 1*, *First Aid Cases for the USMLE Step 1*, and *First Aid for the Basic Sciences: General Principles*, as well as the *USMLERx Step 1 Qmax* test bank. He will begin fellowship training at Brigham and Women's Hospital in 2013. His academic interests include medical education and evidence-based medicine practices.

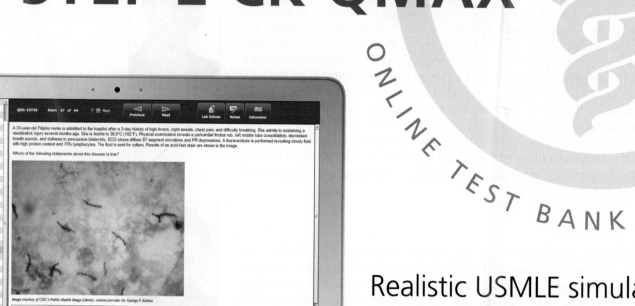